FUNDAMENTALS OF AAC

A Case-Based Approach to Enhancing Communication

FUNDAMENTALS OF AAC
A Case-Based Approach to Enhancing Communication

Nerissa Hall, PhD, CCC-SLP, ATP
Jenifer Juengling-Sudkamp, PhD, CCC-SLP
Michelle L. Gutmann, PhD, CCC-SLP
Ellen R. Cohn, PhD, CCC-SLP, ASHA Fellow

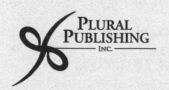

PLURAL
PUBLISHING
INC.

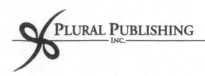

5521 Ruffin Road
San Diego, CA 92123

e-mail: information@pluralpublishing.com
Website: https://www.pluralpublishing.com

Typeset in 10.5/13 Garamond by Flanagan's Publishing Services, Inc.
Printed in the United States of America by Integrated Books International
25 24 23 22   2 3 4 5

Library of Congress Cataloging-in-Publication Data:
Names: Hall, Nerissa, editor. | Juengling-Sudkamp, Jenifer, editor. |
  Gutmann, Michelle L., editor. | Cohn, Ellen R. (Speech therapist), editor.
Title: Fundamentals of AAC : a case-based approach to enhancing
  communication / [edited by] Nerissa Hall, Jenifer Juengling-Sudkamp,
  Michelle L. Gutmann, Ellen R. Cohn.
Other titles: Fundamentals of augmentative and alternative communication
Description: San Diego, CA : Plural Publishing, Inc., [2023] | Includes
  bibliographical references and index.
Identifiers: LCCN 2021055246 (print) | LCCN 2021055247 (ebook) | ISBN
  9781635503531 (paperback) | ISBN 1635503531 (paperback) | ISBN
  9781635501391 (ebook)
Subjects: MESH: Communication Aids for Disabled | Speech Therapy--methods |
  Needs Assessment | Case Reports
Classification: LCC RC428.8 (print) | LCC RC428.8 (ebook) | NLM WL 340.2
  | DDC 616.85/503--dc23/eng/20211124
LC record available at https://lccn.loc.gov/2021055246
LC ebook record available at https://lccn.loc.gov/2021055247

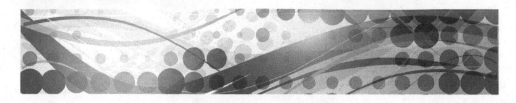

CONTENTS

Section III. AAC Assessment, Intervention, and Implementation for Infants, Toddlers, and School-Aged Individuals   137

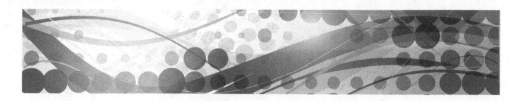

PREFACE

As an editorial team, we feel the ultimate goal of supporting communication and advancing language is core to Augmentative and Alternative Communication (AAC). However, this goal can only be realized if AAC is embedded in the needs of individual learners as they interact within their families and communities.

While there are strong foundational concepts that underlie the field at large, the practice of AAC (the way in which we assess, intervene, and implement it) has to be co-constructed between individuals (as members of a community or multiple communities), their communication partner(s), and the professional(s) with whom they work.

There is no single, one-size-fits-all way to "do" AAC. Instead, each assessment, treatment, and/or implementation plan is unique to the individual, and arises from their cognitive-linguistic profile, physical abilities, sense of self, their psychosocial make-up, their family, and their community.

The field of AAC has grown and evolved tremendously based on an understanding of what AAC is. Its application has become more widespread, and the AAC technology has advanced. The AAC tools are always changing, but the task of supporting an individual's ability to communicate fully and independently in a manner that is meaningful to them remains constant, irrespective of who they are and how they are supported. Each AAC system represents a product wherein language, vocabulary, and access features are shaped by the individual's unique abilities and challenges, as well as by their various community affiliations.

This text is written for preprofessional and professional clinicians interested in learning how to support individuals with complex communication needs (CCN) in need of, and benefiting from AAC, in a range of clinical settings. Each chapter is structured such that fundamental concepts and principles are presented first. Each chapter also contains a relevant case study that presents the concepts and principles "in action" so that the reader is guided through the use of clinical decision making in AAC. Every case study is designed to underscore the cultural, linguistic, and social variability inherent to the fields of AAC and communication disorders, and how each individual influences the manifestation of the AAC system, treatment, and implementation plans.

Online ancillary materials are available on a PluralPlus website that contains an Instructor's Manual, videos, and tutorials.

We invite you to explore the content herein and hope you will find it informative, thought provoking, and enjoyable to read. Further, we hope you find that the multinational and multicultural perspectives contained in chapters and essays enhance your clinical practice. Most of all, we hope it inspires you to engage with people who use AAC who are our greatest inspiration. It has been our privilege to learn from them and to aim ever higher in service provision.

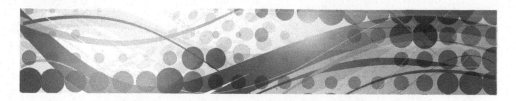

ACKNOWLEDGMENTS

As an editorial team we have been fortunate to be able to bring together the perspectives and expertise of our contributors to co-construct this expansive description of AAC. Sixty-four people authored content in this text, and even more shared their research, ideas, and experiences. This text represents the synthesis of lived experiences, data, practice, and love for the field, and we are so thankful for the time and effort spent by our contributors to bring this book to life.

A huge thanks to the team at Plural, especially Christina Gunning, who kept this project in motion and on track amidst a global pandemic.

To our families and friends who saw us through the authoring of *Tele-AAC: Augmentative and Alternative Communication Through Telepractice,* and then watched us take on a project of astronomically larger scope, we thank you and promise to take a little more time off before the next authoring project.

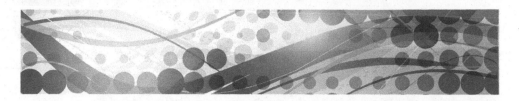

ABOUT THE EDITORS

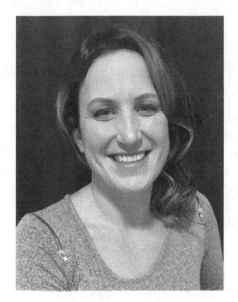

Nerissa Hall, PhD, CCC-SLP, ATP

Dr. Nerissa Hall is co-founder of Commūnicāre, LLC and co-director of the Speech, Language, and Literacy Center at Tate Behavioral, Inc. Her work concentrates on augmentative and alternative communication, assistive technology, and tele-AAC, and she works primarily with school-aged individuals, providing specialized, evidence-based intervention, assessment, and consultation services. Dr. Hall received her Masters and Doctorate degrees from the University of Massachusetts-Amherst, focusing on augmentative AAC skill advancement and implementation, as well as tele-AAC. She has presented nationally regarding these and other related topics. Dr. Hall has served as a LEND Fellow, adjunct faculty at Elms, Cambridge College and the University of Massachusetts-Amherst. She is part of the team that edited *Tele-AAC: Augmentative and Alternative Communication Through Telepractice* and is passionate about advancing the fields of AAC and AT to ensure meaningful outcomes for individuals using AAC and AT and the teams that support them.

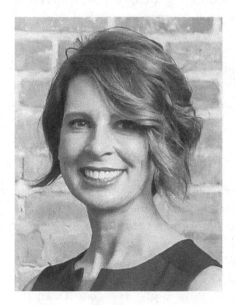

Jenifer Juengling-Sudkamp, PhD, CCC-SLP

Dr. Jenifer Juengling-Sudkamp is a speech-language pathologist who provides augmentative and alternative communication consultations, assessments, and interventions across multiple medical settings to adults with complex communication needs that are often a result of acquired neurodegenerative disorders and/or traumatic brain injury. She has a passion to improve people's access to AAC consultative, evaluation, and/or interventions, and joined a team of talented editors and authors to contribute to the resourceful clinical book, *Tele-AAC: Augmentative and Alternative Communication Through Telepractice*. Dr. Juengling-Sudkamp is a clinical instructor in the Department of Orthopaedics at Tulane University School of Medicine, where she teaches combined undergraduate and graduate courses in applied neuroscience that are specific to the clinical management of athletes with sport-related brain injuries. She also served as the program manager and a consultant for the Sport Concussion Clinic, the NFLPA's Trust Brain and Body, and the Milestone Wellness Assessment programs at Tulane University. She has co-authored publications and co-presented nationally and internationally on topics including AAC, tele-AAC, and the management of cognitive-communication deficit and dysphagia among adolescents and adults with acquired neurological disorders.

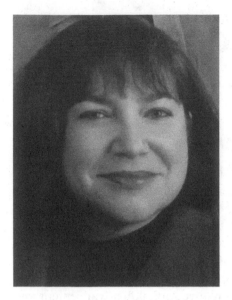

Michelle L. Gutmann, PhD, CCC-SLP

Dr. Michelle L. Gutmann is a clinical professor at Purdue University Department of Speech, Language, and Hearing Sciences, where she teaches a variety of graduate courses including AAC, Counseling in Communication Disorders, and Motor Speech Disorders. After completing her doctoral studies and prior to coming to Purdue, she served as a clinical assistant professor and the Speech-Language Pathologist for the ALS Clinic at Vanderbilt University Medical Center. Prior to returning to doctoral studies, she worked clinically for approximately a decade with both children and adults who needed AAC. She is part of the team that edited *Tele-AAC: Augmentative and Alternative Communication Through Telepractice* and is passionate about working with adults with acquired and/or neurodegenerative communication disorders who need AAC. Dr. Gutmann has served as the Professional Development Manager for ASHA's SIG 12 (AAC) since 2017. She is also active in both research and clinical endeavors related to the application and implementation of AAC for adults with acquired neurological disorders. Her interests include telepractice, interprofessional education, clinical education in speech-language pathology, implementation science, and health literacy. She has published and presented nationally and internationally.

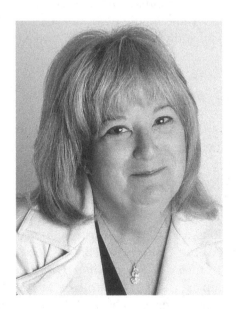

Ellen R. Cohn, PhD, CCC-SLP, ASHA-F

Dr. Ellen R. Cohn is an adjunct faculty member in the Department of Communication and Rhetoric in the Dietrich School of Arts and Sciences and the College of General Studies at the University of Pittsburgh, and is an adjunct Professor at the University of Maryland Global Campus, where she teaches distance education health communication and a variety of other applied communication courses. She has held secondary appointments in Pitt's School of Dental Medicine and in the Clinical and Translational Science Institute, and as a Faculty Fellow, University Honors College, and an affiliated faculty member of Pitt's University Center for International Studies. Dr. Cohn has co-authored books on the topics of videofluoroscopy/cleft palate; communication as culture; diversity across the curriculum in higher education; telerehabilitation; a casebook in communication science and disorders; tele-AAC; and two programs at the University of Pittsburgh's School of Law: Certificate Program in Disability Law, and the first MSL with a Concentration in Disability Law. Dr. Cohn is a past investigator for a Department of Education-National Institute on Disability and Rehabilitation Research, Rehabilitation Engineering Research Center on Telerehabilitation. She served as Professor in the Department of Communication Science and Disorders School of Health and Rehabilitation Sciences, University of Pittsburgh, Associate Dean for Instructional Development (2007–2015), Assistant Dean for Instructional Development (2002–2007), and Director of Instructional Development (1999–2002), School of Health and Rehabilitation Sciences, University of Pittsburgh. Cohn was designated a Diversity Champion, American Speech-Language-Hearing Association (2009), and was a Provost's Office, Diversity Seminar Fellow (2005). Her interests span the areas of telerehabilitation/telehealth/telemedicine; interprofessional education; cleft palate, dentofacial, and craniofacial disorders; clinical training in speech-language pathology; and healthcare communication. She is the Founding Editor (2008–present) of the *International Journal of Telerehabilitation* (a PubMed indexed electronic journal). In 2013, Dr. Cohn was named a Fellow of the American Speech-Language-Hearing Association. In 2006, she received the Honors of the Southwestern Pennsylvania Speech-Language and Hearing Association. In 2020, she and co-author Dr. Jana Cason received the American Speech-Language-Hearing Association's Editor's Award, for Ethical Considerations for Client-Centered Telepractice, *Perspectives of the Special Interest Groups.*

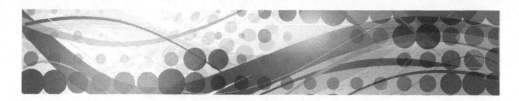

CONTRIBUTORS

Tami Altschuler, MA, CCC-SLP
Speech-Language Pathologist
Clinical Specialist in Patient-Provider
    Communication
Rusk Rehabilitation
NYU Langone Medical Center
New York, New York
Chapter 17

Mary Andrianopoulos, PhD, CCC-SLP
Associate Professor
Department of Communication Disorders
University of Massachusetts
Amherst, Massachusetts
Chapter 26

Meher Banajee, PhD, CCC-SLP
Associate Professor and Program Director
Speech-Language Pathology
School of Allied Health Professions
Louisiana State University Health Sciences
    Center
New Orleans, Louisiana
Chapter 8

Matthew R. Baud, CCC-SLP/L
Assistive Technology Coordinator
Niles Township District for Special Education
Morton Grove, Illinois
Chapter 34

Michelle Boisvert, PhD, CCC-SLP
Speech-Language Pathologist
WorldTide, Inc.
Williamsburg, Massachusetts
Chapters 35 and 36

Mario C. Browne, MPH, CDP
Director
Office of Health Sciences Diversity, Equity, and
    Inclusion

Interim Associate Dean for Equity, Engagement,
    and Justice
School of Pharmacy
University of Pittsburgh
Pittsburgh, Pennsylvania
Essay 2

Diane Nelson Bryen, PhD
Professor Emerita
Temple University
Philadelphia, Pennsylvania
Chapter 14

Craig Burke
Chapter 1

Maria Burke
Chapter 1

William Burke
Chapter 1

Vanessa L. Burshnic-Neal, PhD, CCC-SLP
Advanced Fellow in Geriatrics
Geriatric Research, Education, and Clinical Center
Durham VA Medical Center
Durham, North Carolina
Chapter 29

Telina Caudill, MS, CCC-SLP, ATP
Speech Pathologist
James A Haley VA Hospital
Tampa, Florida
Chapter 27

Shelly Chabon, PhD, CCC-SLP, F-ASHA
Past President, ASHA 2012
Vice Provost for Academic Personnel and Dean
    Interdisciplinary General Education
Portland State University
Portland, Oregon
Essay 7

Mai Ling Chan, MS, CCC-SLP
Director, Growth and Achievement
Cognixion
Exceptional Leader Podcast Host
Lead Author and Publisher
Becoming an Exceptional Leader Book Series
Phoenix, Arizona
Essay 1

Brittney Cooper, MS, CCC-SLP
Joint Special Education Program
San Francisco State University
University of California, Berkeley
Chapter 7

Paula K. Davis, MA, CDE
Associate Vice Chancellor for Health Sciences
    Diversity, Equity, and Inclusion
University of Pittsburgh
Pittsburgh, Pennsylvania
Essay 4

**Kimberly A. Eichhorn, MS, CCC-SLP,
BC-ANCDS, ATP**
Program Supervisor, Speech Pathology Department
VA Pittsburgh Healthcare System
Pittsburgh, Pennsylvania
Chapter 28

Elena M. Fader, MA, CCC-SLP
Director of Assistive Technology Services
New England Assistive Technology, an Oak Hill
    Center
Hartford, Connecticut
Chapter 3

John W. Gareis, M-Div, PhD
Senior Lecturer (Retired)
Department of Rhetoric and Communication
University of Pittsburgh
Pittsburgh, Pennsylvania
Essays 3, 8, and 9

**Karen J. Golding-Kushner, PhD, CCC-SLP,
F-ASHA**
The Golding-Kushner Speech Center and
    Golding-Kushner Consulting, LLC

Consultant
The Virtual Center for VCFS and Other
    Craniofacial Disorders
East Brunswick, New Jersey
Essay 10

Kate Grandbois, MS, CCC-SLP, BCBA, LABA
Owner and Managing Director
Grandbois Therapy and Consulting, LLC
Co-Founder, Co-Host, and Writer
SLPNerdcast
Concord, Massachusetts
Chapter 12; Essay 15

Sarah Gregory, MS, CCC-SLP
Speech-Language Pathologist and Assistive
    Technology Consultant
Ithaca City School District
Ithaca, New York
Chapters 10 and 23

Stacey Harpell, MS, CCC-SLP, RSLP
Client Services Manager
CAYA
Vancouver, BC, Canada
Chapter 15

Katya Hill, PhD, CCC-SLP
Associate Professor
AAC-BCI Innovation Laboratory—iLab
Department of Communication Science and
    Disorders
University of Pittsburgh
Pittsburgh, Pennsylvania
Chapter 21; Essays 13 and 16

Richard R. Hurtig, PhD, F-ASHA
Professor Emeritus
Department of Communication Sciences &
    Disorders
The University of Iowa
Iowa City, Iowa
Chapter 17

Hillary K. Jellison, MS, CCC-SLP, ATP
Founding Partner
Commūnicāre, LLC

Southwick, Massachusetts
Chapters 1 and 22

Jeeva John, MS, CCC-SLP
Speech-Language Pathologist
Oakland Unified School District
Oakland, California
Chapter 19

Tabitha Jones-Wohleber, MS, CCC-SLP
Communication AACtualized, LLC
AT Team Member
Frederick County Public Schools
Shepherdstown, West Virginia
Chapters 32 and 33

Catherine Kanter, MS, CCC-SLP
Clinical Speech-Language Pathologist
Augmentative and Alternative Communication
    (AAC) Programs
Waisman Center UCEDD
University of Wisconsin–Madison
Madison, Wisconsin
Chapter 16

Marika King, PhD, CCC-SLP
Assistant Professor
Department of Communicative Disorders and
    Deaf Education
Utah State University
Logan, Utah
Chapter 6

Chris Klein, MDIV
AAC United, Halakah
Freelance Speaker, Teacher, and Writer
Holland, Michigan
Essay 13

Laura P. Klug, MA, CCC-SLP, CBIS
TBI/Polytrauma Program Manager
Cincinnati VA Medical Center
Cincinnati, Ohio
Chapter 25

Emily Kornman, MCD, CCC-SLP
Clinical Speech-Language Pathologist
The Gleason Foundation

New Orleans, Louisiana
Chapter 16

Rebecca M. Lavelle, MA, CCC-SLP
Speech-Language Pathologist
South Hadley, Massachusetts
Essay 18

Dorian Lee-Wilkerson, PhD, F-ASHA
Associate Professor and Department Chair
Department of Communicative Sciences and
    Disorders
Hampton University
Hampton, Virginia
Essay 7

**Paula Leslie, PhD, MA Bioethics, FRCSLT,
CCC-SLP**
Consultant Scholar
Preston, United Kingdom
Essays 12 and 19

Amal M. Maghazil, MS, CCC-SLP
Head, Speech & Language Unit
Communication & Swallowing Disorders
    Department
King Fahad Medical City
Riyadh, Saudi Arabia
Chapter 2; Essay 11

Sarah Marshall, MA, CCC-SLP
Clinical Speech-Language Pathologist
Communication Aids and Systems Clinic (CASC) |
    Neuromotor Development Clinic
Waisman Center Clinics UCEDD
University of Wisconsin–Madison
Madison, Wisconsin
Chapter 30

Abygail E. Marx, MS, CCC-SLP
Clinical Speech-Language Pathologist
Augmentative and Alternative Communication
    (AAC) Programs
Waisman Center Clinics UCEDD
University of Wisconsin–Madison
Madison, Wisconsin
Chapter 30

MariaTeresa "Teri" H. Muñoz, SLPD, CCC-SLP
Clinical Assistant Professor
Department of Communication Sciences and
     Disorders
Florida International University
President/Founding Board Member
St. Therese's Roses of Hope, Pediatric Center, Inc.
Miami, Florida
Chapter 7

Tannalynn Neufeld, MS, CCC-SLP
Assistant Teaching Professor
Department of Communication Sciences and
     Disorders
University of Washington
Founder and Director
AACcessible Foundation
Seattle, Washington
Essay 20

Gazit Chaya Nkosi, MA, CCC-SLP
Speech-Language Pathologist
Amherst, Massachusetts
Essay 6

Lesley Quinn, MS, CCC-SLP
Language, Literacy, and AAC Specialist
Commūnicāre, LLC
Southwick, Massachusetts
Chapters 22 and 24; Essay 14

Lindsay R. James Riegler, PhD, CCC-SLP, CBIS
Innovation Specialist/Research Speech-Language
     Pathologist
Cincinnati VA Medical Center
Cincinnati, Ohio
Chapter 25

Jeffrey K. Riley, MSc, RSLP
Program Manager–Retired and Co-Founder
CAYA—Communication Assistance for Youth and
     Adults
Vancouver, BC, Canada
Chapter 15

**Kathryn D'Agostino Russo, MS, CCC-SLP,
TSSLD**
Speech-Language Pathologist

New York City Department of Education District
     75
New York, New York
Chapter 5

Rachel Santiago, MS, CCC-SLP
Clinical Coordinator; Speech-Language
     Pathologist
Inpatient Augmentative Communication Program
Department of Otolaryngology and
     Communication Enhancement
Boston Children's Hospital
Boston, Massachusetts
Chapter 13

Tanushree Saxena-Chandhok, MSc (SLP)
Speech-Language Therapist
Specialised Assistive Technology Centre (SATC),
     SPD
Singapore
Chapter 20

Jill E. Senner, PhD, CCC-SLP
Owner and Director
Technology and Language Center, Inc.
Evanston, Illinois
Chapter 34

Julia Serra, SLP-A
Clinical Team Member
Commūnicāre, LLC
Southwick, Massachusetts
Chapter 1

Erin S. Sheldon, Med
Special Education Lead
AssistiveWare
Kingston, ON, Canada
Chapter 31

Amanda Soper, MS, CCC-SLP
Owner
AACreAtively Communicating, LLC
Assistive Technology Specialist
St. Coletta of Greater Washington
Adjunct Professor
Gallaudet University
Washington, DC
Chapter 11

Gloria Soto, PhD
Professor
Department of Speech, Language and Hearing
  Sciences
Department of Special Education
San Francisco State University
San Francisco, California
Chapters 6 and 7

Amanda Stead, PhD, CCC-SLP
Associate Professor
Pacific University
Forest Grove, Oregon
Chapter 18

Annette M. Stone, MA, CCC-SLP
Senior Clinical Speech Pathologist and Director
  of CASC
Waisman Center
University of Wisconsin–Madison
Madison, Wisconsin
Chapter 16

Glen M. Tellis, PhD, CCC-SLP, F-ASHA
Professor and Chair
Department of Speech-Language Pathology
Misericordia University
Dallas, Pennsylvania
Essay 5

Sarah Miriam Yong Oi Tsun, MA, SLP, ATP
Clinical Manager–Specialised Assistive Technology
  Centre (SATC), SPD
Singapore
Chapter 20

Lois Turner, MS, RSLP, CCC-SLP, ATP
Program Manager and Co-Founder
CAYA–Communication Assistance for Youth and
  Adults
Vancouver, BC, Canada
Chapter 15

Danielle A. Wagoner
Agawam, Massachusetts
Essay 17

Barbara Weber, MS, CCC-SLP, BCBA
Private Practice
Hershey, Pennsylvania
Chapter 9

Oliver Wendt, PhD
Director of the Research Lab on AAC in Autism
  and Developmental Disorders
School of Communication Sciences and Disorders
University of Central Florida
Orlando, Florida
Chapter 4

Elisa Wern, Med, OTR/L, ATP
Lead Occupational Therapist and Local Assistive
  Technology Specialist (LATS)
Alachua County Public Schools
Owner
AT and OT Consulting and Coaching
Gainesville, Florida
Chapter 23

Amy Wonkka, MA, CCC-SLP
Speech-Language Pathologist
Public School AAC Specialist – Massachusetts
Co-Founder, Writer, Co-Host
SLPNerdcast
Shirley, Massachusetts
Chapter 12; Essay 15

**Deborah Xinyi Yong, BHSc (Hons) Speech
Pathology, ATP**
Speech-Language Therapist
AAC Specialist
Your Communication Matters Speech and
  Language Therapy
Kuala Lumpur, Malaysia
Chapter 20

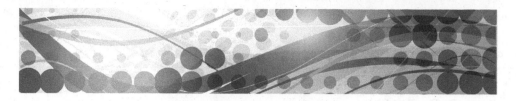

REVIEWERS

Plural Publishing and the authors would like to thank the following reviewers for taking the time to provide their valuable feedback during the manuscript development process.

Karen Copple, PhD, CCC-SLP
Assistant Professor
Eastern New Mexico University
Portales, New Mexico

Katherine M. Czelatdko, MS, CCC-SLP
Clinical Assistant Professor
Marquette University
Milwaukee, Wisconsin

Elena Dukhovny, PhD, CCC-SLP
Associate Professor
Speech, Language and Hearing Sciences
California State University, East Bay
Hayward, California

Jamie D. Fisher, PhD, CCC-SLP
Adjunct Professor
Jackson State University
Jackson, Mississippi

Nicole W. Gallagher, MS, CCC-SLP
Associate Clinical Professor and Speech-Language
    Pathologist
University of Connecticut
Mansfield, Connecticut

Vicki L. Haddix, MS, CCC-SLP
Clinical Associate Professor
University of Memphis
Memphis, Tennessee

Hesper Holland, MS, CCC-SLP
Assistant Professor
Department of Speech-Language Hearing
    Sciences
Texas Tech University Health Sciences Center
Lubbock, Texas

Christina Loveless, MS, CCC-SLP
Assistant Clinical Professor
Communication Sciences and Disorders
    Department
St. Louis University
St. Louis, Missouri

Jyutika Mehta, PhD, CCC-SLP
Professor
Department of Communication Sciences and Oral
    Health
Texas Woman's University
Denton, Texas

Diane C. Millar, PhD
Professor
Radford University
Radford, Virginia

Nikki Murphy, MS, CCC-SLP
Lecturer and Speech-Language Pathologist
Department of Speech Pathology & Audiology
University of Nevada, Reno School of Medicine
Clark County, Nevada

Laura E. Smith, MA, CCC-L/SLP, TSHH
Clinical Assistant Professor and Supervisor for
    Speech-Language Pathology
Department of Communicative Disorders and
    Sciences
University at Buffalo, State University of New York
Buffalo, New York

Margaret Vento-Wilson, PhD, CCC-SLP
Assistant Professor
Department of Speech-Language Pathology
California State University–Long Beach
Long Beach, California

Bruce Wisenburn, PhD, CCC-SLP
Associate Professor
Marywood University
Dunmore, Pennsylvania

SECTION I
AAC System Fundamentals

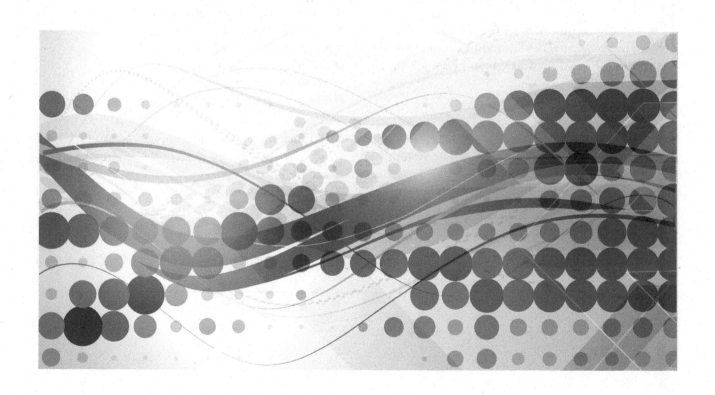

Section I includes five chapters and one essay. The first chapter emphasizes the connection between the person using augmentative and alternative communication (AAC), their communication partners, and their community in the development of meaningful AAC systems. Chapters 2 and 3 discuss AAC system features and detail no-tech AAC systems, as well as mid-tech and high-tech tools. Chapter 4 reviews mobile technology, while Chapter 5 introduces how these AAC systems can be used by persons with different physical abilities and sensory needs through alternative access methods. The essay in this section introduces the combination of brain-computer interfacing and artificial intelligence, and the impact these types of technology have on the field of AAC.

While not the focus of this section, ways of supporting persons who use AAC (PWUAACs), such as aided language stimulation and AAC modeling, start to emerge within the content of the chapters and their respective case studies. These strategies and other concepts (like communicative competence) are discussed in the sections that follow.

Key Terms Reviewed in This Section

- Aided Communication
- Alternative Communication
- Augmentative Communication
- Unaided Communication

- Display representation (schematic, semantic-syntactic, taxonomic, alphabetical, chronological, and Pragmatic Organization Dynamic Display)[1]

- Iconity
- No-tech AAC
- Picture Exchange Communication System (PECS)
- Visual Scene Displays

- Digitized Speech
- High-tech AAC
- Language System

- Mid-tech AAC
- Synthesized Speech
- Voice Output

- Functional communication
- Generative language
- Language intervention
- Mobile technology
- Software design
- Speech-generating devices

- Acquisition of Learning Process (ALP) for access
- Calibration
- Direct access
- Dwell
- Indirect access
- Infrared
- Scanning patterns

---

[1]http://podd.dk/eu-wp/?page_id=33

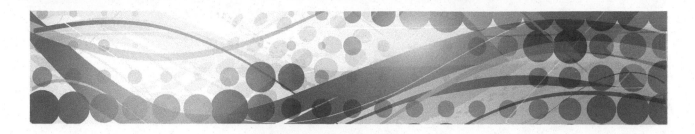

Chapter 1

A CO-CONSTRUCTED DESCRIPTION OF AAC

Nerissa Hall, Hillary K. Jellison, Maria Burke,
William Burke, Craig Burke, and Julia Serra

Introduction

William Burke is 17 years old. He has used augmentative and alternative communication (AAC) in various ways since he was 5 years old. His parents, Maria and Craig Burke (as pictured alongside Will in Figure 1–1), along with speech pathologists/AAC consultants, Hillary Jellison and Nerissa Hall, and speech-language pathology assistant/graduate student, Julia Serra, authored this chapter collaboratively. AAC ensures that an individual has a voice and can be understood. It also serves to connect people with one another, and within their communities. Through synthesis of the perspectives of various stakeholders, one can better understand the power of AAC.

Fundamentals

AAC refers to ways of supporting existing speech and communicating using means other than verbal speech. AAC includes intrinsic, unaided forms of communication (such as facial expressions, gestures, body posturing, and sign language), as well as extrinsic, aided methods (like use of objects, pictures, writing, and typing). AAC is symbolic in that the form or method of AAC represents a letter,

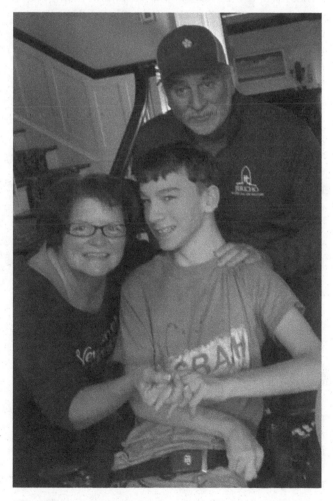

Figure 1–1. Will and his family at the time of authoring this chapter.

word, phrase, or sentence that could otherwise be verbalized.

While AAC is often considered a system involving a carefully organized set of words, icons, letters, and/or phrases, it is important to note that AAC is far more than just a system. AAC establishes a way to communicate and share information between two or more individuals. AAC serves to make meaning. It serves to supplement and augment an individual's existing speech or as an alternative for someone who is nonverbal, aphonic, or hard to understand. AAC creates a connection and allows for meaningful engagement and participation.

For AAC to be efficient, it needs to be relevant and accessible to the individual, with the ability to change and evolve over time, as does the PWUAAC. Adjustable features mean that practitioners and consumers can customize the vocabulary, language, and visual and auditory presentation of the systems (as detailed in the chapters of the first section of this text) to accommodate an individual and personalize the tool that represents their voice. Technological advancements mean that most anyone can use AAC tools through access to manipulative objects or icons, capacitive screens that are responsive to the electrical properties of human touch, the extensive array of switches to account for limited movement, eye-gaze access options, brain-computer interfaces (BCIs) that detect neural signals (Brumberg et al., 2018), or artificial intelligence (Cognixion, 2021), for example. These programming and technological features help ensure the efficiency of the AAC system.

For AAC to be effective, it needs to empower an individual to express themself in an authentic way that is understood and serves to connect them with their communication partner(s). Both the partner and the community need to be taken into consideration for this connection to be genuine. AAC represents an intersection between an individual with complex communication needs (CCNs), the people with whom the individual communicates, and their environment(s). The AAC system arises from the interplay between these elements, evolving as these elements change over an individual's life span.

While there are strong foundational concepts that guide the field, the practice of AAC (the way in which we assess, intervene, and implement it) has to be co-constructed between individuals, their communication partner(s), and their respective communities. The professional(s) with whom they work add to and facilitate this co-constructed communication, rather than dictate it. The role of the speech-language pathologist (SLP) is to establish a foundation for collaborative and transdisciplinary work where the individual and their communication partners are involved in truly meaningful ways. There is no single, one-size-fits-all way to "do" AAC. Instead, each assessment, treatment, and implementation plan must be unique to the individual, and arises from their cognitive-linguistic profile, physical abilities, sense of self, their psychosocial makeup, their family, and their community.

A Change in Focus

"Doing" AAC work means embracing a mindset of discovery, where one is open to and seeking to understand what is important to the individual far beyond the confines of the clinical environment. This involves careful integration of what one knows about the field of AAC with the unique information presented by the individual themself. It means to establish a space and time for genuine involvement of the individual and their family members, caregivers, and important communication partners. For SLPs, this means orchestrating the involvement of various stakeholders and empowering the influence of their input in the ways in which an AAC system is established and subsequently implemented. This is meaningful work that changes lives.

Authentic, family-centered work, by its very nature, ensures generalization into an individual's everyday life and is therefore effective and "supportive of change" (Luterman, 2021). This clinical direction is particularly important when considering AAC, as the burden of responsibility most often falls on familiar communication partners to make sure an individual can communicate effectively and have their needs met, especially in the absence of AAC. Additionally, AAC has the potential to enhance the connection between an individual and their most important partners through shared understanding and meaning. Luterman suggests that by involving the parent or family member, we, in turn, improve the outcomes for the individual (2021); intervening at the level of the caregiver can help to reduce caregiver distress (Maresca et al., 2019; Ncube et al., 2018), which can also lead to improved outcomes and quality of life (QoL). Our pull-out, outpatient, and school-based models of care do not necessarily make space for authentic intervention that emphasizes the family and communication partners (but they can!).

Further highlighting the connection between the individual and their most important communication partners within various environments is the development of friendships. AAC can positively impact QoL by supporting an individual's ability to participate more independently in social exchanges and activities. This also serves as a connection to one's community and "circles" of family, friends, colleagues, professionals, and even unfamiliar partners (Blackstone, 1999). One's community influences our way of thinking, is closely tied to an individual's identity, and is interwoven with the words used and the ways in which people engage, interact, and communicate. To know about one's community means to better understand what is consequential and pertinent for the individual and their social position. This informs the vocabulary and language adjustments necessary to make the AAC system meaningful.

AAC offers access to language, which is an "instrument of communication . . . [and constitutes] a means of asserting one's identity or one's distinctiveness from others" (Jaspal, 2009, p. 17), and is more than words programmed to support participation and overcome barriers. To afford this, AAC must be designed and individually tailored to meet and exceed the needs of the individual; to try to best reflect their uniqueness while creating space for novelty and spontaneity, as well as syntactic, semantic, and pragmatic advancement, self-expression, and the development of their character.

Digitized (voice recorded) and synthesized (computer generated) voices need to match the individual as best possible, and the individual should be involved in making this selection. Collectively, these factors allow AAC to serve as an individual's voice.

A Co-Constructed Understanding of AAC

AAC can be and can mean something different to different stakeholders. By listening to the stakeholders and letting their input carry weight and meaning, the SLP facilitates this process of collaboration and co-development of meaningful AAC.

For the individual with CCNs, AAC means having a voice, being heard, and being understood. However, it also means hard work, where the purpose and reward of the effort may not be easily discernible. While regular practice using a specific set of target vocabulary or word combinations in a prescribed context will help build upon a skill, for an individual this might need to be balanced with AAC "downtime" where using the prescribed system is not always expected. With the ultimate goal being to engage in a manner that is understood, it is important to "hear" from the individual how this can be done most effectively. With the mindset of discovery, and through the use of active listening strategies, AAC practitioners can adjust the AAC system and clinical approach to ensure meaningful connection and authentic representation of the individual.

For parents and caregivers, AAC can mean less guessing and less frustration. It can provide a shared medium for problem-solving and can foster a trusting relationship based on the premise that "we will figure this out." When well-designed and available, and tailored with linguistic and conceptual growth in mind, AAC can pave the way for opportunities and interactions not yet imagined. "Just give me some words" can set in motion a process of co-construction between a caregiver and their child that creates new conversations, new ideas, and new connections.

Maria reflects on a moment with Will and writes:

So, Will's adopted as you know. When the talker (AAC system) was still exciting to him, and finally attached to his chair so he could access it at all times, we were driving together, and he asked me, "what's my Mom's name?" I answered, "Maria," but he then said "no, my other Mom." I totally didn't expect that comment but shared her name with him, and he immediately created a button for her and asked me what she looked like so he could select the best icon for her. I'd never have known he was thinking about her if not for the talker . . . and without the talker he may have been really hesitant to talk with me about what some might think are difficult issues.

AAC can offer the opportunity to establish a real relationship with others. It can empower an individual to explore and express thoughts and feelings they may otherwise not be able to, and creates space for laughter, love, and a more enriched connection. It can also influence the communication of the caregiver and communication partner. Using AAC is significantly slower than using verbal speech (although this is constantly changing with advancing technology). Meaningful incorporation of AAC means making the time for novelty and creating the opportunities for spontaneity. It means exploring the system together or when the individual is asleep or not using it to get a sense of the potential offered within the system. It also means ensuring there is access to vocabulary and linguistic concepts that allow for the actualization of what is not yet realized.

For the individual and their caregivers as a unit, AAC can represent safety in having access to a method of communication that can be understood by people outside of their small and intimate network. AAC can mean less guessing for caregivers (the people who know the individual best and are most equipped to anticipate unmet needs and wants) as well as for less familiar communication partners. AAC can mean improved self-advocacy. By "giving some words," an interplay between the individual and their partner is established, and the PWUAAC can better advocate for themselves.

For the practitioner and communication partner more familiar with AAC systems, AAC means a medium for shared engagement. By pointing to letters, words, or icons on an individual's AAC system or comparable AAC system (strategies known as aided language stimulation [Goossens', 1989] and AAC modeling [Binger & Light, 2007], which are discussed in subsequent chapters), the practitioner can support language development and meaningful communicative exchanges by using AAC as they communicate themselves. This demonstration of multimodal communication involving AAC establishes an environment of respect and acceptance where AAC is available, visible, and incorporated into one's own communicative exchanges. These actions empower **the practitioner to set the tone for success**. By striving for meaningful and motivating connection, the "hard work" inherent to learning and using AAC in a verbal world can be "good work," and fun as well. The seasoned AAC practitioner can take what is almost second nature to them (creating opportunities for modeling and using AAC and multimodal communication) and extend this comfort to others, empowering more widespread acceptance and understanding of AAC leading to immersion of AAC into a way of being.

In Conclusion

The field of AAC is one that has grown and evolved tremendously as our understanding of AAC has broadened, the application of AAC has become more widespread, and AAC technology has advanced. The AAC tools are always changing, but the task of facilitating an individual's ability to communicate fully and independently in a manner that is meaningful to them remains constant, irrespective of who they are and how they are supported. Each AAC system represents a product where language, vocabulary, and access features are shaped by the uniqueness of the individual. This is consistent with the International Classification of Functioning, Disability, and Health (ICF) model developed by the World Health Organization that emphasizes collaborative practice with a focus on an individual's functioning in contexts and environments that are relevant to them (American Speech-Language-Hearing Association [ASHA], 2021). With a mindset of discovery, SLPs working in the field of AAC serve as catalysts for improved communication, meaningful connections, and truly authentic self-expression, where the AAC systems used may change and evolve based on this ongoing interplay between the individual, their partners, and their community.

Case Study: WB

As a group of authors, we use the story of Will, Maria, and Craig to bring to life "the big picture" of AAC. In truth, it is our story and a story of a shared journey influenced by Will, his parents, the communication partners, and environments experienced along the way.

Clinical Profile and Communication Needs

The Individual

At the time of writing this, Will is 17 years old and in 11th grade at a community high school. Will presents with complex communication needs due to his diagnosis of schizencephaly (a rare congenital malformation of the brain that results in a range of cognitive and motor deficits) and has been involved in intensive speech-language, occupational, and physical therapy from a very young age. Will uses a motorized wheelchair and is skilled in accessing technology via direct selection using his dominant hand. Will is a good student and has a small circle of close friends who, like most teenagers, engage with one another via texting. Proloquo4Text® on an iPhone is a backup tool to repair communication breakdowns when his verbal speech is not fully understood. "I can talk like

normal now and I love it," Will adds, but we are all aware that early access to AAC has a lot to do with why we are all here sharing what we know of AAC.

Their Communication Partners

Maria and Craig, Will's parents, along with Uncle Owen are Will's closest communication partners. Will, Maria, and Craig have worked together with Hillary and Nerissa since Will was 5 years old in outpatient, school-based, and recreational environments. In the 12 years of this partnership, there have been very many communication partners that have also been part of this journey. Maria and Craig are strong advocates for Will, sometimes in agreement and disagreement with Will (as parents can be). They push Will to be his best self, both as a person and within school. This has facilitated Will's current successes and has also fostered and developed his determination and inner perseverance.

Will has a large extended family, has friends at school, as well as many friends met through online gaming platforms. Additionally, Will and his family connect with a number of professionals in academic and medical settings. Will is active in his interactions with these communication partners.

Their Environment

As a family, the Burkes are social and have family and friendship circles that are broad, loving, and accepting. At home, Will's family has made many renovations to their house to make it accessible for Will and to support his independence in maneuvering within his home. The Burkes often entertain family and guests (and host fantastic, themed events). Communication, connection, and laughter are extremely important to this family and their circles.

Additionally, Will is an active member of his school community. He attends grade-level and honors classes, with one being English. This is something he and his team are quite proud of. Will recently took a computer-aided design (CAD) class and enjoys art classes when they fit in his schedule. Will is more of an active participant in class within small-group or project-based tasks. However, since being in school remotely (due to the COVID-19 pandemic), most classroom participation occurs via typing and using the chat, and Will is able and willing to be more active. Will is very much a member of his high school community. He is included and appreciated, especially given his awesome sense of humor and inquisitive ideas.

Will is also active in the online gaming community. Within this environment, the playing fields are even. He is not first noticed by his wheelchair, but rather as a gamer (and a good one at that). He has met and interacted with people all over the United States and Canada through online gaming.

The AAC System

When Will first started with AAC, he used a Vantage Plus (shown in Figure 1–2) from Prentke Romich

Company with the 45 One-Hit vocabulary overlay. He quickly switched to a 45 Sequenced overlay where he had access to more vocabulary, various parts of speech, as well as tensing and pluralizing options. Will's language exploded at this point, and it was clear his communication partners were no longer teaching Will about the system but rather learning about it from him. To foster Will's exploration, access to the more complex 84 Sequenced vocabulary was linked directly within the overlay (rather than within the system's programming and operational tools). Will was able to alternate between the overlays, teaching himself where to find familiar words and also being able to revert to his more familiar overlay when he could not find a word in the 84 set.

Will transitioned to Prentke Romich's Accent device (shown in Figure 1–3) with the 84 Sequenced as his main overlay. This was then linked to Word-Power (a word-based rather than icon-based overlay) with the keyboard on his main page. Ready access to the keyboard empowered Will to refine his spelling and keyboarding skills, and he developed his use of word prediction as a rate enhancement technique. Both the Vantage Plus and the Accent 1000 were able to be mounted to Will's wheelchair or could be positioned on his desk or

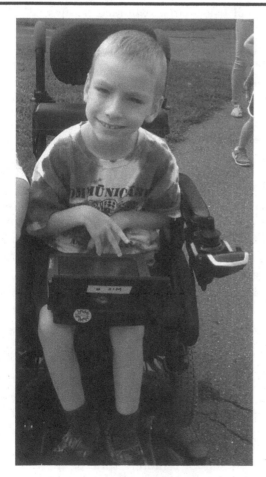

Figure 1–2. Will with his Vantage Plus.

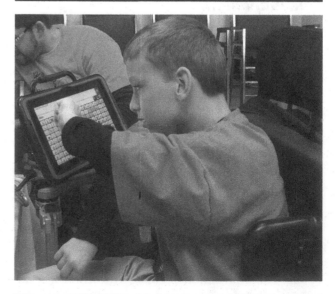

Figure 1–3. Will with his Accent 1000 mounted to his power wheelchair.

table so that the devices were always available and accessible.

Throughout his time working with a voice output device, Will was also working on his speech. He was always encouraged to use multiple methods of communication. As Will's intrinsic methods of communication advanced (such as his verbal speech and gestural communication), he became less reliant on his voice output AAC tools. With the switch to using AAC to repair communication breakdowns rather than his primary mode of communication, and his improved typing skills, Will also switched to using Proloquo4Text on an iPad (which was later added to his iPhone). Now, Will is predominantly verbal, which he loves, and uses texting and Proloquo4Text in certain environments and as a backup when not understood (shown in Figure 1–4).

The AAC Process

The historical review of Will's use of AAC clearly highlights how the AAC tools change over time (and as shown in Table 1–1). This process is not unique to Will but is more reflective of how AAC accommodates the needs of the individual as the individual evolves and progresses over time. The way the AAC systems developed had to do with Will, what was important to him and his family, as well as what was needed based on who he was, with whom he needed to communicate, and the places and environments in which this needed to happen. His clinical team was essentially "along for the ride," inviting input from Will and his family (by honoring their wishes and measuring his performance) and using this input to guide high-level clinical decision-making about AAC selection and customization, communication partner training, and implementation.

Next Steps

This shared journey will continue to evolve in ways not yet discovered. Currently, AAC goals are focused on refining independent communication skills, talking on the phone, applying to colleges, introducing oneself to unfamiliar communication partners, fully engaging in an interview, and ordering pizza. College will bring new priorities and new goals where Will, his parents, and his SLP will come together to co-construct the next phase of the AAC plan.

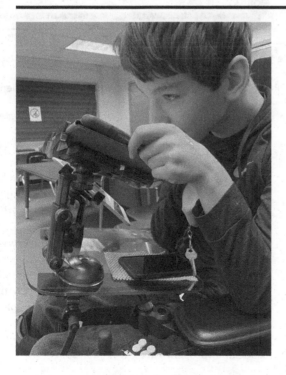

Figure 1–4. Will with his iPhone on his wheelchair tray for ready access to repair communication breakdowns.

Table 1–1. Images of the Main Pages of Will's 45 One-Hit, 84 Sequenced, WordPower, and Proloquo4Text Systems

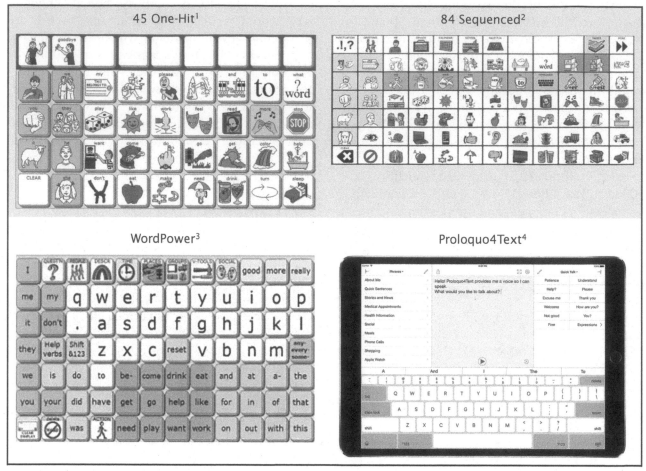

[1]©2021 PRC-Saltillo. Used with permission.

[2]©2021 PRC-Saltillo. Minspeak® symbols used under exclusive license from Semantic Compaction Systems, Inc. Used with permission.

[3]Unity 45 One-Hit and Unity 84 Sequenced are trademarks of PRC-Saltillo. © 2021 PRC-Saltillo. WordPower is a trademark of Inman innovations, Inc.

[4]Proloquo4Text® is an AssistiveWare® product. Used with permission.

References

American Speech-Language-Hearing Association (ASHA). (2021). *International Classification of Functioning, Disability, and Health (ICF)*. https://www.asha.org/slp/icf/

Binger, C., & Light, J. (2007). The effect of aided AAC modeling on the expression of multi-symbol messages by preschoolers who use AAC. *Augmentative and Alternative Communication, 23*(1), 30–43.

Blackstone, S. (1999). Communication partners. *Augmentative Communication News, 12*(2), 1–6.

Brumberg, J. S., Pitt, K. M., Mantie-Kozlowski, A., & Burnison, J. D. (2018). Brain-computer interfaces for augmentative and alternative communication: A tutorial. *American Journal of Speech-Language Pathology, 21*(1), 1–12.

Cognixion. (2021). *AI-powered people*. https://www.cognixion.com

Goossens', C. (1989). Aided communication intervention before assessment: A case study of a child with cerebral palsy. *Augmentative and Alternative Communication, 5*, 14–26.

Jaspal, R. (2009). Language and social identify: A psychosocial approach. *Psych-Talk*, 17–20.

Luterman, D. (2021, April 9). *Counseling parents at the time of diagnosis: Getting beyond informational counseling* [Conference presentation]. UMass Amherst 2021 Communication Disorders Professional Conference, Amherst, MA.

Maresca, G., Pranio, F., Naro, A., De Luca, R., Maggio, M. G., Scarcella, I., . . . Calabrò, R. S. (2019). Augmentative and alternative communication improves quality of life in the early stages of amyotrophic lateral sclerosis. *Functional Neurology, 34*(1), 35–43.

Ncube, B. L., Perry, A., & Weiss, J. A. (2018). The quality of life of children with severe developmental disabilities. *Journal of Intellectual Disability Research, 62*(3), 237–244.

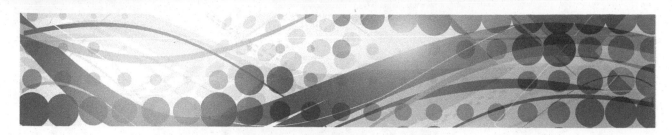

Chapter 2
NO-TECH AAC

Amal M. Maghazil

Fundamentals

AAC references a broad range of methods and systems of communication designed to support individuals from any age, ethnic, racial, or socio-economic group, who are unable to effectively speak either temporarily or permanently. AAC is distinguished into two main categories, unaided and aided systems. Aided AAC systems vary in design based on symbols, organization, and their display. These "no-tech systems" are also known as paper-based, low-tech, or lite-tech (sometimes spelled as light-tech) AAC. They do not involve any form of technology and therefore do not have a battery and do not offer voice output. No-tech AAC systems provide visual referents that can be used to better express oneself. Examples include communication boards, Picture Exchange Communication System (PECs; Bondy & Frost, 2001), and alphabet boards.

No-tech AAC can be an effective means of communicating for a variety of individuals in many different settings. Words, pictures, or phrases placed strategically within an environment can serve as prompts for a person who uses augmentative and alternative communication (PWUAAC) but can also be used to communicate meaningfully in a given context (such as "let's go out" placed by a door in a classroom, like shown in Figure 2–1, that one can point to before exiting the room). A single piece of paper (a language board), like the one shown in Figure 2–2, with words and icons organized in a

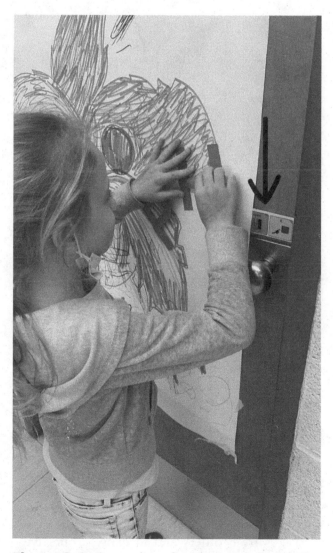

Figure 2–1. Examples of AAC positioned in the environment.

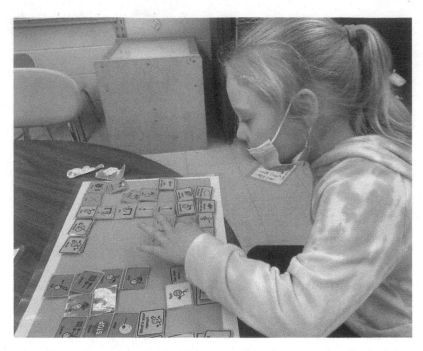

Figure 2–2. Example of a language board.

particular way, can be used by pointing to icons in sequence to build phrases such as "I read it," "you read it," and "make it go," for example. These single pages or language boards can be adhered to furniture (like a cafeteria table) or placed with specific items (like a board game, beside the TV remote, or next to a book) to help support communication in a given context. A series of such pages can comprise a book to offer an individual a rich set of vocabulary and phrases that can be taken with them wherever they go. An alphabet board with (or without phrases), like the one shown in Figure 2–3, is another example of no-tech AAC appropriate for literate individuals.

Unaided AAC

Unaided AAC includes gestures, facial expressions, body language, signs, eye blink, and vocalizations; all-natural nonverbal forms of communication. We use nonverbal communication to interpret messages from others and to express ourselves. Research estimates that two thirds of human interaction is conveyed via nonverbal communication

(Burgoon et al., 2016), which speaks to the effectiveness of unaided AAC.

Unaided AAC is the use of the individual's own body and does not require any external supports. Gestures are fine motor movements of the extremities used to communicate a message (e.g., pointing, thumbs down, head nod). Representational gestures reference objects or actions that people typically develop at a young age (e.g., using one hand and moving it on the hair to resemble "brushing"). Gestures can be used alone or accompanied by facial expressions (e.g., pointing to a person while smiling). Since many individuals commonly use gestures and facial expressions, they are socially and culturally acceptable to many. This makes gestures accessible and easy to use by individuals who require an alternative or augmentative way to communicate. However, gestures alone are oftentimes not enough to meet an individual's communication needs due to the limited number of messages conveyed.

Sign language is also a type of unaided AAC. American Sign Language (ASL) differs from spoken English language due to its unique language systems, which have different morphology, syntax,

Hey!	How are things?	Give me an update on things	Ask me some questions	Tell me something new	I'm in the mood for something good
I want to talk about...	you	the kids	what's new	how things are	something completely different
How was the day?	How was work?	Did you figure out anything?	What are you planning for the day?	Anything exciting happening?	What's the horoscope?
This sucks!	I've been better	How do I look?	What you've been doing?	Will you....	May I please have...
I have an itch, give me scratch	in need of a massage/rub			I appreciate it	Thank you!

q	w	e	r	t	y	u	i	o	p	
a	s	d	f	g	h	j	k	l		
z	x	c	v	b	n	m				
starts with	no!	that's wrong		space			that's it	thank you	yes!	
								someone else		

Hey!	How are you?	Give me an update on things	Ask me some questions	Tell me something new	I'm in the mood for something good
How was the day?	How was work?	Did you figure out anything?	What are you planning for the day?	Anything exciting happening?	What's the horoscope?
This sucks!	I've been better	How do I look?	I'm tired	Will you....	May I please have...
I have an itch, give me scratch	in need of a massage/rub	Feeling better	I'm not feeling great	I appreciate it	Thank you!

Figure 2–3. Example of an alphabet board with phrases (showing the back and front).

semantics, and pragmatics. (It is important to note that native ASL speakers are not considered to be using AAC.) Key word signing and Baby Signs are manual signing systems that sign the main key words in spoken phrases and sentences. For example, a person says, "Do you want a cookie?" and a sign for a cookie is provided simultaneously. Sign language provides access to a wide range of vocabulary that can be used for many communication functions. However, most people do not use or know these signs, so people might be limited in being able to express their wants in unfamiliar environments or in the absence of a sign language interpreter.

Aided AAC

Aided AAC uses external supports or equipment to represent messages for the purposes of communication. Aided AAC includes no-tech, mid-tech, or high-tech. No-tech aided AAC systems are explained in this chapter, whereas mid- and high-tech AAC are discussed in Chapter 3.

Symbols

Aided AAC symbols include real objects, partial objects, associated objects, photographs, line drawings, and traditional orthography, including both concrete and literal representations. Choosing AAC symbols depends on the complexity of the individual's needs considering their cognitive, comprehension, physical, and sensory skills. Real objects are the most concrete and easily accessible in the individual's environment. Associated/partial objects are used when the whole object is unavailable or inaccessible (e.g., using a student's bus ticket to represent the arrival of the bus). Artificially associated objects are used to link specific textures or materials with their referent (e.g., using a small squishy ball to represent break time). Even though these objects offer concrete or abstract meaning to the messages, oftentimes the associations need to be taught to the PWUAAC. Objects can help individuals with complex communication needs to communicate, especially those with severe cognitive and sensory impairments. They can be used alone or displayed on a communication board (like the one shown in Figure 2–4). However, disadvantages include inconvenience, difficulty carrying/transporting objects, limitations in the messages available, and challenges with replicating the object if misplaced.

Photographs represent less concrete messages than objects and can be conveniently found in print or digital formats. High-quality photographs offer representations of objects, people, actions, places, and meaningful events for the PWUAAC. Research has shown that it is easier for individuals with intellectual disabilities to correlate photographs to their referents when compared to line drawings (Beukelman & Light, 2020; Mirenda & Lock, 1989; Sevcik & Romski, 1986). Additionally, for some individuals with visual processing difficulties, photos with nothing in the background or high-contrast coloring may be easier to make sense of, and therefore use to communicate.

Line drawings also provide a variety of symbols to represent a wide range of vocabulary and concepts. Many line drawing sets are available, allowing users to choose sets depending on the number/type of symbols present, language used, concepts represented, symbol customization options (editing, color adjustments, combining symbols), color contrast, high-tech device compatibility, and sharing features. Two commonly used symbol sets are Picture Communication Symbols (PCS) (Tobii Dynavox, LLC, 2021) and SymbolStix (N2Y, LLC, 2021). Both sets can be purchased and have generic, template communication boards ready for immediate use. Other symbol sets available are Widgit symbols (Symbols Worldwide, Ltd., 2019), Pics for PECs, and Pictographic Communication Resources (PCR) (Aphasia Institute, 2015), among others.

An icon's meaning and how it relates to its referent is known as "iconicity," and icons/symbols can vary depending on how easy their meaning is to discern (Bloomberg et al., 1990). This relationship can be clear when the referent is something tangible and observable (like a picture of an apple means "apple"). Such symbols are known as transparent, and their meaning can be identified quickly. In contrast, translucent symbols need a little more information to explain the connection (like a picture of a bed means "sleep" rather than "bed"), and opaque symbols do not clearly repre-

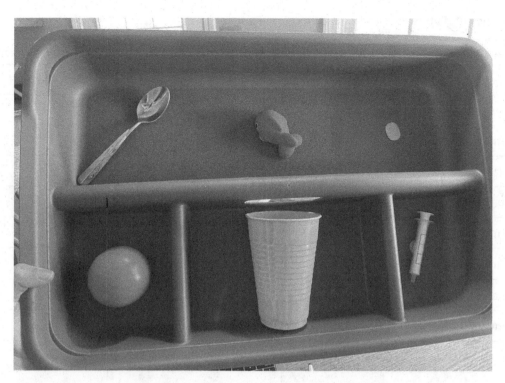

Figure 2–4. Example of an object communication system.

sent their referent (like fireworks meaning "awesome"). Offering a robust vocabulary often means using translucent or opaque symbols to represent adjectives, prepositions, and other more abstract words and concepts.

Individuals may demonstrate variability in their ability to determine an icon's meaning, may find one symbol set more meaningful than another, or may express a preference for a particular symbol set. After taking into account the iconicity, vocabulary selection is critical to truly represent the individual and their needs, as well as support their engagement with their communication partners and their community (see Chapter 7 for details). The communication partner's involvement is key in this stage to help identify the individual's most desired messages. It is essential to start intervention with those highly motivating messages in order to demonstrate effective use of AAC, and establish strong buy-in from the individual and their closest communication partners. This will also impact their commitment to therapy. Furthermore, vocabulary

must be used for various communication functions to ensure its effective usage. If the individual only has an AAC board to get their basic needs met but the vocabulary does not offer them the ability to ask questions, greet others, or make comments, the AAC system will not be functional. Table 2–1 details a variety of communication functions that can be used as a checklist for current and future or desired communication needs and wants.

Designing the display is also critical when creating a no-tech AAC system. A thorough feature-matching process is needed to decide on the number and size of the icons the individual can visually identify, visually discriminate, comprehend, and point to or look toward. Once a template is established, the no-tech AAC system should be set up to allow for adjustments as well as vocabulary and language expansion. For example, if the PWUAAC was able to visually identify a single image within a 20-icon grid, but only visually discriminated an image accurately among three icons (i.e., selected the correct image from a field of three

Table 2–1. Current, Future/Desired Communication Functions

Communication Functions	Current	Future/Desired
Get basic needs met		
Request desired items, activities, people		
Offer greetings, partings		
Ask questions		
Answer questions		
Make comments		
Continue an activity		
Terminate an activity		
Initiate conversation		
Repair communication breakdowns		
Other:		

images), then the grid display should have space for 20 icons, with only three images displayed at once, leaving room for more images to be added on the same grid over time. In contrast, if the individual has a progressive medical diagnosis, like Parkinson's disease, the AAC system should serve their current communication needs while offering the flexibility to be adjusted when needed (such as increasing the size of the icon or adjusting the display to account for reduced range of motion).

Display

Communication boards can be designed in various ways depending on the individual's cognitive-linguistic skills, communication environments, their partners, age, vocabulary, and frequency of use. There are various grid display representations: schematic, semantic-syntactic, taxonomic, alphabetical, chronological, and Pragmatic Organization Dynamic Display (PODD; Porter, 2014). Schematic displays are organized by a specific activity or event

and contain only related vocabulary. For example, a board for "Watching TV" will contain actions, objects, and descriptors needed by the PWUAAC to engage in that task. Semantic-syntactic displays are organized according to parts of speech and spoken word order (pronouns, verbs, describing words, and nouns, etc.) and are designed to support language learning (Beukelman & Light, 2020, p. 209). Taxonomic displays include symbols organized by categories (e.g., places, people). Alphabetical displays are organized by alphabetical order, and chronological displays by the sequence of events or activities (e.g., daily schedule). PODD represents a combination of display options with the first page of the book usually displaying phrase starters ("I have something to say," "something hurts," or "let's play," for instance) paired with a number representing the number of the next page to turn to in order to complete the phrase with more specific choices. For example, the page to turn to after selecting "something hurts" would display words pertaining to one's body.

The background of the icons or words can be color-coded to group different kinds of words. For example, the Modified Fitzgerald key (McDonald & Schultz, 1973) and Goossens', Crain, and Elder key (1992) are both semantic-syntactic grid displays, where vocabulary is organized using specific background colors to distinguish different parts of speech from one another (where pronouns are colored with a yellow background, verbs in green, adjectives in blue, for example). These tools can support grammatical skill development, provide cues for literate individuals, and help highlight specific symbols. Limited evidence is available regarding the most effective grid display organization and background color for individuals with complex communication needs (Thistle & Wilkinson, 2015); however, no-tech AAC systems should be designed to correlate with the individual's unique presentation and communication needs, partners, and environments.

Alphabet boards are another type of no-tech AAC system where letters are alphabetically organized or alphabetized within categories. There are also eye-transfer boards (e-Tran), which are discussed in greater detail in Chapter 5. These include specific groupings of letters and numbers, designed for people with the ability to spell but significantly limited use of their body, therefore warranting the use of their eyes. Alphabet systems can be accessed directly or indirectly through partner-assisted scanning (PAS). For example, the partner starts by saying the letters in alphabetical, QWERTY, or grouped order and then waits for the PWUAAC to indicate which letter (or within which group) the first letter is of their intended word/message. This process continues until the full word is spelled or guessed correctly by the partner. These no-tech systems are used by literate individuals, offer access to novelty and a wide range of expressions, and are easy to use. These boards can be beneficial for individuals with tracheostomies in the intensive care unit (ICU) who need a temporary way to communicate, and for children and adults with the necessary literacy skills for spelling messages to repair verbal communication breakdowns or to communicate. A disadvantage of these display options is that it is time consuming and can be challenging for individuals who have difficulties attending or quickly get fatigued.

PECS (Bondy & Frost, 2001) is another type of no-tech AAC that uses a specific and clearly defined systematic approach to teach individuals with complex communication needs (often individuals with autism) to exchange icons/phrases with their communication partner. It teaches individuals to discriminate icons and communicate by using these icons individually or in combination to form phrases and sentences. It consists of six phases (How to Communicate, Distance and Persistence, Picture Discrimination, Sentence Structure, Responsive Requesting, and Commenting) and works up from using single words to word combinations for a variety of purposes like making requests, asking questions, commenting, and so on.

Last, lite-tech, paper-based (nonelectronic) visual scene-display books (Muttiah et al., 2019; Samarasinge & Muttiah, 2018) are tools that are interactive and contextual. These tools are picture-based and display a scene/context with salient elements that can be pointed to or are manipulative (i.e., can be removed from the base picture and exchanged with a communication partner). These tools can be used for the purposes of communication, especially for individuals benefiting from context, and have been shown to support reciprocal communicative exchanges with young children (Muttiah et al., 2019). Digitized visual scene displays are also available and are reviewed in Chapter 3.

Using No-Tech AAC

Individuals can use no-tech systems directly by pointing to letters, words, pictures, or phrases with their fingers, with their eye gaze, or via lights/lasers (that can be attached to the individual's head or glasses in order for them to be able to shine a light on their intended target). Some individuals might require accessibility modifications like using a touchguide to raise the borders of the grid surface to support accuracy. For example, if an individual has difficulty keeping his finger pointed toward the target, a touchguide made of soft textured material (around each icon) can be helpful in maintaining their position. Or, increased padding (increased space between icons) can enhance the accuracy of the individual's selections. Alternatively, an individual can indirectly access no-tech AAC through PAS, as described earlier. A more in-depth discussion regarding physical access of AAC is presented in Chapter 5.

A well-designed no-tech AAC system can serve as a stand-alone system or can complement a mid- or high-tech system, depending on the needs of the PWUAAC, their partners, and their environments. For example, a PWUAAC may benefit from an alphabet board with phrases or may have a semantic-syntactic language board for communicating in the park or printed on a shirt for when in the pool or during sporting events (as shown in Figure 2–5). When using mid- and high-tech AAC, it is suggested that there also be a corresponding no-tech backup for use in different environments or to be available when a battery-operated tool is being charged or repaired. If an individual is using both no-tech and high-tech AAC, both systems should follow the same organization and color-coding whenever possible to support learning and/or to offer consistency.

Some advantages of no-tech AAC over mid- or high-tech AAC systems include accessibility, versatility, cost-effectiveness, low maintenance, waterproofing, and customizable grid displays. It is easy to print multiple versions to ensure they are available when needed. Some disadvantages include lack of audio output, weight (if containing multiple pages), and being time-consuming to make. See Table 2–2 for more pros and cons.

In Conclusion

No-tech AAC is powerful and can effectively support communication for individuals depending on their strengths and areas of need, their partners, and their environments. There are various ways no-tech AAC systems can be designed with respect to display, the icons used, organization, and color-coding; many of these features can support engagement with a range of partners (i.e., enlarged font to support communication with a partner who may have visual acuity challenges, or icons for partners who cannot read). Similarly, no-tech AAC systems can be printed on various materials, laminated, enlarged, or adapted depending on the environments in which they need to be used. Generic or customized no-tech systems can also be available around the environment to support communication in a given context when AAC may not be available. This is essential to promote immersion of AAC into the environment. Additionally, no-tech AAC offers immediate access to a way to communicate and can also help people determine whether or not AAC can be effective and therefore whether or not additional mid- and high-tech AAC systems should be explored.

It is important to note that decisions about no-tech AAC options should be driven by the individual's needs and not by service limitations (Iacono et al., 2013), and if high-tech AAC is not available, then no-tech systems should be made available and designed to best meet the individ-

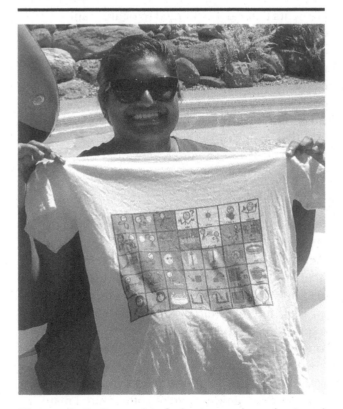

Figure 2–5. Example of a language board printed on a t-shirt for swimming.

Table 2–2. Advantages and Disadvantages of No-Tech AAC

Pros	Cons
Accessible/easy to make	No audio output
Easily duplicated/multiple copies	Multiple pages, can get heavy
Cost effective	Nondynamic display, limited options on single page
Adjustable size (can be as big as a poster)	Slow access, if multiple pages
Ability to use concrete objects/textures	Time consuming to make, print, laminate
Can be printed on different surfaces/materials	Mistakes not quickly adjusted by "edit button"
Waterproof if laminated	Not universally understood if one cannot read
Compatible to all languages, easy to adjust text	
Easily maintained, nonelectrical	
No battery, no need to be charged	
Backup to any mid- or high-tech device	
Can be more efficient	
Supports the engagement of the communication partner	

ual's communication needs. Facilitators and barriers of using unaided and no-tech AAC systems should be identified. Understanding what makes use of AAC work and what hinders effective use is essential to minimize the likelihood of abandonment of the system and increase the success and effective use of AAC. According to Moorcroft and colleagues (2019), barriers fall within all the International Classification of Functioning, Disability, and Health (ICF) domains, and included factors related to personal (health, attitude, and motivation), environmental (caregivers' attitudes, support, services), and body functions (cognition and movement), and that "the onus of responsibility for the successful introduction of AAC systems falls on the professional involved" (p. 727). By understanding these barriers, SLPs can address them to help support successful use of AAC.

Expert Tips or Practical Advice

■ When introducing no-tech AAC systems, start with activities or conversations related to the individual's interests instead of starting with basic wants/needs. This will increase AAC acceptance and functional usage while highlighting the importance of communication for individuals with complex communication needs.

■ When assessing an individual for AAC, think about their strengths (what the individual is doing well) before thinking about their challenges, and design the system around what they can do.

Case Study: PG

Clinical Profile and Communication Needs

The Individual

PG is a 34-year-old male with a history of hypertension who was admitted to an acute inpatient hospital to manage multiple strokes. He was transferred from his hometown to a tertiary care hospital in another city. Magnetic resonance imaging (MRI) revealed posterior circulation ischemic strokes in the cerebellum, brainstem, left thalamus, and left occipital lobe. He also had cardiac thrombosis and pulmonary embolism and required a tracheostomy tube insertion. PG stayed in the ICU before transferring to a medical ward. He had quadriparesis (weakness in all of his four limbs) and limited head and neck control (moving his head slightly from right to left). A modified barium swallow (MBS) study revealed severe oropharyngeal dysphagia, and a nasogastric tube (NGT) was inserted. Then, a couple of weeks later, a percutaneous endoscopic gastrostomy (PEG) tube was inserted.

PG is right-handed, holds a bachelor's degree, and works as a full-time teacher. He is married, has two young children, and is the breadwinner of the household. He resides in Saudi Arabia, and his primary language is Arabic. The caregiver reported that the client was independent with activities of daily living (ADLs) and presented with no communication, hearing, or vision concerns before hospital admission. Currently, PG communicates with his family by eye blink and occasionally laughs/cries in response to conversations or when watching TV.

When assessing PG, it was essential to establish a reliable yes/no response to help determine his language and cognition. Since he was only using eye blink to express "yes" and looking away to express discomfort, another type of unaided AAC needed to be determined. PG occasionally moved some of his fingers spontaneously, but not on demand. He presented with slight head/neck control and approximated a head shake for "no." After PG was trained on these two responses (eye blink for "yes," head shake for "no"), he answered complex yes/no questions with 100% accuracy. His short-term and episodic memory were informally assessed, and he recalled events, people, and procedures from the past week when asked in yes/no format. He presented with variable inattention but was quickly redirected. PG maintained eye gaze toward the person speaking to him and occasionally smiled/laughed in response to humor. He sometimes looked away and seemed frustrated when asked about certain information that he knew.

Their Communication Partners

PG's younger brother was the primary caregiver during the hospital stay. He had a close relationship with PG and had high respect for his older brother. This sometimes affected the partner's attitude toward motivating PG to participate in therapy or try AAC when he was uninterested.

Communication partners at the hospital included doctors, nurses, respiratory therapists, physical therapists, speech-language pathologists, case managers, and social workers. At the time of PG's hospital stay, visitors were not allowed, so he communicated with his family members via video calls. At home, PG's communication partners included his wife, two young children, mother, father, sisters, and brothers. At work, his partners included the school principal/administrators, teacher assistant, students, and parents of students. Other communication partners included his two close friends, ranchers, farmers, store clerks, waiters, baristas, and cashiers.

Their Environment

PG's primary communication environments were his home and school. He visited his parents, sisters, and brothers weekly at their homes or family ranch. At the ranch, he communicated with ranchers and farmers. He worked full time at a school and was a home teacher for elementary school students. On weekends, he went out with his friends to their homes, restaurants/cafes, or the family ranch.

The AAC System and Service Considerations

Based on PG's medical condition, caregiver interview, and background, an aided AAC system is required to express his needs/wants during his hospital stay. AAC is emerging where he lives, so there are limitations to accessing various AAC systems and assistive technology. Since he is at the hospital, he mainly communicates with his brother only by answering yes/no questions or looking to the side to express discomfort/refusal. He requires an AAC system to expand his communicative repertoire and get his basic needs met, request, ask/answer questions, and continue or terminate an activity. These various communication functions are necessary to express pain/discomfort, ask for clarification, respond to healthcare workers, request, refuse, and engage in conversation.

The vocabulary needed was gathered from PG in collaboration with his brother through asking questions about PG, his interests, people in his life, and more. When presented with line drawings accompanied by single words, PG identified icons by holding his eye gaze and confirming with an eye blink when asked if this was his selection. Regarding the size and number of icons, a nine-icon grid display was presented, but PG visually discriminated target icons with 50% accuracy. When the grid display was reduced to six icons 3 × 3 inches in size, he discriminated with 80% accuracy. His performance was consistent when presented with one to two written words only (and without line drawings). When his responses were slow, a repetition of the question was given.

In addition to an alphabet board, a couple of paper-based communication boards were developed to meet various communication functions. Schematic grid displays containing line drawings with written words were used for pain, basic needs, greetings/conversation, and social media (#1 to #4 of Figure 2–6). English text was added to the icons used for expressing pain and requesting to move any of his body parts due to English being the primary language of his nurses. A taxonomic grid display containing names of his family members and friends was developed using text only (Figure 2–6; boards 5 and 6 were omitted due to client confidentiality). All these boards were laminated and attached with Velcro on a large poster board due to PG's performance on the visual discrimination tasks described previously.

PG used partner-assisted scanning along with an eye gaze/blink to use his AAC system. His partner was trained to hold the board in front of PG while looking through the middle at him, and to say the boards' titles, wait for PG to look at the board he needs, and then confirm the selection by asking a yes/no question. Once the target communication board was identified, the partner removed the chosen board and repeated the scanning steps until PG expressed his message.

At the beginning of training, the partner was hesitant and not convinced that PG needed AAC. He believed that PG would medically improve and then would express his needs verbally. When not in therapy sessions, the communication board was not placed near to PG, and it was evident that the partner was not motivated to use AAC. This also affected PG, where he would show decreased motivation during direct training. Therefore, therapy focused on PG's successful use of the AAC system in expressing his thoughts and emotions and participating in conversations about topics of his interest, and involving PG's brother in the success. Additionally, the clinician talked to the brother about helping PG communicate now and assured him that using AAC would not affect his ability to speak. For the majority of sessions, only an alphabet board was used to talk about TV shows, movies, and soccer matches, which were his main topics of interest. Even though the alphabet board was time consuming, it allowed PG the freedom to access a wider range of vocabulary to express himself and engage in a meaningful conversation. Both PG and his partner participated well during training. The other boards were gradually introduced and focused on PG being able to share whom he had called or where he had pain. PG was discharged to an inpatient rehab facility where he continued his AAC intervention.

Next Steps

Despite the type of AAC system chosen, it should be applicable to be used in a variety of communication environments. Due to the PG's extended hospital stay, the AAC system had been designed to support his communication in that specific environment,

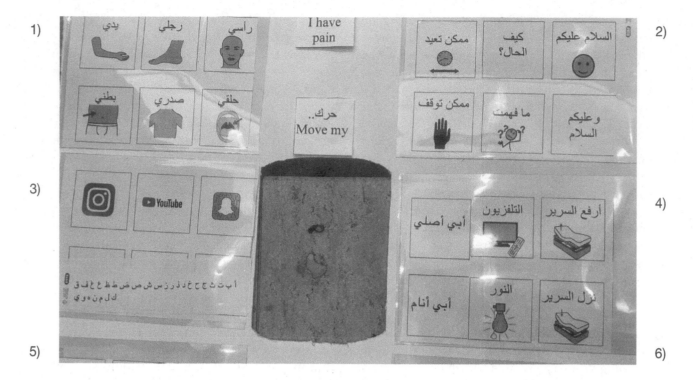

From right to left:
1) Pain board: head, leg, arms, throat, chest, stomach.
2) Greetings/conversation: Salam, How are you? please repeat, Salam to you, I don't understand, please stop.
3) Social media: Instagram, YouTube, Snapchat, Arabic Alphabets.
4) Basic needs: raise bed, TV, I want to pray, lower bed, lights, I want to sleep.
5) & 6) Names of all family members, text only.

Figure 2–6. PG's communication board.

and the application was limited to one setting. Also, due to the emerging AAC services where he lives, access to other technology options (which might assist in increasing the speed and accuracy of his eye gaze responses) was not available for inpatients at the facility at which he stayed. Given this, no-tech AAC systems were adjusted to meet PG's needs in settings other than the hospital, and others needed to be developed to allow PG to express himself for a variety of purposes with his communication partners in various settings. Continuous client and partner training along with consistent monitoring of PG's progressing physical/motor skills are essential in modifying the system to meet his changing needs.

References

Aphasia Institute. (2015). *Pictographic Communication Resources (PCR)*. https://www.aphasia.ca/shop/pictographic-communication-resources-binder-pcr/

Beukelman, D. R., & Light, J. C. (2020). *Augmentative & alternative communication: Supporting children and adults with complex communication needs*. Paul H. Brookes.

Bloomberg, K., Karlan, G., & Lloyd, L. (1990). The comparative translucency of initial lexical items represented in five graphic symbol systems and sets. *Journal of Speech and Hearing Disorders, 33*, 717–725.

Bondy, A., & Frost, L. (2001). The Picture Exchange Communication System. *Behavior Modification, 25*(5), 725–744.

Burgoon, J. K., Guerrero, L. K., & Manusov, V. (2016). *Nonverbal communication*. Routledge.

Goossens, C., Crain, S., & Elder, P. (1992). *Engineering the preschool environment for interactive, symbolic communication*. Southeast Augmentative Communication Conference Publications.

Lacono, T., Lyon, K., Johnson, H., & West, D. (2013). Experiences of adults with complex communication needs receiving and using low tech AAC: An Australian context. *Disability and Rehabilitation: Assistive Technology, 8*(5), 392–401.

McDonald, E. T., & Schultz, A. R. (1973). Communication boards for cerebral-palsied children. *Journal of Speech and Hearing Disorders, 38*(1), 73–88. https://doi.org/10.1044/jshd.3801.73

Mirenda, P., & Locke, P. (1989). A comparison of symbol transparency in nonspeaking persons with intellectual disabilities. *Journal of Speech and Hearing Disorders, 54*, 131–140. https://doi.org/10.1044/jshd.5402.131

Moorcroft, A., Scarinci, N., & Meyer, C. (2019). A systematic review of the barriers and facilitators to the provision and use of low-tech and unaided AAC systems for people with complex communication needs and their families. *Disability and Rehabilitation: Assistive Technology, 14*(7), 710–731.

Muttiah, N., Drager, K. D. R., Beale, B., Bongo, H., & Riley, L. (2019). The effects of an intervention using low-tech visual scene displays and aided modeling with young children with complex communication needs. *Topics in Early Childhood Special Education*. https://doi.org/10.1177/0271121419844825

News-2-You, N2Y-LLC. (2021). *SymbolStix Prime*. https://www.n2y.com/symbolstix-prime/

Porter, G. (2014). *Pragmatic Organisation Dynamic Display*. http://podd.dk/eu-wp/?page_id=33

Samarasinge, S. I. S., & Muttiah, N. (2018). *Effectiveness of shared book reading to increase receptive vocabulary skills of 3- to 4-year-old children with autism* [Undergraduate thesis, University of Kelaniya].

Sevcik, R., & Romski, M. A. (1986). Representational matching skills of persons with severe retardation. *Augmentative and Alternative Communication, 2*(4), 160–164.

Symbols Worldwide Ltd. (2019). *Widgit*. https://www.widgit.com/

Thistle, J. J., & Wilkinson, K. M. (2015). Building evidence-based practice in AAC display design for young children: Current practices and future directions. *Augmentative and Alternative Communication, 31*(2), 124–136.

Tobii Dynavox, LLC. (2021). *Picture Communication Symbols*. https://www.tobiidynavox.com/software/content/pcs-classic-symbols/

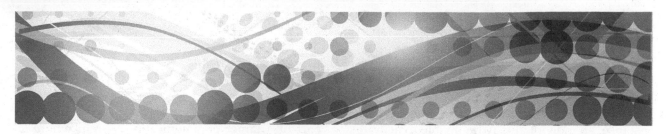

Chapter 3
MID- AND HIGH-TECH AAC

Elena M. Fader

Fundamentals

Mid-tech and high-tech augmentative and alternative communication (AAC) systems represent aided systems that are external to the individual. They are mechanical buttons (not to be confused with switches that are used to support alternative access, as discussed in Chapter 5) or tablets that are generally called "devices." More specifically, mid-tech AAC devices are battery operated, offer voice output, and require minimal training and programming to use them. In contrast, high-tech AAC devices include software or apps (hereafter referred to as "software") displayed on either tablet- or computer-based hardware. Both categories of devices offer voice output, but their displays, the ways they can be used, and the ways in which they can be programmed and customized vary. Both mid-tech and high-tech AAC devices can help supplement or augment an individual's existing speech or act as an alternative mode of communication. These devices can therefore benefit individuals of all ages presenting with various linguistic and physical needs.

Mid-Tech AAC

Mid-tech AAC includes devices offering digitized voice output through voice recording a single message or multiple messages depending on the type of tool. A gender- and age-matched peer should be asked to record the messages on the devices for the voice output to sound appropriate for the given user. These messages can be activated via direct (pressing the device with a body part) or indirect selection (whereby the person presses an external capability switch to trigger the device), as discussed in detail in Chapter 5. A symbol, photograph, and/or text can be adhered to the device and paired with target messages to facilitate the individual's awareness and understanding of them.

Mid-Tech Device Hardware Features

A variety of mid-tech devices exist. These vary by size, the number of messages available, the ways in which they can be activated, and whether or not they can interface with other tools (i.e., have a switch port). For example, mid-tech devices vary in size and subsequent surface area, which are important factors for portability and for physical access. An individual's gross and/or fine motor status may impact whether a small versus a large device is easier to activate (i.e., BIGmack[1] vs. TalkingBrix2[2]). Similarly, the sensitivity, or amount of physical pressure required to activate the button(s) on the device, as well as the angle at which the device can be presented, impact mid-tech selection. Mid-tech devices often have switch ports that

1 AbleNet. (2021). Retrieved from https://www.ablenetinc.com/bigmack/
2 AbleNet. (2021). Retrieved from https://www.ablenetinc.com/talkingbrix-2/

allow for a connection with an additional tool. For instance, an individual may be unable to activate a LITTLEmack[3] with their hand given its size and presented angle but can consistently and effortlessly activate it with a slight finger swipe when a flat Pal Pad[4] capability switch (as shown in Table 3–1) is connected to it.

Mid-tech AAC systems vary in the availability of a single versus multiple message option, along with the maximum recording time. Some devices, such as the GoTalk One,[5] allow for only one message to be recorded onto it, while others, such as the iTalk2 with Levels[6] and the GoTalk 32+,[7] include multiple buttons onto which messages can be recorded (as can be seen in Table 3–1). Some devices, including the GoTalk 32+ and the LITTLE Step-by-Step,[8] also include several recording levels to allow for the recording of multiple messages. To put this feature into perspective, with 32 buttons available and five levels of recording options, the GoTalk 32+ can provide a person who uses augmentative and alternative communication (PWUAAC) with access to up to 160 messages. Table 3–1 shows a range of mid-tech AAC tools, as well as the Pal Pad switch.

Other hardware components to consider are volume controls and mounting capabilities. Having control of the volume is important for use in loud environments and to facilitate conveyance of the message for individuals with hearing impairments, including the person who uses the AAC device along with their communication partner. Additionally, some individuals benefit from having the AAC device secured to a wheelchair mount, table mount, or other customized setup to ensure comfortable and efficient access (and not all devices are designed for mounting). In general, the mid-tech AAC device features listed and described are typically available within the device's technical specifications.

Mid-tech AAC can be a stand-alone system or primary mode of communication for some, can supplement existing speech or support activity-specific participation for others, or can be one part of a larger communication system where an individual has no-tech, mid-tech, and/or high-tech systems depending on specific contexts and communication partners. There are many different ways mid-tech AAC devices can be used. For example, recording questions and comments to be expressed during routine activities can foster engagement and conversational exchanges within group activities. Another example is mid-tech AAC being incorporated into a Functional Communication Training program (a systematic approach to providing easy access to methods of communication to reduce challenging, disruptive, or nonpreferred behaviors [Ghaemmaghami et al., 2021]) where the message "I need help" can be recorded onto a BIGmack, and the individual can systematically be taught to activate the device in lieu of demonstrating negative behaviors.

Repeated opportunities to use mid-tech AAC can help to establish communication skills for individuals with complex communication needs (Romski & Sevcik, 2005). This can be a meaningful way to teach an individual the cause-and-effect nature of communication, wherein a message is shared and a subsequent action results. Additionally, an emerging and developing communicator can explore and use mid-tech AAC prior to using high-tech. However, it is important to note that it is *not* a requirement to follow such an order, and the myth that a user *must* follow a progression of using no-tech AAC before being introduced to mid-tech, and "mastering" mid-tech before being given access to a high-tech device, has been dispelled.

High-Tech AAC

High-tech AAC systems are computers/tablets offering a wide range of visual, auditory, and access features that can empower individuals with very varied profiles to have a voice. While high-tech

[3]AbleNet. (2021). Retrieved from https://www.ablenetinc.com/littlemack/

[4]Adaptivation. (2021). Retrieved from https://www.adaptivation.com/product-page/pal-pads

[5]Attainment. (2021). Retrieved from https://www.attainmentcompany.com/gotalk-one

[6]Adaptive Tech Solutions. (2021). Retrieved from https://www.adaptivetechsolutions.com/italk2-with-levels/

[7]Attainment Company. (2021). Retrieved from https://www.attainmentcompany.com/gotalk-32

[8]AbleNet. (2021). Retrieved from https://www.ablenetinc.com/little-step-by-step/

Table 3–1. Examples of Mid-Tech AAC Systems and an External Switch

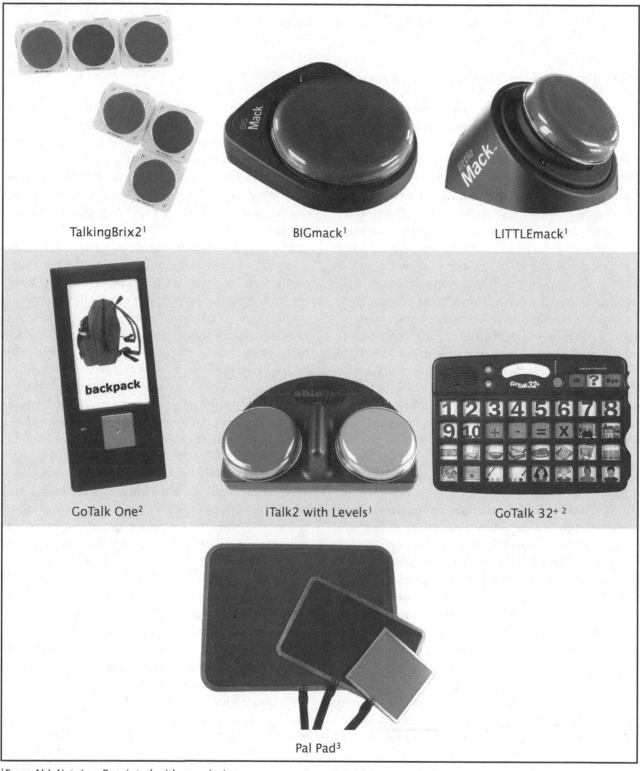

TalkingBrix2[1]   BIGmack[1]   LITTLEmack[1]

GoTalk One[2]   iTalk2 with Levels[1]   GoTalk 32+ [2]

Pal Pad[3]

[1]From AbleNet, Inc. Reprinted with permission.
[2]From Attainment Company. Reprinted with permission.
[3]From Adaptivation Incorporated. Reprinted with permission.

AAC can also offer digitized voice capabilities, what distinguishes these systems from mid-tech devices is that they have synthesized voice options and extensive software features.

High-Tech Device Hardware Features

High-tech devices can vary by their size, weight, alternative access capabilities, portability, mounting options, touch screen sensitivity, and additional features. The size of these devices can range from the size of a cell phone (i.e., approximately 6 inches diagonally) to roughly 13 to 14 inches diagonally, or more (like the size of a laptop). Many have cases or wraps that embed external speakers to offer powerful voice output capabilities. Some systems have eye-gaze attachments with optical sensors to support this access method. Many high-tech AAC systems have a mounting plate so that they can be secured to different mounts, and many vary in the kinds of ports that are available to support connectivity with external accessories such as switches, speakers, a microphone, or storage tool (like an SD card or USB drive, for example). A lot of hardware features are related to physical access and alternative access, both of which are discussed in Chapter 5.

High-Tech Device Software Features

High-tech AAC devices include sophisticated software or apps for programming, customizing, and organizing vocabulary in various display formats (introduced in Chapter 2), offering voice output, supporting navigation within a display, and more. High-tech devices generally come preprogrammed with various vocabulary sets that vary in features and complexity. Many high-tech devices offer "robust" language options that lend themselves to spontaneous novel utterance generation ("SNUG," a term coined by Katya Hill) given the large number of words available representing all different parts of speech, which supports phrase and sentence generation, commenting, requesting, protesting, arguing, joking, questioning, and more. Having access to a way to create novel messages, rather than relying on prerecorded messages, is important for many individuals to share their unique ideas. As

such, high-tech AAC devices typically utilize synthesized speech (the artificial production of human speech based on inputted text), which is universally known as text-to-speech, and there is a range of voice offerings (male, female, child-like or more mature, with the ability to vary volume, pitch, and rate, for example).

In addition to synthesized speech, many high-tech devices can support digitized speech as well. This can be helpful for recording meaningful sounds (i.e., laughing) or even one's voice (which is important for people who may be likely to lose their voice or exhibit reduced intelligibility due to a degenerative condition). Digitized speech can also be incorporated into phonics pages wherein an individual can learn to combine speech sounds to create words, an essential literacy skill. Regardless of the form of voice output, upon selecting a single button on the screen, the corresponding letter, word, or phrase is said aloud and/or transferred to a message window for later expression. Each button can include a symbol, a symbol paired with text, or text exclusively depending on the individual's literacy skills. Incorporating symbols paired with text is preferred and recommended for preliterate and emergent literate individuals using AAC, offering consistent exposure to text.

Robust AAC software offers extensive customization options, which allow it to be set up in accordance with an individual's preferences and needs. Font type/size, button color, background color, grid size, button spacing, voice type, voice rate, grammar support, and the capability to hide buttons (visibility) are adjustable features available in most high-tech AAC systems. Many high-tech systems also offer different languages with extensive vocabularies and various voice options to support bilingual speakers. Having control over these settings is important to ensure that they match an individual's needs in domains such as vision, hearing, sensory, cognitive, and linguistic skills. Given the complexity of many AAC software options, the individual and their communication partners should be trained in using it. Direct instruction and training are critical for ensuring that the individual can maximize the benefits of the device and use it consistently to its full potential (thereby reducing device abandonment).

High-tech AAC devices traditionally present language software in a grid-based layout, wherein symbols, letters, words, and/or phrases are displayed on buttons within a grid of rows and columns. The way in which the messages are organized differs across software (schematic, semantic-syntactic, taxonomic, alphabetical, chronological, as previously detailed in Chapter 2). An alternative format to grid-based layouts is a visual scene display. As discussed in Chapter 2, a visual scene display (VSD) presents a photograph or picture that is meaningful to the individual, often capturing an interaction or familiar activity within a known context. With high-tech systems, "hotspots" with voice output messages, often paired with text, are embedded into different areas of the photograph. Upon selecting a hotspot, the corresponding message is played aloud (Light et al., 2019). This type of vocabulary organization, compared to grid-based, offers rich visual context and can support language development and/or create meaning for people with different needs and profiles. The presentation of an image triggers natural, concrete, and realistic connections to purposeful communication (Light et al., 2019). Examples of software that present AAC in a VSD format are Snap Scene from Tobii Dynavox and GoVisual from Attainment Company, and they can be seen in contrast to grid-based displays in Table 3–2.

Table 3–2. Examples of Grid-Based and VSD Display Options

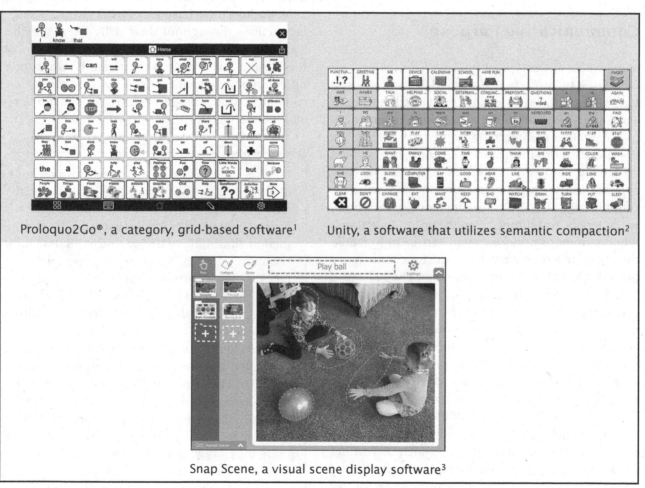

Proloquo2Go®, a category, grid-based software[1]

Unity, a software that utilizes semantic compaction[2]

Snap Scene, a visual scene display software[3]

[1]Screenshot from Proloquo2Go. Proloquo2Go is an AssistiveWare® product. SymbolStix symbols © N2Y, LLC. Used with permission.

[2]Screenshot from Unity® © Prentke Romich Company. Minspeak symbols © Minspeak. Reprinted with permission.

[3]From Tobii Dynavox, LLC © 2021 Tobii Dynavox. All rights reserved. Reprinted with permission.

Regardless of the type of vocabulary organization and display method, high-tech AAC can provide an individual with access to both functional and meaningful communication. In many cases, the goal of high-tech AAC is to provide the individual with a means to communicate for *all* communicative functions, with *all* communication partners, and within *all* contexts. Smaller, milestone objectives must often be met before this larger goal is accomplished. Nonetheless, achieving these objectives can be an effective way to enhance an individual's independence, participation in society, and overall social-emotional well-being. Attaining these targets necessitates that the AAC device contains appropriate vocabulary options (which is discussed in Chapter 7).

Communicative Purpose

Irrespective of the type of system an individual has, whether it be no-tech, mid-tech, high-tech, or a system with multiple devices, an individual must have access to AAC at all times, as needed, to communicate with their communication partners. The places PWUAACs communicate, the individuals with whom they communicate, and the reasons they communicate comprise an individual's "Communication World." Locations may include home, school, work, stores, restaurants, medical offices, and more, while communication partners can include family members, teachers, caregivers, doctors, emergency personnel, and community workers. The reasons a person may be communicating in these situations can include participating in decision-making, initiating interactions, making requests, engaging in conversations, gaining access to medical care, and sharing information. By taking time to think about a person's "Communication World," implementation of AAC devices into this world becomes more natural and powerful (Fader, 2020).

For young children, embedding AAC devices into daily routines and activities, such as reading books, playing games, and engaging in mealtimes, organically leads to repeated opportunities for use of AAC. For students, implementation should not only occur within the speech therapy room but within the regular education classroom, special education classroom, cafeteria, nurse's office, gym, and on field trips as well. School-aged children must also have access to their AAC system in community locations, such as during extracurricular activities and while at restaurants. Utilizing AAC at home is also critical. Family members, or familiar communication partners, often can interpret an individual's vocalizations, word approximations, and gestures to understand what they want and need. Honoring these communication attempts and also encouraging individuals to more independently convey their ideas via AAC can enhance their skills with using the device and subsequently ensure more effective and multimodal communication with both familiar and unfamiliar communication partners. For adults, access to AAC in all environments continues to be critical. As with children and young adults, adults must have a means of participating in interactions throughout their daily lives. Whether it be to perform at work, to engage socially with friends and loved ones, to participate in meaningful community activities, or to guide medical care, communication remains essential for self-advocacy and independence.

For everyone, access to AAC provides a means of fostering healthy relationships, a critical factor in reducing the sexual assault epidemic for individuals with intellectual and developmental disabilities (IDDs) and concomitant communication differences. This population faces a risk of sexual assault at a rate seven times higher than individuals without disabilities (Shapiro, 2018). Several factors contribute to this statistic, including limited to no instruction on sexual health and healthy relationships, and the culture of compliance that many societies have built which demands that individuals obey the expectations of caregivers; individuals with IDD are more likely to be assaulted during the daytime and by somebody they know. Another contributing factor to the disheartening #SevenTimes (a social media campaign that has been developed to spread awareness) statistic is a lack of access to, and direct instruction of, communication for self-advocacy and reporting purposes. Sadly, when people with IDDs face incidences of sexual abuse, they either have no way to report it or they disclose the incident but then are not believed due to their communication challenges. Providing an individual with AAC can help them to learn about this critically important topic, self-advocate for prevention, and successfully report unfortunate incidents of abuse when they do occur.

In Conclusion

Mid-tech and high-tech AAC systems provide an individual with a voice output solution. They vary with respect to how they can be accessed, the voice output options, the vocabulary, and the vocabulary organization. Many features can be customized to meet the unique needs and preferences of the individual, support their interactions with their communication partners, as well as support their involvement in their community. Regardless of whether a person benefits from a device to augment their verbal speech or whether the individual requires an alternative means of communicating, these two types of devices have the potential to drastically enhance an individual's independence and quality of life, and to ensure that they are universally understood.

Case Study: RA

Clinical Profile and Communication Needs

The Individual

RA is a 10-year-old boy with Down syndrome and medical complexities. He attends public school where he receives special education services to support his development in the domains of academics, activities of daily living, fine motor functioning, and speech-language skills. RA has difficulty

sustaining attention and benefits from the use of visual tools (i.e., token boards, visual schedules) to maintain focus and complete tasks. His vision and hearing are deemed to be within normal limits. RA presents with a relative strength in sight word recognition, and his team describes him as a child who is motivated to communicate and extremely eager to be included in social interactions.

RA presents with communication challenges concomitant with his diagnosis of Down syndrome. He uses word approximations, short phrases, and gestures to interact, and tends to guide others toward items he wants as an additional means of communication. He has an articulation disorder that compromises his speech intelligibility. Familiar partners understand him 50% to 75% of the time, while unfamiliar partners generally understand him 25% to 50% of the time. RA has a relative strength in receptive language, demonstrating skills such as following one- to two-step directions, comprehending basic language concepts (i.e., in, then, before), and understanding the meanings of a broad range of vocabulary words. A significant gap exists between his receptive and expressive language skills, with his expressive skills characterized by utterances that are shorter and less complex than his age-matched peers. RA typically communicates to convey general wants/needs, to request recurrence of an item or task, to answer basic questions, and to greet others. He does not communicate for more complex functions such as summarizing information or telling/retelling stories. Initiating and maintaining conversations in a back-and-forth manner is challenging for him. RA becomes frustrated when he is not understood or when he is not sure of the words to use to express himself. Such frustration is manifested in yelling and aggressive outbursts.

RA uses verbal and nonverbal language to communicate, but his speech intelligibility is significantly compromised. He can sometimes be understood by unfamiliar communication partners, but familiar partners are better able to interpret and comprehend his messages. Overall communication partner understanding also increases within known contexts. This presentation suggests that RA is a context-dependent communicator. It is important to note that this communication level is designated to describe his current skills for the purposes of identifying appropriate AAC interventions and strategies. It is *not* an indicator of his communication potential. Some individuals move toward, and achieve, communicative independence while others remain successful, context-dependent communicators (Blackstone & Hunt Berg, 2003).

Their Communication Partners

At home, RA's communication partners include his mother, father, sister, and grandparents. They all report that while RA can be difficult to understand at times, they can generally interpret his needs and wants. The educational team is working to help the family understand the importance of RA having an augmentative mode of communication to support his interactions with those who do not understand him, and to facilitate the advancement of his speech-language skills to more complex levels.

His school-based communication partners consist of his general education teacher, special education teacher, speech-language pathologist, occupational therapist, adapted physical education teacher, music teacher, and nurse. RA also has a one-to-one paraeducator who has worked with him for the last 4 years. He is eager to interact with his peers and has a particularly strong relationship with his classmate, JF (who will play an important role in the implementation of RA's AAC).

Within the community, RA participates in adapted swim lessons and therapeutic horseback riding. His instructors in both programs often have difficulty understanding his expressive communication. Peers that are of a similar age to RA attend these activities as well. However, RA's interactions with them are limited given his difficulty maintaining conversations and his reduced speech intelligibility. RA's mother attends all sessions and often serves as the "interpreter" to help the group understand RA's messages. RA's engagements with doctors, health professionals, and emergency personnel are important to consider as well given his medical profile. His mother serves as an "interpreter" during these appointments, too. RA's independence with managing his medical care is thus compromised, which will become a more significant issue as he gets older.

Their Environment

RA's primary environments within his Communication World are his home and his school. RA lives in a single-family home. Communication occurs among his family members in all areas, both indoors and outdoors. RA enjoys playing in his backyard. His AAC system must be functional in all spaces, so specific considerations must be made. For example, having difficulty seeing the backlit screen of a tablet-based device outside in the sunshine may become a barrier to communication, so a backup system may be required in such situations.

While at school, RA participates in activities within the regular education classroom, special education classroom, related service spaces, music room, gymnasium, cafeteria, nurse's office, and outdoor playground. Any AAC system that is recommended for RA must be available in all these contexts throughout his school day. Such consistency is critical for helping him learn the reasons and the ways for using the device in a generalized manner. Above all else, access to communication is a basic human right that must be supported (Brady et al., 2016).

RA also needs to access his AAC system at his grandparents' house, local stores, his two favorite restaurants, and the community center where he participates in extracurricular activities. Additional locations include health care facilities and hospitals, as needed, given RA's medical profile.

The AAC System

Despite ongoing speech therapy, RA's speech sound development has remained compromised, and he is unable to communicate for a broad range of functions. He does not have a way to communicate safety and medical information, particularly if he is not with a familiar caregiver. His social interactions, behaviors, and overall development are impacted. As such, his communication needs must be met by an augmentative mode that supplements his verbal speech and facilitates his global language development.

Based on RA's individual profile, RA's preferences, conversations with his family and school team members, and assessment results, he would benefit from a high-tech device for primary use, a mid-tech device for secondary functions, and a no-tech (paper-based) board for environmental modeling and use within water-based or messy activities, (i.e., swimming lessons). This no-tech system will also serve as a backup system that RA can use in situations when his high-tech device is not available, such as when the battery is charging or is accidentally left at home when he goes to school.

Exclusive use of no-tech AAC systems as well as mid-tech AAC devices is limiting for RA because he requires a system with voice output and extensive vocabulary to maximize his participation and engagement in interactions, as well as his continued language and literacy development. No-tech/lite-tech AAC does not contain voice output and instead relies on the communication partner to interpret a selected message. Reliance on the prerecorded digitized speech characteristic of mid-tech AAC would be limiting for RA given his relative strength in receptive language along with his strong desire to communicate with others.

When used in isolation, lite-tech and mid-tech AAC would not sufficiently facilitate his language development, and subsequently his social, academic, and behavioral development would also be inhibited. The robust vocabulary, customization options, and synthesized speech characteristic of high-tech devices will support his global development and interactions. However, to maximally support RA's access to communication, the team should consider providing him with an AAC system that includes no- and mid-tech supports to supplement the high-tech device. When a system, rather than only one tool, is made available to an individual, he is provided with multiple modes of communication that can be utilized in isolation and in combination with one another. This system allows the individual to have access to the most efficient communication modes within varying communication contexts and while interacting with different communication partners.

The features required of RA's mid-tech device include multimessage capabilities and a small surface area to offer message variety and given his fine-motor abilities. By having more than one message, RA will have access to multiple functional, high-frequency expressions in moments of escalation. The device can be preprogrammed with phrases such as, "Can I have a break?" or "I need help, please!" to support Functional Communication Training. By having immediate access to relevant messages, rather than having to navigate through the dynamic display pagesets of a high-tech device, RA can utilize them quickly instead of resorting to challenging behaviors.

The TalkingBrix2 is a mid-tech device that contains the necessary features for RA. A BIGmack was ruled out because RA does not require such a large surface activation area for physical access, and this larger device would compromise portability. The TalkingBrix2 device was compared to an iTalk2, but the flexibility of being able to attach and detach individual Brix to one another was engaging and meaningful for RA, and he really enjoyed working with this system.

The features of a high-tech device that were identified as being necessary to match RA's needs are listed and described in Table 3–3.

In accounting for these features that are critical for RA's communication success, specific high-tech AAC devices can be ruled in and out of the consideration process. Given that RA demonstrates fine and gross motor skills sufficient for accessing a touch screen device via traditional direct selection, an iPad platform is appropriate. No alternative access methods need to be considered.

Given his stage of language development and literacy levels, he would benefit from symbols paired with text on individual buttons. As such, text-based AAC apps including Grid for iPad,[9] AlphaCore,[10] Predictable,[11] and Proloquo4Text®[12] must be ruled out. That being said, RA must nonetheless be given access to a keyboard to continue to develop his emerging reading and writing skills.

[9]Smartbox Assistive Technology. (2021). Retrieved from https://thinksmartbox.com/product/grid-for-ipad/
[10]Talk To Me Technologies. (2021). Retrieved from https://www.talktometechnologies.com/pages/alphacore
[11]Therapy Box Limited. (2020). Retrieved from https://therapy-box.co.uk/predictable
[12]AssistiveWare. (2021). Retrieved from https://www.assistiveware.com/products/proloquo4text

Table 3–3. Features of a High-Tech Device Identified as Being Necessary for RA

Feature	Rationale
Voice output	Provide auditory feedback; improve conversational skills
Synthesized speech	Allow all words to be produced without needing to record button messages
Message window	Encourage creation of phrases and sentences
Extensive symbol set	Allow access to vocabulary without limitations
Core/fringe template	Follows a preset, structured system for using high-frequency words; enhances language development
Grammar support	Support learning of syntax and morphology
Color coding	Learn parts of speech/word types for enhanced communication efficiency
Preprogrammed phrases	Ensures quick access to high-frequency messages
Keyboard with word prediction	Generate messages using a standard QWERTY keyboard with word prediction to enhance the rate
Dynamic display	Navigate to a robust language system
Overlay backup	Prevent pageset from being deleted or lost; create copies for lite-tech boards

Efficient communication is important for RA; thus, access to a word prediction tool will be helpful. As such, pagesets within TouchChat HD[13] other than WordPower[14] must be ruled out. While apps such as LAMP Words for Life[15] and Proloquo2Go®[16] contain a keyboard with word prediction, RA exhibited a more efficient rate of icon selection and a higher level of independence when using a keyboard with symbolated word prediction.

Symbolated word prediction is a feature wherein a symbol is paired with the text within the word prediction bar. For example, if an individual begins typing "mon-" on the keyboard, words such as "Monday," "Money," and "Monkey" may appear. By having a picture of a monkey paired with the word, RA can more quickly select it after visually scanning the word prediction bar as compared to if just the text had been visible.

The Super Core 50[17] pageset of Grid for iPad and Snap Core First[18] are two high-tech AAC apps that encompass the benefit of symbolated word prediction along with the other features identified as being critical for RA. In trialing and exploring these two apps, Snap Core First was selected as the most appropriate app to meet RA's unique needs.

In conjunction with the mid-tech device and the high-tech device, the team should create lite-tech, paper-based versions of the high-tech device pagesets. These versions can be laminated for use during his swimming lessons, at times when the

---

[13]PRC-Saltillo. (2021). Retrieved from https://touchchatapp.com/apps/touchchat-hd-aac

[14]Inman Innovations. (2021). Retrieved from http://www.inmaninnovations.com/index.php

[15]PRC-Saltillo. (2021). Retrieved from https://aacapps.com

[16]AssistiveWare. (2021). Retrieved from https://www.assistiveware.com/products/proloquo2go

[17]Smartbox Assistive Technology. (2021). Retrieved from https://grids.thinksmartbox.com/en/sensory-software/super-core-50-pcs

[18]TobiiDynavox. (2021). Retrieved from https://us.tobiidynavox.com/pages/snap-corefirst

high-tech device is not available (i.e., not charged, or when the high-tech screen cannot be viewed due to sunlight glare), and for modeling purposes. They can be secured to various locations around the environment for ongoing exposure to communication. One option is to take screenshots of RA's different Snap Core First pages directly from the iPad. Printable, lite-tech Snap Core First boards are also available online from TobiiDynavox.

Next Steps

All teachers, support staff, and paraprofessionals who work with RA should be trained in using the AAC system. RA's family should receive training as well to ensure that AAC is embedded throughout all environments. Dr. Janice Light (1989) combined with Blackstone and Wilkins (2009) identified that successful AAC use is based on one's own operational (use of device components), linguistic (knowledge of language), strategic (use of compensatory strategies), social (consideration of pragmatics), and emotional (i.e., awareness of emotions, self-regulation) competence (which is discussed in more detail in subsequent chapters, and is revisited throughout the book as foundational to successful AAC use and service delivery). These five competency domains must be integral to RA's treatment plan.

Additionally, the school team and family should become knowledgeable about Snap Core

First, in regard to both technical competencies and implementation strategies. A number of resources are available from the manufacturer. The individual's entire team should also receive training on executing research-based best practices for effective AAC implementation. The team should collaboratively devise an AAC Implementation Plan that includes delegated responsibilities among individual team members (i.e., family charges high-tech device daily and returns mid- and high-tech device daily, SLP compiles editing suggestions from others and executes customizations). The plan should also detail the short-term goals for RA's use of the device and the strategies for supporting achievement. Table 3–4 offers sample goals to consider.

These goals will best be met in an individual treatment setting in combination with support to directly embed and integrate the AAC system within RA's natural environments. To foster RA's motivation and desire to use AAC, his peers should be encouraged to explore, learn, and use the Talking-Brix2 and Snap Core First alongside him. Incorporating RA's close friend, JF, as a peer model in the implementation process may be key. Integrating games and challenges into direct instruction and social interactions can keep engagement with AAC fun, interesting, and meaningful. Notably, RA's communication partners should obtain his permission before using his system, though, as it is his personal voice. The lite-tech boards can be a helpful

Table 3–4. Sample Goals

Functional Communication Goal	Estimated Completion Time	Short Term	Long Term
Express feelings or state of being	2 weeks	Yes	No
Call for help from an unfamiliar person	1 month	Yes	No
Engage in social communication exchanges with a familiar person	1 month	Yes	No
Communicate physical needs and emotional status to a support person	>3 months	No	Yes
Convey a functional message in lieu of a challenging behavior	>3 months	No	Yes

tool for communication partners to utilize in lieu of, or in conjunction with, the high-tech device.

All primary communication partners must establish an understanding of the AAC prompting hierarchy for providing an appropriate level of support. RA significantly benefits from visual point prompts as well as from being given extended wait time. Specifically, it is important that his communication partners give him additional time to process a message he wants to say and then figure out the motor plan for conveying that message via his AAC system before an adult intervenes to help him. This strategy applies when he is working to say something spontaneously as well as when he is expected to answer a question or respond to a probe. Overcueing early on can lead to prompt dependence—remember, "stop before you prompt!" A balance must be made between supporting RA's success and challenging him to reach independence. A sample AAC prompting hierarchy is as follows:

I/Independent: AAC user able to perform the task on their own

Vpp/Visual Point Prompt: Communication partner (CP) points to the vicinity of the target or directly at the target

Vb/Verbal Prompt: CP describes target/tells user/encourages device use

Wv/Written Visual Prompt: CP uses printed words or pictures to show target

M/Modeling: CP shows the user the target location

Ppa/Partial Physical Assistance: CP provides minimal support (i.e., guiding at the elbow)

HuH/Hand Under Hand: CP provides full physical assistance

As RA's language and communication skills develop, the AAC system must be concurrently customized to meet his growing needs. His educational team, with input from his family, should conduct regular reassessments of his skills and identify new communication functions (i.e., asking ques-

tions, answering questions, commenting, describing, protesting, etc.) to target. The device should be designed to provide RA with the appropriate vocabulary and grammar to fulfill these functions.

References

Blackstone, S., & Hunt Berg, M. (2003). Social networks: *A communication inventory for individuals with severe communication challenges and their communication partners.* Augmentative Communication, Inc.

Blackstone, S., & Wilkins, D. (2009). Exploring the importance of emotional competence in children with complex communication needs. *Perspectives on Augmentative and Alternative Communication, 18*(3), 78–87.

Brady, N. C., Bruce, S., Goldman, A., Erickson, K., Mineo, B., Ogletree, B. T., . . . Wilkinson, K. (2016). Communication services and supports for individuals with severe disabilities: Guidance for assessment and intervention. *American Journal on Intellectual and Developmental Disabilities, 121*(2), 121–138.

Fader, E. (2020, July 16). AAC implementation from a "Communication World" Perspective. *PrAACtical AAC.* https://praacticalaac.org/praactical/aac-implementation-from-a-communication-world-perspective/

Ghaemmaghami, M., Hanley, G. P., & Jessel, J. (2021). Functional communication training: From efficacy to effectiveness. *Journal of Applied Behavior Analysis, 54,* 122–143. https://doi.org/10.1002/jaba.762

Light, J. (1989). Toward a definition of communicative competence for individuals using augmentative and alternative communication systems. *Augmentative and Alternative Communication, 5,* 137–144.

Light, J., McNaughton, D., & Caron, J. (2019). New and emerging AAC technology supports for children with complex communication needs and their communication partners: State of the science and future research directions, *Augmentative and Alternative Communication, 35,* 26–41. https://doi.org/10.1080/0743461.2018.1557251

Romski, M. A., & Sevcik, R. A. (2005). Augmentative communication and early intervention: Myths and realities. *Infants and Young Children, 18*(3), 174–185.

Shapiro, J. (2018). The sexual assault epidemic no one talks about. *npr.* https://www.npr.org/2018/01/08/570224090/the-sexual-assault-epidemic-no-one-talks-about

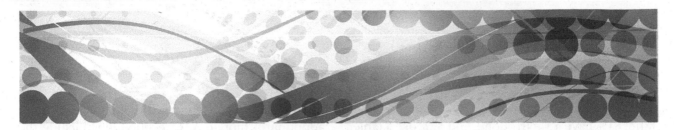

Chapter 4
MOBILE AAC

Oliver Wendt

Fundamentals

Introduction: What Are Mobile Technologies?

Mobile technology refers to portable electronic devices that incorporate a liquid crystal display (LCD) to project digital images which can be manipulated by gestures on the screen using one's fingers, by using a stylus, or by typing or selecting characters from a digital keypad (Fietzer & Chin, 2017). In general, mobile devices include tablet computers (e.g., Android™ tablets, Apple iPad®, Microsoft® Surface,® among others), smartphones (e.g., Apple iPhone®, Samsung Galaxy®), and laptop computers. A newly emerging category of mobile technology is wearable technology (also known as "Wearables"). These hands-free gadgets can be worn as accessories, woven into clothing, or implanted in body parts; wearable devices are typically powered by high-speed microprocessors and provide capabilities to send and receive data via an Internet connection (Hayes, 2020). Popular examples of wearable technologies include the Apple Watch®, Fitbit Versa™ Smartwatch, or Google Glass.

Mobile computing application software that enable access to, sharing of, and interaction with information on mobile devices have been known as "apps" and are typically distributed through "app stores" such as the Amazon Appstore, Apple App Store, or Google Play® Store, among others. The most common operating systems (OS) for mobile devices to run these applications are Apple's iOS® (formerly iPhone OS) and Google's Android™ platform.

Many specialized apps are available to promote augmentative and alternative communication (AAC) for users with complex communication needs. When mobile devices are equipped with AAC apps, they take on the function of a speech-generating device (SGD), a technology that affords the use of digitized or synthesized speech output (Schlosser & Koul, 2015). The difference to dedicated SGDs lies in the fact that the mobile platform typically offers a wide range of functions in addition to communication purposes (e.g., access to multimedia content, social media applications, photo/video producing capabilities, etc.). In terms of AAC taxonomy, mobile (AAC) technologies are all examples of aided communication—that is, a communication mode requiring equipment external to the user's body (Lloyd et al., 1997), and as discussed in the previous chapters.

The Mobile Technology Revolution in AAC

Mobile devices, most commonly produced as smartphones or tablet computers, represent the most prevalent digital technology in our society:

96% of U.S. adults possess a cell phone of some kind, 81% have a smartphone, and 52% use a tablet computer, with each ownership category steadily increasing over the last 5 years (Pew Research Center, 2021). This proliferation of mobile technology is astonishing in the face of a concurrent declining trend in ownership of desktop or laptop computers, a decline that was as large as 73% only a few years ago (Anderson, 2015). Typically developing children nowadays spend on average 2.3 hr per day interacting with digital technologies, and the percentage of time using mobile devices has tripled over the last 10 years, from 15 to 48 min daily (Bernacki et al., 2020). This rapid rise and scope of mobile technologies also left an impact on the field of AAC, causing a development that McNaugthon and Light (2013) coined the "mobile technology revolution": Tablet devices such as the Apple iPad® moved AAC closer to the mainstream. Individuals who require AAC are no longer limited to the use of specific dedicated SGDs, they can simply obtain mainstream technologies "off the shelf" to cover their communication needs. McNaughton and Light (2013) notice greater consumer empowerment through mobile AAC technology. The broader availability of mobile devices, the ease of downloading AAC applications, and the decreased cost of such solutions compared to dedicated SGDs have led to significant changes in the processes of how individuals with complex communication needs and their families obtain AAC technology. In the past, traditional SGDs were usually distributed to users through a clinical pathway of service delivery, starting from AAC assessment by licensed AAC specialists, subsequent prescription of equipment as specified by a clinical team, and finally many follow-up supports to optimize intervention outcomes. This traditional distribution model has changed to a new consumer-driven approach; the relatively low cost of mobile devices equipped with AAC apps enables more families, school districts, and related entities to acquire AAC technology on their own without depending on third-party funding (McNaughton & Light, 2013). In a survey by Meder (2012), nearly 30% of families indicated that affordability was the key influential driver when purchasing a mobile device over a dedicated solution for AAC purposes.

Further critical factors driving the increased adoption of mobile AAC technologies include the ease of use, social acceptance, and ubiquitous nature of such devices. In the past, parents and clinicians were often confronted with a certain learning curve when dealing with new technical operations on traditional SGDs; the learning demands on communication partners were substantial (Light & McNaughton, 2012). The operational competencies for AAC apps on mobile devices, however, seem to be easier to understand for end users who are already familiar with operating similar interfaces on their own mobile devices. Shane and colleagues (2012) observed that even laypeople with little or no technical expertise can create personalized content for AAC purposes with relative ease; major reasons lie in the simple interfaces provided by mobile apps and increasing general familiarity with mobile technology. In a similar vein, mobile AAC technologies promote social acceptance. Mobile devices are a popular element of mainstream culture and are socially valued; there is less of a stigma for the end user as is often the case with traditional forms of assistive technology. Last, mobile AAC solutions are an example of ubiquitous computing: applications that easily integrate with daily life in a transparent fashion with little or no need for attention. Contemporary mobile AAC solutions are integrated with the entire suite of applications on the device platform creating a system that offers enhanced functionality and interconnectivity to support everyday activities (McNaughton & Light, 2013). Beyond the mere purpose of communication, such a ubiquitous system provides access to cell phone, videoconferencing, and social media capabilities to promote social connections, access to the Internet for information gathering, access to a variety of multimedia content applications, and access to productivity tools for educational and work-related tasks. The impact of such ubiquitous computing solutions is best illustrated with a statement by the computer scientist Marc Weiser who wrote in his seminal paper on "the computer for the 21st century": "The most profound technologies are those that disappear. They weave themselves into the fabric of everyday life until they are indistinguishable from it." (Weiser, 1991, p. 94)

Principles in Mobile Technology Application Design

Creating well-designed mobile applications in general is a challenge for developers and vendors of mobile solutions, and this is particularly true in the field of AAC, where such solutions are supposed to serve a very heterogenous population of end users, all of which differ widely in their motor, cognitive, and sensory perceptual skills. Beneficial user experiences are largely determined by the usability of mobile applications. Usability is defined as the degree with which a mobile application can be meaningfully used by a targeted user group to accomplish certain goals with effectiveness, efficiency, and satisfaction within a particular context of use (Venkatesh & Ramesh, 2006). Reaching high degrees of usability is challenging in the mobile technology space because many devices such as smartphones, ultraportable tablets, and wearables have relatively small screens and input mechanisms that do not leave much room for error (Chen et al., 2010). To create high-quality and user-friendly mobile applications, developers and vendors ideally adhere to application development guidelines as provided by operating system (OS) inventors including Apple, Google, and Microsoft, and they also pay attention to present-day principles of mobile application design to optimize usability. People with complex communication needs aiming to use mobile devices and their caretakers should be familiar with the most common design approaches to understand their various intentions and purposes. A brief overview follows.

Gamification

Gamification refers to a relatively recent design approach with the intent to optimize human-computer interaction. The major notion behind gamification is to embed game-like elements in the interface to make electronic transactions more engaging and interesting to the end user (Marczewski, 2015). The approach has become increasingly popular to enhance skill development and retention. By providing rewarding experiences to users and motivating them to reach the next level or goal

within a gaming context, users end up spending more time interacting with the technology. Basically, gamification identifies the most appealing elements of games and integrates these elements with non-game components and contexts to increase the user's motivation to engage in a target behavior (Goethe, 2019). The higher level of user engagement leads the user to aim for better performance relative to learning, socializing, achievement, mastery, and status. Practicing skills and behaviors that typically seem challenging, tedious, and boring are now turned into fun and engaging exercises (Hamari, 2017). An example for gamification in an AAC context is the SPEAKplay! app designed by our research lab to train the motor skills in prospective AAC users to adequately access and operate AAC applications on mobile devices (Wendt et al., 2020).

Just-in-Time Learning and Programming

The concept of "just-in-time" (JIT) originally referred to a business strategy focusing on targeting needs as they appear (Schlosser et al., 2016). Related to AAC intervention, JIT holds great promise to improve learning with and programming of mobile AAC technologies. Contemporary features of mobile devices such as improved portability, onboard cameras, and intuitive user interfaces allow AAC content on such devices to be created and modified during daily interactions, in responsive ways right at the very moment when new needs emerge. Well-designed AAC applications will allow for such JIT capabilities. Holyfield et al. (2019), however, still note that many clinicians are not aware of the advantages of JIT programming and still take considerable time to proactively program vocabulary into devices that they likely believe will be needed in the near future. But the programmed vocabulary may or may not emerge during the anticipated activity, and more importantly, new items of interest may surface which have not been preprogrammed into the device. JIT capabilities help to resolve such scenarios instantaneously by allowing the clinician or communication partner to create and add new vocabulary items when new context and new needs start to unfold (Holyfield et al., 2019).

User-Centered Design

User-centered design refers to a process of product design that involves user-centered activities to drive the development process. In the beginning, the envisioned end users are identified alongside their capabilities, needs, and expectations. Subsequently, user-centered design tries to create a clear understanding of the larger goals that the users would want to accomplish through interactions with the software. The process identifies the tasks that are leading up to the larger goals, in addition to the physical and social environments in which the interactions occur so that the users achieve their goals. To generate this level of insight, the intended end users must actively contribute to the development process by engaging in design and testing activities (Hall, 2001; Lubas et al., 2014).

Another key element of user-centered design is prototyping. Ongoing prototype creation is an efficient way to integrate user feedback into the design process. User-centered design approaches do not specify how many and what kind of prototypes are necessary, but the general requirement is to have some level of user involvement at every major step of the product development process.

Participatory Design

Similar to user-centered design, this approach puts a lot of emphasis on direct involvement of end users in the design process. These are taking an active role in the processes of designing, developing, and evaluating the technology (Brosnan et al., 2016). It is particularly important to assign the envisioned end users a responsibility for co-creating or co-designing the technology; for their own benefit and empowerment, they are supposed to contribute meaningfully to the final outcome. For individuals with special needs, in our case individuals with complex communication needs, there are four distinct roles they can take on during co-designing activities: user, tester, informant, and design partner (Druin, 2002; Frauenberger et al., 2011). The first two roles lead to more passive involvement, while the latter two are associated with more active participation. As informants, individuals with complex communication needs can make more specific contributions during certain stages, for example, providing feedback to concept design and input on design decisions. The role of design partner provides even more recognition as an equal collaborator during all phases of the design process. This role allows for a maximum of participation; final decision-making on design issues becomes more of a collaborative process between developers and end users. Deciding which role is most appropriate and beneficial can be a challenge: The impact on product development and empowerment of the end users can be significant, at the same time it is important not to overburden them with too many tasks and responsibilities (Frauenberger et al., 2011).

Research Evidence and Funding Issues Related to Mobile Technology

As with all AAC modalities, interventions based on mobile AAC technology should be supported by scientifically valid evidence. It is important in this context to realize that a mobile device equipped with an AAC app does not function differently from an SGD. Many currently available dedicated SGDs incorporate a tablet computer as their hardware platform; the AAC software or app enables that hardware to function as a communication aid. Various SGD manufacturers provide their AAC app as a stand-alone product serving as an entry point for the consumer into the larger product suite. The consumer can initially download the app onto their mobile device and after successful initial use migrate to the fully equipped SGD running the same app, but now with access to a wider range of additional features such as better speakers, a rugged case, switch access, longer-lasting battery, and advanced tech support, among others. The benefits of using SGDs during AAC interventions have been documented through a variety of systematic reviews in recent years (e.g., Alzrayer et al., 2014; Schlosser & Koul, 2015), which included both traditional, dedicated SGDs and tablet-based devices turned into dedicated SGDs. For these reasons, it would be misleading to say that mobile AAC technologies do not have a strong evidence-base. The entire notion of mobile AAC technology being a distinct category to SGDs can lead to serious implications from a funding perspective: As AAC advocate Lew Golinker points out, as more labels are applied to the same technology, the more confusing this can be for insurance agencies and funding bodies (L. Golinker, personal communication, October 16, 2020). Funding stakeholders may come to think of a mobile AAC device as a different type of SGD and as such, it may not be accepted for funding purposes. Instead, mobile AAC devices should be seen as examples for the existing and recognized class of SGDs that is fundable through Medicare code E 2510.

The need to reference an existing code for funding purposes is a second reason to be cautious about introducing a new label of mobile technology (L. Golinker, personal communication, October 16, 2020). If insurance agencies are given the impression that mobile devices are different from the technology fundable under existing Medicare codes, they may demand a new code created for their coverage. In the meantime, funding requests may be denied until such new codes have been established, which in return would be counterproductive to serving prospective users of mobile AAC technology.

Case Study: LM

Clinical Profile and Communication Needs

The Individual

LM is a school-age child with minimally verbal autism spectrum disorder (ASD). LM was 10 years and 3 months old at the time of intake and was diagnosed with ASD, a severe neurodevelopmental condition characterized by deficits in social communication, social interaction, and restricted and repetitive patterns of behavior or interests (American Psychiatric Association, 2013). Individuals with ASD typically show a documented language disorder with an onset before age 3 years. This

language disorder can occur at varying levels of severity ranging from mild impairment to more profound expressive, receptive, and pragmatic disorders. Recent surveys suggest that about one third to one half of individuals on the autism spectrum have little to no functional speech and need ongoing AAC intervention to participate in educational, home, and community settings (Rose et al., 2016; Tager-Flusberg & Kasari, 2013).

A similar situation presented itself with LM. According to parent report, LM was a perfectly normal child until about 18 months of age when he started to regress into autism. He stopped engaging in reciprocal interactions with his family and showed no interest in humans. He seemed to consider other people as tools that he would only use when he needed something. In addition, a variety of further ASD characteristics became evident: LM's stereotypical behaviors included frequent hand-flapping and jumping up and down, particularly when being excited about an event or object of interest. He had developed a very focused interest in Disney movie DVDs and would regularly arrange and sort the DVD cases in a particular sequence. Certain sensory responses included a sensitivity for loud noises to which he would typically react by covering his ears with his hands. LM was a picky eater and reluctant to try new foods; because of sensory issues he would often consume food items that produce a strong sensation in the oral cavity (e.g., smoked bacon, crunchy chips, mint lollypops). From time-to-time LM would also put objects in his mouth to chew on them and experience their taste or texture. His motor development was within normal limits, but the parents reported many difficulties with toilet training which occurred much later than usual.

In terms of his communication profile, LM's early speech and language milestones were severely delayed. Starting at 18 months, LM would not react to his name when being called, would not wave his hand for hello or goodbye, barely used gestures such as pointing to objects, and remained nonverbal until the age of 7 years. His communicative repertoire consisted mainly of prelinguistic behaviors such as reaching and grabbing for items. He would demonstrate some maladaptive behaviors (e.g., escaping, having tantrums, screaming) as a means of communicating and expressing frustration. At around 7 years of age, some speech started to emerge in the form of delayed echolalia, stereotypical vocalizations, and jargon. Echolalic utterances would often relate to content from his Disney movies. LM remained at a level of less than 10 functional spoken words while intelligible, spontaneous utterances were generally lacking. One particular strength, however, was his ability to make eye contact with communication partners. During communicative acts, LM consistently used eye-gaze shifts to socially reference his objects of interest or to express his need for the communication partner.

Their Communication Partners

LM resided at home with his mother, father, and older brother. His brother, too, was diagnosed with ASD, but at a mild severity level. Under the previous *Diagnostic and Statistical Manual of Mental Disorders, Fourth Edition* (*DSM-IV*) criteria (American Psychiatric Association, 1999), his brother's condition was determined as Asperger Syndrome. The family lived in a college-town neighborhood, and both parents were employed at the local university. English was the language spoken at home. LM did not have a childhood friend or social contacts outside of school. He enjoyed trips with either one of his parents to local stores and larger buildings, such as university halls or hotels where he could engage in locating and counting rooms or specific items of interest.

The Environment

LM attended a public school where he was placed part-time in a regular education elementary-grade classroom with some sessions in a special education pull-out room. He was taught at grade level by a regular education classroom teacher and was accompanied for the entire day by a paraprofessional. His speech-language therapy sessions were limited to one session of 30 min/week. The speech-language pathologist observed that LM seemed to acquire a sight word vocabulary and was occasionally able to speak one-word utterances when prompted, for example, during a labeling task. In his home environment, LM stayed mostly

in his bedroom or in the living room, lining up his DVD collection among other collectibles, engaging with construction toys, and watching his favorite movies.

AAC Considerations

LM was referred to our research lab for evaluation to identify AAC strategies that would enhance his ability to communicate in educational, home, and community settings while also addressing the acquisition of verbal speech. To confirm his autism diagnosis and severity level, our team administered two standardized ASD assessments, the Autism Diagnostic Observation Schedule™-Second Edition (ADOS™-2) (Lord et al., 2012) and the Childhood Autism Rating Scale-Second Edition (CARS-2); (Schopler et al., 2010). The ADOS-2 represents the current "gold standard" in autism diagnostics and consists of a series of structured and semi-structured tasks that involve social interaction between the examiner and the child; its first module specifically addresses individuals who are at the preverbal/single-word stage. The CARS-2 is an observation-based instrument that can be completed by a clinician, teacher, or parent; it asks for ratings in 15 distinct categories of behaviors to describe the individual. An ADOS score of 8 out of 10 confirmed a high level of autism spectrum–related symptoms; difficulties included the items of nonechoed spoken language, frequency of spontaneous vocalizations directed to others, immediate echolalia, and stereotyped use of words or phrases. A CARS-2 score of 35 put LM at a moderate-to-severe level of autism and revealed particular problems related to verbal communication, abnormal use of, and response to, taste, smell, and touch, plus severely inappropriate interest in, or use of, toys and other objects.

The parents' desire was to give LM more control over his environment and better means to indicate basic wants and needs, which, in turn, may lead to better social interaction. Another concern was to improve natural speech production in terms of the amount and quality of spoken one- or two-word utterances. School records revealed that LM had received some AAC intervention using the Picture Exchange Communication System® (PECS®).

PECS intervention uses principles of applied behavior analysis and a set of distinct teaching, reinforcement, and backward chaining strategies to teach functional communication (Bondy & Frost, 1994, 2002). In his school-based sessions, LM had started to communicate via PECS but had not surpassed Phase 2 of the PECS protocol. For these reasons, LM was enrolled in a research project aiming to create a prototype of an AAC application that would be tailored to the learning characteristics of individuals with severe ASD and that would allow individuals to carry out common instructional protocols, such as PECS, on a digital platform. In a nonresearch context, the assessment process would end in a feature-matching process to compare the suitability of different app and/or dedicated SGD solutions using the guidelines by Gosnell, Costello, and Shane (2011)—see assessment Chapters 8, 10, and 15 for more information.

The AAC System or Service

Targeted intervention outcomes for LM included (a) requesting for preferred items on his iPad and (b) acquisition of natural speech related to the requesting activities. Requesting was defined as activating one or more graphic symbols to obtain items from three different classes of stimuli including sensory materials, snacks, and toys. Natural speech acquisition was defined as intentional speech productions that were related to the items of interest. Intentional speech was recorded as any vocalization, word approximation, or complete word utterance intended to convey a meaningful communicative message.

Because LM was already familiar with the traditional PECS and had mastered PECS Phase 2, our research team developed a modification of the PECS protocol to allow the infusion of an AAC application. Instead of physically taking a graphic symbol card and exchanging it with a partner, the new protocol would allow LM to drag and drop graphic symbols onto a sentence strip created by the application. The details of the modified PECS protocol are described in Boesch et al. (2013a, 2013b) and Wendt et al. (2019), the major phases for LM can be summarized in the following paragraphs.

Modified PECS Phase III. The goal of this phase was to teach discrimination between graphic symbols on the screen, so that LM could create specific messages (Bondy & Frost, 1994). Initially, LM was taught to discriminate between two items, and upon mastery, more and more items were added onto the display to continually grow vocabulary. A correspondence check was performed to ensure that LM selected the correct item. If necessary, an error correction procedure was implemented.

Modified PECS Phase IV. LM now used an "I want" symbol to start a sentence followed by a symbol for a preferred item. The goal was to build sentence structure. During this stage, the clinician started to work with LM on speech elicitation; initially, the sentence strip would be read back to LM while pointing out each word. This would be repeated but with a time delay of 1 to 2 s between the "I want" and providing the item, motivating LM to finish the sentence using his own speech utterances.

Modified PECS Phase V. In the beginning of this phase, the clinician started with the prompt "What do you want?" Subsequently, the prompt was faded out to encourage LM to produce more spontaneous sentences. Toward the end of this phase, the clinician added a set of attributes to the graphic symbol vocabulary to enhance LM's ability to describe his preferred items and understand semantic relationships. The attributes chosen included "big vs. small," "few vs. many," "long vs. short," "round vs. square," plus the colors "blue," "red," "green," and "black."

To encourage generalization of newly acquired skills, the modified protocol was implemented across three different settings with different preferred items in each: food snacks in the university clinic, toys in the family home, and sensory materials in the school classroom.

The protocol was carried out using a prototype of the SPEAKall!® application that was specifically designed around the learning characteristics of individuals with severe ASD. (Figure 4–1 presents a screen image of the app designed to address attribute-object relationships.) SPEAKall! creates a very intuitive interface: The upper portion of the screen allows one to select graphic symbols and photographs, and the lower portion contains

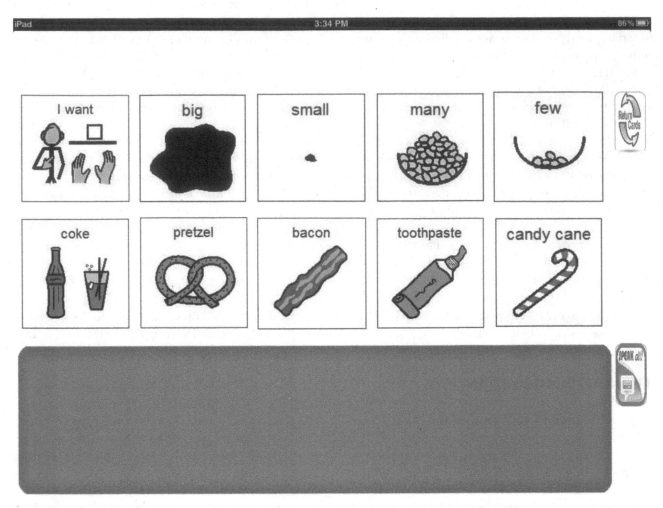

Figure 4–1. An example for a communication display on the prototype of the "SPEAKall!" application to teach attribute-object relationships. (Copyright SPEAK MODalities LLC, 2013; evaluation version available from the author upon request.)

a storyboarding strip where users can drag and drop symbols to compose sentences. Learners with motor control issues can make symbol activations with a simple touch gesture. The app also provides the capability to add photos to the existing repertoire of symbols, creating relevant and recognizable content for daily activities. Once a learner has constructed an utterance on the sentence strip, a push on the "Speak All" button reads the sentence out loud. The generation of voice output occurs via prerecorded speech from caretakers or via Apple's synthetic Siri® voice.

Our team engaged in the user-centered and participatory design approaches outlined earlier to obtain feedback from major stakeholders in LM's life and to tailor the application to the needs of clients with more severe ASD characteristics. The following features were added to the application, differentiating it from other products on the market while making it a very "autism-specific" solution.

The user interface was kept as simple as possible to avoid cognitive overload and reduce operational constraints to successful iPad use. All backgrounds, colors, and stimuli were kept free of disturbing visual or sound effects that might elicit autistic symptoms; major interface components were designed in clearly distinguishable styles with calming colors. A "hidden lock" button was added to keep the learner within activities. Options also included the choice between prerecorded speech or a variety of synthetic voices that may be preferable over the human voice for some learners with autism because of auditory comprehension difficulties.

Using this treatment package of modified instructional protocol plus autism-specific mobile app, LM significantly increased his ability to request preferred items using "I want" sentences in conjunction with a variety of attributes to describe the item. He reached mastery of Phase V after 19 sessions in the clinic, after 17 sessions in the school, and after 16 sessions in the home environment. Maintenance probes taken after 6 to 8 weeks showed continued performance at mastery criterion after the intervention was completed. In terms of natural speech acquisition, LM reached a level of producing single-word utterances as well as full sentences using his own voice. On average, his productions of meaningful, intentional speech utterances occurred 24 times during a 20-trial session in the clinic, 28 times in the school, and 29 times in the home environment.

Next Steps

After functional communication (LM's ability to make his immediate wants and needs known) had been established and LM was demonstrating improvement in natural speech acquisition, next steps focused on broadening communicative functions beyond requesting and working on early language goals. LM had already demonstrated success in constructing sentences that associated an attribute with a noun. Our subsequent goals for him were focused on expanding his communicative repertoire by learning how to combine words (i.e., graphic symbols), building his vocabulary, and enhancing his ability to generalize newly learned language forms. Once a client with complex communication needs has acquired single-word utterances and masters an initial communication repertoire (with or without speech), it is important to make the transition from single- to multiple-word utterances to produce two-term semantic relationships (e.g., such as action+object,

agent+action, possessor+possession, etc.; Brown & Leonard, 1986). In LM's case, we decided to target action-object combinations, as he had already produced some adjective-object phrases. Our intervention approach to teach two-symbol combinations incorporated mobile AAC technology with an evidence-based instruction known as matrix training (Wetherby & Striefel, 1978). Matrix training uses linguistic elements (e.g., nouns, verbs, etc.) presented in systematic combination matrices, which are arranged to induce generalized rule-like behavior. The clinician models combining a limited set of words in one semantic category with another set in a related semantic category to facilitate the individual's ability to combine lexical items (Nelson, 1993).

To carry out matrix training on mobile devices, our research lab developed an iOS application titled "SPEAKmore!®" (Figure 4–2 presents an example of a 6 × 6 action-object matrix.) The application emulates a communication board on the screen displaying the items from each semantic category (in our example the actions on the left side and the objects on the right side). A stimulus is shown adjacent to the communication board. This stimulus is a videorecording of a scenario to be described by a symbol combination. Upon stimulus appearance, the learner will have to produce the correct symbol sequence to describe the stimulus. If the learner produces an error, the application applies a least-to-most prompt procedure (i.e., graying out parts of the possible selections, and highlighting others) to guide the learner in constructing the correct response.

The design of the learning scenario follows the principles of gamification outlined earlier. To keep the learner engaged and motivated to stay within the activity, the app creates a gaming experience by awarding stars for correct responses. A progression bar displays the number of stars earned and how many attempts are left within a session. The learner works toward earning a big star creating a special effect at the very end. In LM's case, the app was programmed to teach a 6 × 6 action-object matrix using vocabulary appropriate for emerging communicators: The six actions included "point to," "drop," "take-out," "put-in," "shake," and "wipe"; the six objects included "ball," "cup," "spoon," "fork,"

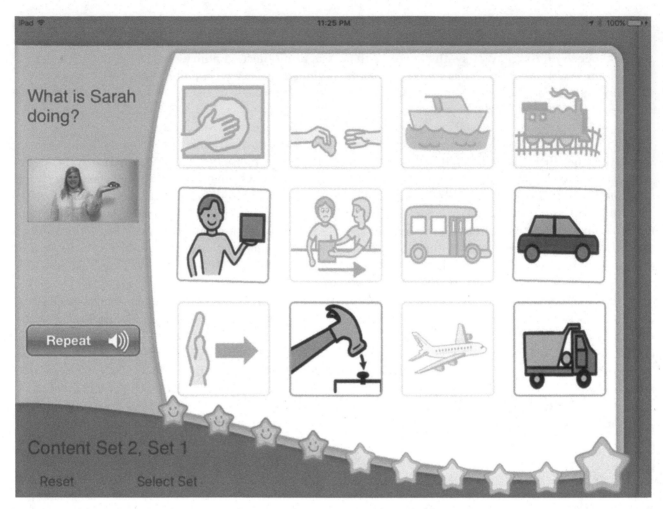

Figure 4–2. An example of a 6 × 6 action-object matrix taught through the iOS app "SPEAKmore!" (Copyright SPEAK MODalities LLC, 2013; evaluation version available from the author upon request.)

"apple," and "car." From the total pool of 36 possible symbol combinations, the SPEAKmore! application actively taught 12 combinations. After each intervention session, the app can switch into a generalization mode to test generalization on the remaining 24 symbol combinations. LM reached mastery on the entire pool of 36 possible symbol combinations after six intervention sessions.

Future intervention efforts can now expand the matrix training by teaching more of a variety in semantic relations (e.g., agent+action, attribute+entity, possessor+possession, etc.) and by moving from two-term to three-term combinations (e.g., agent-action-object, agent-action-locative). This allows for the development of linguistic compe-tence and systematic advancement of language (and expressive output) using design features of mobile technology.

References

Alzrayer, N., Banda, D. R., & Koul, R. K. (2014). Use of iPad/iPods with individuals with autism and other developmental disabilities: A meta-analysis of communication interventions. *Review Journal of Autism and Developmental Disorders, 1,* 179–191. https://doi.org/10.1007/s40489-014-0018-5

American Psychiatric Association. (1999). *Diagnostic and statistical manual of mental disorders* (4th ed.).

American Psychiatric Association. (2013). *Diagnostic and statistical manual of mental disorders* (5th ed.). https://doi.org/10.1176/appi.books.9780890425596

Anderson, M. (2015, October 29). *U.S. technology device ownership 2015*. Pew Research Center: Internet, Science & Tech. https://www.pewresearch.org/internet/2015/10/29/technology-device-ownership-2015/

Bernacki, M. L., Greene, J. A., & Crompton, H. (2020). Mobile technology, learning, and achievement: Advances in understanding and measuring the role of mobile technology in education. *Contemporary Educational Psychology, 60*, 101827. https://doi.org/10.1016/j.cedpsych.2019.101827

Boesch, M. C., Wendt, O., Subramanian, A., & Hsu, N. (2013a). Comparative efficacy of the Picture Exchange Communication System (PECS) versus a speech-generating device: Effects on requesting skills. *Research in Autism Spectrum Disorders, 7*, 480–493. https://doi.org/10.1016/j.rasd.2012.12.002

Boesch, M. C., Wendt, O., Subramanian, A., & Hsu, N. (2013b). Comparative efficacy of the Picture Exchange Communication System (PECS) versus a speech-generating device: Effects on social-communicative skills and speech development. *Augmentative and Alternative Communication, 29*, 197–209. https://doi.org/10.3109/07434618.2013.818059

Bondy, A. S., & Frost, L. A. (1994). The Picture Exchange Communication System. *Focus on Autistic Behavior, 9*(3), 1–19. https://doi.org/10.1177/108835769400900301

Bondy, A., & Frost, L. (2002). *A picture's worth: PECS and other visual communication strategies in autism*. Woodbine House.

Brosnan, M., Parsons, S., Good, J., & Yuill, N. (2016). How can participatory design inform the design and development of innovative technologies for autistic communities? *Journal of Assistive Technologies, 10*(2), 115–120. https://doi.org/10.1108/jat-12-2015-0033

Brown, B. L., & Leonard, L. B. (1986). Lexical influences on children's early positional patterns. *Journal of Child Language, 13*(2), 219–229. https://doi.org/10.1017/S0305000900008023

Chen, T., Yesilada, Y., & Harper, S. (2010). What input errors do you experience? Typing and pointing errors of mobile web users. *International Journal of Human-Computer Studies, 68*(3), 138–157. https://doi.org/10.1016/j.ijhcs.2009.10.003

Druin, A. (2002). The role of children in the design of new technology. *Behaviour & Information Technology, 21*(1), 1–25. https://doi.org/10.1080/01449290110108659

Fietzer, A. W., & Chin, S. (2017). The impact of digital media on executive planning and performance in children, adolescents, and emerging adults. In F. C. Blumberg & P. J. Brooks (Eds.), *Cognitive development in digital contexts* (pp. 167–180). Academic Press. https://doi.org/10.1016/B978-0-12-809481-5.00008-0

Frauenberger, C., Good, J., & Keay-Bright, W. (2011). Designing technology for children with special needs: Bridging perspectives through participatory design. *CoDesign, 7*(1), 1–28. https://doi.org/10.1080/15710882.2011.587013

Goethe, O. (2019). *Gamification mindset*. Springer. https://doi.org/10.1007/978-3-030-11078-9

Gosnell, J., Costello, J., & Shane, H. (2011, April). There isn't always an app for that! *Perspectives in Augmentative and Alternative Communication, 20*, 7–8. https://doi.org/10.1044/aac20.1.7

Hall, R. R. (2001). Prototyping for usability of new technology. *International Journal of Human-Computer Studies, 55*(4), 485–501. https://doi.org/10.1006/ijhc.2001.0478

Hamari, J. (2017). Do badges increase user activity? A field experiment on the effects of gamification. *Computers in Human Behavior, 71*, 469–478. https://doi.org/10.1016/j.chb.2015.03.036

Hayes, A. (2020, August 28). *The ins and outs of wearable technology*. Investopedia. https://www.investopedia.com/terms/w/wearable-technology.asp

Holyfield, C., Caron, J., & Light, J. (2019). Programing AAC just-in-time for beginning communicators: The process. *Augmentative and Alternative Communication, 35*(4), 309–318. https://doi.org/10.1080/07434618.2019.1686538

Light, J., & McNaughton, D. (2012). The changing face of augmentative and alternative communication: Past, present, and future challenges. *Augmentative and Alternative Communication, 28*(4), 197–204. https://doi.org/10.3109/07434618.2012.737024

Lloyd, L. L., Fuller, D. R., & Arvidson, H. H. (1997). *Augmentative and alternative communication: Handbook of principles and practices*. Allyn & Bacon.

Lord, C., Rutter, M., DiLavore, P. C., Risi, S., Gotham, K., & Bishop, S. (2012). *Autism diagnostic observation schedule: ADOS™-2*. Western Psychological Services.

Lubas, M., Mitchell, J., & De Leo, G. (2014). User-centered design and augmentative and alternative communication apps for children with autism spectrum disorders. *SAGE Open, 4*(2), 215824401453750. https://doi.org/10.1177/2158244014537501

Marczewski, A. (2015). *Even ninja monkeys like to play: Gamification, game thinking, and motivational design*. Gamified UK.

McNaughton, D., & Light, J. (2013). The iPad and mobile technology revolution: Benefits and challenges for individuals who require augmentative and alternative communication. *Augmentative and Alternative Communication, 29*(2), 107–116. https://doi.org/10.3109/07434618.2013.784930

Meder, A. (2012). *Mobile media devices and communication applications as a form of augmentative and alternative communication: An assessment of family wants, needs, and preferences* [Master's thesis, University of Kansas]. University of Kansas ScholarWorks. http://hdl.handle.net/1808/10676

Nelson, N. W. (1993). *Childhood language disorders in context: Infancy through adolescence.* MacMillan.

Pew Research Center. (2021). *Mobile fact sheet.* https://www.pewresearch.org/internet/fact-sheet/mobile/

Rose, V., Trembath, D., Keen, D., & Paynter, J. (2016). The proportion of minimally verbal children with autism spectrum disorder in a community-based early intervention programme. *Journal of Intellectual Disability Research, 60*(5), 464–477. https://doi.org/10.1111/jir.12284

Schlosser, R. W., & Koul, R. K. (2015). Speech output technologies in interventions for individuals with autism spectrum disorders: A scoping review. *Augmentative and Alternative Communication, 31*(4), 285–309. https://doi.org/10.3109/07434618.2015.1063689

Schlosser, R. W., Shane, H. C., Allen, A. A., Abramson, J., Laubscher, E., & Dimery, K. (2016). Just-in-time supports in augmentative and alternative communication. *Journal of Developmental and Physical Disabilities, 28*(1), 177–193. https://doi.org/10.1007/s10882-015-9452-2

Schopler, E., Van Bourgondien, M. E., Wellman, G. J., & Love, S. R. (Eds.). (2010). *Childhood Autism Rating Scale* (2nd ed.). Western Psychological Services.

Shane, H. C., Laubscher, E. H., Schlosser, R. W., Flynn, S., Sorce, J. F., & Abramson, J. (2012). Applying technology to visually support language and communication in individuals with autism spectrum disorders. *Journal of Autism and Developmental Disorders, 42*(6), 1228–1235. https://doi.org/10.1007/s10803-011-1304-z

Tager-Flusberg, H., & Kasari, C. (2013). Minimally verbal school-aged children with autism spectrum disorder: The neglected end of the spectrum. *Autism Research, 6*(6), 468–478. https://doi.org/10.1002/aur.1329

Venkatesh, V., & Ramesh, V. (2006). Web and wireless site usability: Understanding differences and modeling use. *MIS Quarterly, 30*(1), 181–206. https://doi.org/10.2307/25148723

Weiser, M. (1991). The computer for the 21st century. *Scientific American, 265*(3), 94–104. https://doi.org/10.1038/scientificamerican0991-94

Wendt, O., Allen, N. E., Ejde, O. Z., Nees, S. C., Philips, M. N., & Lopez, D. (2020). Optimized user experience design for augmentative and alternative communication via mobile technology: Using gamification to enhance access and learning for users with severe autism. In C. Stephanidis, M. Antona, Q. Gao, & J. Zhou (Eds.), *HCI International 2020—Late breaking papers: Universal access and inclusive design. [Lecture Notes in Computer Science: Human-Computer Interaction, Vol. 12426]* (pp. 412–428). Springer. https://doi.org/10.1007/978-3-030-60149-2_32

Wendt, O., Hsu, N., Simon, K., Dienhart, A., & Cain, L. (2019). Effects of an iPad-based speech-generating device infused into instruction with the Picture Exchange Communication System (PECS) for adolescents and young adults with severe autism. *Behavior Modification: Special Issue on Communicative Interventions, 43*, 898–932. https://doi.org/10.1177/0145445519870552

Wetherby, B., & Striefel, S. (1978). Application of miniature linguistic system or matrix-training procedures. In R. L. Schiefelbusch (Ed.), *Language intervention strategies* (pp. 317–356). University Park Press.

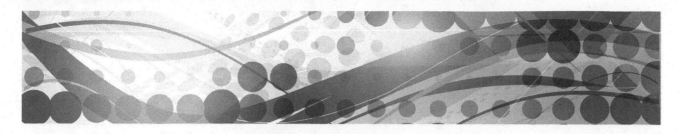

Chapter 5
PHYSICAL ACCESS FEATURES OF AAC

Kathryn D'Agostino Russo

Fundamentals

What Is Alternate Access and Who Is It for?

AAC is not a "one-size-fits-all" area of practice, especially when it comes to assessment and intervention for individuals with severe and complex physical disabilities who may not be able to use their fingers or hands to access AAC. Instead, these individuals may need alternative access methods to access both low- and high-tech communication options. Access refers to the means by which an individual interacts with and makes a selection on their AAC system.

Alternative access methods include options such as eye gaze, head tracking, brain-computer interfaces (BCIs) and scanning. These access methods allow individuals with complex communication needs (CCNs) and physical impairments to access AAC and participate more fully in every aspect of life—communication, community, education, and vocation. These access methods may also support an individual's use of other assistive technologies, such as power wheelchairs or other adapted equipment. Individuals who use AAC may use a variety of access methods across their life span, and it is important that speech-language pathologists (SLPs) employ a collaborative approach and ongoing assessment to determine what is the best access method and AAC system for an individual at any given time.

Types of Alternate Access

There are two main means of access—direct selection and indirect selection or scanning, both of which are discussed in this chapter.

Direct Access Methods

Direct selection involves direct indication of one's desired target (e.g., message, symbol, letter, or whatever the selection set is) in one of four main ways: physical contact (i.e., touching or pointing to the target), physical pressure (i.e., pressing on or depressing the desired target), no contact pointing (i.e., where pointing is carried out without actually touching the surface of the device such as with eye-tracking technology), and speech recognition (i.e., for people who can speak but who cannot use their hands, fingers, or other options to make selections). In addition to these, a relatively newer direct selection technology is BCIs.

A variety of direct access options are currently available, each of which has its own associated specifications. One of the most ubiquitous is eye-gaze technology, and it can be found in a number of different AAC systems (as shown in Table 5–1). To use eye-tracking or eye-gaze technology, the reflection of a light source (e.g., ambient lighting) is captured by a camera attached to the AAC device. The camera communicates with the device's internal computer, and the computer tracks the reflection of the light from the eye. Software correlates reflected infrared (IR) light and mouse movement

Table 5–1. Eye-Gaze Options

Tracker	Manufacturer	Works With	Calibration and Other Features
Look	Prentke Romich https://www.prentrom.com	PRC Accent devices	• 0, 1, 2, 5, or 9 calibration points • Replaces NuEye
PCEye	Tobii Dynavox https://www.tobiidynavox.com	TobiiDynavox ISeries devices Windows computers and tablets	• 1, 2, 5, or 9 calibration points • Ability to improve calibration for select points instead of recalibrating entirely
Hiru	Irisbond https://www.irisbond.com	PC computers and tablets iPadOS (macOS and Android coming soon)	• 0, 1, 5, 9, or 16 calibration points
Eyegaze Edge	Eyegaze Inc. https://www.eyegaze.com	Eyegaze Edge tablet, but can also be used to control Windows and Mac computers	• 5, 9, or 13 calibration points • Do not need to recalibrate if user moves away
Skyle	Inclusive Technology https://www.inclusivetlc.com	iPad Pro with the Skyle application	• 5 or 9 calibration points • User can use any AAC or iPad application

with information from an initial calibration. Selections are made when the user focuses their gaze on a specific icon or cell for a select length of time, known as dwell time, or by a purposeful blink, or some combination of blink and dwell time (Fager et al., 2012a, 2012b; Koch Fager, 2018). Before an individual can successfully use eye tracking, they must go through a calibration procedure. During calibration, the user focuses on one or more fixed points on a monitor in order to confirm that the IR light is reflecting and capturing eye gaze correctly. Eye and vision disorders, such as cortical visual impairment (CVI), nystagmus, amblyopia or strabismus, and even presbyopia may affect an individual's ability to calibrate and use eye gaze as an access method; however, there are a variety of settings that can be adjusted to allow for successful and accurate use. These include changing the size or color of icons, increasing the dwell time, adjusting the acceptance rate for blinking, choosing to

track the dominant eye only rather than both eyes, and applying cursor adjustments. For individuals who wear prescription progressive glasses (i.e., in which the bifocal part of the lens is not visibly obvious to the viewer), some adjustments may need to be made with respect to the distance between the device and the user. In addition to collaborating with occupational therapists (OTs), physical therapists (PTs), and caregivers for appropriate positioning, SLPs can consult with ophthalmologists and teachers of the visually impaired (TVIs) to determine what adjustments may be necessary for use of eye gaze.

Eye-gaze technology is beneficial for individuals with severely limited physical movements due to congenital disorders, such as cerebral palsy (CP), Rett syndrome or genetic disorders, or acquired neurodegenerative disorders such as amyotrophic lateral sclerosis (ALS) and brainstem or spinal cord injuries (SCIs). Typically, the AAC system must be mounted between 18 and 24 in. from the individual's face in order for the eye-tracking module to work successfully.

Head tracking is similar to eye tracking in that it is also a direct selection method that uses IR technology. However, in head tracking, the user wears a reflective dot on their forehead, hat, bridge of their nose, or glasses to reflect the IR light (Koch Fager, 2018) presented by a small camera positioned above or near the top of the device monitor. As with eye gaze, when using head tracking, the individual selects their intended message by aligning the reflective dot with the target and dwelling on the target for a predetermined length of time. The camera registers the position of the reflective dot with respect to the screen and the user's head, and the selection is made. This access method is better suited for individuals with the ability to move their head and neck, such as some individuals with CP or people with SCIs below the level of the neck. Teams can consider relative or absolute tracking depending on the individual's range of motion (Fager et al., 2012b).

It is important to differentiate between eye tracking and head tracking. Eye-tracking technology does not require any head movement to potentiate selections, whereas head tracking capitalizes on the user's ability to make fine but deliberate head movements to potentiate selections.

BCIs are a newer technology that allows for direct selection on a keyboard by interpreting a person's brain signals in response to a specific display (Huggins & Kovacs, 2018). They may be invasive, with electrodes implanted directly on the brain's cortex, or noninvasive, with electrodes placed on the scalp (Fager et al., 2012b). Currently, BCIs are separate systems typically used for computer access and do not yet interface well with AAC systems. Many BCIs are spelling interfaces, such as the BCI2000 with P300 Speller (Oken et al., 2014). In spelling interfaces, a display of letters is presented, and characters flash randomly. The brain elicits a P300 wave when the target character is highlighted. Communication using this method is generally slow due to low rates of characters per minute. The rapid serial visual presentation (RSVP) keyboard is a BCI that aims to improve speed and accuracy of typing and communication by using a predictive language model (Oken et al., 2014; Orhan et al., 2012). The RSVP keyboard displays characters in a sequence, and after the user selects a character, generates a second sequence based on the high probability that certain letters would follow the first using a predictive algorithm. There is growing evidence that BCIs may be an appropriate access method for individuals with locked-in syndrome (Fager et al., 2012b), a condition of complete paralysis of just about all voluntary muscle movements aside from movements of the eye, or other disorders where motor movement is negligible or severely limited and who may not be able to use or sustain eye gaze. As with all access methods, it is important for SLPs, persons who use augmentative and alternative communication (PWUAAC) and other team members to review current research in order to determine whether a BCI will meet a person's communication and participation needs.

Indirect Access Methods

If direct selection is not an option, often due to motor control issues, the person must use indirect selection to choose their desired target on an AAC system. Indirect selection can take a number of forms, all of which involve presentation of the choices or targets—or the array—in some manner, either by a person or by the technology. To drive the technical presentation of potential targets in an organized and predetermined manner, and to indicate selection of a desired target once presented, all targets must be scanned.

Indirect selection includes switch scanning and partner-assisted scanning (PAS), where options are presented to a user either visually or auditorily (or both). To begin the presentation of options, the user activates a switch or the communication partner begins presenting potential messages. To select the desired message, the user then activates a switch. To use scanning methods, the person using AAC does not directly interact with their AAC system and must use an external tool, such as a switch or communication partner, to access the AAC system. Many individuals and professionals prefer direct access methods because these are faster than using indirect access, the motor movements tend to be more natural and easier for individuals to learn (Fager et al., 2012a), and the cognitive load tends to be less. Whether a direct or indirect access method is chosen, SLPs and other professionals must continually assess how sensory, physical, language, and cognitive abilities influence performance (Chen & O'Leary, 2018). Table 5–2 offers a side-by-side comparison of direct and indirect access methods.

Scanning is often accomplished by use of a switch that serves as an interface between the speech-generating device (SGD) and the person. Switches differ across many parameters such as size, shape, and the manner in which they are activated (as introduced in Chapter 3). There are two major types of switches: mechanical switches (which require pressure for activation and some travel, or excursion of the switch) and electrical switches (which do not require pressure for activation but may require travel, or excursion of the switch). Mechanical switches often provide some type of activation feedback (e.g., a click or some other sound associated with activation), whereas electrical switches do not always provide activation feedback. Within each of the two major types of switches, there are myriad examples of switches. For example, there are mechanical switches that vary with respect to their thickness, shape, size, and the amount of pressure and travel required for activation. Similarly, electrical switches vary with respect to size, shape, and the method of activation. Table 5–3 provides a brief overview of some switch manufacturers and types of switches.

Newer to the marketplace are electromyographic (EMG)-based switches that capture small electrical signals from muscle activity. The EMG signal then wirelessly activates electronic assistive technology such as AAC devices. Importantly, this class of switch uses newer materials that do not rely on gels or other skin preparation, which were problematic for earlier EMG-based switches.

Interprofessional teams may consider switch scanning for individuals who cannot use direct selection methods. The most frequently used type of indirect selection is scanning. To scan, an individual uses a switch to scroll sequentially through a visual or auditory display of potential messages to locate their intended target. A person may use one or two switches, different scanning modes, and different scanning patterns depending on their motor and cognitive abilities and their communication needs.

When using a single switch, the scanning mode can be automatic or inverse. In single-switch automatic scanning, the user activates the switch to initiate the scan and then activates it a second time when the visual cursor or auditory cue reaches the intended message or group of messages. In an inverse scanning mode, the individual maintains pressure on the switch until the desired target is reached before releasing the switch. In two-switch step scanning, the individual uses the first switch to advance the cursor and the second switch to select the chosen message. Each mode requires different concentration and precise motor timing paired with specific body movements. Table 5–4 summarizes the main scanning modes.

Scanning Patterns

Scanning patterns are configurations in which the representations (e.g., vocabulary, messages, icons) on a user's SGD are presented to them. The main scanning patterns include linear scanning, grouped scanning, and circular scanning. Circular scanning is a relatively simple scanning pattern in which items are situated in a circle (often in a clockwise layout) and are scanned one at a time. Items are highlighted either with the sweeping motion of a pointer (e.g., an arrow or something resembling the minute hand on an analog clock) or with a small light at each point. Circular scanning is limited in terms of the number of items that can be

Table 5–2. Direct and Indirect Access Methods

Direct Access—User can directly choose	Indirect Access—User must use external tool to choose
• Touch	• Switch scanning
• Eye gaze	• Partner-assisted scanning (PAS)
• Head pointing	
• Speech recognition	
• Brain-computer interface (BCI)	

Table 5-3. Some Switch Manufacturers and Sample Switches

Manufacturer	Switch	Features
AbleNet https://www.ablenetinc.com	Jelly Bean Switch	■ Pressure switch ■ Provides auditory and tactile feedback through a click when pressed ■ Mounting plate included
	Candy Corn Switch	■ Proximity switch ■ Provides visual and auditory feedback when activated ■ Requires user to move within 0.5 in. of the switch
	Micro Light Switch	■ Pressure switch ■ Provides auditory and tactile feedback through a click when pressed ■ Requires 0.4 oz of force
	BIGmack or LITTLEmack	■ Pressure switch ■ Single message voice output ■ Output for toy or tool
Enabling Devices https://www.enablingdevices.com	Jumbo Switch	■ Pressure switch ■ Provides auditory and tactile feedback through a click when pressed
	Plate Switch	■ Pressure Switch ■ No batteries needed ■ Positioned at an angle so that it requires less force
PRC-Saltillo https://www.prc-saltillo.com	AeroSwitch	■ Pressure switch ■ Connects to PRC-Saltillo devices using Bluetooth
Adaptivation, Inc. http://www.adaptivation.com	PalPad	■ Pressure switch ■ Completely flat ■ Requires only 2 oz of force

Table 5-4. Scanning Modes

Scanning Mode	How It Works	Number of Switches
Automatic	Activate switch to initiate scan, activate switch again at desired target	1
Inverse	Maintain pressure on the switch until desired target and then release	1
Step scanning	Activate the switch to initiate each step along the scan (There is a 1:1 relationship between each activation and each advance of the scan.)	1
Two-step scanning	Activate first switch to advance the scan; activate second switch at desired target	2

represented (i.e., usually up to 12 items) and is relatively easy to learn. This type of scanning pattern may be used as an introduction to scanning.

Linear scanning is the slowest pattern because the user must scan linearly through every item. Grouped scanning is sometimes referred to as block scanning and is faster because vocabulary or symbols are organized into groups, and the user scans to the desired group before scanning through items within that group. Once a group of vocabulary or symbols is selected, a linear scan pattern begins. Within grouped or "group-item" scanning, row-column scanning is the most commonly used scanning pattern. In row-column scanning, the scan is set to scan row by row until the user indicates the row in which the desired target is located, and then the scan continues column by column until the desired target is reached. Some AAC vocabularies specifically designed with switch scanning in mind, such as Prentke-Romich Company's CoreScanner™, are arranged to optimize communication for people who use scanning as a method of access.

A person using scanning may rely on visual or auditory prompts to indicate they have scanned to their desired target. Visual prompts allow the individual to see what icons, letters, or groups of items are being scanned by using a cursor or highlighted box to surround the scanned items. If the person who uses AAC cannot use visual scanning (e.g., due to visual impairment) but their hearing is intact and functional, auditory scanning may be an option. In auditory scanning, the individual relies on auditory prompts as the items are being scanned. The auditory prompt may be a phonemic cue or a whole-word prompt that is topically related to the target, usually in a different voice than the user uses when communicating. When the user hears the prompt they want, they select that target using a switch, and the full message is spoken aloud. Some people who use auditory scanning choose to wear an earpiece (e.g., earbud) or use a small speaker by their ear so that only they can hear the private auditory prompt voice. For instance, someone using auditory scanning may be listening to one-word prompts about various dinner options. Once they hear the prompt for the intended target, they would select that target, and the public message would be spoken (Table 5–5). During training or therapy sessions, it is often helpful for the individual and communication partners to hear the auditory prompts so that the association between the prompt, its selection, and the full message can be made clear.

In addition to customizing by scanning mode and scanning pattern, switch use can be further adjusted by modifying some or all of the following parameters: the speed or rate of scanning, activation feedback associated with switch use (a visual or auditory cue that a switch activation has been registered), message feedback (when a message is spoken), the color of highlighting of the scan pattern, changing the shape or boldness of the cursor, and/or adjusting the auditory prompts. These parameters are adjustable on almost all communication devices.

Table 5–5. Sample Private and Public Auditory Prompts

Private Auditory Prompt	Public Message to be Spoken
Spaghetti	I want spaghetti & meatballs.
Hot dog	One hot dog with mustard and relish please.
Omelet	I'd like a cheese omelet with hash browns.
Pizza	I want a thin crust Margherita pizza.
Burger	I'd like a burger and fries, no onion on the burger.

The rate of communication when using switch scanning tends to be slow, so SLPs must consider which settings can be adjusted so that a user can scan their AAC system as efficiently as possible (Fager et al., 2012a).

Assessment for Alternate Access

The determination of the best access method for an individual is a critical aspect of assessment for AAC and should be made by an informed team of professionals from disciplines such as occupational and/or physical therapy in addition to speech-language pathology. In cases where access is extremely complex, a biomedical engineer may provide insights and ideas, as might a TVI. It is critical that assessment for alternate access is carefully conducted since many other decisions about AAC and other assistive technologies (ATs) are associated with a user's method of access. Similarly, if access is not working well for an individual, they may not be able to readily use their SGD and may abandon the technology (Johnson et al., 2006; Waller, 2019).

Switch Site Assessment

Switch site assessment is an important part of AAC assessment for individuals who need to use indirect selection as a method of access. Switches can be placed at or near a variety of body parts, such as the hands, feet, fingers, knees, elbows, head, or even the cheek or mouth. Angelo (2000, p. 591) outlined the following 11 considerations essential for single switch site assessment:

- reliability of motor movements
- volitional nature of movement
- safety
- movements that are easily performed
- endurance
- activities and positions the client assumes throughout the day and evening
- efficiency of movement
- previous successful movements
- ability to perform timed response

- ability to activate the access device within a given time frame
- time between switch closures

Switch site assessment is an iterative process in which the individual's physical abilities are matched to various switch types to see which can be used deliberately and efficiently. For children, switch games are often used during trials with various switches to make what is sometimes a long process fun and engaging. For adults, switch games may be replaced by various on-screen targets that the person has to select to incentivize the process.

Switch technology is constantly evolving, and there are a myriad of types and sizes of switches that can be activated by different amounts of pressure or different types of movement (Koch Fager, 2018). For example, proximity switches allow a user to move a body part near the switch to activate it. In contrast, microswitches allow activation with the lightest of pressure. Sip and puff switches require pneumatic activation (i.e., sucking and blowing through a narrow tube for activation). There are even switches that can be activated through tiny muscle movements such as blinking or moving the cheek muscles (such as the masseter muscle). Importantly, when selecting an access site, if a healthy, volitional body movement is not immediately apparent, working toward identification of an access site may become the goal.

If a Switch Site Is Not Identified Right Away

SLPs can still build an individual's language through aided language stimulation (ALgS) or modeling different phrases and communicative functions by using the communication system, while the interdisciplinary team works to determine a suitable switch site and to train the user to access the switch(es). Not only does ALgS support a person learning new words to express themselves, it supports continued development of their receptive language and provides a model for use of AAC. In this way, a person may simultaneously learn language and motor automaticity. Switch access for AAC may be considered for people with concomitant physical and visual impairments, for individuals who will gradually lose all vision abilities, or for individuals who are unable to control their eye or head movements.

Multimodal and Low-Tech Access for Communication

When working to determine an access method and communication system for a person with CCNs, it is important to consider multimodal, low-tech, and backup systems for environments or situations when it may be difficult or impossible for a person to access their high-tech AAC system, as discussed in Chapters 2 and 3. PWUAAC may benefit from learning to use multiple alternative access methods so that they may communicate when their usual AAC system cannot be used in a specific environment, when using different positioning equipment, or when there are changes in medical status. For example, it is sometimes difficult to access eye gaze outdoors because of sunlight or glare, or a person may be unable to use head tracking when they are lying down. There are also emergency situations (e.g., natural disasters) where equipment may not be readily available and/or charging of an AAC system may not be feasible. In other cases, an individual's abilities may fluctuate throughout the day due to fatigue or effects of medications. Learning new body movements and using alternative access methods can be tiresome, especially for newer users, so it is important that the team and individual work together to determine a secondary system to use if the individual becomes fatigued. PAS or an e-Tran board may be an appropriate method for communicating in scenarios where a person cannot use their SGD.

As reviewed in Chapter 2, PAS is an important scanning option that can be used on its own with a low-tech communication board and/or with a communication board being used for an SGD. Importantly, to use PAS successfully, the user must have an agreed upon signal to indicate their choice or a reliable way to indicate "yes" and "no" so that they can signal when the desired target has been reached or when the facilitator should continue scanning. The signal could be a gesture

(e.g., thumbs up), eye movement (e.g., blink), activation of a single-message SGD (e.g., a LittleMack programmed to say "that's the one"), or any other behavior that the user and communication partners agree on.

In PAS, a communication partner provides choices in an established and systematic scanning pattern that is often closest to row-column scanning. The communication facilitator starts the scan by asking the user if their desired target is in row one or group one and points at the row or group being referenced on the communication board. If the user indicates "no," then the facilitator continues the scan by asking "is it row two? Row three?" and so on until the user indicates that the desired target is in the row indicated by the facilitator. The scan begins again from the beginning until the message is spelled out. To conserve energy and effort, some users of PAS prefer to only indicate "yes" rather than indicating "no" for each row or group in which the intended target is not located. This way of using PAS is common but requires that the system be agreed upon, in advance, by all participants. In that way, the scanning can proceed quickly and efficiently. PAS can be used when an SGD is not available or easily accessible, such as during transport or when in alternative seating positions; or if vocabulary specific to the communicative context is not available on the person's dedicated SGD.

A related option is partner-assisted auditory scanning (PAAS) in which the same principles as PAS apply. However, in PAAS, no visual stimuli are used. Rather, the stimuli are presented auditorily, and the user indicates "yes" when the intended target is reached. This option may be used with the alphabet when the layout is well known by both the user and the communication partner. This might be helpful for people who are literate and want to spell words but who may have difficulty keeping their eyes open or who need to rest frequently. If the alphabet layout has a vowel on the left, at the beginning of each row, and the consonants that follow the vowel in alphabetical order (Figure 5–1), then the communication partner could ask the user "Is it in row one (A to D)," wait for response, "row two (E to H)," wait for response, and so on. This AEIOU layout is one option for use with PAAS.

Row 1: **A** B C D

Row 2: **E** F G H

Row 3: **I** J K L M N

Row 4: **O** P Q R S T

Row 5: **U** V W X Y Z

Figure 5–1. AEIOU layout for use with partner-assisted auditory scanning.

An e-Tran, or eye transfer board, is a communication board that allows a person to use eye gaze without technology. Made of clear plastic or acrylic, e-Tran boards have picture symbols or letter groups placed at intervals around the frame (e.g., at the corners and at the top middle and bottom middle of the frame, depending on the person's field of vision). It is important that whatever groupings are on the side facing the user are replicated and in the same position facing the communication partner so that the communication partner knows what the user is referring to in terms of direction of gaze. The e-Tran board can be placed in front of a person, or a communication partner can hold it up where both the person and their communication partner can see it. In this way, the communication partner can see what symbols or letter groups the PWUAAC is gazing at, indicating their message. After gazing at a letter group or group of symbols/pictures on an e-Tran board, PAS is often used to determine the exact letter or symbol the person is indicating. e-Tran boards with letter groups are a viable low-tech option for individuals who can spell. e-Tran boards with symbols are useful when vocabulary specific to the communicative context is not available on a person's dedicated SGD or is not frequently used. SLPs and caregivers can also quickly create e-Tran boards using laminating sheets or PVC-piping picture frames.

Considering Multiple Methods of Access

Regardless of whether a different access method or communication system is selected in conjunction with a user's current SGD or as a backup method for when the SGD is unavailable, it is crucial that the team work together to train the PWUAAC and their communication partners on multiple access modalities. Determining multimodal access allows PWUAAC the ability to communicate with multiple communication partners in multiple communication settings, and to access a variety of assistive technologies that will allow them to fully participate in their community (Fager et al., 2012a). Additionally, there are some PWUAAC who prefer to use two or more modalities together to access their communication system (Koch Fager, 2018), such as using head tracking to highlight the intended icon and using a switch to select the intended icon. Many SGDs support the use of multiple access methods.

Although an SLP must consult with an OT and PT to determine optimal positioning of the user and AAC equipment, including any switches, the SLP can make recommendations about which access method will best fit an individual's current communication needs while taking into consideration the person's concomitant physical or sensory impairments. This information will help guide the SLP about what access methods may be viable, such as recommending eye gaze as a tool for individuals with limited movement and control of their extremities, or auditory scanning for individuals who have no functional vision. If direct selection using the hands, eye gaze, or head pointing is not possible, the SLP can consider different switch sites based on cephalocaudal (from head to tail) and proximodistal (from central to peripheral) development patterns. This means that individuals often develop motor control from head to toe and from the center of the body to the extremities. Using this knowledge, the SLP can try to switch placements at the head and upper extremities before trying lower extremities or feet.

It is also important to consider the trajectory of the person's primary diagnosis. While all PWUAAC will require minor adjustments to their systems over time, such as increasing the display size or adjusting the rate of scanning, or the placement of the switch with respect to their bodies, there are other considerations as well.

Considerations for Individuals With Chronic Conditions

For individuals with chronic conditions, access methods may be stable for long periods of time, barring unforeseen changes due to aging and/or postural issues related to seating. That is, these individuals may continue to use prescribed access options until such time that they need help with their assistive technology—be it wheelchair, or AAC device, or other technology.

Considerations for Individuals With Progressive Conditions

For individuals with progressive conditions, access is a critical consideration in terms of selection of an SGD. Knowing the trajectory of the disease from the outset is important so that the clinician considers SGDs that support a variety of access options. In this way, when a different access method is required due to progression of the disease, new learning is minimized because the SGD and the representation set remain the same. Although moving from direct selection to alternate access may necessitate changes to the layout to optimize efficiency, familiarity with the device may facilitate transition between different access options. Whenever possible, it is best to avoid a point of crisis in terms of the necessity of learning and acclimating to a new method of access. Thus, knowing the trajectory of the disorder and monitoring progress on a regular basis may preclude the need for urgent intervention that can add stress to an already stressful situation.

Another facet to consider is that some people prefer to have more than one access method so that if they fatigue from use of one option, there are others available to them. This can be the case for people with progressive conditions where the effects of fatigue and exertion may render one access method unusable at certain times of day. Having another access mode readily available mitigates the effects of lack of access to the SGD.

Access and Mobile Tablets

When considering an access method, the SLP and the individual should discuss whether a dedicated device or mobile tablet is the best option. As technology and accessibility solutions advance, it is becoming increasingly easier to use switch scanning, eye gaze, and head tracking with mobile tablets, like those discussed in Chapter 4. This typically requires external hardware, such as Bluetooth switches or an eye-gaze bar. Because add-on switches and other external hardware are not made by the companies that design mobile tablets, they do not always interface smoothly and may require extra adjustments. The SLP and the user can work together to create "recipes," which are a sequenced series of actions assigned to complete a specific function, such as using operational features, which may make using a mobile tablet easier. Dedicated devices tend to be more durable and interface directly with the alternative access methods, but some individuals may prefer mobile tablets for portability, funding, or leisure reasons. Apps may also be able to be installed on a phone, iPad, and/or secondary iPad, making AAC more readily and generally available.

Learning Language and Access Skills

Learning to use AAC is a complicated process that involves "developing motor automaticity, learning the access method, expanding language skills, and juggling social and cognitive demands" (Burkhart, 2018, p. 33). It is the task of the SLP to support language development and learning, but this can be strongly impacted by the individual's motor abilities. People with CCNs must simultaneously learn language and how to move their bodies to access AAC, and this learning may not occur at the same rate. SLPs should constantly evaluate how linguistic abilities are different from the motor automaticity needed for use of an AAC system (Chen & O'Leary, 2018). In supporting an individual who uses alternative access methods to use AAC, SLPs must collaborate with OTs and PTs to confirm that body movements are volitional, nonfatiguing, efficient, and healthy, so as not to cause stress injuries (Angelo, 2000; Fager et al., 2012a). When first introduced to an alternate access method, a PWUAAC will need specific instruction and practice in how to use the method, whether that be how to move their eyes, head, or other body part. This could be using eye gaze to participate in a cause-and-effect game on an SGD or using two switches to operate an adapted pourer and switch-adapted blender during a cooking activity. Targeted activities such as these allow individuals to experience motor success and build the motor abilities to access an AAC system without the added stress of learning language at the same time (Burkhart, 2018). It is critical that SLPs balance their therapy sessions with practice aimed at increasing linguistic skills and practice aimed at increasing motor automaticity of the access method, in order for the PWUAAC to become a proficient communicator to fully participate in their community.

The Acquisition of Learning Process (ALP) for AAC Access (Clarke et al., 2018) is a useful tool for SLPs and other team members when they consider the balance between linguistic and motor skills that is necessary for successful use of an AAC system. OT Lisbeth Nilsson originally developed the ALP to use with people learning to use powered mobility, and it has been adapted for use with people learning to use AAC by SLPs Chip Clarke and Sarah Wilds. It describes what movements, understanding, attention, social interaction, and emotions of the individual learning to use AAC might look like across three stages (introvert/exploring functions, difficult transition/exploring sequencing, and extrovert/exploring performance) and eight phases ranging from novice to expert. As an individual using alternative access methods progresses through the stages and phases, they move from focusing on their body and the access method with a vague understanding or awareness of how to use them together, to integrated use across all settings with a focus on the communication output.

Not only is the ALP important for helping an SLP support a PWUAAC's linguistic and motor learning, it is a vital tool for measuring progress using AAC over time.

In Conclusion

Communication is a fundamental human right, and alternative access methods, such as eye gaze, head tracking, and switch access, make communication possible for people with complex communication needs and complex bodies. SLPs and other professionals must work together to determine what access methods support an individual's skills and needs not only across the day, but across the life span. As technology continues to advance, SLPs and other professionals should continue to advocate for these technologies to be accessible to all individuals by interfacing with and supporting alternative access methods. With the help of alternative access methods and collaborative therapies to learn the motor skills necessary to access AAC, people with CCNs can use a variety of AAC systems and other assistive technologies to fully participate in all aspects of life.

Case Study: JB

Clinical Profile and Communication Needs

The Individual

JB is a 5-year, 7-month-old male diagnosed at birth with spastic quadriplegic cerebral palsy (CP) due to a prenatal stroke. Due to hypertonia, contractures, and lack of volitional movement of upper and lower extremities, he uses a wheelchair and wears orthotics on his wrists and ankles to prevent further contractures. JB has limited movement of his neck and head, and typically presents with his neck in full flexion with his chin resting on his chest. JB is able to perform full neck extension, but this requires extended response time, and he fatigues when maintaining neutral neck positioning or with repeated neck extension. He presents with limited lateral range of motion (i.e., bringing head down to touch ear to shoulder) and rotation (i.e., turning head to look to the side) of his head, with greater lateral flexion and rotation to the right side than to the left. When his head is resting on his chest, JB's eyes are typically closed. JB was recently assessed by a multidisciplinary team and was diagnosed with CVI. He scored a 2.5 to 3 on The CVI Range (Roman-Lantzy, 2007), placing him in Phase I. JB consumes a modified diet and eats limited amounts of pureed foods and pudding-thick liquids. Due to limited oral intake, JB also receives feedings via a gastrostomy tube.

According to The Communication Matrix (Rowland, 2021) completed by his parents and school-based team before his AAC evaluation, JB demonstrated emerging communication skills at Level 3—Unconventional Communication. He typically uses body movements such as stiffening his body, facial expressions such as smiling or furrowing his brow, and early sounds such as cooing, laughing, or whining to protest, request recurrence, and attract attention. He is beginning to make choices by smiling when a preferred item is named or brought into his visual field. All team members agreed that a multidisciplinary AAC assessment was necessary to support JB's communication.

Their Communication Partners and the Environment

JB lives with his parents, one grandparent, and two older siblings. Their extended family lives in the same neighborhood, so they frequently attend barbecues and family meals on the weekends. JB enjoys reading and literacy activities, as his family routine includes nightly bedtime stories where each child chooses a book to read. JB also enjoys music and vestibular input, such as rocking or swinging. He attends kindergarten in a full-time special education program in his district's public school, in a classroom with 1 teacher, 4 paraprofessionals, and 11 other students. As per his individualized education program (IEP), JB receives speech-language therapy, occupational therapy, physical therapy, and vision services. JB rides a school bus to school, and his family has a wheelchair-accessible van.

AAC Considerations

Due to the limited range of motion of his head, neck, and extremities, the team initially recommended trialing a static display speech-generating device (SGD) accessed via eye gaze. JB's flexed neck position made it difficult to position the SGD directly across from his line of vision, so the PT recommended the use of a neck cuff to facilitate a neutral head position. JB was observed to open his eyes and use his vision more often when wearing the neck cuff. During the first few trials, JB was unable to calibrate the eye-gaze sensor, demonstrated difficulty selecting icons, and was observed to scan the screen without focusing on any quadrant and then moving his eyes to the side. This behavior was also observed when targeted activities to develop eye-gaze skills were introduced, such as games with fixed or moving targets. The SLP consulted the ALP for AAC, and even after several trials, JB was at the Novice phase of Stage 1. The team agreed to trial other access methods while also working to develop his visual behaviors in case eye gaze should become a viable option in the future. The SLP also continued to provide aided language stimulation using the SGD or e-Tran board to build JB's receptive language, and to continue to expose him to eye-gaze access.

JB trialed accessing an SGD using a switch mounted on his wheelchair's headrest at various locations around his head. Switch access at his hands, elbows, feet, or knees was ruled out due to lack of volitional movement of these body parts. JB's most purposeful movement was extending his neck to activate a switch located behind his head when he was not wearing his neck cuff; however, the neck cuff impeded his range of motion. He was inconsistently able to activate a switch located on the right side of his head by turning his head and was unable to access a switch located on the left side of his head. When the SLP consulted the ALP for AAC, JB was at the Curious Novice Phase, as he quickly understood that his head was activating the switch and continued to attempt activations by turning his head to operate a toy or use a single-message SGD to request preferred music.

Following Linda Burkhart's Stepping Stones to Switch Access protocol (a systematic way of teaching switch use; Burkhart, 2018), the SLP trialed two switch sites for two-switch step scanning: one behind and one on the right side of his head. Despite multiple trials, JB had difficulty sequencing the movements necessary to operate two different switches to scan through potential messages or to select his intended message. When the scanning switch was placed in either position (behind his head or on the right side of his head), he was observed to initiate the scan pattern, but stopped and discontinued his communication attempt without scanning further or selecting a message using the second switch. When participating in activities to develop motor automaticity of using two switches, JB was only able to activate one switch and demonstrated difficulty using another head movement to activate the second switch. Additionally, he was unable to time his movements to use one switch for automatic or inverse scanning at either site. JB was also observed to fatigue after repeatedly moving his head to the switch in either location, typically after about 30 min of use.

The team recommended an extended trial of PAS using a single-message SGD connected to a proximity switch mounted on the right side of his head, while team members continued to work on improving visual skills needed to use eye gaze and determining other volitional movement patterns. A proximity switch was chosen because JB's ability to reach the switch on the right side of his head varied throughout the day due to fatigue, fluctuations in tone, and whether or not he was wearing the recommended neck cuff. The proximity switch allowed him to be less precise in turning his head so he could reach the switch more easily. The single-message SGD was programmed to say "hey" so that JB could initiate a communication exchange by activating the switch. The SLP trained communication partners to ask, "Do you have something to say?" when JB activated his single-message SGD. The SLP also trained communication partners to then initiate PAS and to provide choices with appropriate extended response time. When initially learning to activate the switch behind his head, JB benefited from tactile cues at the back of his head when he used facial expressions and early sounds to attract attention. The SLP and other team members also provided targeted switch acti-

vation practice to develop JB's switch access skills using switch-activated toys and appliances, as well as using the switch to activate a single-message SGD programmed with a repeated line from favorite books. Additionally, the SLP continued to introduce activities that required two switches, while the OT and PT worked on developing healthy neck movements, so that two-switch step scanning might be a viable access method as JB developed more skills.

While JB was developing motor automaticity using one switch in the hopes that a second switch location could be developed, the SLP introduced a low-tech communication book with core vocabulary presented in a specific order so that JB could expand his language beyond choice-making. This allowed communication partners to provide aided language stimulation and build JB's receptive and expressive language while he learned to use switch access.

Initially, JB could only attend to two choices presented auditorily via PAS (i.e., one option and the choice of "something different") and required almost 30 s of extended response time to indicate his choice using the switch-activated SGD or facial expressions and early sounds. With repeated practice and aided language stimulation, JB learned to scan through four choices (i.e., three options and "something different") with only 10 to 15 s of extended response time. Additionally, he was able to visually attend to the presentation of familiar objects on a dark background as they were named in the PAS sequence. The SLP trained communication partners to look and listen for JB's smiling and vocalizations to indicate his intended message, in addition to his use of the single-message SGD. This allowed JB to use PAS to communicate in positions where he could not turn his head to access the switch. Given access to PAS and a single-message SGD combined with aided language stimulation and modeling of the switch access method helped JB to advance from the Novice phase to the Beginner phase of the ALP for AAC.

As other team members such as the vision specialist continued to work on developing JB's visual behaviors, the SLP regularly exposed JB to SGDs and activities accessed through eye gaze, while providing aided language stimulation to encourage his linguistic development. After repeated exposure and modeling, JB was able to calibrate the eye-gaze sensor, participate in simple cause-and-effect games with fixed targets, and follow direct models of core vocabulary. In between short periods of targeted practice to develop eye-gaze access, the SLP modeled language on a static display SGD with 28 high-contrast icons. JB began to imitate modeled words and phrases and generate novel utterances via SGD. During the second trial of eye gaze as an access method, JB quickly moved from the Novice phase to the Beginner phase on the ALP for AAC Access. When provided with consistent aided language stimulation and natural responses, JB's AAC access and use improved to the Advanced Beginner phase of the ALP's Stage 2. He demonstrated consistent use of core vocabulary and communicative functions that had been consistently modeled across all modalities, such as protesting using the word "stop."

The AAC System or Service

After experimenting with multiple vocabulary settings, static and dynamic displays, and different dwell times, cursor movements, and color settings, the SLP recommended that JB would be most successful using eye gaze as an access method with a static display SGD with a 28-icon core vocabulary with motor planning. JB benefited from high-contrast icons that inverted in contrast when the cursor highlighted them and a dwell time of 0.2 s. Initial therapy goals included expanding JB's expressive communication from using unconventional communication behaviors to using abstract symbols to request and protest objects and activities. The SLP and communication partners continued to provide aided language stimulation of different words, phrase types, and communication functions, such as commenting and asking questions.

Although the team agreed that an SGD accessed using eye gaze was the best fit for JB's present and near-future communication needs, they continued to develop his use of no-tech and low-tech AAC systems. JB is not able to access his SGD when seated in positioning equipment, when riding the bus to school, and when traveling in his family's

wheelchair-accessible van. The SLP recommended the use of PAS in these scenarios or when his SGD did not have vocabulary for a specific communication situation. Additionally, the SLP taught JB to use an e-Tran board to communicate during those circumstances where access to his SGD was neither possible nor safe. Due to his CVI, JB sometimes had difficulty perceiving the icons on his e-Tran board but is continuing to develop his visual skills with the help of the interdisciplinary team.

Next Steps

It is important to note that the SLP consistently assessed JB's access skills using the ALP for AAC Access with the help of interdisciplinary team members, as well as continued to expand JB's language and vocabulary. The SLP can incorporate preferred activities, such as reading and music, into therapy sessions while modeling different communicative functions. Although a static display SGD with 28 icons accessed via eye gaze is a good fit for JB's current communication needs, he will likely need a larger vocabulary as his visual skills and access abilities develop and his language needs increase. The SLP should regularly trial increased display sizes that still allow for motor planning and introduce dynamic displays to provide a more robust vocabulary. In addition to collaborating with JB's OT and PT to confirm safe positioning for eye-gaze access and healthy movement patterns for switches for PAS and other assistive technologies, the SLP should continually consult with the vision specialist to determine whether and how JB's CVI is changing and how he is developing new visual characteristics. This will impact his ability to access a larger vocabulary display. The SLP will have to train JB's family with respect to SGD setup and maintenance, as well as in the use of strategies that scaffold communication for JB. Additionally, the SLP and family should closely work together to support JB's ability to communicate across a variety of communication environments, since activities in which JB wants to participate will likely change as he gets older. In this way, the SLP and JB's team can support JB in becoming a proficient communicator and AAC user and in participating in his community.

Expert Tips and Practical Advice

- When working with people with complex access needs, it is crucial that the SLP consult with other team members about seating and positioning as well as motor, sensory, and visual abilities.
  - These areas are not within an SLP's scope of practice, so although the SLP may identify an alternative access method, it is important that a team approach is used to make sure the method and access site are both safe and viable.
- Always plan for the scenarios when low-tech or a different access method might need to be used.
  - Work with the individual and their communication partners beforehand

to develop a plan for environments or scenarios when using their high-tech SGD is not possible, so no one is left without the ability to express themselves.

- The SLP should always keep in mind that the individual's language abilities may not be at the same level as the motor skills needed to access the SGD. These differences can sometimes make it seem like a person does not have the expressive language necessary for an interaction or that they cannot use a particular access method.
  - The SLP should use ongoing assessment tools, such as the ALP for AAC Access to support the development of language and motor automaticity.

References

Angelo, J. (2000). Factors affecting the use of a single switch with assistive technology devices. *Journal of Rehabilitation Research and Development, 37*(5), 591–598.

Burkhart, L. (2018). Stepping stones to switch access. *Perspectives of the ASHA Special Interest Groups, 3*(12), 33–44. https://doi.org/10.1044/persp3.sig12.33

Chen, S. K., & O'Leary, M. (2018). Eye gaze 101: What speech-language pathologists should know about selecting eye gaze augmentative and alternative communication systems. *Perspectives of the ASHA Special Interest Groups, 3*(12), 24–32. https://doi.org/10.1044/persp3.sig12.24

Clarke, C., Wilds, S., & Nilsson, L. (2018, November 15–17). *Facilitating AAC access ability: Moving forward with the assessment of learning process (ALP) for AAC* [Conference session]. American Speech-Language Hearing Association (ASHA) Convention, Boston, MA. https://plan.core-apps.com/asha2018/event/f39c09c41e6792679c3752f3d04de09d

Fager, S., Bardach, L., Russell, S., & Higginbotham, J. (2012a). Access to augmentative and alternative communication: New technologies and clinical decision making. *Journal of Pediatric Rehabilitation Medicine: An Interdisciplinary Approach, 5*, 53–61. https://doi.org/10.3233/PRM-2012-0196

Fager, S., Beukelman, D. R., Fried-Oken, M., Jakobs, T., & Baker, J. (2012b). Access interface strategies. *Assistive Technology, 24*(1), 25–33. https://doi.org/10.1080/10400435.2011.648712

Huggins, J. E., & Kovacs, T. (2018). Brain–computer interfaces for augmentative and alternative communication: Separating the reality from the hype. *Perspectives of the ASHA Special Interest Groups, 3*(12), 13–23. https://doi.org/10.1044/persp3.sig12.13

Johnson, J. M., Inglebret, E., Jones, C., & Ray, J. (2006). Perspectives of speech language pathologists regarding success versus abandonment of AAC. *Augmentative and Alternative Communication, 22*(2), 85–99. https://doi.org/10.1080/07434610500483588

Koch Fager, S. (2018). Alternative access for adults who rely on augmentative and alternative communication. *Perspectives of the ASHA Special Interest Groups, 3*(12), 6–12. https://doi.org/10.1044/persp3.sig12.6

Oken, B. S., Orhan, U., Roark, B., Erdogmus, D., Fowler, A., Mooney, A., . . . Fried-Oken, M. B. (2014). Brain-computer interface with language model-EEG fusion for locked-in syndrome. *Neurorehabilitation Neural Repair, 28*(4), 387–394. https://doi.org/10.1177/1545968313516867

Orhan, U., Hild, K. E., II, Erdogmus, D., Roark, B., Oken, B., & Fried-Oken, M. (2012). RSVP keyboard: An EEG-based typing interface. *2012 IEEE International Conference on Acoustics, Speech and Signal Processing*

(ICASSP) (pp. 645–648), Kyoto, Japan. https://doi
.org/10.1109/ICASSP.2012.6287966

Roman-Lantzy, C. (2007). *Cortical visual impairment: An approach to assessment and intervention*. AFB Press.

Rowland, C. (2021). *Communication Matrix*. Communication Matrix Foundation. https://www.communicationmatrix.org

Waller, A. (2019). Telling tales: Unlocking the potential of AAC technologies. *International Journal of Language and Communication Disorders, 54*(2), 159–169.

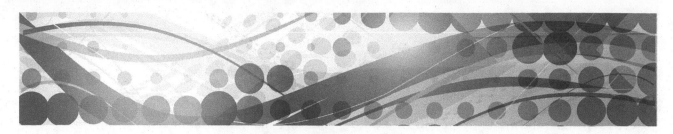

Essay 1

CLINICAL CONSIDERATIONS AND AAC: THE FUTURE OF AAC

Mai Ling Chan

What is on the horizon for augmentative and alternative communication (AAC)? Think *gaming technology*. It makes sense that the continued evolution of AAC devices would build on available technology and find ways to incorporate the most successful features in order to increase accessibility, user satisfaction, and the most desired outcome—rate enhancement.

Advances in gaming technology have surpassed the expected *amazing graphics* and have moved to an immersive experience. What does this mean? Instead of manipulating the world in front of them on the screen, the gamer feels like they are physically within the environment of the game thanks to visual, audio, and haptic (technology that uses touch and proprioception) inputs that create a spatial presence for the player. It makes them *feel like they are there and really doing the actions*.

The level of immersion depends on the gaming system utilized. These vary in terms of the types of controls and consoles used to interact with the game. There are also a myriad of controllers now available including variations of keyboards, joysticks, paddles, and game pads. Whatever the access method, every player is given the same baseline skills as every other player once they enter the game. Depending on the type of game, this means they begin at a certain "level" and can "advance" based on their ability to manipulate the features available to them. This is where people with disabilities have had the opportunity to not

only compete on an equal playing field regardless of physical limitations, but they have also been able to rise to the top of major competitions and establish themselves as esports celebrities.

As people with disabilities grew in number and notoriety, they also gained attention and were sought after for their input, feedback, and opinions as they related to the development of new, more accessible controllers, systems, and ultimately, the entire user experience. I have had the honor of interviewing several key people for my Xceptional Leaders podcast who have worked directly with Microsoft. For example, Erin Hawley, a young woman and accomplished writer from my hometown, Keyport, New Jersey, served as a direct consultant on the development of the Xbox Adaptive Controller. She shares her experience in her podcast interview as well as her chapter of my book, *Becoming an Exceptional Leader*. Erin is joined by many other people with disabilities who have paired their love for technology with product development. This has become essential when developing for the disability community, following the guideline of "by us—for us."

In addition to accessible controllers, video games have also incorporated augmented reality (AR), an interactive experience where the real-world experience is enhanced by computer-generated information. If you followed the 2016 worldwide Pokémon Go sensation, you will recall the mobile game activated people of all ages into a frenzy to find imaginary creatures strategically "placed" in geographic locations around the world. The technology utilized location-based and AR technology—two features that have not been used in current AAC software . . . yet.

When Andreas Forsland's mother required ventilator support following an aggressive case of pneumonia (2012), he immediately recognized the need for her to be able to communicate basic messages while intubated. Forsland, the founder of Cognixion (a Santa Barbara, California–based software company that is on the cutting edge of AAC technology), put his lifelong technical design experience for global companies like Philips, IBM, Apple, and Citrix to work and created Smartstones® Touch™, a palm-sized stone controlled through simple touch and motion gestures to wirelessly control apps on mobile devices that send messages, reminders, and location-based alerts to family and friends. Since then, Cognixion has developed the Speakprose app that utilizes the Apple front-facing TrueDepth camera and created custom facial recognition technology to provide hands-free access to AAC software on the iPhone X and the iPad Pro 4th Generation and newer models. In the Speakprose app, the technology allows head movements to control the selection of communication and control tiles on the screen—acting as a mouse controller.

Unveiled in 2020, Cognixion ONE, the world's first brain-computer interface (BCI) combined with AR AAC applications emerged as the first-ever Wearable Speech™ generating device for communication and environmental controls. "A BCI, sometimes called a neural control interface (NCI), mind-machine interface (MMI), direct neural interface (DNI), or brain-machine interface (BMI), is a direct communication pathway between an enhanced or wired brain and an external device. BCIs are often directed at researching, mapping, assisting, augmenting, or repairing human cognitive or sensory-motor functions" (Krucoff et al., 2016).

Research on BCI began in the 1970s and has been focused on acquiring brain signals, analyzing the information, then controlling a desired action on an external device. The goal has been to "replace or restore useful function to people with neuromuscular disorders" (Shih et al., 2012), and

for communication, BCIs provide an access method utilizing changes in brain activity.

The Cognixion ONE headset utilizes noninvasive (like mentioned in Chapter 5), dry electrodes positioned at the back of the head to capture electroencephalogram (EEG) reported brain activity localized in the visual cortex. In order to create the brain activity, letters, words, phrases, and app commands are presented to the AAC user via AR through the lens on the front. The user can see their environment, and they can also see the app options in a slightly transparent overlay—much like the Pokémon Go experience but in a hands-free, heads-up (rather than looking down at a device) display. This enables eye contact with communication partners and a greater sense of integration with the world around them.

Ever-changing advancements with mobile technology (Chapter 4), natural language processing (essentially a computer's processing of human language; Higginbotham, 2003, 2012), BCI, and AR all represent evolving avenues for increased AAC access. Although the future of AAC may be cutting edge and exciting, the most important aspect is that it is individualized to the user. One shoe does not fit all when it comes to communication. It is important to note that one system is not better than the other. As an evaluator for AAC, all available options must be considered and trialed in the best interest of the person being served. Ultimately, it is essential that the user is in control, allowing the technology to adapt to them—making every message unique because of the person it is being delivered by. The future will be brighter as a result of a chorus of current and new voices being heard, thanks to continued advancement in passionate and mindful access to technology that enables individuals' own personalities to emerge.

References

Higginbotham, J., Lesher, G. W., Moulton, B. J., & Roark, B. (2012). The application of natural language processing to augmentative and alternative communication. *Assistive Technology, 24,* 14–24.

Krucoff, M. O., Rahimpour, S., Slutzky, M. W., Edgerton, V. R., & Turner, D. A. (2016). Enhancing nervous system recovery through neurobiologics, neural interface training, and neurorehabilitation. *Frontiers in Neuroscience, 10*, 584. https://doi.org/10.3389/fnins.2016.00584

Shih, J. J., Krusienski, D. J., & Wolpaw, J. R. (2012). Brain-computer interfaces in medicine. *Mayo Clinic Proceedings, 87*(3), 268–279. https://doi.org/10.1016/j.mayocp.2011.12.008

Wolpaw, J. R., Birbaumer, N., McFarland, D. J., Pfurtscheller, G., & Vaughan, T. M. (2002). Brain-computer interfaces for communication and control. *Clinical Neurophysiology, 113*(6), 767–791.

SECTION II
AAC Language Fundamentals

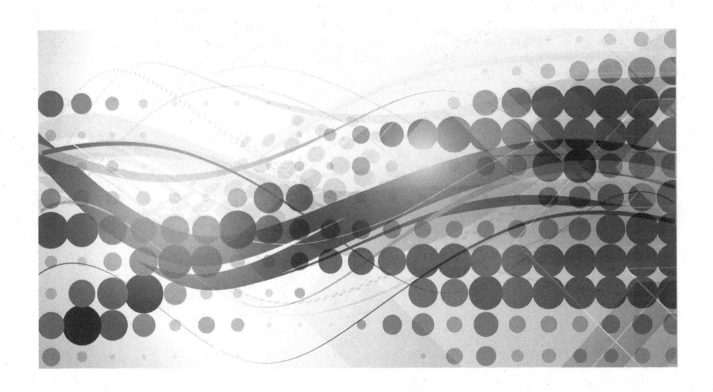

Section II is composed of a series of essays and chapters that emphasize the impact of the physical, social, and cultural environment on the development and implementation of augmentative and alternative communication (AAC) systems. The first essay of the section, Essay 2, establishes our understanding of social determinants of health, and the interplay between one's social environment, physical environment, and available health services. Chapter 6 speaks to cultural and linguistic responsivity and the importance of affirming home language and culture and understanding linguistic and nonlinguistic forms of communication and how these influence meaningful use of symbols as well as culturally appropriate vocabulary and strategies for functional AAC use. Chapter 7 speaks to vocabulary and how the specific words and messages selected on an AAC system should reflect the individual's age, culture, linguistic background, and personality, reiterating the connection between AAC and one's identity, as introduced in Section I.

Essay 3 is the first of nine essays on topics of culture and other considerations important for communicating value and respect, and for AAC design and implementation. The essays represent various vantage points and build on one another to offer rich and diverse perspectives with practical suggestions for clinicians and communication partners. Essays 6, 9, 10, and 11 provide specific guidance regarding vocabulary.

Key Terms Reviewed in This Section

- Additive environments
- Culturally and linguistically diverse
- Self-reflection
- Subtractive environments

- Cognitive framework
- Core vocabulary
- Developmental framework
- Fringe vocabulary
- Functional framework
- Personalized vocabulary
- Relational basic concepts

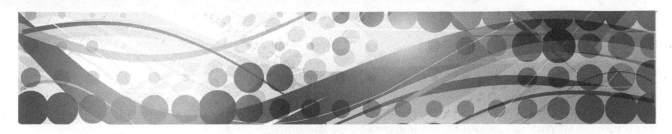

Essay 2

CULTURAL CONSIDERATIONS AND AAC: CULTURE AND SOCIAL AND ECONOMIC DETERMINANTS OF HEALTH AND THE USE OF AAC

Ellen R. Cohn and Mario C. Browne

Understanding the challenges of a person who uses augmentative and alternative communication (PWUAAC) within the context of their cultural attributes and knowledge of their social and economic status is necessary. Research suggests that social determinants of health (SDOHs) can have a profound impact on a person's health and predicted longevity (Braveman & Gottleib, 2014). It makes sense that social and economic challenges can also affect a family's ability to function as active participants in the clinical process that is requisite to achieve augmentative and alternative communication (AAC) adoption.

What Are Social Determinants of Health?

According to the Office of Disease Prevention and Health Promotion, social determinants of health (SDOH) can be defined as follows:

[T]he conditions in which people are born, grow, live, work and age as well as the complex, inter-related social structures and economic systems that shape these conditions. Social determinants of health include aspects of the social environment (e.g., discrimination, income, education level, marital status), the physical environment (e.g., place of residence, crowding conditions), built environment (i.e., buildings, spaces, transportation systems, and products that are created or modified by people), and health services (e.g., access to and quality of care, insurance status). (ODPHP, 2021)

Deficits in SDOHs can have a profound impact because they are as follows:

[L]inked to a lack of opportunity and to a lack of resources to protect, improve, and maintain health, and taken together, these factors are mostly responsible for health inequities—the unfair and avoidable differences in health status seen within and between populations. (Centers for Disease Control and Prevention [CDC])

The effects of SDOHs are so well defined that even the zip code one lives within, and whether a child grew up in a home owned by the family, can be predictive of the child's future health and life span. Some suggest that SDOHs contribute more to an individual patient's health than their genetic code or medical care (HIMSS, n.d.).

Consider the following two examples: How do socioeconomic circumstances influence a family's ability (but not necessarily their desire or motivation) to attend appointments, acquire AAC equipment, or serve as communication partners for a PWUAAC? Which of the two families do you think suffers the most chronic stress, potentially leading to health problems? Which of the two families do you predict might have the most difficulty attending appointments to acquire and learn how to use AAC equipment?

Scenario 1: A Family Suffering From Societal and Economic Stressors

As an example of one end of the socioeconomic spectrum, the pediatric child has a severe communication disorder that requires a speech-generating device (SGD). The child and their African American family live in an apartment within a low socioeconomic status (SES) neighborhood. There are no local grocery stores to buy fresh fruits and vegetables. At the end of each month, the family suffers from food insecurity and sometimes hunger. The parents work in low-paying part-time jobs in which they have little autonomy or stability, and for which there are no associated benefits or health care. Thus, the parental stress level is perpetually high. The family does not have the means to take a vacation or time off. If they must attend numerous appointments for their child who requires AAC, they sacrifice income and could even lose employment. The neighborhood suffers from violence and adversarial relationships with local law enforcement. The parents share one old and unreliable car, and therefore largely rely upon public bus transportation. Family medical history includes Type 2 diabetes, high blood pressure, and depression. The ever-present unrelenting stress, some of which they attribute to the racism they encounter (an SDOH), and their environmental challenges are contributory to their chronic health challenges. The family cannot afford Internet service and except for

a smartphone, does not have computing devices in the home.

Scenario 2: A Family With Superior Resources

On the other end of the spectrum, a pediatric PWUAAC and their family live in a home that they own in a high SES neighborhood. The Caucasian (white) family has little contact with persons of color in their neighborhood. They live within a gated community guarded by a caring professional security force. Both parents are professionals and hold high administrative positions in which they supervise many others. While their job responsibilities are not without stress, the parents largely control their own schedules and work tasks. They can take time off from work to take their child to appointments and attend school functions. Nearby, there are local food markets for take-out and large grocery stores with healthy fruits and vegetables. The parents have time to prepare healthy meals. There are trails and parks to enjoy the outdoors, and to engage in exercise. The family takes several vacations a year and employs a full-time nanny. They, including the nanny, drive reliable vehicles. A well-trained dog provides affection and is a walking companion. As a result, their stress levels and health are significantly better than the family described previously. The family has many electronic devices and excellent Internet service.

Of course, a great many families fall somewhere between these two extremes of Scenarios 1 and 2. Furthermore, neither challenging nor privileged socioeconomic circumstances should presume inferior or superior levels of motivation to care for their child.

Digital Resources and Social Determinants of Health

It is paradoxical that while Americans (even those with lower incomes) enjoy increasing access to the Internet, broadband adoption, and smartphone ownership, the digital lives of lower- and higher-income Americans can be markedly different. The results of a Pew Research Center Survey of U.S. adults reported by Vogels (2021) found that

> Roughly, a quarter of adults with household incomes below $30,000 a year (24%) say they don't own a smartphone. About four-in-ten adults with lower incomes do not have home broadband services (43%) or a desktop or laptop computer (41%), respectively. And a majority Americans with lower incomes are not tablet owners. By comparison, each of these technologies is nearly ubiquitous among adults in households earning $100,000 or more a year.

Higher-income Americans are likely to have both numerous devices and access to broadband. However, such is not the case for many lower-income families. Termed "smartphone-dependent" Internet users, they own a smartphone but do not have broadband Internet in the home. During the COVID-19 pandemic, the lack of in-home Internet service greatly disadvantaged students who were only able to participate in remote education via their smartphones.

Stark differences exist in the employment rates of individuals who have a disability and those who do not. In 2020, only 17% of disabled persons were employed compared to 61.8% of people without a disability (U.S. Bureau of Labor Statistics, 2021). These disparities (i.e., SODH and the digital divide) as well as the economic challenges caused by high levels

of unemployment faced by persons with disabilities can profoundly affect the use of AAC. It is therefore vital that professionals recognize and attempt to overcome the social and economic challenges faced by many of their clients and their families.

References

Braveman, P., & Gottlieb, L. (2014, January–February). The social determinants of health: It's time to consider the causes of the causes. *Public Health Reports, 129*(2), 19–31. https://doi.org/10.1177/00333549141291S206

Centers for Disease Control and Prevention. (n.d.). NCHHSTP Social Determinants of Health. https://www.cdc.gov/nchhstp/socialdeterminants/index.html

HIMSS. (n.d.). *Social determinants of health: Can ZIP codes influence health outcomes?* https://www.himss.org/resources/social-determinants-health-can-zip-codes-influence-health-outcomes

Office of Disease Prevention and Health Promotion. (2021). *Social determinants of health*. https://www.healthypeople.gov/2020/topics-objectives/topic/social-determinants-of-health

U.S. Bureau of Labor Statistics. (2021, February 24) News release, U.S. Department of Labor. https://www.bls.gov/news.release/pdf/disabl.pdf

Vogels, E. (2021). *Digital divide persists even as American with lower incomes make gains in tech adoption.* Pew Research Center. https://www.pewresearch.org/fact-tank/2021/06/22/digital-divide-persists-even-as-americans-with-lower-incomes-make-gains-in-tech-adoption/

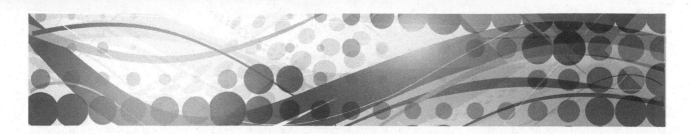

Chapter 6

CULTURAL AND LINGUISTIC RESPONSIVITY IN AAC

Gloria Soto and Marika King

Fundamentals

Shauna is a speech-language pathologist (SLP) specializing in augmentative and alternative communication (AAC) at a large urban school district in the United States. She has 15 years of clinical experience and is regarded as an AAC expert by her colleagues. However, like many clinicians, Shauna has more questions than answers when it comes to providing AAC services to children from culturally and linguistically diverse (CLD) backgrounds. In a recent e-mail to one of the authors, Shauna wrote the following:

We are told here that because the language of instruction is in English, our therapy sessions should be completed in English, as well. Now, given that we have been virtual since March 2020, one of the silver linings is that many of us are able to connect with families we didn't get to within the past. Whenever possible, I have used interpreters through the District (mostly in Spanish) to attend my teletherapy sessions to help parents participate for my bilingual families, as many of my students have complex communication needs and need adult assistance to participate in therapy sessions virtually. However, I am thinking to the future when we are back in-person, should all attempts be made to provide therapy exclusively in the home language?

Just English? A combination of both? (Personal communication with an SLP specializing in AAC from a large urban district, November 2, 2020)

Questions like this resonate among many professionals serving clients from families who speak languages other than English at home. Like Shauna, most clinicians find that their language and cultural background do not match their clients. Yet, like Shauna, these clinicians want to know how best to support their clients from CLD backgrounds using evidence-based practice. There is no recipe book to dispense straightforward directions for providing evidence-based AAC services to children from CLD backgrounds. However, in this chapter, we draw from best practices in bilingualism, AAC, and communication disorders to offer a road map for providing culturally and linguistically responsive AAC services. Our goal is to demonstrate that as an SLP, assistive technology (AT) specialist, or educator, you are uniquely positioned to advocate for your clients and to support their communication in a way that builds on their cultural and linguistic identity.

Culturally and linguistically responsive AAC services start with reflection. Self-reflection is an ongoing exercise and involves recognizing one's own beliefs, biases, and ideas about multilingualism, culture, disability, and AAC. These conscious and unconscious ideologies and attitudes permeate our well-intentioned therapeutic decision-making and interactions with our clients and their families. Thus, it is critical that as educators and clinicians, we continue to practice critical self-reflection—contemplating how our decisions and behaviors are influenced by our own culture, values, and attitudes.

However, reflection goes beyond the individual level because organizational or administrative policies and guidelines often influence our decisions and practices. Clinical practice is not delivered in a vacuum but within an inequitable system that grants access to those with the "social capital" to navigate it. Consideration of how these systemic and structural factors (e.g., disparity) may privilege some clients over others and influence our professional practice and our relationship with our clients and their families is an essential aspect of culturally and linguistically responsive AAC service provision.

In terms of multilingual and multicultural support, educational and therapeutic environments can be characterized as additive or subtractive. In additive environments, home language and culture are viewed as assets and are supported and maintained. Minority families are seen as resourceful and resilient, and their culture and language are strengths to capitalize on. In subtractive environments, families' home language and culture are either ignored or viewed as barriers to social/educational access and participation that must be overcome. As described later, inherent biases and permeating beliefs as well as structural and policy factors and lack of training and resources foster a subtractive language environment and can lead to long-term adverse outcomes for children and families from CLD backgrounds.

Consequences of Subtractive Bilingual Environments for AAC Users

A persistent myth in education and health care is that, despite evidence to the contrary, exposure to more than one language will cause children with disabilities to be confused or experience further developmental delays. As a result, health care and education professionals often advise parents to speak only English at home, even when they are not fluent. A message such as this carries an enormous amount of power among families for whom professionals can be absolute authorities. Many of these families are at the intersection of multiple marginalizing and disempowering factors such as ethnicity, language, culture, immigration history, socioeconomic status, and disability. Faced with overwhelming pressures such as the fears ahead of their child's diagnosis and a push for linguistic and cultural conformity, families from "minority homes" often make the difficult decision to give up their home language (Tönsing & Soto, 2020).

Parents play an indispensable role in supporting language development, whether their child has typical or atypical development and regardless of the communication modality they use. Stopping the use of home language can cause a major disruption to the child's participation within family routines and can affect parent-child relationships and parents' sense of self-efficacy for supporting their child's learning and development (Yu, 2018). When a child's ability to communicate with their own family is compromised, they will stand at the margins of family interaction. The socioemotional and linguistic effects of family alienation for children who use AAC is still unknown. We know that for children without disabilities, losing proficiency in their home language means much more than just a loss of a linguistic system; it is a separation from their roots, a denial of their cultural identity, and a dismissal of their potential as a bilingual and bicultural member of society, with adverse implications in academic achievement and social participation.

Building Additive Bilingual Environments for AAC Users

Promoting additive bilingual environments can counter the detrimental effects of home language loss. Home language maintenance leads to linguistic, academic, and socioemotional benefits for bilingual clients with and without language disorders. Our responsibility as AAC professionals is to do everything in our power to minimize our clients' marginalization within their families and communities due to their communication impairment, while providing evidence-based interventions to support optimal access to the same academic, vocational, and social opportunities as their bilingual "typical" peers. If AAC is going to help our clients reach their greatest potential, maintaining their home language and culture has to be part of that. By maintaining their home language, our clients can participate in an enriched environment that builds on their cultures. Professionals can play an important role in calming parents' fears and misapprehensions about bilingualism and second language learning as they consider their language of choice for their child with AAC needs. Yet, we must respect parents' language choice, whatever that might be.

As the population of students growing up in homes where English is not spoken continues to increase, it is imperative to develop AAC systems and practices that affirm home language and culture. In AAC service delivery, affirming home language and culture cannot be the family's sole responsibility. Clinicians and teachers can play a critical role in shaping families' attitudes toward maintaining their home language regardless of whether they speak it themselves. Persons who use augmentative and alternative communication (PWUAACs) spend a large portion of their day at school. When clinicians express interest in their clients' home language, affirm the importance of home language proficiency in their clients' lives, value it publicly, and find ways to integrate it into their practice, families and clients' desire and motivation to maintain it increases.

Culturally and Linguistically Responsive Assessment

As described in Chapters 8, 10, and 15, AAC assessment is a dynamic process designed to gain information to aid the design of an appropriate and effective AAC intervention plan. The complexity of this process calls for a collaborative team of professionals and caregivers who, using a variety of assessment tools and procedures, determine an individual's communication strengths and needs within family, school, and vocational contexts. In addition to the information collected for monolingual children, the assessment of a bilingual child must include a comprehensive language profile of expressive and receptive skills in both languages.

This will allow clinicians to set appropriate goals and develop the most appropriate intervention strategies for each language. Through assessment, it is important to find out whether the child was exposed to two languages from birth, or learned their home language before entering school. A family language practice questionnaire can be utilized to describe the age at which the child was exposed to each language, the amount of exposure to each language on a typical day, the people who speak each language to the child, the different contexts for each language use, and the child's preferred and dominant language. It is important to recognize that language dominance is a dynamic construct that changes with age, context, modality, and communication partner.

Standardized Assessment

Assessing the abilities and needs of individuals whose speech is severely limited can be a difficult task. Standardized test performance can be influenced by sensory/motor access limitations or limitations imposed by a discrepancy between the communicative abilities of the client and the response modalities required by the test. Assessing the abilities and needs of individuals who are bilingual can be further complicated by linguistic and cultural biases. Often, standardized and formal tests do not provide a valid assessment of linguistic competence in bilingual clients because test results may be biased by a discrepancy between the linguistic and cultural behaviors expected by the testing instrument versus those of the actual test taker, as well as by the lack of normative data from participants. Before using any test, the service provider should examine it to evaluate whether the client has had access to the information being tested, can comprehend what is being asked, and has a reliable means to respond. If the test is biased in any of these areas, testing procedures should be modified. Modifications will vary depending on the source of bias, but they may include providing more time to complete the task, rewording or translating items, and/or providing for alternative means of responding. All modifications must be documented and described on the test protocols and assessment report. Adapting tests nullifies standardization although the findings can still be clinically informative.

Although standardized bilingual language assessments may be unavailable or may require modification, language assessment for bilingually exposed children should always attempt to measure the child's receptive and expressive language abilities in the languages they are regularly exposed to. A basic understanding of how bilingual language is organized in the bilingual brain is necessary to provide informed evidence-based assessment. On a neural level, the languages of a bilingual child are separate yet interacting systems that are intrinsically connected. Although underlying linguistic proficiency contributes to abilities across languages, for the most part, bilingual children's language skills in each language appear to be language specific (e.g., DeAnda et al., 2016). Another feature of bilingual communication is the ability to alternate between languages within or across utterances and speakers (i.e., code-switching). Bilingual PWUAACs are unique because they may express more than one spoken language across multiple modalities (e.g., speech approximations, speech-output device). Therefore, language profiles should be documented in each language, and expressive language assessment should allow for the formulation of meaning in any language and in any modality that is produced.

Clinicians and educators continue to rely heavily on standardized and formal tests to identify disabilities, make educational placement decisions, and design AAC systems and intervention programs. In cultural and linguistic responsive assessments, even adapted standardized tests must be combined with information obtained through the use of comprehensive qualitative approaches such as observation, inventories, and interviewing.

Observation

Consistent with the assessment approaches presented in Chapters 8, 10, and 15, observation should be conducted in environments where the client typically participates, such as home, school, after-school programs, community, and vocational settings. Parameters of observation should include (a) quality and quantity of communicative inter-actions, (b) partner expectations and demands on the client's communicative performance, (c) partner use of language facilitation techniques and communication breakdown repair strategies, and (d) variation across situations in which different communicative functions are emphasized.

Before making an observation, the AAC service provider must understand not only the linguistic but also the nonlinguistic forms of communication that are meaningful to the client in the relevant cultural contexts, because (a) nonverbal and nonlinguistic forms of communication are a critical component of the communicative repertoires of individuals with complex communication needs, and not being aware of culturally meaningful forms of nonverbal communication would lead to misinformation about an individual's current communication skills; (b) AAC intervention builds on existing communication skills, both verbal and nonverbal; and (c) AAC intervention should not only respect but also enhance culturally appropriate ways to communicate.

Participation inventories can be used to collect information to analyze an individual's level of functioning and participation in typical activities and environments. When making observations and creating inventories, service providers must be sure that they have a clear understanding of the activities being observed and analyzed if they are unfamiliar with them.

Interviewing

A strength-based assessment is critical in assessing our client's strengths and needs. In a strength-based assessment, caregivers are encouraged to share what is unique about their child, and provide insight into their child as a whole. Therefore, finding ways to involve and communicate with caregivers (as introduced in Chapter 1), who know our client best, is a critical component of AAC assessment. Ethnographic interviewing differs from traditional interviewing in that the practitioner does not presume that they know in advance what is important to the client and their family. The ultimate goal of ethnographic interviewing is to elicit rich descriptions from clients and their families of their life experiences. A key technique in ethnographic interviewing is the use of open-ended questions that allow the interviewee to set the agenda. The practitioner's job is simply to listen and to understand. Service providers should use the "safest" communication style, in which they use a tone of absolute and genuine respect for the client and the family, and avoid the use of technical jargon, which often alienates the family from participating in the assessment process. Soto and Yu (2014) described some strategies that AAC service providers can use to elicit family participation during the assessment process. These include the following:

1. Listen to parents' priorities, their expectations, and preferences regarding communication with their child, and act on this knowledge by designing an intervention plan that addresses them.

2. Ask parents about their family structure and roles, and act on this knowledge by inviting and including input from other influential family members as appropriate. This is particularly important when working with clients for whom the extended family is the acting family unit. In some families, young parents may be considered too inexperienced to make major decisions on behalf of their children. Key decisions may need to be made in consultation with older relatives within the larger family unit. Care, assistance, and financial support may also come from the extended family network.

3. Recognize and respect that other family priorities at particular times may take precedence over educational concerns.

4. Respond to family needs for flexible meeting times and other logistics.

5. Avoid the use of technical jargon that may be a barrier to understanding.

6. Present results and recommendations clearly so parents understand and can become actively involved in the provision of services.

Culturally and Linguistically Responsive Intervention

Broadly speaking, the ultimate goals of AAC intervention are (a) improving the communicative effectiveness of our clients in a range of settings; (b) improving the autonomy, social participation, and integration of our clients in the same academic, social, vocational, religious, etc., communities as their peers with typical development; and (c) improving the overall well-being of our clients and their families (Enderby, 2014). In setting a culturally and linguistically responsive plan of action, professionals need to include the family's input about their preferred language and communication needs, their views on the child's communicative disability, and the level of engagement they are able to sustain. In order to make intervention relevant to any family, it is important to elicit family members' perceptions of meaningful intervention goals. Professionals should explore different ways to provide caregivers with an opportunity to share their ideas. Professionals who do not speak the family's language will need to use bilingual and bicultural interpreters and/or cultural brokers (who bridge or link different cultures) that can indicate to families that they are valued members of the intervention team.

Providing a Culturally Appropriate Means to Communicate

When the client is a member of a bilingual (e.g., Spanish and English) or bidialectal (e.g., African American English and Mainstream American English) family, professionals can accommodate the linguistic preferences of the family by developing a bilingual/bicultural AAC system. A bilingual/bicultural AAC system should include culturally appropriate vocabulary (accommodating the primary language or dialect of the client's immediate cultural group), culturally appropriate and meaningful means of representation (i.e., symbols), and culturally appropriate strategies for functional AAC use. Culturally appropriate vocabulary could be gathered by sampling the language and/or dialect of siblings and peers and consulting developmentally appropriate vocabulary inventories (see Chapter 7 and the subsequent cultural essays for a more thorough discussion of vocabulary selection and for relevant examples). The vocabulary should allow the child to communicate about things considered important in their cultural contexts. Vocabulary and symbol selection should always be reviewed by the family and a person highly familiar with the client's native language and cultural practices. Language is one of the most critical elements by which individuals are socialized into their culture. As discussed earlier, not having access to a bilingual/bicultural AAC system may further our clients' cultural/social isolation, identity conflicts, and increase their sense of being "different."

Family members are the client's most significant communication partner and as such they are key informants for selecting vocabulary and messages that are relevant to their child. Tools such as vocabulary checklists (in the home language) and family interview guides can facilitate vocabulary selection for bilingual children and identify messages that are important to daily routines and meaningful activities. The way that vocabulary messages are represented and displayed on the AAC system is another important consideration as families are more likely to adopt AAC systems that include culturally relevant symbols and messages. Thus, consulting with families regarding symbol representation is critical.

Professionals should partner with caregivers to develop AAC systems that include culturally germane symbols and messages that facilitate our clients' participation in culturally relevant and meaningful family activities. This will require systems that have the ability and flexibility to switch quickly and easily between languages. Several AAC apps and software programs include vocabulary and corresponding speech output in various languages and dialects. Some of these programs also allow the user to code-switch or alternate between language layouts. However, many languages and dialects are not yet available on high-tech AAC systems. Alternatively, supporting home language access may require the use of light-tech systems in the home language (e.g., communication boards or books). Family members may also help to record and store analog messages in the home language to an AAC device. Decision-making regarding AAC devices should always involve collaboration and consultation with the client and/or their family and should consider the family's goals for their child, their views on the child's disability, and level of comfort with AAC. Furthermore, for bilingual children, AAC goals should consider the individual's language development and communication needs across contexts and communication partners. Supporting communication across contexts and languages requires creative AAC solutions across AAC modalities.

A common misunderstanding among professionals is that only those who are proficient in their clients' home language can support it. To work competently across cultures and languages, it would be ideal if the clinician's cultural and linguistic backgrounds matched those of their client; however, it is not essential to speak our clients' languages. In fact, given the linguistic diversity found in our public schools, this would be totally impossible. Rather, cultural competence requires a basic level of understanding of the client's culture, and the basic features and structures of the client's language, and how these may interact with the learning of English as represented and organized in their AAC system. When the clinician does not speak the client's home language, intervention in the home language can be delivered through an interpreter. The American Speech-Language-Hearing Association provides best practice guidelines for working with interpreters. Another possible scenario is the coaching and training of communication partners (through an interpreter if the communication partner is monolingual and in English if the communication partner is bilingual) on language facilitation strategies that can be delivered in the home language.

Facilitating Parent and Family Participation

The introduction of an AAC system and the strategies to support its use will affect not only our clients but also their families. Some families may welcome AAC within their family system, while others may have competing needs, priorities, or stressors that leave them unable to do so. Research indicates that when families are involved in the decision-making process, there are positive consequences for both the child and the family, including greater family satisfaction with and participation in AAC programs and services, increased family sense of empowerment, and improved child behavior and well-being.

Cultural responsiveness requires professionals to understand and respect the diversity of families in terms of family structure, socioeconomic status, religion, language, and culture, even when these differ substantially from their own. Families have often reported feeling a lack of respect from professionals who hold a stereotypical and deficit view of families from minoritized backgrounds. Involving families in culturally and linguistically responsive practice goes beyond providing the family with information about AAC services in their language, and obtaining family consent and compliance in collaborative events through interpreters. A culturally and linguistically responsive professional recognizes the centrality of the family and contributes to strengthening the family's capacity to enhance the child's language and communication.

The introduction of AAC creates changes and requires adaptation within the family system. The degree to which families can engage in the AAC process is dynamic and may fluctuate over time. Professionals need to consider a family's appraisal of their child's disability, as well as the resources and social supports families use to mitigate the effect of stressors. Families' levels of involvement are closely tied to the degrees to which they have access to the linguistic, cultural, and economic capital necessary to navigate the service provision system. Culturally responsive AAC intervention should take into account the social and communicative interaction patterns valued by our clients' families and target (a) culturally meaningful nonverbal forms of communication, (b) communicative functions most frequently used at home and other relevant social networks, (c) primary language used, and (d) discourse strategies most commonly used by family members. To increase the use of the AAC system, AAC intervention should enhance cultural communication styles and communicative functions most often used with the children by their families. For example, if collaborative prayer is a valued activity within the family, then it should be prioritized as an intervention target.

Parents from CLD backgrounds may hold different perceptions of their child's disability than those held by service providers, view themselves as inadequate to the task of collaborating with professionals, perceive parent participation as intim-

idating or inappropriate, may have overwhelming life circumstances, and/or may be disillusioned with clinical/educational programs. Parent disillusionment is often followed by decreasing levels of participation and noncompliance. Perceptions of being provided inadequate and unsatisfactory services and of being looked down upon or not being acknowledged as legitimate participants in the intervention process may elicit noncompliant behaviors that, in turn, engender nonsupportive responses by service providers. As AAC service providers plan for family collaboration, they must understand the values, beliefs, child-rearing practices, parent-child interaction styles, interpersonal styles, attitudes, and behaviors of the families that they serve. The degree to which an intervention will be effective is a function of the nature and quality of the interaction between the family and the professional institutions that serve them.

Case Study: JR

The following sections of this chapter present a clinical case study illustrating a culturally and linguistically responsive intervention designed to support the development of bilingual language proficiency in a child who uses AAC. Specifically, the case study is designed to illustrate the strategies used by the educational team to (a) affirm the child's home language and culture, (b) empower parent participation as key members in their child's educational team, (c) assess the child's communicative competence in both languages, and (d) design interventions that meet the family's communicative needs.

Clinical Profile and Communication Needs

The Individual

JR is a 10-year-old girl who attends a fifth-grade classroom for students with complex communication needs. JR has a primary diagnosis of severe verbal apraxia and a secondary diagnosis of developmental delay. JR is a member of a large multigenerational

Spanish-speaking family. When JR entered school, the team, in collaboration with the parents through an interpreter, filled out a Home Language Survey and an Informal Assessment of Primary Language Proficiency form (California Department of Education, 2021) to understand the language practices of the family. Prior to entering school, JR was immersed in a Spanish-speaking family and community. JR's parents, grandparents, aunts, and uncles speak only Spanish to each other and to the children, so Spanish was JR's first language. However, upon entering school, JR's siblings and cousins began to use English with each other and reserved Spanish to use with their elders (i.e., sequential bilingualism).

JR began receiving speech and language services at 3 years of age. In the beginning of kindergarten, the team completed Social Networks (SN): A Communication Inventory for Individuals with Complex Communication Needs–Revised version (Blackstone & Hunt Berg, 2012). The SN provided critical information on the communication modes JR used in different contexts and with different communication partners. Parents sent videos of JR in different activities with different family members. The results of the SN and the videotaped observations indicated that at home JR relied mainly on vocal word approximations (in English and Spanish) and natural gestures. The SN deemed that these unaided modes of communication mainly served to request and respond to yes/no questions, and were insufficient to meet JR's increasing communication needs at home. The conversation that followed the administration of the SN pictured JR as a lovely, chatty, and playful girl who loved Reggaeton, Taylor Swift, Ariana Grande, and Justin Bieber; playing with her siblings and cousins; watching cartoons; and cooking with and listening to family stories from her maternal grandmother. The team concluded that the introduction of a speech-generating device with bilingual capabilities in both English and Spanish was necessary to meet JR's communication needs at school, home, and community.

Like many bilingual children, JR presents an uneven profile in her two languages. She uses Spanish only at home to "converse" with her parents and elders. Her Spanish skills are typical of the earlier stages of Spanish language development.

JR's language proficiency in Spanish was assessed using the MacArthur Inventarios del Desarrollo de Habilidades Comunicativas (IDHC; Jackson-Maldonado et al., 2003). As instructed in the manual, JR's parents reported on the words that JR understood and produced in Spanish. Using the IDHC, JR's parents realized that JR understood much more than she was able to express. Increasing her expressive vocabulary, and being able to "converse" about topics of personal relevance are two of her long-term goals in Spanish.

JR's expressive English proficiency was assessed using the expressive vocabulary subtest of the CELF-5 (Clinical Evaluation of Language Fundamentals-4; Wiig et al., 2013). She responded with English and Spanish verbal approximations, gestures, and her SGD. JR uses gestures to gain attention, and with access to an SGD is able to produce one- to five-word comments, respond to questions, transfer and share information, participate in class activities, and express ideas and feelings. To examine JR's receptive language in English, the SLP administered an adapted version of the TACL-4 (Test for Auditory Comprehension of Language, 4th edition; Carrow-Woolfolk, 2014). Like in Spanish, her receptive language skills in English are stronger than her expressive ones. JR presents with difficulties using pronouns, verb morphology and complex sentences including negatives, and interrogatives. Addressing these targets within the context of the academic curriculum is one of her long-term goals. According to the AAC Profile, an assessment tool that measures functional skills for developing communicative competence, JR demonstrates a Level II in operational, linguistic, social, and strategic competence when using her SGD in Spanish, and a Level III when using it in English (Kovach, 2009). The AAC Profile includes an inventory of skills that can be used to describe the functional level of the client in four areas of communicative competence (i.e., operational, linguistic, social, and operational) and along a developmental continuum.

Their Communication Partners and Environment

JR's dad was born in Texas to a family of Mexican descent with a long history in Texas predating statehood. JR's mom was born in Guatemala and immigrated with her mother into the United States as a young woman. Both mom and dad work long hours outside of the home to make ends meet. JR's maternal grandmother is the children's primary caregiver. When JR entered the Special Education (SPED) system, mom and dad felt overwhelmed by JR's diagnosis and disempowered by the professional jargon and a service delivery system that seemed to place an unusual high level of responsibility on "parental participation." Not knowing anything about JR's diagnosis and prognosis or the SPED system procedures, JRs parents leaned on the professionals as the "experts" and yielded their authority to make school decisions. Misguided by professional advice, JR's mom feared that speaking Spanish with JR would "confuse" her. She believed that speaking English to JR (a language she did not speak well herself at all) would be the fastest way to help her learn English and access the programs and services that were available only in English. It took the team time, professional development, and parent coaching to build mom's confidence in her ability to parent a bilingual child with complex communication needs.

AAC Systems

At this point, the goals of JR's AAC bilingual intervention are (a) improving JR's ability to tell personal stories and build strong relationships with family and friends, (b) increasing JR's integration in family events (JR's family members are active participants in their church), and (c) increasing JR's academic participation at school. JR's bilingual system includes software in both Spanish and English with developmentally appropriate vocabulary. JR's is a true bilingual system, which means she can switch between languages within a single sentence. The SLP, who is not fluent in Spanish, has trained a paraprofessional in basic programming and on explicit vocabulary instruction. She also has worked closely with several members of JR's immediate family through an interpreter on language facilitation strategies. The team has also added vocabulary in English and appropriate icons that represent topics of great importance to the family in school (e.g., church, Quinceañeras, extended family events such as birthdays and weddings).

JR now can spontaneously generate novel utterances of one to three words to respond to questions, transfer information, express feelings and needs, participate in classroom academics, and share news from home in English. She requires moderate adult facilitation to use S+V+O constructions. A sentence construction strip is always Velcroed onto her SGD to cue accurate simple syntactic constructions. She frequently uses vocabulary in the categories of proper nouns, people words, drinks, calendar, foods, toys, clothing, body parts, feelings, holiday words, exclamations, some spatial/positional prepositions, places, occupations, vehicles, animals, actions words (categorized by body part), numbers, and the alphabet. She is currently learning how to use function words in English (articles, prepositions, conjunctions, pronouns) that build complete, syntactically correct sentences: "a," "the," "to," "at," "for," "from," "in," "and," "went," "with." Her novel constructions in Spanish are mostly noun phrases or verb phrases with limited verb morphology.

Next Steps

The next steps for JR's team are (a) to build a responsive infrastructure for positive, active, and responsive relationship with JR's family; (b) to continue to affirm JR's home language and culture; (c) to continue empowering JR's parent participation; (d) to describe JR's language proficiency in her two languages; and (e) to design interventions that are responsive to JR's communicative needs in her family context and meet the increasing demands of the curriculum.

(a) To build a responsive infrastructure for positive, active, and responsive relationship with JR's family:

- The team is looking to recruit a member as a family liaison who is proficient in both languages and has strong competence in SPED and AAC issues. The liaison's primary responsibility is to ensure that JR's family has the needed information and resources to actively and successfully participate in JR's educational program.

■ The team is working on finding explicit ways to empower JR's parents to be advocates of AAC and bilingualism to other families in the district. With support from the district, the team is working on developing meaningful family learning activities that develop other families' understanding of and support for AAC and the program's goals. The learning activities address issues of disability, AAC and bilingualism, as well as best practices and specific program features such as the dual language intervention plan. The activities are designed to support equitable participation by all families (e.g., varying the time and location, providing child care, and using community-building and family-friendly activities).

(b) To continue to affirm JR's home language and culture:

■ The team is creating materials (e.g., Google slides/visual schedules; adapted books, and premade digital worksheets) that are in the home language and build on concepts and vocabulary that JR has already learned in English.

■ The SLP is conducting therapies bilingually, with support of a bilingual paraprofessional. The SLP provides direct instruction, modeling, and corrective feedback in English, and the aide translates to the family. The SLP promotes JR's metalinguistic awareness by highlighting linguistic variation.

■ The SLP is learning social greetings in the home language.

■ The SLP models core language in Spanish on the device throughout the session and uses printed icon sequences from JR's device as visual supports.

(c) To continue empowering JR's parent participation:

■ The team wants to increase the use of parent/child routines as a basis for intervention. The SLP is coaching JR's mom to use language elicitation strategies (e.g.,

aided input, pause and expectant looking) in the context of shared book reading to elicit the language goal.

■ The SLP is working toward feeling more comfortable asking JR's mom questions directly when she does not understand something. Sometimes JR will refer to a song, or make a request that the SLP or the paraprofessional does not recognize or understand. The SLP then asks the mom directly.

■ The SLP is coaching JR's mom in basic programming of JR's device, such as adding new vocabulary, as needed, and ensuring the device is up to date with needed language beyond the therapy session.

(d) To assess JR's AAC communicative competence in both languages:

■ The team is working on a data management system for tracking JR's data overtime, and working to determine whether linguistic, social, strategic, and operational goals have been met. They are using the AAC Profile to help identify JR's level of communicative competence in both languages. The team will use two forms of the AAC Profile: one for JR's AAC competence in English, and the other for Spanish.

■ The team is collecting language samples in Spanish. They are using the Protocol for the Analysis of Spanish Language Samples with AAC (Soto, 2020) to describe JR's current level of Spanish language proficiency and set up new linguistic goals.

(e) To design interventions that are responsive to the family's communicative needs:

■ JR's mom is very good at advocating for her child by communicating items or goals she would like to see represented in therapy. The entire team wants to capitalize on this by incorporating some of JR's mom's goals into the therapy sessions. For example, JR's mom expressed interest in creating a project to educate JR's school community about how she communicates (i.e., disability awareness in Spanish and English). The team is fully supportive of this project and helping JR's mom with materials and content.

■ As JR's mom is becoming more comfortable providing ideas and feedback about home or school routines that need a particular language support, the team is ensuring that mom knows how they are responding by having a consistent mode of communication with her. Recently mom reported that they need help repairing communication breakdowns across the day. This requires deliberate and explicit question-asking and scheduling time to address all her concerns.

References

Blackstone, S., & Hunt Berg, M. (2012). *Social networks: A communication inventory for individuals with complex communication needs and their communication partners—Revised version*. Attainment Company.

California Department of Education. (2021). *English learner forms*. https://www.cde.ca.gov/ta/cr/elforms.asp

Carrow-Woolfolk, E. (2014). *Test for Auditory Comprehension of Language* (4th ed.). Pro-Ed.

DeAnda, S., Poulin-Dubois, D., Zesiger, P., & Friend, M. (2016). Lexical processing and organization in bilingual first language acquisition: Guiding future research. *Psychological Bulletin, 142*(6), 655–667. https://doi.org/10.1037/bul0000042

Enderby, P. (2014). Introducing the therapy outcome measure for AAC services in the context of a review of other measures. *Disability and Rehabilitation: Assistive Technology, 9*, 33–40. https://doi.org/10.3109/17483107.2013.823576

Jackson-Maldonado, D., Thal, D. J., Fenson, L., Marchman, V., Newton, T., & Conboy, B. (2003). *El inventario del desarrollo de habilidades comunicativas: User's guide and technical manual*. Paul H. Brookes.

Kovach, T. (2009). *Augmentative and alternative communication profile: A communication of learning*. Pro-Ed.

Soto, G. (2020, December). *The Protocol for the Analysis of Aided Language Samples in Spanish: A tutorial* [Paper presentation]. La Fabrica de Palabras, Spain.

Soto, G., & Yu, B. (2014). Considerations for the provision of services to bilingual children who use augmentative and alternative communication. *Augmentative and Alternative Communication, 30*(1), 83–92. https://doi.org/10.3109/07434618.2013.878751

Tönsing, K. M., & Soto, G. (2020). Multilingualism and augmentative and alternative communication: Examining language ideology and resulting practices. *Augmentative and Alternative Communication, 36*(3), 190–201.

Wiig, E. H., Semel, E., & Secord, W. A. (2013). *Clinical Evaluation of Language Fundamentals* (5th ed.). Pearson.

Yu, B. (2018). Bilingualism and autism: A summary of current research and implications for augmentative and alternative communication practitioners. *Perspectives of the ASHA Special Interest Groups, 3*(12), 146–153.

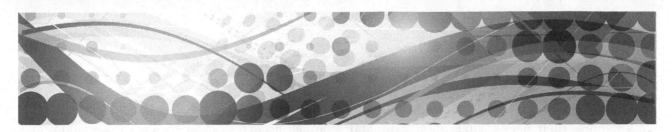

Chapter 7
LANGUAGE AND VOCABULARY FEATURES OF AAC

Brittney Cooper, MariaTeresa "Teri" H. Muñoz, and Gloria Soto

Fundamentals

If you have ever struggled to retrieve a word in conversation, due to a memory lapse or limited proficiency in a second language, you can attest to the necessity of vocabulary for expressing messages. The ability to map ideas onto words and articulate those words to others is the foundation of communication. Typically developing toddlers acquire new words at an incredible rate with minimal direct instruction, and vocabulary is the only language domain that continues to develop throughout the life span. For most, new vocabulary arises spontaneously from unique, socially mediated life experiences. When individuals, especially children who are in the early stages of language development and unable to spell, are introduced to augmentative and alternative communication (AAC), they depend on others to supply them with the words they will need to voice their thoughts. Communication service providers are tasked with the decision about which words and messages to include. In the case of communication software with extensive word libraries, professionals have to decide which words to target in instruction and intervention as well as how to organize words and messages to meet their clients' needs. Although resources and training around vocabulary selection have evolved in promising ways, the provision of adequate and appropriate vocabulary continues to be an area of concern for persons who use augmentative and alternative communication (PWUAACs) and their communication partners.

This chapter briefly discusses the purposes of communication and some characteristics of individuals that are important to consider when selecting vocabulary. The following section describes three vocabulary selection frameworks (i.e., functional, developmental, and cognitive) that should be interwoven throughout the selection process to help guide decisions on a case-by-case basis. Next, we describe three types of words that are relevant to AAC, followed by vocabulary selection resources and strategies. Although this chapter presents numerous elements, we hope to underscore three overarching principles to lean on when embarking on the journey of choosing vocabulary for PWUAACs: (a) there is no singular approach that can be applied to every client; (b) clinicians must consider the whole person, regardless of their clinical setting; and (c) you cannot and should not go at it alone.

General Considerations

As introduced in Chapter 1, the purpose of AAC is to assist people with profound speech and/or language challenges to participate in their various social settings (home, school, recreation, work, etc.), form and maintain their relationships, perform in their social roles (parent, employee, student, etc.), express their needs, guide their care, and develop their capacity for language and learning (Beukelman & Light, 2020). In order to determine the most useful vocabulary for achieving these goals, it is important to think about the ways people use language in their daily lives.

Pertinent to each of these objectives is the capacity to share information with others. Formulating requests is a form of information sharing that is often prioritized for beginning communicators with AAC. Although it is an important speech act, humans use communication to share so much more than wants and needs. Recounting events and storytelling are important parts of communication that foster interpersonal connection for both adults and children. Those using AAC should have vocabulary and messages that allow them to talk about mundane situations, special events, autobiographical stories, and fables. Consider how each of these capabilities can foster a relationship between a grandparent and grandchild, for example, as well as how their absence can hinder the growth of such a relationship. For children, being able to tell fantasy stories, learn story structure, and sequence events has obvious social and educational implications.

People who use AAC also need to have appropriate vocabulary and messages to permit information sharing regarding their care and safety. Unfortunately, both adults and children who use AAC need to have a vocabulary that allows them to report abuses fully and clearly. In addition, Beukelman and Light (2020) point out the importance of including procedural descriptions in AAC systems. These messages may be preprogrammed to share detailed and time-sensitive information, such as giving instructions for preparing medication or driving directions home. Preprogrammed procedural descriptions can also be used to give instructions for a favorite recipe or to give directions in the workplace.

Of course, back-and-forth conversation is a huge part of all of our lives. The ability to engage in conversation is invaluable for keeping us connected to people. Importantly, in the context of early conversations with young children, adults deploy a range of strategies to scaffold their child's participation and model conventional uses of language. In addition, greetings and small talk are all needed to meet society's expectations and maintain social interactions. Including words and messages to initiate interactions, respond to salutations, express interest (e.g., wow, cool, great, I bet, etc.), and exit conversations is an important part of supporting a client's participation in their communities. The specific words and messages selected for each of these speech acts should reflect the individual's age, culture, linguistic background, and personality; a young user of AAC today may prefer to say something is *lit*, as opposed to *great* in certain contexts. Just like oral speakers, those using AAC need options for different social situations, such as dialogue with friends, family, professionals, younger people, elders, and strangers.

It is crucial to remember that a client's cultural background will influence the vocabulary that is needed and appropriate. For example, in the United States and other Western cultures, the ability to say "no" reflects a value of self-determination. However, in some cultures, "no" is considered harsh and confrontational. Indirect refusals like "maybe," "I'll try," or "I don't know," on the other hand, are considered more socially acceptable. In Spanish, adding diminutives, such as *-ito* or *-ita* to the end of a noun signals a register used by and directed toward children (e.g., muñeca/muñequita; [little] doll). Even within the same geographic region, families can maintain different social expectations, such as insisting on "yes, ma'am/no, sir" responses or cringing at "I want" phrases.

Certain aspects of conversation, like greetings and farewells, are fairly predictable, but the bulk of conversation involves a give and take of information that requires novel messages and the ability to transition from one topic to another. Individuals using AAC will require context-specific vocabulary for a range of settings (home, school, girl scout meetings, doctor's office, place of worship, transit, restaurant, work, etc.) as well as topics of interest (hobbies, movies, etc.). For culturally and linguistically diverse clients, certain life domains may require vocabulary in their heritage language (such as is detailed in the essays included in this section, Section II). Every individual and family is multidimensional, so it is essential that clinicians avoid making decisions based on assumptions regarding age, gender, culture, or anything else, even if done with the best intentions.

In order to select a robust and meaningful vocabulary, clinicians must explore multiple sources and solicit suggestions from the client, their communication partners, peers, teachers, community members, and care providers. In addition, clinicians, *along with their clients and stakeholders*, should consider the individual's overall communication abilities and their priorities for AAC. Factors such as age, literacy level, and cognitive ability are critical elements that will influence vocabulary and message decisions.

We now discuss three broad frameworks that can help guide the vocabulary selection process. Importantly, these approaches should not be thought of as mutually exclusive. In order to support the whole client, a singular approach should not be adopted. Instead, the three frameworks should be uniquely combined to best meet the needs of each individual.

Vocabulary Selection Frameworks

We demonstrated the importance of recognizing that people use communication in innumerous ways and that PWUAACs need to be afforded the tools to participate in all of them. Drawing on a functional, developmental, and cognitive framework throughout the process can facilitate the selection of resources as well as a range of vocabulary and messages that can enable communication in multiple domains.

Functional Framework

A **functional approach** to vocabulary selection emphasizes essential vocabulary or messages that an individual needs either within specific situations or to meet specific needs. For example, a client who uses medication requires easy access to their medication names as well as words like *pills* and *insulin*. Those requiring assistance for toileting or eating need to be able to communicate those needs. Certain messages require a quick and timely execution to be effective yet may take too long to produce using letter-by-letter or word-by-word selection; STOP THAT HURTS or I HAVE SOME-THING TO SAY, for example. Other examples of functional vocabulary include preferred items, regulatory messages (e.g., *I need a break, I want more*) or state words (e.g., sick, hungry, mad, tired).

When selecting functional vocabulary, it is important to identify words that will support participation in subject-specific (or context-specific) situations, such as art class (e.g., cut, glue, paint, glitter), on the playground (e.g., slide, sandbox, etc.), or at work. Selecting functional vocabulary based on each environment (e.g., grandma's house) or activity (e.g., math lesson) utilizes an **environmental approach.** Analyzing a person's routine, environment, and frequent communication needs can guide decision-making for an initial lexicon as well as accelerate the process of retrieval and expression for individuals with proficient language and spelling abilities. Literate individuals who are able to generate any message they like through letter-by-letter spelling do not rely on others to provide them with vocabulary; however, they often benefit from some preprogrammed words and messages that enhance the timing, speed up production, and reduce fatigue, which may be experienced by those with co-occurring motor impairments (Beukelman & Light, 2020).

For example, someone who uses public transportation may benefit from messages that can inform the bus driver of their stop. A person who frequents an office may need to express PLEASE HIT NUMBER FOUR every time they use the elevator. Programming a student's class schedule with messages like I HAVE SCIENCE THIRD PERIOD WITH MISS SMITH can aid in several situations. Similarly, words that are used frequently can be programmed or coded with shortcuts to speed up letter-by-letter message construction. Can you imagine a high school math student having to spell out math formulas or words like *circumference, hypotonus,* and *parenthesis,* while doing group assignments? Thinking from a functional framework can also help identify situations that are most impacted by fatigue and attempt to remedy them. For example, a student who primarily uses letter-by-letter spelling at school may be tired by their last period. This client can be supported by identifying words and messages necessary for participation during that portion of the day.

Developmental Framework

A central element of the developmental framework is that AAC is a tool for language learning. Thus, vocabulary should not be limited to things the child can communicate now but should support their growing linguistic abilities. Clinicians utilizing a developmental approach select and teach vocabulary concepts that (a) are appropriate based on age and developmental level and (b) foster further linguistic and literacy development. A developmental approach requires that professionals familiarize themselves with words and concepts that are used by typically developing children, because evidence suggests that the first words produced by children with disabilities are similar to the first words of children without disabilities (Laubscher & Light, 2020).

In addition to the careful selection of first words, the developmental approach calls for vocabulary selection that is guided by principles of typical language development (Beukelman & Light, 2020). All children go through a basic sequence in language acquisition: first, they babble, then produce single-word utterances, and only after they begin to combine words into longer utterances, and they begin to use grammar (Brown, 1973; Nelson, 1973). When they start using language, children begin using words to *refer* to objects, activities, events, and properties that are salient and they can experience (i.e., referential style). As the language skills of the child improve, they transition from a referential style to a predicate style of communication, which allows them to *describe* the relationships among those objects, activities, events, and properties (e.g., from "baby" to "baby crying"). Vocabulary selection has to account for and enable children who use AAC to make those transitions, too. The composition of vocabulary should allow for children to shift from reference (nouns) to predication (verbs, adjectives, etc.) and then to grammar (i.e., function words and bound morphemes).

To support early word combinations, it is important to include words from a variety of word classes. Commonly, early developing verbs, such as *eat, go, fall*, and *sleep*, are especially important because children begin to produce subject-verb and subject-verb-object sentences around 2 years of age. These foundational sentence frames lend

to the use of morphological elements; in fact, verb diversity is a predictor of grammatical outcomes among typically developing toddlers and verbal toddlers with language impairment (see Bean et al., 2019). When using this approach, new vocabulary and morphosyntactic structures should be added and modeled frequently, and intervention should focus on eliciting increasingly complex language.

A developmental framework is critical when working with children who are acquiring language and literacy, but it should not be limited to young children. When thinking developmentally, clinicians are not only observing current needs, but they also anticipate future hindrances or learning opportunities and introduce tools to approach them. For example, a young man transitioning to a community-based program for adults with cognitive impairments should be provided with the new vocabulary he will need and opportunities to practice using them as early as possible. We can also revisit the hypothetical math student introduced in the previous section; once her speech-language pathologist (SLP) learned about her upcoming geometry class, the student and SLP met with the teacher and reviewed the course textbook to identify vocabulary words that were long, frequently occurring, and likely to present a challenge. After reviewing the list with the student, the SLP supported her in programming the words with shortcuts (e.g., cir+4 for CIRCUMFERENCE).

Cognitive Framework

Finally, a **cognitive approach** recognizes the impact of language on cognitive and conceptual development. Just like those who use verbal speech, PWUAACs use language to learn, reason, and discuss complex ideas. PWUAACs need vocabulary to express cognitive activities, such as comparing, describing, evaluating, measuring, and categorizing. When we perform these tasks, we often use non-object words (e.g., *same, different, longer, wrong, less*) and words that refer to our thought processes (e.g., *I think, maybe, seems like*) to express our conclusions.

Exercising a cognitive approach to vocabulary selection can support concept development, further vocabulary learning, and maintain cognitive function. Those making vocabulary choices for emergent communicators should select words that describe basic cognitive situations that young children are known to attend to. For example, the very first words that typically developing children produce often point out cognitive-conceptual features of their environment, such as recurrence (more, again), existence (there), and nonexistence (gone; Bloom, 1976). Even before they begin speaking, infants demonstrate an understanding of concepts like containment (in), support (on), and movement (go), and they show the ability to make spatial comparisons (Bowerman & Choi, 2001).

It is essential to provide vocabulary that allows children to share their observations about the world with others. This approach is especially relevant for school-aged children, because their academic success requires that they learn new words, ask questions, and share what they know. Imagine a student who wants to respond to his teacher's request to define a *lagoon* but is unable to utilize concept vocabulary, such as *bigger, smaller, next to, shallow,* or *separated.* In this case, having access to the words *lagoon* and *lake* is not helpful without the conceptual words needed to compare them. Drawing on a cognitive framework can support aging populations as well. Older adults who may be at risk for cognitive decline benefit from verbal reasoning and other cognitive tasks. Thus, clinicians should ensure that they have access to the vocabulary needed to perform these mental functions and express their conclusions.

It should be noted that, in many cases, words can fall at the intersection of two or more approaches, depending on a client's unique situation. For example, when choosing an emergent vocabulary for a toddler, the word *more* satisfies all three approaches. Similarly, if a child with a cognitive impairment is using an activity board to participate in a science lesson about lagoons, providing words like *shallow* and *separated* would be functional (activity-based) as well as supportive of cognitive development.

It cannot be overstated that these three frameworks must be intertwined in order to provide a robust vocabulary. No single approach can produce a sufficiently diverse and useful lexicon. When clinicians are making choices about vocabulary

selection for those developing language, decisions should be guided by two principles outlined by Beukelman and Light (2020): the need to convey essential messages and the eventual development of language skills. Furthermore, PWUAACs need to have a blend of content words (words that possess salient meaning, such as nouns, verbs, adjectives, and adverbs) and function words (words that permit grammaticalization, such as articles, determiners, pronouns, and auxiliary verbs) in order to be effective communicators. The next section describes three categories of vocabulary words that should be considered during the vocabulary selection processes. Exercising each vocabulary selection framework for every client can help professionals choose appropriate words from each category.

Types of Vocabulary

Choosing words that are developmentally appropriate, motivating, and useful for the client is no small task. Bean et al. (2019) synthesized recommendations provided by the American Speech-Language-Hearing Association (ASHA) to put forth four variables that can facilitate vocabulary selection: (a) the context/environment in which the vocabulary can be used, (b) the length of time the word will be relevant, (c) whether it can elicit and maintain interaction with people, and (d) whether the word will facilitate the development of grammatical structures. We choose to add an additional variable: (e) whether the word supports the acquisition or expression of new concepts. When choosing vocabulary for clients using AAC, clinicians typically draw from three categories of words, recognizing that a robust vocabulary requires a mix of all three.

Personalized Vocabulary

Words that are uniquely relevant to a specific person are known as personalized vocabulary. Everyone uses words to name people, places, pets, objects, and actions that are important to them. Sometimes, a client may require special items (e.g., wrist brace) or actions (e.g., suction) that they need to talk about. Including personalized words is not only functional, it serves to customize the communication system and allows the user to engage in conversations about things that are motivating and special to them. Words that express personal interests will likely be used over a long period of time and with multiple partners. Talking about preferred things can also motivate an individual to practice and expand their language expression.

Fringe vocabulary is a term used to refer to words that are context-specific, such as words for a particular class (e.g., paintbrush for art class) or activity (e.g., spinner while playing a game). Incorporating fringe and personalized vocabulary is important because they have the potential to be functional, motivating, and facilitative of participation and social connection. However, an AAC system that leans too heavily on personalized and fringe vocabulary risks limiting the person's communications, often restricting their participation to answering simple questions or making requests. A word's contribution to overall communication competence will be limited if it is not useful in a variety of contexts or if its relevance is short term, such as those added for a particular theme, like *turkey*, *cornucopia*, and *pilgrim* during the month of November.

Core Vocabulary

AAC intervention should not be limited to the execution of specific communication behaviors, but to develop a level of linguistic competence that will allow clients to communicate unlimited novel ideas. To this end, researchers have strived to identify a core set of vocabulary that can be used to generate diverse messages across varied contexts. Core vocabulary is commonly defined as a relatively small set of high-frequency words that are used by a variety of people in numerous settings.

Core words are typically identified by collecting natural language samples of multiple speakers over a period of time or in more than one setting (e.g., school and home). The words are analyzed in order to identify those that overlap across all or most of the speakers or across settings. Usually, the words are also ranked according to how frequently they were produced. Core word lists have been developed for various populations, such as toddlers, preschool-, and school-aged children,

in order to inform word selection for comparable nonspeaking children; see van Tilborg and Deckers (2016) for an extensive review. Core lists have also been created by analyzing frequently occurring words found in written text, used by naturally speaking adults, and adults with disabilities who communicate by spelling. This type of analysis consistently shows that a small number of words make up a large proportion (70%–80%) of the total words spoken. Many core lists include words from several grammatical classes; however, core lists privilege closed-class function words (i.e., pronouns, auxiliary verbs, determiners, copula, prepositions, articles) and a small number of high-frequency content words (e.g., want, more, eat, good, make). Because of this limitation, core lists should be supplemented with vocabulary that is relevant to each client's interests, needs, and contexts (Laubscher & Light, 2020).

Drawing on core words for vocabulary selection and intervention for people using AAC has numerous benefits. A small number of words can be used across activities, settings, communication partners, and speech acts. They can be displayed in a consistent location on a communication device, which can support the development of a motor plan to increase the speed of activation. Importantly, a small number of core words can be combined to produce numerous messages that facilitate participation, and they are building blocks for generative language, thus supporting syntactic development.

For children learning to use language, incorporating core words is vital for paving the way toward grammatical speech. However, relying solely on core word lists is problematic. Because these lists represent words that overlap across speakers and settings, they do not capture important content words that are a necessary part of children's vocabulary, such as personalized vocabulary and basic concepts words, which we discuss in the next section. Referencing core word lists can be an effective strategy for locating developmentally appropriate words that are highly functional, and facilitative of linguistic and cognitive advancement. However, clinicians must make case-by-case decisions and refrain from adopting a singularly "core approach." A system containing only core words would not sufficiently address anyone's communication needs.

Furthermore, many function words that typically appear on core lists may not be developmentally appropriate or functional, especially for early communicators with small productive vocabularies.

Basic Concepts and Relational Vocabulary

Basic concepts are fundamental, early developing words made up of colors, letters, numbers, shapes, size/comparison words (e.g., big, different), directions/positions (e.g., in front of, over), self-/social awareness words (e.g., happy, sad), texture words (e.g., smooth, wet), quantity words (e.g., more, full), and time/sequence words (e.g., new, slow; see Bracken & Crawford, 2010 for a list of early basic concepts). A subset of these concepts is known as *relational basic concepts*. Relational basic concepts deal with size, distance, amount, spatial location, and time (Boehm, 2000). Relational basic concepts differ from other words, including nonrelational basic concepts (i.e., colors, letters, shapes, numbers, emotions, and some adjectives), because their meaning can only arise by attending to the *relationship* between objects, events, and conditions in the world. For example, the meaning of words like *same* or *next* depends on a comparison between two or more things.

Relational basic concepts, and the more inclusive category of basic concepts, are pervasive in early education classrooms. Preschool teachers use them frequently, and they are represented in curriculum standards for prekindergarten through first grade in all 50 states (Bracken & Crawford, 2010). Acquisition of basic concepts is correlated with overall vocabulary, language development, literacy, and academic achievement. Preschool children with stronger concept knowledge are better at learning new words (Booth & Waxman, 2002) and grouping words into categories (Mintz, 2005), supporting the notion that basic concepts are the foundation for cognitive and conceptual development.

In addition, basic concepts and relational words are frequent and highly functional, as they allow children to tell stories, recount events, describe objects and situations, share their observations, comment on activities, and direct the actions of others. Concept words, which include both basic concepts and relational words, can be incorporated into a variety of activities and support social interactions. For example, instead of targeting nouns like *turkey* and *pilgrim* during a Thanksgiving-themed lesson, spatial and temporal words like *first, after,* and *together* can be the focus of intervention; these words will retain their relevance long after the holiday season. The child can also be supported to use concept vocabulary as a word strategy to give a classmate directions or make comments. Incorporating relational and nonrelational basic concepts is important for increasing the complexity of utterances. When combined with core and personalized vocabulary, the potential for novel utterances is limitless, even at the two-word stage (e.g., *eat later, red table, want big, mom gone*). Activities involving basic concepts and preferred items can motivate practicing grammatically correct sentences and provide opportunities to practice cognitive skills like measuring, comparing, and qualifying.

Typically developing children begin to express concept words soon after they start speaking and demonstrate mastery of most basic concepts by age 6 years. Some high-frequency concepts like *gone, more,* and *up* are found on core word lists developed for young children, but many more are not. In fact, many developmentally appropriate concept words are at risk for being overlooked during vocabulary selection because they do not meet the criteria for personalized or core vocabulary, and some may not be included in communication software libraries at all. McCarthy et al. (2017) investigated the presence of basic concept words in eight widely used AAC communication programs. They report that the inclusion of basic concepts varied greatly, especially words related to comparison, size, and sequence. For example, *before, last,* and *shallow* were all missing in at least half of the programs. Exercising a cognitive approach to vocabulary selection can assist providers in identifying appropriate conceptual words that will support the client in multiple domains.

Vocabulary Selection Tools

Clinicians have several tools and strategies that can be applied to the task of choosing vocabulary.

Each resource lends itself to one or more of the selection frameworks and vocabulary types (i.e., personalized, core, basic/relational); thus, providers will need to draw upon more than one source depending on the client's characteristics and goals. Consulting with the client and those who know them well is always best practice and is useful for including personally meaningful and motivating vocabulary (i.e., topics of interests, preferences). Parents, caregivers, and teachers are common informants, but siblings, friends, and coworkers can also suggest useful vocabulary because they can reveal topics that are relevant to the client's social group.

To add more structure to the process, clinicians can elicit words by category like food, toys, places, names of people, and so on. Fallon, Light, and Paige (2001) developed a parent questionnaire that combines vocabulary checklists and open-ended questions by categories. For children, vocabulary inventories such as the MacArthur-Bates Communicative Development Inventories (MB-CDI; Fenson et al., 2006) can offer additional suggestions. These approaches are valuable for identifying both functional and personalized vocabulary; however, clinicians may need to work with families to prioritize words that will be useful in multiple settings long term.

Core word lists are another important resource for vocabulary selection, providing the function words needed for grammaticalization as well as other high-frequency words that may not be captured on inventories or reported by informants. When using lists and inventories, clinicians need to ensure that the list is appropriate for the client in terms of age and developmental level. For culturally and linguistically diverse clients, resources that reflect the individual's heritage should be utilized whenever available. For example, Soto and Cooper (2021) produced a list that can aid in the selection of initial vocabulary for Spanish-speaking children under 30 months of age. Also, Boenisch and Soto (2015) published a list of high-frequency words spoken by school-aged children who speak English as a second language.

For school-aged children and young adults, consultation with educators, curriculum materials, and grade-level standards can help clinicians anticipate the vocabulary a student may need to be successful and participate meaningfully in class. Understanding curriculum expectations can help clinicians prioritize concepts that are likely to be reinforced for a long time. For example, Common Core standards expect kindergartners to be able to retell stories, explain similarities and differences between events, and name the author and illustrator of a book with support. Informants, inventories, and core lists may not provide sufficient vocabulary to engage in these activities. Reviewing lists of basic concepts, including assessments, can help identify important words. Schwarz and McCarthy (2012) created a basic concept vocabulary database by compiling all of the words from the Wiig Assessment of Basic Concepts (WABC; Wiig, 2004), the Boehm-3 (Boehm, 2001), and the Bracken Basic Concept Scale–Receptive (BBCS-R; Bracken, 1998). These three basic concept assessments are frequently used to assess school readiness for preschool and early elementary students.

Relying on checklists, inventories, or informants outside of the client's actual communication contexts will pose limitations. Clinicians need to work with others in examining all of the client's environments to ensure they have access to the words they need. As much as possible, the team should anticipate the vocabulary that will be needed in order to maximize learning and participation during language-rich activities (e.g., *planets, stars, gas, ticket, light-year, orbit*, before a field trip to a planetarium). Ecological assessments in the form of observations and task analyses can underscore vocabulary and messages that are needed for successful communication in a given domain. For example, Downing (2009) suggests observing school-aged clients and their typically developing peers in the classroom to identify communication behaviors that are needed for each step of an activity. Structuring an observation in terms of specific steps (e.g., greeting, getting to their seat, group work) can highlight the language practices expected and demonstrated by peers, as well as the barriers impacting the client. Such an analysis can suggest words or messages the student needs to be successful within each step of a daily routine. Clinicians can also support family members and other caretakers to keep a communication diary where they document communication breakdowns and suggest words that can prevent a similar breakdown in the future. Since there is no one-size-fits-all approach, strategies should be combined in nuanced ways depending on the needs of each client.

In Conclusion

When introducing AAC as an intervention, the vocabulary selected will have significant implications on the types of communicative acts a person will be able to engage in. In this chapter, we present several considerations as well as types of vocabulary and vocabulary selection tools. In order to facilitate decision-making regarding resources and words, we suggest utilizing three selection frameworks—functional, developmental, and cognitive—for every client throughout the process. In the following section, we present a case study to demonstrate how the three vocabulary selection frameworks, along with the capabilities, characteristics, and needs of the client coalesce to ensure the most meaningful and useful vocabulary is provided.

Case Study: AN

Clinical Profile and Communication Needs

The Individual

AN is a bicultural 3-year, 8-month-old female recently diagnosed with autism. She enjoys Disney movies, toys with lights and sounds, and visiting the playground close to her home. AN has a moderate visual impairment and wears corrective lenses, which she frequently removes. AN has an expressive vocabulary of approximately 12 to 15 words. She demonstrates communicative intent throughout the day using nonverbal behavior, such as pointing, bringing objects to adults, crying, turning away, jumping up and down, and using a few manual baby signs (e.g., more, give me, open). When AN is happy or excited, she wiggles her fingers in front of her mouth and eyes while smiling. AN sometimes engages in self-injurious behavior

(SIB), such as biting the skin around her fingers and the back of her hand and hitting her thigh with her fist. Her family and teachers report that these behaviors occur during undesirable tasks or when she is unable to do what she wants. AN appears to get frustrated when adults do not understand what she wants or when her requests are denied.

Due to her limited vocabulary and increasing occurrence of SIB, the family pediatrician referred AN for a comprehensive communication assessment by a bilingual SLP. AN was evaluated in both Spanish and English to assess her total communication repertoire. To assess her receptive and expressive language skills, the Spanish and English versions of the Preschool Language Scale, Fifth Edition (Zimmerman et al., 2011) were completed. The comprehensive evaluation also consisted of a parent intake interview, a language sample, and observations during free play with toys. The results of the Spanish and English versions of the PLS-5 revealed that AN's composite standard scores in Spanish and English were comparable. In Spanish and English, respectively, her receptive language standard scores (SS = 70; 70) were higher than her expressive language standard scores (SS = 64; 67), which supports her diagnosis of autism and confirms that her language delay is affecting both of her languages.

Throughout the assessment, AN identified body parts (eyes, ears, hair, hand, feet), clothing items (shirt, shorts, shoes), primary colors, items presented in photographs (bird, shoe, cookie), and objects (cup, spoon, ball) in both Spanish and English. She also understood the verbs "eat," "drink," and "sleep." Expressively, AN did not use words to greet, answer yes/no questions, or make requests. She was observed to sign "more" one time to request animal crackers and verbalized "no" one time in protest. She enjoyed carrying toys over to her mother. However, she would get upset when her mother or the SLP attempted to play with them. Although her spontaneous speech was very limited, she labeled several pictures, switching between Spanish and English. AN labeled "house" and "bear" in Spanish (/kæ ə/ and /ɔsə/, respectively). She produced the following words in English "cat" /kæt/, "cup" /kʌ/, "brush" /bʌ/, and "spoon" /pu/. AN presents with articulation errors in both languages, resulting in highly unintelligible speech. Further language sample analysis indicated that AN had a mean length of utterance (MLU) of 1.75, which is significantly below average for a child AN's age.

AN's mother, Mrs. N, provided information regarding AN's communication at home that corroborated the evaluation results. She shared that AN seems to know a variety of words in Spanish and English. She is able to locate things like her shoes and other household items when requested in either language but does not otherwise follow directions without help. She does understand simple commands in Spanish like *ven* (come), *dame* (give me), *pon* (put), *dormir* (sleep), *para* (stop), *bailar* (dance), and *comer* (eat). She will also point to pictures in books and on iPhone games. AN uses a few words at home. Her functional vocabulary in Spanish includes *tete* for milk, *awa* for water, *titi* for her sister, *Aba* for her grandmother, *mio* (mine). In English, she sometimes says *juice, cat, night* (for sleep), *shoes*, and *Elsa* (her favorite movie character). She can also say *one, two*, and *three* in both languages. Mrs. N shared that she can sometimes get her to repeat words, but she typically uses nonverbal communication, vocalizes, and produces jargon. Mrs. N said she had an easier time understanding AN's nonverbal communication. However, recently AN has been getting increasingly irritable at home and school when she is not understood right away.

Their Communication Partners and Environment

AN lives with both of her parents and a 6-year-old sister in a multicultural and bilingual home. The family lives in Miami, Florida, a city with a large Spanish-speaking population. Her mother was born in the United States and speaks Spanish and English. AN's maternal grandparents immigrated from Havana, Cuba, and live close to the family. AN's father was born in Asturias, a northern region of Spain, and is fluent in Spanish and English. AN's parents use English more frequently when speaking to their children, although both languages are used equally in the home. Spanish is used exclusively around the children's maternal grandparents, who routinely come over for visits and support the

family by providing childcare. The children also FaceTime weekly with their paternal grandparents who live in Spain. These grandparents are monolingual Spanish speakers and visit the family for a month every year.

AN's parents have expressed their desire to pass on their heritage language to their children so that they can remain connected to their grandparents and other relatives in Spain and Cuba. Her parents would have liked to enroll AN in a dual-language school that her older sister attends. However, due to her diagnosis of autism and communication challenges, school personnel suggested they enroll her in a monolingual-English, prekindergarten inclusion classroom. AN participates in a general education PreK class with peers who are either typically developing or diagnosed with a disability. AN's teacher, Ms. Smith is a monolingual English speaker. English is the language of instruction at school; however, some of AN's communication partners, including Ms. Hernandez, her SLP, Ms. Arroyo, a paraprofessional in her classroom, and a few of her classmates, are bilingual. In this inclusion class, AN's family members (parents and grandparents), teacher (Mrs. Smith), and SLP (Mrs. Hernandez) comprised the Interprofessional Practice (IPP) team. This IPP team collaborated to select a method of intervention that would facilitate AN's communication development.

The AAC System

The IPP team agreed that functional communication, bilingual language development, and literacy are priorities for AN. The team decided to implement an intervention utilizing aided AAC to support her expressive communication and overall language growth. The SLP recommended using a speech-generating device (SGD) programmed with the Language Acquisition through Motor Planning (LAMP) software. LAMP was suggested for multiple reasons. First, the vocabulary is displayed on the device in a consistent location to facilitate selections (Bedwani et al., 2015). This display supports learning by maintaining a consistent motor plan. A consistent motor plan is necessary for helping AN become autonomous since she has a vision impairment and benefits from a clear organizational structure. Second, the LAMP approach is a robust language representation and organizational system that can facilitate AN's vocabulary acquisition and the emergence of inflectional morphemes necessary for linguistic development. Third, the system is available in both English and Spanish and allows the user to toggle between languages easily and even code-switch within the same utterance when needed. Since the location of words remains constant regardless of the language being used, the SGD with LAMP can encourage dual-language learning.

The team discussed the operational and attentional demands that the new system may place on AN. To reduce frustration and encourage early independence, the team decided to display 20 words or fewer on each page while temporarily hiding words and pages that would be made accessible later as AN gains operational and linguistic competence. (Fortunately, AN's system offers *babble mode*, giving her the means to explore her system and play with icons that are normally hidden.) The team also decided to support AN's communication skills with various no-tech communication boards to supplement her SGD in the classroom.

Vocabulary Selection. After selecting the AAC system, the IPP team considered various factors to identify the vocabulary that AN would need on her SGD. These factors included her multicultural background, capabilities, personality, academic and home settings, and routines. As a first step, the SLP worked with AN's parents to complete the Vocabulary Selection Questionnaire for Preschoolers Who Use AAC (Fallon et al., 2001) to identify words that are functional and developmentally appropriate. They were also asked to think about the words and messages AN might need for her regular activities. The team decided to include words for important people (i.e., me, mom, dad, sister, Abuela Carmen, Abuelo Jorge, Ms. Hernandez, Ms. Arroyo, Ms. Smith, and her classmates). They also customized the names of her maternal grandparents, whom she and her sister affectionately refer to as Abo and Aba. They included places, such as Aba's house, school, bathroom, and playground. Both of her parents and teachers agreed that "playground" was a necessary word since previously, AN had attempted to leave the classroom when her request

to go to the park was not understood. A few familiar household items were included, such as a few clothing items, ball, iPad, cup, and spoon. However, her mother felt that household items were not a priority since AN is fairly independent in attaining household things that are typically accessible. Mrs. N also did not think that AN would be motivated to use these words. Mrs. N suggested items that were not always accessible, such as her favorite light-up toy at school, three beloved Disney movie options, and some preferred food and drink options.

AN's teacher provided input as well. She felt it was important to include places within the classroom (e.g., blocks center, library center, tabletop center) since the children chose their centers each morning. She also suggested including the days of the week since AN loves the calendar portion of the morning routine and always gets very excited. The team agreed that the days of the week and the months of the year should be included because they are personally motivating for her, they support her cognitive development and access to the general education curriculum, and they allow her to participate in a daily routine. The team also agreed to leave the colors, shapes, letters, and numbers pages accessible, since they are commonly used in the classroom, developmentally appropriate, and can be used outside school. When prompted to think about AN's activities at school, Ms. Smith suggested several nouns that are applicable to each center (e.g., animals, dress-up items, art supplies). The team recognized the utility of those items at school; however, they worried that it could be overwhelming and not useful in other contexts. Ms. Hernandez, the SLP, agreed to work with Ms. Smith to create a one-page no-tech communication board for each center that could be laminated and kept at each location. These communication boards can enable participation and requesting without having to navigate through her SGD. The team agreed to transfer the relevant vocabulary to the SGD once she gains more operational competence.

Although the team thought of many more potentially useful nouns, they were conscientious that verbs and nonobject words are necessary for providing AN with a robust communication system that will facilitate word combinations and eventually syntax development. To identify early developing verbs, the SLP referenced the MB-CDI (Fenson et al., 2007) and a Spanish frequency list for children (Soto & Cooper, 2021). The team included familiar words (i.e., *eat*, *drink*, *sleep*), as well as frequent and early developing verbs like *put*, *play*, *want*, *come*, *go*, *stop*, *help*, *open*, *hug*, and *give* in both languages. AN's dad suggested including verbs relevant for a park (i.e., *swing*, *climb*, *slide*, *push*, *jump*) to motivate AN to use the SGD. Ms. Hernandez suggested some early developing relational concepts that are commonly found on core word lists for preschool children, including prepositions (i.e., *in*, *on*, *out*), and other nonobject words (i.e., *done*, *gone*, *up*, *down*, *this*, *that*, *more*, *again*, *next*, *no*) that could be used across contexts to form combinations.

AN's mother expressed her wish for AN to greet and say goodbye, something she rarely does. The team agreed that social words like *hi/hola* and *bye/adios* were needed in both English and Spanish. AN's parents requested *thank you/gracias* and *please/por favor,* as well. Ms. Smith felt AN should have a way to greet her classmates that would be fun for AN and easy for other children to understand. They decided to program the following message on the home screen: *Do you want a high-five?* The team also considered other preprogrammed messages to facilitate interactions with peers. They added *Do you want to play? Watch this!* and *I don't like that.*

Finally, Ms. Hernandez and AN's parents reviewed the LAMP system's translations to make sure they were appropriate for AN and her family. The LAMP program has a button on the top left that switches the display between English and Spanish while maintaining the vocabulary's position. Ms. Hernandez showed Mr. and Mrs. N how to add words to the system. The icon for "Aba's house" was programmed to function as a noun word and also as a folder. They added a few objects, games (*dominos*), food items (*galleticas, pastelitos*), the names of her grandparents' two pets, and *patos* (ducks) because AN and her grandmother enjoy feeding the ducks that live around their community.

The IPP team decided on the following initial goals for AN: to use the device for various functions (i.e., requesting, greeting, commenting, answering a question) throughout the day in at least three different settings (e.g., home, school, outside, grandma's house) with encouragement and help as needed. A second goal was to form various two-word combinations including nouns, relational words, and basic concepts. Soon after receiving her SGD, AN appeared to enjoy the system's cause-and-effect display (pressing of an icon that activates speech production); thus, she quickly met her goal of using the SGD for various functions. Her favorite speech acts included asking for high-fives, stating the day of the week, and telling her dad PUSH and STOP while on the swing.

In order to meet her second goal, AN required intervention targeting her operational and linguistic competence. To facilitate ANs operational competence, Ms. Hernandez helped AN identify vocabulary by directing her with "show me" paired with a word. This supported AN's ability to locate words and navigate through pages. The SLP also coached other IPP team members to model two-word combinations using the SGD and reformulate AN's one-word utterances into two- to three-word phrases. Her parents were encouraged to model switching the system between languages and forming one- and two-word utterances in English and Spanish. During speech sessions, Ms. Hernandez scaffolded AN's use of basic concepts, relational words, and core vocabulary during sensory-rich activities and supported Ms. Smith in generalizing those words to the classroom. The availability of core words, verbs, basic concepts, and personalized vocabulary facilitated innumerable word combinations for a variety of activities.

Over the next several months, AN appeared to benefit from the LAMP's visual and motor structure. She demonstrated automaticity in producing frequently occurring two-word combinations, such as making requests in English and Spanish (*want juice, quiero aqua, Ama ven* [*come*]), commenting on her schedule (*school done, voy* [*go*] *playground*), greeting (*hola Abo, Hi Ms. Smith*), and terminating activities (*no more*) with minimal to no support since her SGD displays the vocabulary in a consistent location, elicits a consistent motor pattern, and provides auditory feedback.

As the months continued, she became increasingly independent at producing novel two-word combinations. As AN's linguistic and operational competence improved, her expressive communication and utterance length gradually increased to 2.0 to 2.5. She used a wide range of word types, including colors, sizes, location words, verbs, environmental nouns, and personalized vocabulary to independently produce spontaneous and generative communication for various speech acts.

The IPP team recognized the importance of adding vocabulary and morphosyntactic structures to AN's SGD frequently to ensure continued language development. Ms. Hernandez, the SLP, regularly visited AN's classroom, met with Ms. Smith, and spoke to her mother over the phone. Ms. Hernandez encouraged Mr. and Mrs. N to keep a communication diary at home where they recorded communication breakdowns and communication opportunities, along with suggestions for words. Ms. Hernandez also placed a clipboard near AN's cubby so that adults in the classroom can write down ideas for new vocabulary. Because AN was demonstrating success, the team imported the center-based words that were originally on laminated language boards/communication sheets. However, Ms. Smith kept the paper versions to use as backups.

In addition to increasing AN's noun repertoire, which was largely made up of environmental and personalized items, Ms. Hernandez reviewed the Boehm Test of Basic Concepts and the Wiig assessment to identify and incorporate concepts that are important for preschool success. Finally, the team agreed that AN should be encouraged to produce longer utterances as well as morphosyntactic elements.

Next Steps

Moving forward, the IPP team will focus on (a) expanding AN's MLU, (b) fostering her bilingual development, (c) regularly evaluating and updating her vocabulary, and (d) supporting her family to independently manage her SGD. In order to facilitate longer utterances, the IPP team will continue to work toward increasing the length and complexity of AN's productions throughout her daily activities. After considering developmental norms regarding morphology and syntax, the team will

write short- and long-term objectives to teach AN the following skills using her SGD with LAMP:

- AN will combine three words to produce the following syntactic structures: Subject + Verb + Object, Verb + Adjective + Object, and Adjective + Subject + Verb.
- AN will answer questions, describe situations, or comment by producing 3+ word utterances including spatial-relational words (e.g., *together, up, down, outside, etc.*) or prepositions.
- AN will use the following morphemes: present progressive (-ing), regular past tense (-ed), regular plural (-s), and the superlative form (-er).

As AN gains competence in using morphemes, the IPP team will continue to use the functional, cognitive, and developmental frameworks to facilitate the emergence of function words, such as determiners, pronouns, and auxiliary verbs, to support the development of morphosyntactic skills.

In order to support AN's bilingual development, all of her goals will be targeted in Spanish as well. As AN's MLU gradually increases, the following function words and concepts will be targeted in both her languages: definite and indefinite articles [Spanish (S): "la," "el"; English (E): "the," "a," "an"], demonstratives [(S): "este," "esa"; (E): "this," "that"], possessive determiners [(S): "mio,""tuyo"; (E): "my," "your"], pronouns [(S): "el," "ella," "ellos"; (E): "him," "her," "them"], and auxiliary verbs [(S): "ser," "estar"; (E): "is," "are"]. Given the mix of content and function words on her SGD, AN will have the vocabulary she needs to produce unlimited, grammatically correct utterances in both English and Spanish. Because Ms. Hernandez is bilingual, she will encourage AN to produce utterances in both languages during therapy sessions. Her parents will focus on providing models in Spanish and encourage AN to use Spanish at home as much as possible.

Because vocabulary is constantly expanding, the IPP team will need to create a consultation schedule to ensure that AN's vocabulary is evaluated on a routine basis. Ms. Hernandez will teach Ms. Smith how to program new vocabulary but will also provide ongoing support. Ms. Hernandez will collect the words and topics from the clipboard in AN's cubby biweekly and check in with Ms. Smith after AN's speech sessions. The IPP team will also need to plan for the following school year. When the end of the school year approaches, the IPP team will schedule a meeting with the receiving kindergarten teacher and SLP to determine needed vocabulary and prepare for anticipated communication demands. They will also discuss strategies to maximize meaningful communication and language-learning opportunities throughout the day. The receiving SLP, teacher, and AN's parents will need to assess AN's new school environment using observations, task analysis, and environmental inventories as early as possible. As AN moves into higher grades, her education team will need to focus on vocabulary that allows her to benefit from and engage with grade-level curriculum.

Finally, AN's parents need to be empowered and supported so that they can continue to drive their daughter's dual-language development. Although Mr. and Mrs. N know how to program vocabulary, Ms. Hernandez will set up a regular meeting time to review the communication diary and work together to make decisions for new vocabulary that will be functional as well as beneficial for her cognitive and linguistic development. The team knows it is important to include AN's grandparents and sister in order to maximize use of the SGD in multiple settings outside of school. Ms. Hernandez will invite them to subsequent meetings, but importantly, she will work with Mrs. N so that she can feel confident in her ability to educate her family members and others about AN's communication and SGD.

References

Bean, A., Cargill, L., & Lyle, S. (2019). Framework for selecting vocabulary for preliterate children who use augmentative and alternative communication. *American Journal of Speech-Language Pathology, 28*(3), 1000–1009. https://doi.org/10.1044/2019_AJSLP-18-0041

Bedwani, M. A. N., Bruck, S., & Costley, D. (2015). Augmentative and alternative communication for children with autism spectrum disorder: An evidence-based evaluation of the Language Acquisition through Motor Planning (LAMP) programme. *Cogent Education, 2*(1), 1045807. https://doi.org/10.1080/2331186X.2015.1045807

Beukelman, D. R., & Light, J. (2020). *Augmentative and alternative communication: Supporting children and adults with complex communication needs* (5th ed.). Paul H. Brookes.

Bloom, L. (1976). *One word at a time: The use of single word utterances before syntax.* Mouton. https://doi.org/10.1515/9783110819090

Boehm, A. E. (2000). Assessment of basic relational concepts. In B. A. Bracken (Ed.), *The psychoeducational assessment of preschool children* (3rd ed., pp. 186–203). Allyn & Bacon.

Boehm, A. E. (2001). *Boehm Test of Basic Concepts, Third edition (Boehm3): Examiner's manual.* Pearson.

Boenisch, J., & Soto, G. (2015). The oral core vocabulary of typically developing English-speaking school-aged children: Implications for AAC practice. *Augmentative and Alternative Communication, 31*(1), 77–84.

Booth, A. E., & Waxman, S. R. (2002). Word learning is "smart": Evidence that conceptual information affects preschoolers' extension of novel words. *Cognition, 84*(1), B11–B22. https://doi.org/10.1016/S0010-0277(02)00015-X

Bowerman, M., & Choi, S. (2001). Shaping meanings for language: Universal and language-specific in the acquisition of spatial semantic categories. In M. Bowerman & S. C. Levinson (Eds.), *Language acquisition and conceptual development* (pp. 475–511). Cambridge University Press. https://doi.org/10.1017/cbo9780511620669

Bracken, B. A. (1998). *Bracken Basic Concept Scale—Revised: Examiner's manual.* Psychological Corporation.

Bracken, B. A., & Crawford, E. (2010). Basic concepts in early childhood educational standards: A 50-state review. *Early Childhood Education Journal, 37*(5), 421–430. https://doi.org/10.1007/s10643-009-0363-7

Brown, R. (1973). *A first language: The early stages.* Harvard University Press.

Downing, J. (2009). Assessment of early communication skills. In S. Soto & C. Zangari (Eds.), *Practically speaking: Language, literacy, and academic development for students with AAC needs* (pp. 27–46). Paul H. Brookes.

Fallon, K. A., Light, J. C., & Paige, T. K. (2001). Enhancing vocabulary selection for preschoolers who require augmentative and alternative communication (AAC). *American Journal of Speech-Language Pathology, 10*(1), 81–94. https://doi.org/10.1044/1058-0360(2001/010)

Fenson, L., Marchman, V., Thal, D., Reznick, S., & Bates, E. (2006). *MacArthur-Bates Communicative Development Inventories, Second edition (MB-CDI): User's guide and technical manual*. Paul H. Brookes.

Laubscher, E., & Light, J. (2020). Core vocabulary lists for young children and considerations for early language development: A narrative review. *Augmentative and Alternative Communication, 36*(1), 43–53. https://doi.org/10.1080/07434618.2020.1737964

McCarthy, J. H., Schwarz, I., & Ashworth, M. (2017). The availability and accessibility of basic concept vocabulary in AAC software: A preliminary study. *Augmentative and Alternative Communication, 33*(3), 131–138. https://doi.org/10.1080/07434618.2017.1332685

Mintz, T. (2005). Linguistic and conceptual influences on adjective acquisition in 24- and 36-month-olds. *Developmental Psychology, 41*(1), 17–29. https://doi.org/10.1037/0012-1649.41.1.17

Nelson, K. (1973). Structure and strategy in learning to talk. *Monographs of the Society for Research in Child Development, 38*(1/2), 1–135. https://doi.org/10.2307/1165788

Schwarz, I., & McCarthy, J. H. (2012). *Basic concepts in the classroom: What vocabulary do you hear during a week of instruction?* [Data set]. UTHSC. https://www.uthsc.edu/asp/research/documents/l3-basic-concept-vocabulary-database.pdf

Soto, G., & Cooper, B. (2021). An early Spanish vocabulary for children who use AAC: Developmental and linguistic considerations. *Augmentative and Alternative Communication, 37*(1), 64–74. https://doi.org/10.1080/07434618.2021.1881822

van Tilborg, A., & Deckers, S. R. J. M. (2016). Vocabulary selection in AAC: Application of core vocabulary in atypical populations. *Perspectives of the ASHA Special Interest Groups, 1*(12), 125–138. https://doi.org/10.1044/persp1.sig12.125

Wiig, E. (2004). *Wiig Assessment of Basic Concepts (WABC): Examiner's manual*. Super Duper Publications.

Zimmerman, I. L., Steiner, V. G., Pond, R. E., Karas, G. B., Marshall, J., Boland, J., & Marshall, E. (2011). *Preschool Language Scales, Fifth edition (PLS-5): Examiner's manual*. Pearson.

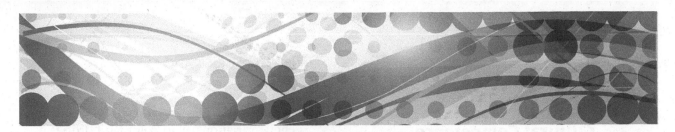

Essay 3

CULTURAL CONSIDERATIONS AND AAC: INTRODUCTION TO MODELS OF CULTURE

Ellen R. Cohn and John W. Gareis

In this first in a series of essays about culture, we need to establish a common understanding of the meaning of "culture." Culture encompasses all aspects of our experiences as human beings in a specific society; as examples, how we dress, what we eat, how we behave, how we worship, how we are treated as babies and raised into adulthood, and how we communicate both verbally and nonverbally. Culture influences how we perceive our physical world, as well as the intellectual, psychological, and social aspects of our lives.

A clinician needs to understand the cultural values of a person who uses augmentative and alternative communication (PWUAAC) and their communication partners. For example, when selecting vocabulary, what subjects are sensitive and to remain unspoken in a culture? How do you address elders in the culture? How does a person's perceived gender influence their communication preferences? For how long do people in the culture grieve the loss of a loved one, and what form does that take? How does a PWUAAC view technology in general, and AAC specifically? Do they celebrate birthdays? How does the culture regard U.S. culture?

As we do a "deep dive" into the cultural preferences of the PWUAAC, can we fully grasp their culture if we are not borne into it? The different aspects of a new culture are so numerous as to

be overwhelming to learn. Many believe that we cannot fully understand a different culture until we fully grasp our own.

That is where models of culture come in. Models help us to organize aspects of culture into schemas that we can research and perceive. As a caution, while we can discern much about a PWUAAC (e.g., by making mistakes, relying on an informant, and researching the culture), it is a matter for debate whether we can fully understand another culture.

This essay describes three consequential models of culture, with the Purnell model described in the most detail. Taken together, they can illuminate our understanding of a specific culture.

Edward T. Hall's Cultural Iceberg Model

Imagine an iceberg floating in the Arctic. Only a small part of the iceberg—the tip—floats above the water and can be easily seen. Edward Hall (1976) described the most obvious external or conscious part of culture. Beneath that surface is a much larger unconscious and hidden culture that is implicitly learned and difficult to change. The model of Purnell that follows provides a structure that is helpful when exploring the hidden aspects of culture.

Purnell's Model for Cultural Competence

The Purnell Model for Cultural Competence was created by Larry Purnell, PhD, RN, FAAN for health care practitioners (Purnell, 2002). Purnell viewed cultural competence as a process, not a destination. Initially, we may not be aware that we lack knowledge of another culture: *unconscious incompetence*. A second step in developing cultural competence is to be aware that we lack an understanding of another culture: *conscious incompetence*. This requires *cultural humility*. A third step is to learn about another culture and provide culturally specific interventions: *conscious competence*. The fourth and final step is when we can automatically provide culturally competent care: *unconscious competence*. The culturally competent clinician adapts their plan of care to the culture of the PWUAAC. In doing so, they do not allow their own experiences and values to influence their perceptions of the other culture.

The Purnell model consists of two characteristics of culture. Primary characteristics of culture are "age, generation, nationality, race, color and religion" (Purnell, 2002, p. 11). Secondary characteristics of culture are "educational status, socioeconomic status, occupation, military status, political beliefs, urban versus rural residence, enclave identity, marital status, parental status, physical characteristics, sexual orientation, gender issues, and reason for migration (sojourner, immigrant, undocumented status)" (Purnell, 2002, p. 11).

Purnell identifies 12 domains of culture and relates each of these domains to the person, the family, and the global society:

1. *Overview/heritage* include residence, topography, economics, education, and occupations.
2. *Communication includes both verbal and nonverbal communication.*
3. *Family roles and organization* include the structure of the family and gender roles, extended family, roles of the aged and social status.
4. *Workforce issues* include acculturation to the work, autonomy and supervisory issues, and language barriers.

5. *Biocultural ecology* includes biological and genetic variations, skin color, and drug metabolism.
6. *High-risk behaviors* include safety, tobacco, alcohol, recreational drugs, and physical activity.
7. *Nutrition* includes common foods, the meaning of foods, deficiencies, and health promotion.
8. *Pregnancy* includes attitudes toward fertility and pregnancy, birthing, and postpartum.
9. *Death rituals include* rituals after death and bereavement.
10. *Spirituality* includes religious rituals and practices, prayer, and the meaning of life.
11. *Health care practices* include traditional practices, pain medication, and sick roles.
12. *Health care practitioners* include gender and health care and perceptions of practitioners and folk practitioners.

Hofstede's Cultural Dimensions Model

Geert Hofstede's model is based on six dimensions that can be used to analyze and compare the cultural values of different countries:

1. *Power distance index (PDI):* Do people question authority and try to distribute power? In contrast, to what degree do they accept that less powerful members of a family or society accept that power is not distributed equitably?
2. *Individualism vs. collectivism:* To what degree does a society support individualism, versus loyalty to a family or group?
3. *Uncertainty avoidance (UAI):* To what extent do people tolerate ambiguity and change in the status quo?
4. *Masculinity vs. femininity (MAS):* Do members of the society embrace traditionally held masculine versus feminine values? (Author's note: This dichotomy contains some out-of-date stereotypes.)
5. *Long-term orientation vs. short-term orientation (LTO):* Are traditions honored and

maintained, or do members of the society (often poorer) value pragmatic, short-term change to adapt to difficult circumstances?

6. *Indulgence vs. restraint (MD):* Does the society allow short-term gratification of human desires or regulate this via restrictive and strict norms? (Hofstede, 2001)

This model reveals the potential impact of a society's culture on the values of its members.

Conclusion

It is incumbent upon clinicians to offer culturally competent care to PWUAACs and their communi-cation partners, and to exercise cultural humility. While each of the three models offers a unique perspective of cultural values, they are best applied in tandem with a clinician's curiosity and non-judgmental acceptance of values that differ from their own.

References

Hall, E. (1976). *Beyond culture.* Anchor Books.

Hofstede, G. (2001). *Culture's consequences: Comparing values, behaviors, institutions, and organizations across nations* (2nd ed.). SAGE Publications.

Purnell, L. (2002). The Purnell Model for Cultural Competence. *Journal of Transcultural Nursing, 13*(3), 193–196. https://doi.org/10.1177/10459602013003006

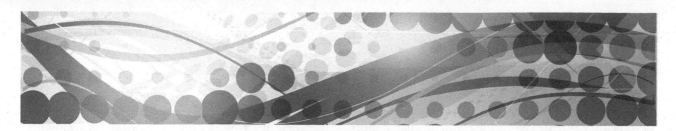

Essay 4

CULTURAL CONSIDERATIONS AND AAC: INTRODUCTION TO AFRICAN AMERICAN CULTURE— CULTURAL VALUES AND COMMUNICATING RESPECT

Paula K. Davis

Understanding cultural norms is critical in relating to and communicating with patients and clients and building bridges to respectful and reciprocal relationships. African Americans' cultural norms vary as they are not a monolithic group in origin, ethnicity, socioeconomic status, and so on. While the U.S. Census uses the collective term "Black/ African American" to categorize peoples from the African diaspora (Gatison, 2017), until recently, African Americans have largely comprised individuals descended from African people brought to America in the slave trade from 1619 to 1859. "African American" typically refers to Black people born in the United States; however, Black people in the United States also include first- and second-generation immigrants from Africa and first- and subsequent-generation immigrants from the Caribbean (also descendants of enslaved Africans) who may refer to themselves according to their family's country of origin (i.e., Haitian, Jamaican). Thus, given immigration and diasporic spread, Black people residing in the United States are a diverse group. This variety in origin also drives variety in experience and perspective. There are two values that persist in the culture of Black Amer-

icans descended from those enslaved in the United States—trust and respect.

Purnell (2003) posits that culture is

the totality of socially transmitted behavioral patterns, arts, beliefs, values, customs, life-ways, and all other products of human work and thought characteristics of a population of people that guide their world view and decision making. These patterns may be explicit or implicit, are primarily learned and transmitted within the family, are shared by most members of the culture, and are emergent phenomena that change in response to global phenomena. Culture is learned first in the family, then in school, then in the community and other social organizations such as the church. (p. 3)

Thus, culture is borne not solely of individual and internal experiences but also of the interplay of varied perspectives including those external to the person or group. American culture was constructed to support a hegemonic structure affording privileges to Whites and denying privileges to Blacks. Jim Crow and other laws codified Black peoples' American existence as "other" and disparities in health care, education, housing, and employment driven by systemic racism persist to this day. Years of medical research that objectified and abused Black bodies (such as the U.S. Public Health Service Syphilis Study, also known as the Tuskegee Syphilis Study; Dr. J. Marion Sims's fistula experiments performed on enslaved women; and the misappropriation of Henrietta Lacks's cells for research) fostered a deep and ever-present mistrust in medical research and health care and those who provide it. As the world combats the COVID-19 pandemic, advances in vaccine research have allowed for rapid development; however, persistent mistrust in medical systems has led many in Black communities to delay or reject vaccination, even as those communities experience disproportionate levels of COVID-19 infection. While levels of medical mistrust by African Americans may vary by age, education, geography, and other factors, practitioners will likely encounter individuals for whom that mistrust persists in their engagement with health care and its systems.

While American culture wrestles with eliminating social injustice and dismantling racism embedded in systems—including health care—providers must work to establish trusting relationships with African American patients. Key to establishing those trusting relationships is ensuring patients feel respected—acknowledged, heard, and valued. According to Briggs and colleagues (2015, p. 270), African American racial respect is defined as "the experience of inherent worth through affirming and nurturing relationships between African Americans and their family, peers, and society," which acts as a counterbalance to persistent social injustice, upholding values of racial resiliency and psychological well-being. This core value persists within African American culture in response to years of infantilization while owned as chattel and

diminution of standing as free, equal Americans during Jim Crow segregation in years following. Thus, having that same respect of self and family reflected by others is critical. Elders are highly regarded and are to be treated as such, addressed formally instead of in the familiar (i.e., Miss Jones, or Miss Rosa—never "Rosa"). Irreparable gaps between provider and patient can develop should patients feel they are not respected as fully formed, contributing citizens.

Providers can mitigate mistrust by first examining their own biases to be certain they do not bring stereotyped views and attitudes into interactions; second, honoring the cultural grounding of clients and patients; and third, listening actively and taking time to have conversation and establish rapport. Understand that your African American patients and clients may have had many clashes with systems and structures that have not afforded them that sense of respect and value so critical to their self-perceptions.

References

Briggs, H., Kothari, B., Briggs, A. C., Bank, L., & DeGruy, J. (2015). Racial respect: Initial testing and validation of the racial respect scale. *Journal of the Society for Social Work and Research*, 6(2), 269–303. https://doi.org/10.1086/681625

Gattison, A.M. (2017) African American Communication and Culture. In M. Allen, *The SAGE Encyclopedia of Communication Research Methods. In the SAGE Encyclopedia of Communication Research Methods*. (pp. 15–19). SAGE Publications. https://doi.org/10.4135/9781483381411

Purnell, L. (2003). Transcultural diversity and health care. In L. Purnell & B. Paulanka (Eds.), *Transcultural health care: A culturally competent approach* (2nd ed., pp. 1–7). F. A. Davis.

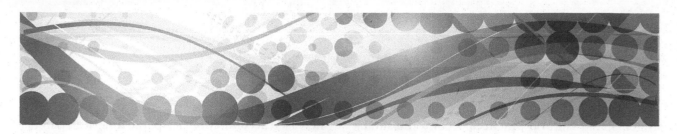

Essay 5

CULTURAL CONSIDERATIONS AND AAC: INTRODUCTION TO HISPANIC CULTURE—CULTURAL VALUES AND COMMUNICATING RESPECT

Glen M. Tellis

The United States is deemed to be a melting pot, where people from various countries and cultural backgrounds apparently live a homogeneous existence; however, the melting pot phenomenon has been supplanted by a pluralistic view of American society (Lynch & Hanson, 2011). Within the Hispanic culture, for example, many individuals in the United States keep their separate identities and maintain their subcultures while contributing to the whole composition of society. Green (1982) suggested that American society is now a transactional entity where individuals identify with certain ethnic and cultural groups but also recognize the larger society. It becomes difficult to categorize these groups as being similar to each other since they maintain their own attitudes, behaviors, beliefs, and lifestyles (Leith, 1986).

By 1970, many immigrants entered the United States from Mexico, South America, the Caribbean, and Central America. With the influx of new arrivals, for the 1970 census, the U.S. government officially created the term "Hispanic" to identify people from these regions or origins—regardless of race (U.S. Census Bureau, 1996). The term "Hispanic" was based on origin, descent, nationality group, lineage, or the country in which a person's ancestors were born; however, many in these communities prefer the term "Latinos" or "Hispanic Americans." For the remainder of this essay, therefore, the term "Hispanic American" or "Latino" will be used.

The estimated population of the United States as of January 1, 2021, was approximately 329.5 million. From this population, 18.5% were of Hispanic origin (U.S. Census Bureau, 2020). Mexicans make up the largest subgroup of Hispanic Americans. By 2050, it is estimated that the Hispanic-origin population will increase to 29%, and the White non-Hispanic population will be about 47% (Passel & Cohn, 2008).

Cultural Values and Communicating Respect

Latino cultural groups usually have their own traits in universal categories of behavior (e.g., values, family structure, communication, world view, learning styles) (Arredondo et al., 2014). The exact rules within these classifications, however, appear to be culture specific. Even though differences occur among various cultural groups, abundant overlaps exist (Banks, 2008). For example, attitudes toward family, roles of individuals in a community, belief systems, and cultural practices seem to be similar in various cultures.

Respect for Authority

In the United States, the traditional patriarchal organization of Latino family life is transforming; however, the family is still very interdependent and supportive (Galanti, 2003). Hispanic American culture traditionally is conservative and has a patriarchal structure. Authority figures, especially the father, are respected. The father or the oldest male in the family expects females to be submissive, provide emotional support, and run the daily activities of the family (Kemp & Rasbridge, 2004). When talking to adults, children may look away or lower their heads because maintenance of eye contact during conversation is considered a sign of disrespect and a challenge to authority. It is expected that older children take care of their younger siblings, but decision-making remains with the parents.

Cultural Values and Other Aspects

The Latino culture is collectivistic in nature. Responsibility is shared, and group activity is the norm where people ask each other for opinions. The goals of the group are important, and the group works hard for the benefit of the community as a whole. Cooperation is central within Hispanic American culture; individuality is not emphasized (Gudykunst, 1998). Cooperation is valued over competitiveness. Success is often attributed to fate or destiny, while a person's academic or technical accomplishments are not as important.

In the Latino culture, standing in close proximity or touching another person during conversations is acceptable. Kissing, hugging, and patting each other on the back are part of the culture. When Hispanic Americans meet someone new, they may kiss the person on the cheek or hug the other person. Building relationships is important within the culture (Truxillo, 1995), and the family unit and the extended family and friends are con-

tinuously evolving because of acculturation. With increased acculturation, Hispanic American parents tend to subscribe to egalitarian gender attitudes (Leaper & Valin, 1996).

Acculturation takes place when attitudes and/or behaviors of persons from one culture change because of exposure to a different culture (Moyerman & Forman, 1992). The process of change is often regarded as a form of adaptation (Berry, 1980). On a daily basis, Latinos are in contact with mainstream cultures in the United States. Because of this contact, it is probable that changes may occur in Hispanic American norms, attitudes, values, and behaviors (Gordon, 2010). When immigrants are exposed to a new group, culture, or nation, a cultural learning process takes place (Berry, 1980). Along with acculturation, generations in the United States (i.e., how many generations of a family has lived in the United States) and the educational level of parents and children are additional factors to consider as families transform, assimilate, and acculturate from generation to generation.

In summary, Latinos in the United States are a fast-growing, vibrant, diverse, and constantly evolving population. Most Hispanic Americans were born in the United States, and a number of the cultural aspects discussed in this essay may not be relevant to these populations because of acculturation, generational shifts, and educational levels. Nonetheless, the information that was provided in this essay can be used as a guide when interacting with Latinos.

References

Arredondo, P., Gallardo-Cooper, M., Delgado-Romero, E. & Zapata, A. (2014). *Culturally responsive counseling with Latinas/os.* American Counseling Association.

Banks, J. A. (2008). *Teaching strategies for ethnic studies.* Pearson.

Berry, J. W. (1980). Acculturation as varieties of adaptation. In A. M. Padilla (Ed.), *Acculturation: Theory, models, and some new findings* (pp. 9–25). Westview Press.

Galanti, G. A. (2003). The Hispanic family and male-female relationships: An overview. *Journal of Transcultural Nursing, 14*(3), 180–185.

Gordon, M. M. (2010). *Assimilation in American life: The role of race, religion, and national origins.* Oxford University Press.

Green, J. W. (1982). *Cultural awareness in the human services.* Prentice Hall.

Gudykunst, W. B. (1998). *Interpersonal comments, bridging differences: Effective intergroup communication* (3rd ed.). Sage Publications.

Kemp, C., & Rasbridge, L. A. (2004). *Refugee and immigrant health: A handbook for health professionals.* Cambridge University Press.

Leaper, C., & Valin, D. (1996). Predictors of Mexican-American mothers' and fathers' attitudes toward gender equality. *Hispanic Journal of Behavioral Sciences, 18*(3), 343–355.

Leith, W. R. (1986). Treating the stutterer with atypical cultural influences. In K. St. Louis (Ed.), *The atypical stutterer.* Academic.

Lynch, E., & Hanson, M. (2011). *Developing cross-cultural competence* (4th ed.). Paul H. Brookes.

Moyerman, D. R., & Forman, B. D. (1992). Acculturation and adjustment: A meta-analysis study. *Hispanic Journal of Behavioral Sciences, 14*(2), 163–200.

Passel, J. S., & Cohn, D. (2008). *U.S. population projections: 2005–2050.* Pew Research Center. https://www.pewresearch.org/hispanic/2008/02/11/us-population-projections-2005-2050/

Truxillo, C. (1995). Hispanic culture. *The Americas, 51,* 421–422. https://doi.org/10.1017/S000316150002263X

U.S. Census Bureau. (1996). Population projections of the United States by age, sex, race, and Hispanic origin: 1995 to 2050. *Current Population Reports* (Series P25-1130). Government Printing Office, Bureau of the Census, Current Population Reports.

U.S. Census Bureau. (2020). *U.S. Hispanic population growth.* https://www.census.gov/library/visualizations/2020/comm/us-hispanic-population-growth.html

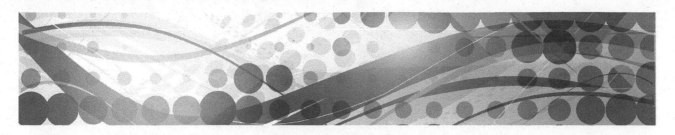

Essay 6

CULTURAL CONSIDERATIONS AND AAC: LGBTQIA+ AFFIRMATIVE PRACTICE: EMPOWERING OUR QUEER CLIENTS AND FAMILIES

Gazit Chaya Nkosi

The Queer community has often been referred to with variations of the acronym LGBTQIA+ (lesbian, gay, bisexual, pansexual, transgender, genderqueer, queer, questioning, intersexed, agender, asexual, and ally) in an attempt to represent the vast diversity of gender identities and sexual orientations within the community. As the acronym has proven insufficient to hold every unique identity represented in the community, many individuals and organizations are embracing the word "queer" as a more inclusive umbrella term that acknowledges a matrix of gender identities, sexual preferences, orientations, and habits. The Queer community is as varied and complex as the entire human population, with significant intersectionality in terms of ability, age, ethnicity, cultural-linguistic identity, race, religion, and socioeconomic status/class. Because queer people exist in every part of the world, in every age group, and across every other identity, speech-language pathologists (SLPs) in every setting will inevitably work with queer clients and colleagues whether they may realize it or not. "SLPs are in a unique position to support clients in expressing their authentic voices. Given that SLPs work in a variety of home- and community-based settings, it is essential that SLPs be ready to empower LGBTQ+ individuals as they develop or regain communication skills within their natural environments" (Taylor et al., 2018, p. 72).

SLPs working with persons who use augmentative and alternative communication (PWUAAC) are even more likely to serve clients with queer identities. "Indeed, there is a significant overlap between the LGBT and disabled worlds, as disabilities are more common among LGBT people than among the general population. The converse is also true: disabled people are more likely to identify as a sexual minority than are abled people." (Noe, 2018, p. 29) Additionally, within communities with individuals who identify as culturally deaf, autistic, and/or neurodiverse, and others with intersecting multiple marginalized identities, there is reported to be increased acceptance and pride in divergence from mainstream cultural norms, including those related to gender and sexuality (Couture, 2016). "Research and anecdote dealing in autistic sexual and gender identities present the picture of a group of people who may not conform to (cis) gender binaries, (hetero)sexual norms, or discrete sexual categories of a 'heterosexual, bisexual, or homosexual' nature" (Jackson-Perry, 2020, p. 221). Queer individuals also experience disproportionately greater risk for health concerns and disability related to chronic stress from institutional reinforcement of heterosexual/cisgender customs, legal and social discrimination, daily microaggressions, disproportionately higher levels of poverty and resulting limits to preventative medicine and healthcare access, and delay of care in order to avoid discrimination (Noe, 2018).

While "LGBTQ+ affirmative practice is within the scope of an SLP's role and is consistent with the American Speech-Language-Hearing Association Code of Ethics," SLPs must be aware that there is often significant risk involved with disclosure of one's queer identity. For most, our identities are a primary source of family, social, and cultural connection and support. However, queer people disproportionately experience rejection or disconnection based on this aspect of their identity from their families of origin, their religious community, their cultural community, the institutional and legal systems, and/or society at large. Worldwide, there continue to be legal and cultural barriers to queer people's ability to live their lives authentically and access health care safely. "LGBT persons face a common set of challenges within the health care system. These challenges range from access to health care coverage and culturally competent care to state and federal policies that reinforce social stigma, marginalization, or discrimination." (Daniel & Butkus, 2015, p. 135)

Revealing one's queer identity can create significant safety risks for individuals in terms of family connection, social standing, legal standing, and housing and job security. Given this, providers should ensure they understand the individual risks for their clients (both personal and legal) and create opportunities for clients and colleagues to understand that they are ready to affirm and empower the individual without relying on the individual to "out" themselves or reveal their queer identity.

Simultaneously, it is vital that providers not "out" their clients or reveal their queer identity without explicit permission, even to the client's parents, family members, and significant others. It is important to ask your client what pronouns, name, or identity they want to use in a specific setting versus others. A client may not be using a specific name or pronoun at home or work due to lack of family acceptance or other form of discrimination. Respecting these choices and ensuring confidentiality in the therapeutic setting may allow for a client to interact authentically.

Additionally, providers should avoid assuming their client's identity based on stereotypes. For example, a client may present with short hair, refer to their "partner," wear a tie and button-down shirt, use she/her pronouns, and identify as a straight, cisgender woman. Another client may appear the same, use they/them pronouns, be referred to as "mom" by their children, and identify as transmasculine. Another client may have a beard along with physical traits typically associated with "women" and identify as a cisgender woman, a trans man, or a nonbinary individual. The combination of physical traits, clothing choices, names, and pronouns are infinite. There are no "signs" or rules of physical presentation or language that can be attributed to any individual queer identity. The prevailing myths and stereotypes around how queer and trans people "look" are misleading and damaging to the community. Using incorrect pronouns (misgendering) or assuming one's gender identity or sexual orientation prior to the individual's disclosure is experienced as a microaggression.

While it is important to avoid explicit or implicit discrimination, it is equally as important to be intentional about using signals in our physical space, the way our forms and materials are set up, and the language we use to clearly indicate that we are an LGBTQ+ affirmative provider. The first step in cultural humility around working with individuals in the Queer community is to do an honest baseline analysis of our current beliefs, physical space, materials, and language practices.

Part of our professional ethics includes a commitment to ensuring that our personal beliefs do not become a barrier to our ability to provide affirmative and empowering care to every client we serve. If our personal beliefs are not affirmative of queer individuals, it is our professional commitment to leave that out of our work life just as we would with any other religious or personal belief. SLPs may need to seek support from their professional advisors, colleagues, and religious or spiritual leaders in navigating this necessary commitment to cultural humility and unbiased care in the workplace.

In our physical space, providers can put up visual indicators to our clients, parents, and colleagues to demonstrate that we are an LGBTQ+ affirmative provider, such as, but not limited to, signs ensuring client confidentiality, "safe space" stickers or signs that incorporate a rainbow flag or transgender pride flag, the "Gender Unicorn" chart (*The Gender Unicorn*, 2015), and pins or name tags that list our name and pronouns (e.g., "Hello my name is ____, my pronouns are they/them/theirs"). In our offices and schools, we can advocate for gender-neutral restroom options and support our clients in their ability to communicate their needs around restroom safety and choice.

In our materials and forms, we can ensure that we provide space for clients to list: legal name along with preferred name, pronouns, sex assigned at birth (male/female) and gender (leave blank for client to fill), parent 1 and 2 (rather than mother/father), siblings/children (rather than sisters/brothers/son/daughter), and include "partnered" as option along with "married, divorced, etc." as some may not have access to or want of legal marriage. On our e-mail signature, we can include our pronouns and encourage everyone in our organization to do the same. Additionally, we can ensure that our books and visuals include stories and depictions of all types of families, individuals, relationships, and children.

For AAC tools and materials, providers should work directly with PWUAAC to include specific vocabulary relevant to gender identity and sexual orientation. PWUAAC may themselves be queer identified; however, they may also need this vocabulary for interacting with and affirming the people in their family, social, and/or professional communities. The vocabulary to be included will be specific to each PWUAAC; however, a brief selection of vocabulary with definitions is included with this essay. These definitions are general and may be different according to the individual. Providers are encouraged to offer these as a starting point and then to follow the guidance of their client as to which items are relevant and appropriate for their individual needs.

In our language, we can explicitly state our pronouns when we introduce ourselves (e.g., "My name is ____, my pronouns are hy, hym, hys."), ask our clients and their support people their pronouns ("What are your pronouns?"), ask our clients if they have a significant other or partner (rather than boyfriend/girlfriend, husband/wife, or asking if they are married, etc.), use the singular "they" to refer to persons who have not yet been identified with pronouns, accept and affirm the grammatical validity of the use of the singular pronouns "they, them, theirs, themself/ves," and explicitly state that all information shared will be kept confidential when asking background and demographic questions. Additionally, providers can check in with pronouns and names, regularly acknowledging that many individuals' identities and expression exist on a continuum, and names, pronouns, presentation, and identities may shift from one meeting to the next or one setting to another. Providers should also avoid stating that the use of affirming language is "hard for them," asking if they can use pronouns or names that the client previously used because "they are used to it," and/or excessive apologizing or drawing of attention to errors with pronouns or other language related to gender identity or sexual orientation. When a mistake is made, the provider is encouraged to apologize briefly, correct the error, and move forward.

All of these practices support us in becoming affirming and empowering providers for our queer PWUAAC and their support community. However, it is essential that providers pursue continuing education; authentic dialogue with queer family members, friends, colleagues, and clients; and professional and civic engagement in removing institutional, legal, and governmental barriers for queer individuals and all peoples. Striving for cultural humility allows us to continue to grow and expand our professional proficiency and efficacy. Cultural humility "is defined by flexibility; awareness of bias; a lifelong, learning-oriented approach to working with diversity; and a recognition of the role of power in health care interactions" (Agner, 2020, p. 1).

Vocabulary and Definitions

Adapted from: Michigan Medicine, Adolescent Health Initiative, 2014.

AFAB: Assigned female at birth.

Ally: A person who is a member of the dominant group who works to end oppression in their own personal and professional life by supporting and advocating with the oppressed population.

AMAB: Assigned male at birth.

Asexual/aromantic: Asexual people experience little to no sexual attraction, aromantic people experience little to no romantic attraction. Some, but not all, asexual people are aromantic.

Biological sex: The sum of the biological (chromosomal hormonal, and anatomical) factors that make an individual male, female, or intersex.

Bisexual/pansexual: Romantic attraction, sexual attraction, or sexual behavior toward both males and females, or to more than one sex or gender. It may also be defined as romantic or sexual attraction to people of any sex or gender identity, which is also known as pansexuality.

Cisgender: Someone whose gender identity is the same as the biological sex they were assigned at birth.

Coming Out: To declare and affirm both to oneself and to others one's identity as queer. Individuals may live with varying levels of "outness" across settings according to the level of safety within each context or personal preference.

FTM: Female-to-male transgender man.

Gay males/men: A person who identifies as a man/male who experiences sexual and/or romantic attraction with other individuals who identify as men/male.

Gender binary: The idea that there are only two genders (male/female).

Gender identity: A person's self-identified sense of being male or female (or neither or both). This term refers to how people think about and express their gender.

Gender identity spectrum: The acknowledgment that, while individuals may choose to self-identify with one specific label or identity; it is healthy for an individual's gender to exist on a spectrum

allowing for identity, expression, presentation, and pronouns to change and shift throughout one's life.

Gender pronouns: Personal pronouns are used in place of nouns referring to people. Some examples include he/him/his, she/her/hers, they/them/theirs/themselves, ze/zie/hir/hirs/hirself, xe/xem/xyr/xyrs/xemself, ey/em/eir/eirs/emself.

Heterosexism: Discrimination or prejudice by heterosexuals against individuals who identify as queer in terms of sexuality.

Homophobia: Thoughts, feelings, or actions based on fear, dislike, judgment, or hatred of individuals who identify as queer in terms of sexuality. Homophobia has roots in sexism and can include prejudice, discrimination, harassment, and acts of violence.

Intersex: A person born with sex chromosomes, external genitalia, and/or an internal reproductive system that is not considered explicitly male or female.

LGBTQIA+: An acronym representing lesbian, gay, bisexual, pansexual, transgender, genderqueer, queer, questioning, intersexed, agender, asexual, and ally.

Lesbian: A person who identifies as a woman/female who experiences sexual and/or romantic attraction with other individuals who identify as women/female.

Medical transition: A part of transition in which a transgender person undergoes medical treatments (gender affirming surgeries and/or cross-sex hormone therapy) so that their sex characteristics better match their gender identity.

MTF: Male-to-female transgender woman.

Nonbinary: Individual who identifies as a gender that is beyond the gender binary. Nonbinary individuals may identify as genderfluid, agender (without gender), genderqueer, or something else entirely.

Partners/significant others: An inclusive term for referring to one's romantic partner, using the plural is inclusive of individuals who may have multiple partners.

Polyamory/polyamorous: The practice of, or desire for, intimate relationships with more than one partner, with the informed consent of all partners involved. It has been described as consensual, ethical, and responsible nonmonogamy.

Queer: An umbrella term that acknowledges a matrix of gender identities, sexual preferences, orientations, and habits not represented by the cisgender-heteronormative culture.

Sexual identity spectrum: The acknowledgment that, while individuals may choose to self-identify with one specific label or identity, it is healthy for an individual's sexuality to exist on a spectrum allowing for identity, expression, partner choice, and sexual practices to change and shift throughout one's life.

Sexual orientation: How a person identifies and interacts with others sexually and/or romantically, meaning the physical and emotional ways we are attracted to or interact with persons of the same gender, another gender, or all genders.

Transgender: Someone whose gender identity is different from the biological sex they were assigned to at birth.

Transphobia: The fear or hatred of transgender people or gender nonconforming behavior. Like biphobia, transphobia can also exist within the Queer community as well as among cisgender, heterosexual people.

Transition: The process a gender diverse person undergoes when changing their body, bodily appearance, pronouns, presentation, documentation, and other aspects of self in relation to the world to be more congruent with the gender/sex they feel themselves to be.

References

Agner, J. (2020). Moving from cultural competence to cultural humility in occupational therapy: A paradigm shift. *American Journal of Occupational Therapy, 74*(4). https://doi.org/10.5014/ajot.2020.038067

Couture, V. G. (2016). Multiple minority identities: Applications for practice, research, and training. *Journal of Rehabilitation, 82*(1).

Daniel, H., & Butkus, R. (2015). Lesbian, gay, bisexual, and transgender health disparities: Executive summary of a policy position paper for the American College of Physicians. *Annals of Internal Medicine, 163*, 135–137.

Jackson-Perry, D. (2020). The autistic art of failure? Unknowing imperfect systems of sexuality and gender. *Scandinavian Journal of Disability Research, 22*(1), 221–229.

Michigan Medicine, Adolescent Health Initiative. (2014). *LGBTQ+ Youth-Friendly Services Starter Guide.*

Noe, D. (2018). Squaring the disability. *Gay & Lesbian Review Worldwide, 25*(3).

Taylor, S., Barr, B-D., O'Neal-Khaw, J., Schlichtig, B., & Hawley, J. L. (2018). Refining your queer ear: Empowering LGBTQ+ clients in speech-language pathology practice. *Perspectives of the ASHA Special Interest Groups, SIG 14, 3*(14), 72–86.

The Gender Unicorn. (2015). Trans Student Educational Resources. http://www.transstudent.org/gender

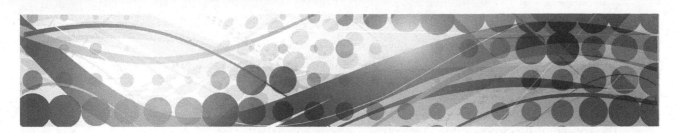

Essay 7

CULTURAL CONSIDERATIONS AND AAC: SELF-EVALUATION OF CULTURAL COMPETENCE

Dorian Lee-Wilkerson and Shelly Chabon

Communication sciences and disorders (CSD) professionals will often evaluate their cultural comfort and knowledge in preparation for and implementation of assessment and treatment, examining whether their clinical interactions are somehow altered when they do not share cultural traits such as race, ethnicity, language, or income with the individuals being served. They may wonder if gender, gender identity, or sexual orientation influences their choice of treatment approaches and treatment materials and the ways in which they interact with those they serve. CSD professionals will evaluate whether age or perceptions of disability and ableness influence levels of participation and use this data to plan activities that would diminish these effects. CSD professionals will consider if their understanding of communication strengths, challenges, and needs align with the perceptions and expectations of individuals served (American Speech-Language-Hearing Association [ASHA], 2017; U.S. Department of Health and Human Services [USDHHS], 2018). This reflective process of evaluating one's cultural competence informs professionals about how and why consideration of cultural differences is an important overarching framework that supports accurate interpretation and good use of clinical data, efficient and effective implementation of assessment and treatment strategies, and the development of clinical innovations that improve clinical outcomes.

There has been some discussion about whether CSD professionals should aspire toward cultural competence, cultural humility, or cultural responsiveness. It is true that how one names an entity and defines it determines how one measures or assesses it. Words can be fateful. Some CSD professionals may use the term "cultural competence" to describe the knowledge and skill used to navigate cross-cultural interactions, and how well they can move in and out of different cultural groups, not allowing their own cultural background to have unwanted effects on their clinical practices (Greene-Moton & Minkler, 2020; Gregory, 2020; Mayfield, 2020). The concept of "cultural humility," as introduced in the essay preceding this, describes a commitment to creating a culture of inclusion in the clinical process through a continuous process of self-evaluation and self-critique (Greene-Moton & Minkler, 2020; Hyter & Salas-Provance, 2019). The concept of "cultural responsiveness" has been used to describe skill in responding to and serving individuals within the context of their cultural background (Gay, 2010). To evaluate your cultural competence, we suggest the following:

1. Examine your cultural humility:
   a. Assess your privilege. Have you benefited from your race, gender, education, height, weight, hair color, your ability to see, hear, walk, talk, swallow, and/or your families' income (Oluo, 2018)?

b. Assess your cultural knowledge and the source of this knowledge. Are you motivated to learn more about unfamiliar cultures? Do you think that learning more about different cultural groups will increase your clinical competence?

c. Assess your explicit and implicit biases. Are you vulnerable to the influences of stereotyping?

d. Assess your prejudices. Do you unknowingly commit microaggressions?

2. Examine your cultural competence:

a. Are you aware of the stereotypes and biases that influence your clinical decision-making?

b. Do you consider the ways your cultural values and beliefs, and the ways the cultural values and beliefs of individuals served influence the conscious and unconscious behaviors that occur during the clinical process?

c. Are you open to new experiences that inform you about the cultural values, beliefs, and practices of others?

d. Do you actively seek to eliminate or reduce bias in your assessment and treatment practices?

e. Do you participate in collaborative partnerships to advocate for diversity, equity, and inclusion?

3. Examine your cultural responsiveness:

a. Do you respect and hold individuals served in high regard, ensuring that their perspectives are valued and integrated into the clinical decision-making process (Royal, 2020)?

b. Do you actively seek to build trusting relationships with individuals served by caring enough to understand and advocate for their interests (Royal, 2020)?

c. Do you use the cultural background of individuals served as the overarching framework when developing clinical practices ensuring that you "do no harm" (ASHA, 2010)?

d. Do you intentionally include culturally relevant knowledge in assessment and therapy practices and materials (Gay, 2010)?

e. Do you acknowledge when you or others commit microaggressions and seek to be an ally to those targeted (Anderson, 2021a, 2021b)?

References

American Speech-Language-Hearing Association. (2010). *Cultural Competence Checklist: Personal reflection.* http://www.asha.org/uploadedFiles/Cultural-Competence-Checklist-Personal-Reflection.pdf

American Speech-Language-Hearing Association. (2017). *Issues in ethics: Cultural and linguistic competence.* https://www.asha.org/practice/ethics/cultural-and-linguistic-competence/

Anderson, N. (2021a). *Combatting microaggressions: How can I help?* ASHA Learning Center (WEB19983). https://learningcenter.asha.org/diweb/catalog/item/id/6276635

Anderson, N. (2021b). *Recognizing microaggressions: Am I doing that?* ASHA Learning Center (WEB19980). https://learningcenter.asha.org/diweb/catalog/item/id/6276597

Gay, G. (2010). *Culturally responsive teaching: Theory, research, and practice* (2nd ed.) [Multicultural Education Series]. Teachers College.

Greene-Moton, E., & Minkler, M. (2020). Cultural competence or cultural humility? *Moving beyond the debate. Health Promotion Practice, 21*(1), 142–145. https://doi.org/10.1177/1524839919884912

Gregory, K. (2020). Moving forward as a profession in a time of uncertainty. *ASHA Leader Live.* https://leader.pubs.asha.org/do/10.1044/leader.FMP.25082020.8/full/

Hyter, Y., & Salas-Provance, M. (2019). *Culturally responsive practices in speech, language and hearing sciences.* Plural Publishing.

Mayfield, V. (2020). *Cultural competence now.* ASCD.

Oluo, I. (2018). *So you want to talk about race.* Seal Press.

Royal, K. (2020). Equity summit, Portland State University. Portland, Oregon, October 30..https://www.pdx.edu/diversity/equity-summit

U.S. Department of Health and Human Services, Office of Minority Health. (2018). *Think cultural health.* https://minorityhealth.hhs.gov/omh/browse.aspx?lvl=2&lvlid=53

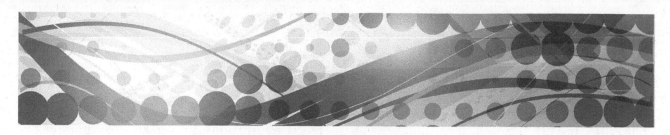

Essay 8

CULTURAL CONSIDERATIONS AND AAC: RELIGIOUS CONSIDERATIONS

John W. Gareis

Whether it is through Shaman and Medicine-men, the latest Papal pronouncement on abortion or stem cell research, or members of a hospital's chaplaincy team, religion and health care have had a unique relationship throughout history. So important is religion to health care, in fact, that Purnell lists it—along with nationality, race, color, gender, and age—as one of the six primary characteristics of culture in his Model for Cultural Competence (Purnell 2002). And while understandable importance is attributed to the other characteristics, the one that is often neglected is religion. Several articles written over the past few years, however, discuss the important connection that often exists for patients between their religious beliefs and health care. As one author writes,

> Healthcare providers should be respectful of a patient's religious and spiritual needs. Many patient's anxieties are reduced when they turn to their faith during healthcare challenges. Because many patients turn to their beliefs when difficult healthcare decisions are made, it is vital for healthcare professionals to recognize and accommodate the patient's religious and spiritual needs. Health professionals should provide an opportunity for patients to discuss their religious and spiritual beliefs and tailor their evaluation and treatment to meet their specific needs. (Swihart et al., 2020, p. 612)

Such reliance on religious beliefs not only provides the patient with much needed comfort and support in difficult situations, but it is often viewed as a stabilizing force in the face of an otherwise confusing and uncertain decision. Indeed, religion and spirituality can impact a patient's decisions regarding treatment procedures and medication. Some of the more common areas of concern include diet, prescription medication, and medical procedures.

Diet

Many religions have very strict restrictions on what may or may not be eaten by adherents. Judaism, for example, forbids the consumption of pork, shellfish, and meat that has not been slaughtered and prepared properly. Hindis do not eat beef but will consume milk and other dairy products; and, although restrictions have loosened in the past few decades, Catholics often give themselves to a fish-only diet on certain days of the week or during special seasons of the church year. Muslims also have dietary restrictions. As one article reporting the eating habits of Muslim students at U.S. universities pointed out, "Muslim students were concerned about consuming Halal food (foods that are allowed under Islamic guidelines). Due to the limited access to the Halal food items in the United

States, they are consuming fewer meats" (Alakaam et al., 2015, p. 112).

Dietary issues not only cover what or what not to eat, but also when food may or may not be eaten. Some observe mandatory fasts that can last for hours or days, depending on the holiday or season of the year. For example, Muslims are expected to fast during the entire month of Ramadan.

Prescription Medication

Another component of health care that is influenced by a patient's religious beliefs is medication. Here the issues range from concerns about how some medicines are manufactured to what they contain. As Joy Ogden states in her article, *Religious Constraints on Prescribing Medication*:

> Many pharmaceutical products have constituents that would have implications for Jewish, Muslim, Hindu and Sikh patients. Those with active ingredients directly derived from animals include: heparin, an injectable anticoagulant, that is commonly extracted from porcine intestinal mucosa or bovine lung; conjugated oestrogens, used in some HRT preparations, derived from pregnant mares' urine; and insulin (bovine or porcine) extracted from the pancreas of cows or pigs. (Ogden, 2016, pp. 48–49)

A more recent concern for some religious groups is the development of medications through stem cell research. The U.S. Roman Catholic bishops oppose the research as "immoral, illegal, and unnecessary" since they believe that life is sacred from the moment of conception. Other groups, however, hold that a fertilized egg does not hold the full status of personhood.

Medical Procedures

Religious objections are fairly well known in regard to such procedures as abortion and organ transplants. Other areas of concern may include blood transfusions, preventative medication like vaccines, and sexual health beyond reproduction. In fact, some religious hospitals disallow sharing information about the use of condoms to prevent transmission of HIV/AIDS and sexually transmitted diseases. Another major area of concern is end-of-life (EoL) decisions.

That there is a wide variety of thought regarding EoL and life-sustaining care among religious groups is not overly surprising, even among physicians. One study reported that physicians in the United States with a Roman Catholic affiliation "were three times more likely to object to withdrawal of life support, compared to Protestants and Jews, and those with no religious affiliation" (Curlin et al., 2008, p. 115). One can only imagine, then, how those numbers look among patients and family members facing EoL decisions. It would seem, then, that having this information in advance could prevent some future clashes or misunderstandings between patients, family members, and health care providers.

For while some cases can be treated with alternative measures, others occasionally require legal intervention to resolve the matter.

Conclusion

There are a myriad of other issues that can be added to the list of concerns for people of faith relating to health care. The three discussed earlier, however, provide ample support for the ongoing need for health care workers to become familiar with their patients' religious beliefs. As the *AMA Journal of Ethics* pointed out in a 2018 article:

> Religion and spirituality will continue to influence health care on both patient and community levels. It is up to the medical community to appreciate this fact and educate trainees on religion and spirituality's role in health care, (and) recognizing the roles of religion and spirituality in medicine can help clinicians approach their patients. (Zaidi, 2018, p. 611)

References

Alakaam, A., Castellanos, D., Bodzio, J., & Harrison, L. (2015). The factors that influence dietary habits among international students in the United States. *Journal of International Students, 5*(5), 104–120. https://files.eric.ed.gov/fulltext/EJ1060049.pdf

Curlin, F. A., Nwodim, C., Vance, J. L., Chin, M. H., & Lantos, J. D. (2008). To die, to sleep: US physicians, religious and other objections to physician-assisted suicide, terminal sedation, and withdrawal of life support. *American Journal of Hospice and Palliative Medicine, 25*(2), 112–120. https://doi.org/10.1177/1049909107310141

Ogden, J. (2016). Religious constraints on prescribing medication. *Prescriber, 27*(12), 47–51. https://doi.org/10.1002/psb.1524

Purnell, L. (2002). The Purnell Model for Cultural Competence. *Journal of Transcultural Nursing, 13*(3), 193–196. https://doi.org/10.1177/10459602013003006

Swihart, D. L., Yarrarapu, S. N. S., & Martin, R. L. (2020, October 6). *Cultural religious competence in clinical practice.* https://www.ncbi.nlm.nih.gov/books/NBK493216/

Zaidi, D. (2018). Influences of religion and spirituality in medicine. *AMA Journal of Ethics, 20*(7), 609–612. https://doi.org/10.1001/amajethics.2018.609

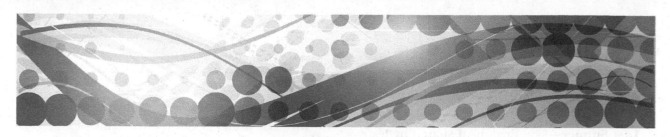

Essay 9

CULTURAL CONSIDERATIONS AND AAC: ESSENTIAL FAITH-BASED VOCABULARY FOR PROTESTANT CHRISTIAN USERS OF AAC

John W. Gareis

Because there are a myriad of vocabulary words that are used by people of faith, this list is an effort to highlight and explain some of the more common expressions that might be used in a health care setting. The list is neither exhaustive nor universal and references only that terminology that may be familiar to Protestant Christians.

Anointing—Ritualistic pouring or dabbing oil onto a person for the purpose of healing. Typically accompanied by prayers of healing.

Atonement—The process of having one's sins forgiven by God via the crucifixion of Jesus.

Baptism—The ritual symbolizing the forgiveness of sins during which the person is immersed in or sprinkled with water.

Born Again—Is a phrase used often by evangelical Christians which refers to their acceptance of Jesus as Lord and Savior.

Christ—Literally "the anointed one" or "Messiah." Used as a designator for the divinity of Jesus of Nazareth.

Circumcision—Removal of the foreskin of the penis not typically seen as a religious procedure among Christians.

Communion—Another name for the Eucharist or Lord's Supper, typically celebrated with bread and wine or juice.

Consecration—To set apart or make holy. Typically accomplished by prayer over the water at baptism or bread and wine for communion.

Eternal Life—Eternal existence with God of the soul or spirit beyond death.

Eucharist—See *Communion*.

Exorcism—The expelling of evil spirits from one who is possessed.

Heaven—The dwelling place of God.

Hell—The place of eternal torment for those who die unforgiven.

Incarnation—The Word of God taking on human form in the person of Jesus of Nazareth.

Jesus Christ—Designator for Jesus of Nazareth who is believed by Christians to be the Messiah, the Son of God in the flesh.

Judeo-Christian—A term used since the 1950s to designate the shared heritage and components of the Jewish and Christian faiths.

Kingdom of God—Heaven.

Last Supper—The final meal shared by Jesus and his disciples where he instituted the Eucharist. See *Communion* and *Eucharist*.

Laying on of Hands—Ritual of placing a hand or hands upon an individual being prayed for. Typically used for blessing or during prayers of healing,

Lord's Day—The Sabbath or Sunday for Christians.

Lord's Prayer—Also known as the "Our Father," it is a prayer attributed to Jesus and repeated universally by Christians.

Messiah—See *Christ*.

New Testament—The 27 recognized books of scripture recognized as being or containing the revelation of God by Christians.

Old Testament—The name Christians assign to the Hebrew scriptures.

Pentecost—Occurs 50 days after Easter to celebrate God sending the Holy Spirit upon the disciples. The birthday of the Christian Church.

Prayer—Conversation with God that typically involves words of Adoration, Confession, Thanksgiving, and Supplication.

Predestination—The doctrine held by many Christians that all of life is predetermined by God, and nothing happens without divine cause or reason.

Resurrection—The belief that as God raised Jesus from the dead, so the power of God raises the souls of believers who have died to eternal life with God.

Sabbath—Seventh day in Hebrew. Celebrated as Sunday among Christians.

Sin—Actions prohibited by or against the will of God.

Supplication—A prayer that requests something of God offered on behalf of another person or one's self.

Trinity—Name given to the three manifestations or experiences of God as Father, Son, and Holy

Spirit—Also referred to as God the Creator, Redeemer, and Sustainer.

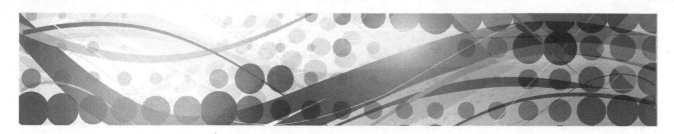

Essay 10

CULTURAL CONSIDERATIONS AND AAC: ESSENTIAL VOCABULARY FOR JEWISH USERS OF AAC

Karen J. Golding-Kushner

How the Deity Is Referred To

God (G-d); Elokim (Elohim); Hashem; Hakadosh Baruch Hu; Adoshem (Adonay); Ribono Shel Olam; Lord

Titles of Religious Leaders and Other Key Figures

Rabbi; Rabba; Rabbanit; Rebetzin; Cantor; Chazan; Shaliach Tsibur (also abbreviated "Shats"); Gabbai; Rebbe; Messiah: Mashiach; Shaliach; Mashgiach

Things We Read and Write

Siddur; Chumash; Talmud; Mishna; Gemarra; Machzor; Haggadah; Megillah; Megilat Esther; Torah; Ketubah; Tikun (two meanings, one is a book that contains Torah readings, the other is an all-night study session done on Shavuot)

Ritual Objects and Related Things

Ark (Aron Kodesh); Yad; Ner Tamid (Eternal Light); Grogger; Bima; Tallit (Tallis) Tzitzit; T'fillin; Mechitza; Menorah (Chanukiah); Dreidel; Shofar; Sukkah; Sheh'aylah (also: Shailah); Tzedakah; Tzedakah Box (Pushka); Magen David; Mezuzah; Hashgacha; Laver; Sermon (Drasha); kippah (yarmulka); shtreimel; kittel

What We Do and Say

Shalom; Shabbat shalom; good Shabbos; good Yomtov, Chag sameach; Kvetch; Kibitz; Nosh; Daven; Pray; Schmooze; shlep; Purim Shpiel; Tikun Olam

Holidays and Celebrations

Rosh Hashana; Yom Kippur (Day of Atonement); Sukkot or Sukkos; Shmini Atzeret; Simchat

(Simchas) Torah; Chanukah; Tu B'Shvat (New Year for Trees); Purim; Passover (Pesach); Shavuot (Shavuos); Tisha B'av; Fast Day; Yom Ha'atzmaut; Yom Hashoah; Oneg Shabbat; Melava malka; Siyum

Praying: Key Prayers, Blessings, and Names of Services

T'fila; Shema: Shema Yisroael Hashem Elokaynu Hashem Echad (Here Oh Israel, the Lord our God, the Lord is One); Amidah (also "Shmonah Esray"); Modeh Ani; Alenu; Tehillim; Kaddish; Hamotzi; Kiddush; Shehechiyanu; Bench Licht; Havdalla; Minyan; Shacharit; Maariv; Mincha; Hallel; Musaf; Kol Nidre; Yizkor; Ne'ilah; Vidui: Halacha; Mitzvah

Where We Go: Houses of Worship, Study, and Gathering

Synagogue; Shul; Temple; Shteeble; Kollel; Yeshiva; Jewish Day School; Chabad House; Hillel; Mikva

Family

Zaidy; Bubbie; Saba; Savta; Ema; Abba

Life-Span Topics

Shalom Zachor; Bris; Simchat Bat; Upshirin; Bar Mitzvah; Bat Mitzvah (Bas Mitzvah); Vort; L'chaim; Kiddushin; Chasuna (Wedding); Chuppah; Breaking the Glass; Seudah; Eulogy (Hespid); Shiva; Shloshim; Unveiling; Yahrzeit

Food

Kosher; Dairy (Chalavi); Meat (Fleishig); Pareve; Cholent; Challah; Kugel; Gefilte Fish; Blintzes; Matza; Matza Ball; Matza Brie; Taiglach; Latkes; Hamantashen; Seder; Charoset; Shwarma; Schnitzel; Kreplach; Falafel; Humus

Who We Are

Reform; Reconstructionist; Humanistic; Conservative; Orthodox; Frum; Yeshivish; Chasid; Chasidic; Zionist; Ashkenazim; Sephardim; Jewish; unaffiliated

Guidance on Use of This Vocabulary

As seen earlier ("Who We Are"), there are many different expressions of Jewish identity, worship, and practice. Variations occur within each of these identities, and among members of different congregations, geographic regions, and families. The wide range of vocabulary presented includes general terms that would likely be used by all of them and also terms that would be used only in specific communities. Therefore, selection of vocabulary to represent the communication needs for a specific Jewish augmentative and alternative communication (AAC) user is best made in concert with the person who uses AAC (PWUAAC), their family, and perhaps with the advice of their spiritual leader or teacher. Some PWUAAC might choose very few of the words, and others, an expansive range; they may have other words to add that were not included here.

Providing definitions of terms beyond a selected few would exceed the space requirements of this book. However, a source of definitions can be found in many Web-based glossaries. The previous list addresses the serious nature of making sure the vocabulary needs are met for PWUAAC; the following in no way is meant to diminish that intent. PWUAAC should also be enabled to express or react to communication that incorporates humor. Therefore, we next point out the role that humor plays for Jews of all denominations. Jewish humor has been used to amplify Jewish values, express the levity in daily Jewish life, and even to celebrate the survival over historical persecution (Friedman & Friedman, 2014). Collections of classic jokes can be found on the Internet by searching "Old Jews Telling Jokes." We look forward to the day when Jewish PWUAAC are more widely represented in such public creative forums.

Reference

Friedman, H. H., & Friedman, L. W. (2014). *God laughed: Sources of Jewish humor.* Transaction Publishers.

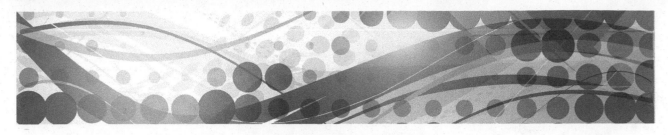

Essay 11

CULTURAL CONSIDERATIONS AND AAC: ESSENTIAL VOCABULARY FOR MUSLIM USERS OF AAC

Amal M. Maghazil

Guidance on Use of This Vocabulary

Islam is a religion practiced by 1.9 billion Muslims worldwide. The largest Muslim population resides in the Asia Pacific, Middle East, Northern Africa, and Sub-Saharan Africa regions (World Population Review, 2021). Due to the wide spread of Islam across continents, Muslims have diverse linguistic, cultural, and social backgrounds. The Quran, Islam's sacred text, and prophetic traditional texts and prayers are in Arabic. Knowing the Arabic language is essential in understanding the religion, but since many Muslims do not speak it, they rely on translating the texts in their mother tongue language. For example, a Muslim prays in Arabic but can learn about Islam in Indonesian. It is impossible to cover all the vocabulary that Muslims use due to the reasons mentioned earlier.

This section includes the most common vocabulary that Muslims use in Arabic. We tried to avoid including any specific cultural vocabulary. Arabic is written from right to left. It is important to note that varieties of the Arabic language are used for different functions (Beeston, 2016). Classical Arabic is the form of language used in the Quran and traditional Islamic texts. Modern Standard Arabic (MSA) is the language used in print, media, academia, and formal speeches, which all Arab speakers understand. Google translate uses this form of Arabic in translations. Vernacular varieties are spoken regional dialects and used informally in writing (e.g., texting). For example, in MSA, a ball means "Kurah," but in other dialects, Egyptian "Koora," and Levantine, "Tabeh."

It is essential to know the linguistic, cultural, and social background of the Muslim who uses augmentative and alternative communication (PWUAAC) and their family to select vocabulary unique to the individual's needs and wants. It is best to always start by asking, "do you speak Arabic?" If they say yes, you ask what dialect they speak. Some can still use the vocabulary mentioned below, even if they do not speak it, but others will want to translate them into their mother tongue. For example, Muslims refer to prayer in Arabic as "Ṣalāh" but in Persian, it is "namāz." So, a PWUAAC might pick either the Arabic or Persian version depending on their preference and exposure. If you search "Colloquial Arabic vocabulary," you will find many books and resources for various dialects like Levantine, Egyptian, Moroccan, and Gulf "Khaliji" dialects that will be helpful in vocabulary selection for PWUAACs.

Deity/God

Allāh; Rabb; Subḥānahū wa-taʿālā.

Religious Texts

Quran (Religious Text); Tafsir; Hadith; As-Sīrah an-Nabawiyyah (Prophetic biography); Qiṣaṣ al-ʾAnbiyāʾ (Stories of the prophets); Adhkar.

Religious Leaders and Other Key Figures

Mohammed alayhi s-salam (Prophet Mohammed, Peace be upon him, often abbreviated as PBUH); Rusul; Anbya; Imam; Sheik; Hafiz; Qāri; Moaʾthen; Khateeb; Alim; Caliph; Mufti; Jibrīl (Gabriel).

Houses of Worship

Masjid; Musalla; Al-Masjid Al-Ḥarām; Al-Masjid Al-Nabawi; Al-Masjid al-ʾAqṣā; Makkah; Medina; Al-Quds; al-Kaʿbah; Qubbat al-Sakhrah; Jabal an-Nūr; Rawḍah ash-Sharifah.

Ritual Objects/Related Things

Mushaf; Misbahah; Subha (prayer beads); Sajjada; Hijab; Nijab; Mabkhara; Kofiya; Abaya; Thob; ʿAmama; Bakhoor.

Actions

Ṣalāh; Wuḍūʾ; Tayammum; Zakat; Sawm; Duʿāʾ; Dhikr; Tasbih; Telawa; Hifz; Ġusl; Tahseen; Tawaf; Saʿi; Sadaqah; Waqf; Hajj; Umrah.

Greetings/Sayings

Salam; As-salāmu ʿalaykum; Wa ʿalaykumu s-salam; Bism Allah; Al-Ḥamdu lillāh; Jazāka llāhu ḫayran; Mā shāʾa llāh; ʾIn shāʾa llāh; Subḥāna llāh; Al-ḥamdu li-llāh; Lā ilāha illā llāh; Allāhu Akbar; Sallā -llāhu ʿalayhī wa-ʾālihī wa-sallam.

Holidays and Celebrations

Eid; Eid AlFitr; Eid AlAdha; Sana Hijriya; Ramadan; Iftar; Suhoor; Laylat al-Qadr; Hajj; Umrah; Arafa; Ruet-el-Hilal; Mawlid.

Prayers and Names of Services

Athan; ʾIqāmah; Qibla; Khutbah; Ṣalāh (prayer); Salat Alfajr; Salat Aldhuhr; Salat AlAsr; Salat AlMaghrib; Salat AlIsha; Salat AlSunnah; Salat AlJumuʾah; Salat al-Eid; Ṣalāt al-Janāzah; Salat al-Istikhaara; Tahajjud, Jumuʾah; Tarawih; Jamaʾah; Halaqa; ʾĀyah; Sūrah; Telawa; Tawaaf.

Family

Abb; Abu (Father of); Umm; Bint; Ibn; Akhi; Okhti.

Life-Span Topics

Aqīqah; Khitan; Nikah; Zawāj; Talaq; Janāzah; Aš-šahādah (Shahadah); Bulugh (puberty); Bāligh; Hajj; Umrah; Khatm al-Qurʾān; Ijazah.

Food

Halal; Haram; Tamra (Date); Tamr (Dates); Zamzam.

Who We Are

Muslims; Sunni; Shia; Sufi.

References

Beeston, A. F. L. (2016). *The Arabic language today*. Routledge.

World Population Review. (2021). *Muslim population by country 2020*. https://worldpopulationreview.com/country-rankings/muslim-population-by-country

SECTION III
AAC Assessment, Intervention, and Implementation Toddlers, Preschoolers, and School-Aged Individuals

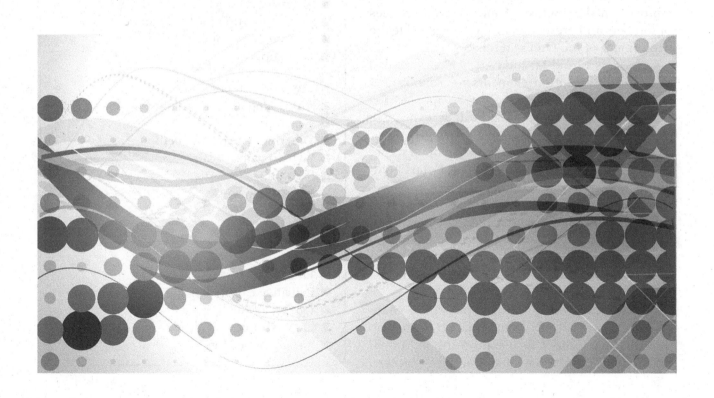

Section III covers content pertaining to service delivery for toddlers, preschoolers, and school-aged individuals seeking or using augmentative and alternative communication (AAC). This section continues the mindset of responsive practice and starts with an essay establishing a framework for ethical communication—a critical extension from Section II as we move from theory to practice. The second essay in this section, Essay 13, co-authored by Chris Klein, an individual using AAC, expands elements of ethical practice to encompass clinical mindset and skills as they relate to supporting acquisition of AAC devices for individuals needing AAC.

Chapter 8 introduces the assessment process using the SETT Framework (Zabala, 2007[1])—a framework that is discussed in many of the chapters that follow, emphasizing the interconnectedness of the **s**tudent/individual, **e**nvironment, **t**asks, and **t**ools in AAC assessment, intervention, and consultative practices. Chapter 9 illustrates this approach in the context of intervention services for toddlers and preschoolers and brings to life the involvement of the family in this process.

Chapters 10 and 11, and Essay 14, cover assessment and intervention elements for school-aged individuals. In these chapters, AAC competence (as detailed by Light, 1989[2]) is more fully explained, as are prompting and modeling strategies. AAC, language, and literacy are further developed within this section, and the involvement of stakeholders (including communication partners in educational settings) is highlighted. Chapter 12 provides important information about data collection and writing goals for AAC services. Essay 15 focuses on visual supports and makes the distinction between visuals used for AAC and those used for participation and behavior modification support.

This section ends with Chapter 13; a chapter that collects all of the information shared up until this point about focusing on the individual and their most important communication partners,

AAC systems, methods of access, and intervention/implementation suggestions in the context of AAC to support the varying needs of children in end-of-life care. We are once again reminded of the role AAC plays in individual expression, meaningful participation, social connection, and the preservation of dignity.

Key Terms Reviewed in This Section

- Early intervention
- Interprofessional teaming
- Natural environment
- Universal Design for Learning

- Modeling
- Predictability
- Prompt fading

- Assessment
- Communication partner training
- Feature matching
- Peer support

- AAC competency
- Aided language stimulation
- Coaching
- Descriptive teaching method
- Five domains of language
- Wait time

- Accuracy
- Reliability
- Validity

- End-of-life
- Palliative care
- Quality of life
- Quality of death
- Social connection

---

[1]Zabala, J. S. (2007). Ready, SETT, go! Getting started with the SETT framework. *Closing the Gap*, *23*, 5.
[2]Light, J. (1989). Toward a definition of communicative competence for individuals using augmentative and alternative communication systems. *Augmentative and Alternative Communication*, 5, 137–144.

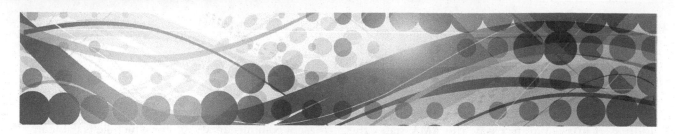

Essay 12

ETHICAL CONSIDERATIONS AND AAC: A FRAMEWORK FOR ETHICAL COMMUNICATION AND PRACTICE

Paula Leslie

Communication is at the heart of everything we do as audiologists and speech-language pathologists. More so, perhaps, than other clinicians for whom effective communication is a means to them being able to provide the specific care of their disciplines. In our world, we are communicating *about* communication (and swallowing of course). What then, do we mean by ethical communication? Surely one would think that as health care professionals, we are never unethical. Let us consider the terminology:

Ethical: an ethical action or behavior is one that follows principles or rules based on ethics.

Ethics: a system of principles relating to good and bad and/or how to live one's life. To be ethical is to follow a moral compass, that is to act for the good, with reference to something outside of the self. This might be religion, law, societal norms. What is good and bad, and what we might have responsibility *for* and *to*.

Communication: the two-way transfer of information and understanding, to inform, to share, to support folk making decisions.

We have professional codes of ethics, but often these read like business missions rather than the moral direction to take in clinical care. For exam-

ple, in the American Speech-Language-Hearing Association (ASHA) Code of Ethics, the preamble states the following:

> The ASHA Code of Ethics is a framework and focused guide for professionals in support of day-to-day decision making related to professional conduct. (ASHA, 2016)

This should not be interpreted as how to avoid litigation but how to act as a competent professional, which in the health care disciplines includes professional duties. Those duties include creating and respecting autonomy, doing good and acting to prevent or remove harm (beneficence), not committing harm (nonmaleficence), treating people fairly, and telling the truth (veracity) (Seedhouse, 2009). The American Medical Association (AMA) Code of Ethics also addresses communication in Principle 5:

> A physician shall continue to study, apply, and advance scientific knowledge, maintain a commitment to medical education, make relevant information available to patients, colleagues, and the public, obtain consultation, and use the talents of other health professionals when indicated. (AMA, 2001)

And in relation to Informed Consent which is addressed in a separate essay, the AMA states the following:

1) Assess the patient's ability to understand relevant medical information and the implications of treatment alternatives and to make an independent, voluntary decision.
2) Present relevant information accurately and sensitively, in keeping with the patient's preferences for receiving medical information. (AMA, 2021)

How do these professional statements link to the use of augmentative and alternative communication (AAC)? The vision of the professional organization (ASHA) that supports people with communication disorders is as follows:

Making effective communication, a human right, accessible and achievable for all. (ASHA, 2021)

We now have access to many forms of AAC across the technology spectrum. Thus, for people who have difficulty with communication on either side of the exchange, there should be no excuse to leave them struggling. Enabling communication is fundamental to the duties of health care professionals, ensuring informed consent can be given by a patient or family member regarding any type of intervention. This is as true today as over 100 years ago when Justice Benjamin Cardozo summed up the court's opinion:

Every human being of adult years and sound mind has a right to determine what shall be done with his own body; and a surgeon who performs an operation without his patient's consent commits an assault for which he is liable in damages. This is true except in cases of emergency where the patient is unconscious and where it is necessary to operate before consent can be obtained. (*Schloendorff v. Society of New York Hospital*, 1914)

A person can only exercise the right to autonomous decision-making if they can understand the information shared with them, consider the costs, benefits, and implications, and communicate that decision to others (Appelbaum & Grisso, 1988).

References

American Medical Association (AMA). (2001). *Code of medical ethics.* https://www.ama-assn.org/about/publications-newsletters/ama-principles-medical-ethics

American Medical Association (AMA). (2021). *Code of medical ethics: Opinion 2.1.1—Informed consent.* https://www.ama-assn.org/delivering-care/ethics/informed-consent

American Speech-Language-Hearing Association (ASHA). (2016, March). *Code of ethics.* http://www.asha.org/Code-of-Ethics/

American Speech-Language-Hearing Association (ASHA). (2021). *About the American Speech-Language-Hearing Association: Vision.* https://www.asha.org/about/

Appelbaum, P. S., & Grisso, T. (1988). Assessing patients' capacities to consent to treatment. *New England Journal of Medicine, 319*(25), 1635–1638. https://doi.org/10.1056/NEJM198812223192504

Schloendorff v. Society of New York Hospital, 105 N.E. 92 (211 NY 125 1914).

Seedhouse, D. (2009). *Ethics: The heart of healthcare* (3rd ed.). John Wiley & Sons.

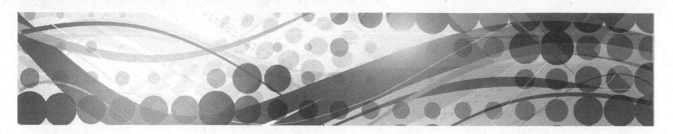

Essay 13

ETHICAL CONSIDERATIONS AND AAC: A CONSUMER'S PERSPECTIVE

Chris Klein and Katya Hill

An expectation of an individual with a disability who needs augmentative and alternative communication (AAC) technology, a parent of a child who needs AAC, or a spouse of an adult with a disability is that the speech-language pathologist (SLP) knows what they are doing. Consumers assume that the SLP is trained and competent in AAC and is not a salesperson representing a product line. We do not think to ask those questions, because we feel that professionals will disclose information and biases that may affect decisions about devices, treatment, and services. However, most AAC consumers learn from unfortunate experiences that their interests may not be paramount to those making AAC. AAC speakers have to protect themselves from conflicts of interests, not fully disclosed information, and bias of those providing clinical, educational, and funding services. As an AAC speaker, a parent, or family member, we approach the topic of ethics and AAC service delivery from different perspectives.

I am regularly approached by families with a version of the following question: "Now that we have an evaluation for an AAC device for our child or my child is receiving AAC therapy, what should we expect from SLPs as the long-term goal?" Mostly, expectations for individuals with complex communication disabilities are set way too low. That means SLPs, other team members, and even parents may be selling them short.

Unfortunately, in many cases, a person is being evaluated by an SLP who is not trained well and has not acquired the necessary AAC knowledge and skills for a thorough evaluation. This is especially true when the SLP forgets that AAC is about achieving language competence above other functional communication goals. AAC is *not* just about what the device does and getting a device funded, it is about ensuring that a robust language system is available for fast and effective real-time communication using the device. When an untrained or undertrained SLP is doing the evaluation, especially when they ask an AAC manufacturers' salesperson to be involved, the discussion often turns to the extra features of the device and buzzwords about the language program. Sometimes, evaluating and measuring language performance gets left out of the discussion and comparison among the various AAC devices.

When language performance is not evaluated (how an AAC device is improving communication), independence and quality of life become much more difficult. If a person is not showing progress on their communication competence, hardly ever is the representation and organization of language discussed. Instead of changing the intervention, the person is most likely assumed not to be able to use AAC technology, or the technology is simplified. This frustrates me tremendously, because I believe everyone has potential to improve their expressive language and literacy using an AAC device. They just have to have the opportunity to do so.

Therefore, the SLP needs to make sure that the person who needs AAC is fully involved in the AAC evaluation process, instead of just being a bystander. The goal for a person who uses augmentative and alternative communication (PWUAAC) is to say anything they want and to say it as fast as possible. They need access to everyday language to do that, and without that AAC really does not help them.

I am sad as it feels that AAC has become more about what the device can do instead of what this device can do to a person's language development, fluent communication, and potential. As a PWUAAC, this is troubling because I am always wanting to make sure I am progressing on my device. This is why I believe more PWUAACs need to be part of the research process as well as the AAC evaluation process. We need to have performance data or evidence that shows us the most useful communication device and the effectiveness of therapy services. With this in mind, SLPs need to think about how to reduce bias and to control the role and responsibilities of the AAC vendor in the evaluation process. SLPs must ensure that the AAC speaker and family members are fully informed of their options. Most importantly, admit when you do not have the experience to lead the AAC evaluation by referring to or seeking the help of an SLP who does.

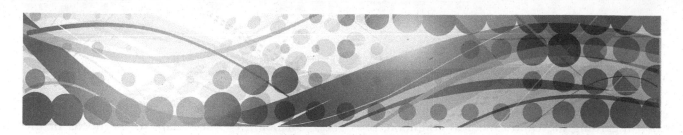

Chapter 8
ASSESSING TODDLERS AND PRESCHOOLERS

Meher Banajee

Fundamentals

Research (Branson & Demchak, 2009; Iacono & Erikson, 2016; Kent-Walsh et al., 2015; Romski et al., 2015) provides evidence that early intervention (including augmentative and alternative communication [AAC]) should be implemented as early as possible. Between 2018 and 2019, 372,896 children were enrolled in early intervention services in the United States. However, a survey of early intervention in 2006 (Dugan et al., 2006) indicated that early intervention providers typically did not initiate AAC options until a child was over 2 years of age (Dugan et al., 2006).

General Principles of Assessment of Toddlers and Preschoolers

This chapter provides some of the beginning principles for conducting an AAC assessment with toddlers and preschoolers. One of the principles for conducting an AAC assessment is the use of the SETT model (Zabala, 2007), which stands for the following: student, environment, tasks, and tools. It includes the child's need to be assessed within the natural environment while performing tasks of daily living in order to determine the ideal AAC tools.

In addition, all assessments should be conducted using the seven "M"s of assessment (Sny-der & Hemmeter, 2018)—that is, the assessment should be

a. multisource (or information for the assessment needs to be gathered from multiple sources, e.g., parents, teachers, grandparents)
b. multidiscipline (or assessments should be conducted by an interprofessional team)
c. multimethod (or different methods including formal and informal methods should be used during the assessment)
d. multicultural (culture needs to be considered while conducting the assessment)
e. multidomain (different domains including fine and gross motor, speech and language, social aspects, and cognition should also be assessed by different disciplines)
f. multicontext (assessment should be conducted within naturally occurring environments such as the home, nursery school, or grandparents' homes)
g. multi-occasion (assessment should be conducted at different times within those environments)

Preparation for the Assessment

Before starting with the evaluation, information regarding the child needs to be collected via a case history or an intake form. Pertinent information regarding the child's medical condition, prenatal, natal, and postnatal history, developmental milestones, as well as current skills needs to be obtained. Past history and current speech and language, cognitive, gross and fine motor and social skills also need to be determined. Status of the child's vision and hearing as well as a detailed feeding history also need to be gathered. A photograph (if available) of the child in their seating system would help to determine the need of positioning and seating during the evaluation. History of use of a low- or high-tech communication system, as well as past speech and language assessment and intervention should be obtained. Interests, likes, and dislikes of the child are important to be determined in order to maintain the child's interest as well as programming of personalized vocabulary, as discussed in Chapter 7, into the communication systems to be used during the assessment.

Assessment

Formal Language Assessment

At the time of the assessment, a brief interview needs to be conducted to obtain any information that has not been collected ahead of time using the intake forms. After a brief interview, communication skills of the student (or child) need to be assessed. Based on the principles of assessment for early intervention (Early Steps, 2021), the assessment needs to be conducted within the child's natural environment (which includes the child's nursery school or daycare, home, and/or places frequently visited by the family) with familiar toys and objects. Formal (criterion-referenced) and informal procedures provide different types of information and therefore both need to be completed.

Criterion-referenced assessments such as (a) Assessment, Evaluation and Programming System (Bricker & Waddell, 2002); (b) Communication Matrix (Rowland, 2011); (c) Rossetti Infant Toddler Scale (Rossetti, 2006); and (d) the Communication and Symbolic Behavior Scale (Wetherby & Prizant, 2001) are among the few assessments that are effective for gathering information about the child.

Criterion-referenced tests have the distinct advantage of being easy to adapt to the needs of the child (who might have motor challenges) following principles of Universal Design for Learning (UDL; CAST, Inc., 2021)—an educational framework designed to support individual learning differences by offering flexibility. The examiner must ensure that test adaptations reflect multiple methods of representation (e.g., enlarging pictures for children who might be visually impaired), multiple means of expression (e.g., using eye gaze as a response method), and multiple means of engagement (e.g., use of breaks and sensory input such as the use of textured seat cushion) (CAST, 2021). In addition, criterion-referenced tests can be administered within the natural environment, during different activities. Assessment can be conducted at home during mealtimes, playing with preferred toys, and during daily routines (e.g., diaper changing and/or bath time).

It is of utmost importance that the assessment is conducted using input from different professionals. Various models are used to obtain input from different disciplines and professionals. These include the following:

- Multidisciplinary model: Professionals from each discipline evaluate the child separately and generate individual reports, which are then sent to a coordinator who integrates them into a single report. A distinct disadvantage here is the family has to have multiple appointments where each professional views the child using a narrow lens of their discipline.
- Interdisciplinary model: Similar to the multidisciplinary model; however, the disciplines come together during grand rounds or a staffing meeting to exchange information. Clearly, there is very little input from the family in this process.
- Transdisciplinary or interprofessional model: Child is assessed simultaneously by multiple professionals. Family is an integral part of the assessment process, and a common sample of behavior is obtained from which all professionals derive their inferences. This model is characterized by role release,

role expansion, and arena-style assessment. An integrated report is developed at the conclusion of the evaluation.

Test Adaptations

Bristow and Fristoe (1987) examined the effect of various response methods on the validity of test results of typically developing children. The study compared scores obtained through the standard administration protocol of the Peabody Picture Vocabulary Test—Revised (PPVT) (Dunn & Dunn, 1981) to scores obtained through alternate response modes, including (a) eye gaze, (b) scanning, and (c) headlight pointing. The authors concluded that, with few exceptions, the results of each assessment version were highly correlated (Beukelman & Mirenda, 2013, p. 169). Test adaptations that follow the principles of UDL, like the adaptations shown in Figures 8–1 and 8–2, a choice board and rotary scanner, empower the individual to engage in the testing procedures in flexible ways.

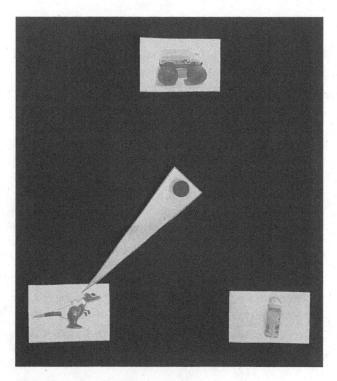

Figure 8–2. Rotary scanner.

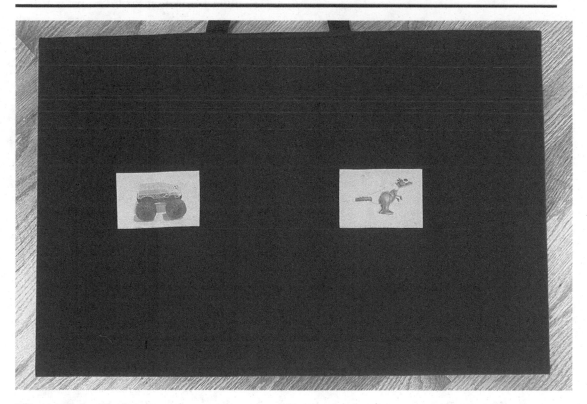

Figure 8–1. Choice board.

Informal Language Assessment

Play is the child's "business." Play is how a child grows. Use of language should be observed ideally during a play routine. Informal procedures for assessment of language involve the use of language during unstructured and structured play situations using preferred toys and materials (books, art materials, playdough, etc.). When you observe that a child has difficulty playing with a toy, use simple adaptations, again, using principles of UDL. Examples of toy adaptations include (a) use of switch-adapted toys (e.g., bubble blowers or mechanical figures that can move, like the one shown in Figure 8–3) and art materials (e.g., spin art); (b) page fluffers to help with turning pages of a book (e.g., staggered use of Velcro dots on book pages, or spacers between pages, like shown in Figure 8–4); and (c) use of pipe insulation or grips to assist with grasping knobs, handles, or items (e.g., like shown in Figure 8–5) for better access.

Receptive, expressive, and pragmatic functions can be assessed using play. Receptive language skills include following directions, identification of names of objects, and knowledge of actions, descriptors (e.g., colors, size, quantity), and locations of objects. Expressive language skills may include use of residual speech, verbalizations, vocalizations, gestures, eye gaze, and yes/no responses. Pragmatic skills include the ability to initiate communication, take turns during conversation, and indicate recurrence and termination of conversations. A significant discrepancy between receptive and expressive language (i.e., the individual understands far more than they are able to express), warrants consideration of AAC to support functional communication, as well as language expansion while the child's verbal speech develops.

An oral mechanism examination can further justify the need for an AAC system. If the child does not demonstrate adequate ability to use their oral structures, then it is assumed that verbal speech

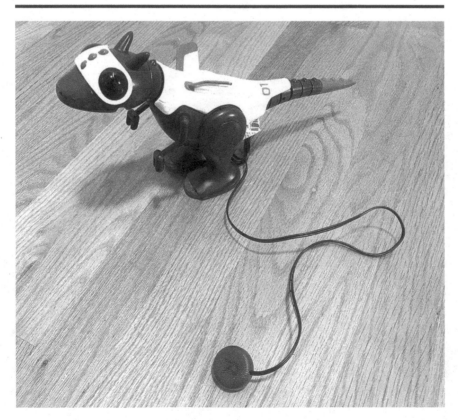

Figure 8–3. Switch-accessible toy.

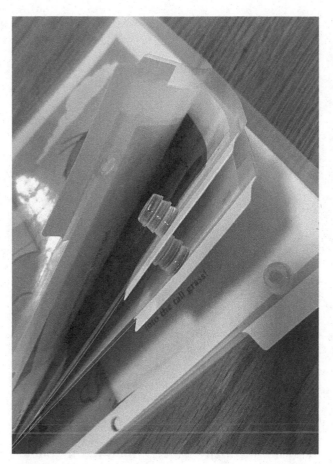

Figure 8–4. Page fluffer.

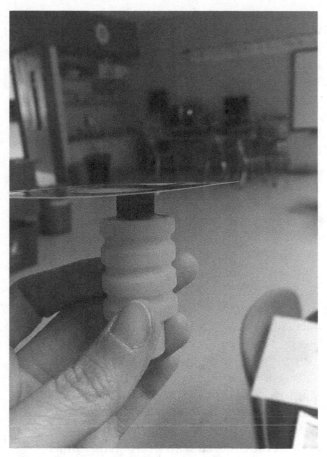

Figure 8–5. Adapted handle.

may not develop in the near future and an AAC system is needed. Symmetry of the oral structures (e.g., lips, cheeks, and face) and mobility of the lips, tongue, and soft palate need to be explored. The configuration and shape of the hard palate should be determined. Finally, functional use of the structures via a feeding examination needs to be completed. Tongue movement (e.g., tongue lateralization and elevation), jaw mobility, and lip movements (e.g., rounding on a straw while drinking) can be assessed during eating finger foods (e.g., crackers) as well as spoon foods (e.g., yogurt).

Augmentative Communication Assessment

Both low- and high-tech AAC systems need to be considered (like those described in Chapters 2 and

3 of this text). Both systems have their advantages and disadvantages; however, a multimodal system needs to be considered. A no-tech system consisting of gestures, facial expressions, vocalizations, and verbalizations is a quick method to be used in the absence of technology; however, a low-tech communication system can be effective in meeting the needs of a child needing AAC and is a great backup for a high-tech system when it needs to be repaired or is not charged.

Low-tech AAC systems (communication books, Pragmatic Organization Dynamic Display [PODD] systems, eye-gaze options) can be uniquely tailored to meet the needs of a toddler or preschooler needing AAC. They can be created to offer a range of vocabulary and can be designed in flexible ways. Additionally, low-tech AAC systems have the advantages of easy replacement, quick access, and are cheaper. However, for some these can be limiting (in terms of breadth of adequate vocabulary), being cumbersome to transport, offering limited independence of access, and lacking voice output. As opposed, a high-tech system has the advantage of having voice output, the ability to communicate on a variety of topics independently, as well as the ability to mirror typical communication using turn-taking.

Whether completing a low- or high-tech AAC evaluation, the following factors need to be considered.

Hearing and vision can be formally and informally assessed. An evaluation from an audiologist and an ophthalmologist can be supplemented with informal observation for functional use of the AAC device. Size of the locations and volume as well as tactile input (use of textures) can be provided if necessary. Larger locations with high contrast (e.g., black background), raised outlines of pictures, as well as tactile symbols can be used with children with vision challenges. Project Core (2020), developed by Karen Erikson from North Carolina Literacy Center, is one example of the use of tactile symbols. Icons that light up or vibrate might be options for children with hearing impairments.

Fine and gross motor skills of the client can be observed informally; however, for a child who has significant motor issues, it might be necessary to obtain assistance from an occupational or physical therapist to assist in the positioning of the child. Principles of positioning (e.g., adequate lateral trunk supports, feet supports, 90-degree angle at the hips, knees, and feet) should be used to seat the child before starting the evaluation. Positioning is especially important when assessing a child who needs switch and head access or eye control access. Fine motor skills (such as pointing) need to be assessed with the help of an occupational therapist and appropriate adaptations (use of a keyguard or stylus, increasing space between the locations and stabilizing the arm using a dowel or weights) need to be in place before the child is assessed for access methods.

Once a child is positioned adequately, it is important to explore access methods for low- and high-tech systems, like those reviewed in Chapter 5.

It is sometimes necessary to think "outside the box"; consideration needs to be given first to least intrusive methods such as direct selection (touch, head pointing, eye gaze, use of a stylus). Other methods such as single-switch scanning (e.g., directed vs. automatic scanning) or dual-switch scanning (e.g., one switch to activate scanning and the second switch to make a selection) or the use of a joystick/mouse might be considered. Computer games such as Look to Learn (Tobii Dynavox, 2021a) can be used to teach access methods in a low-stress and fun activity.

Size, number of symbols, and type of symbols need to be assessed. The size and the number of symbols are related in that if you increase the size of the symbols, the number of symbols that will fit into an AAC system will decrease. Motor planning for accessing symbols should be considered; therefore, it is usually a better idea to start with an AAC system with an ideal number of locations and hide (or not open) all symbols. Once the child has demonstrated that the revealed symbols are used functionally, the rest of the icons can be opened.

Beukelman and Light (2020) proposed the following hierarchy: objects, followed by photographs, followed by line drawings. Although a hierarchy exists regarding cognitive load of different symbols, consistent use of the symbols paired with the appropriate communication function (e.g., using the symbol for "more" with recurrence of an activity) helps the child understand the symbol via a cause-and-effect relationship. Visual scene displays have been found to be of a distinct advantage for use with young children (Light et al., 2004, 2010). Visual scene displays generally provide the user with a large fringe vocabulary pertinent to the particular activity or environment and therefore should be supplemented with core vocabulary (smaller functional vocabulary words used by all users across all activities and environments).

Although tests (e.g., the Test of Aided-Communication Symbol Performance or the TASP; Bruno, 2003) are available that provide a starting point for designing or selecting an appropriate AAC device page set, sometimes the symbol set is determined by the type of high-tech system recommended at the end of the evaluation. For example, Tobii Dynavox (2021b) systems use single-meaning Picture Communication Symbols, whereas the systems developed by Prentke Romich Company use multi-meaning Minspeak symbols (Semantic Compaction Systems, 2018).

The last component (although sometimes thought to be the most important component of an AAC assessment) is the selection of high- and low-tech options. At least three different devices should be considered and prepared for the evaluation. Selection of the devices need to account for different access methods (if necessary), symbol sets (single- vs. multiple-meaning icons), number and size of locations, and need for navigation between pages or sequencing of icons on a single page. Preparation of devices includes programming or making sure vocabulary necessary for desired functional play activities is available on the devices. For example, one device may be programmed for use with stacking Legos, whereas the second device for use during a tea party, and the third device for use during snack time.

Low-tech options might be created using screenshots of the overlays used during the assessment process. Supplemental low-tech systems to the high-tech devices might also be considered. Examples of these systems are "more"/"all done" symbols or switches placed on the lap tray, a single switch to attract attention, or a smaller, more portable low-tech communication board for the playground or to be used while toileting.

The final step in the assessment is to complete a feature match. It is important to see that all the communication needs of the child have been addressed. Which features of the devices tried matched the needs of the child? If prompting was used, which system required the least amount of prompting? A form (such as shown in Table 8–1) can be used to determine the appropriate system for the child.

On most occasions, the child will respond appropriately during the evaluation, and you will be able to determine the optimum device, accessories, and access method for the child. However, there might be times when two devices are used in a similar manner by the child, or the child might

not respond adequately during the evaluation, and a device trial for an extended period of time is necessary. Most manufacturers of high-tech systems will provide free loaners for device trials. At the end of the trials, input from the child's caregivers, teachers, or therapists can be obtained to determine the best device for the child, based on a collective decision.

Case Study: RC

Clinical Profile and Communication Needs

The Individual

Let's meet RC, a 3-year 1-month-old girl. At birth, she was hypoxic due to an emergency cesarean section. She had severe shoulder dystocia, which caused obstructed labor. After delivery of the head, her anterior shoulder was unable to pass below the pubic symphysis which resulted in a brain injury. RC was diagnosed with spastic quadriplegic cerebral palsy and Erb's palsy (paralysis) of her left arm. She spent 5 days in the neonatal intensive care unit (NICU) and underwent surgery for placement of a gastrostomy tube for feeding. In addition, RC was diagnosed with severe epilepsy at 2 years old following a 45-minute and a 20-minute seizure and was prescribed *Kepra* to control her seizures.

Her intake form provided the following information: RC communicated using some one-word approximations. She was reported to have adequate comprehension skills. She started cooing and babbling between 3 and 6 months old. She does not yet hold her head upright independently, nor does she sit or stand without support, or move to desired objects/toys that are out of reach. RC received speech and occupational therapy through Early Steps. RC's patterns of communication include vocalizations, facial expressions, eye gaze, and facial expressions, which she used for requesting objects and actions and expressing feelings (e.g., pain, happiness, or fussing). She was unable to express herself adequately in most situations,

Table 8–1. Sample Table Used To Assess Device Features

Device	Symbol		Visual/Perceptual Skills				Physical Skills			Device Features		
	Object/picture	Number of locations	Size of pictures	Space	Contrast required	Visability range	Most functional position	Activator	Type of scanning	Portability	Expandability	Acceptance

which frustrated her since her preferences are never considered or asked. Recently, she has started to demonstrate challenging behaviors such as throwing herself back to threaten to overturn her wheelchair. This helped her to get attention even though it might result in time out. It also was reported that RC enjoyed watching videos of Dora the Explorer, playing with bubbles, and playing with her baby doll.

RC was fed via a gastrostomy tube. Recently she has started eating two to three spoonfuls of soft foods such as yogurt or pudding. Her hearing was reported to be within functional limits. However, vision issues were reported. RC has delayed visual maturation due to hypoxia at birth—atrophy in her left eye and decreased ability to track consistently. Corrective surgery was performed in both eyes. Surgery proved to be successful on the right eye but not on the left. RC's mother plans to begin patching the right eye in order to strengthen the left starting this month.

RC was referred for the evaluation by her occupational therapist who provided information about her fine and gross motor skills. She reported that RC had limited fine motor skills in that she was unable to hold objects independently and used a slapping movement of her hand to make choices between objects placed on either side of her lap tray. She was unable to cross midline with either hand. RC uses a manual wheelchair for mobility, which has been customized for supporting her trunk, feet, and head. Side bumpers were provided on the lap tray to assist with keeping RC's arms in midline. RC's occupational therapist accompanied her for the evaluation.

Communication Partners and Environment

RC's communication partners are mainly her family which consists of her mother and father. Her paternal and maternal grandparents visit approximately once every other week. Early intervention therapists (occupational therapist, speech-language pathologist, and special instructor come to her house once a week). She also goes to see her primary care physician (once every 6 months), neurologist, orthopedist, and ophthalmologist (usually once a year). RC is enrolled to start in a public school at the beginning of the next school year.

RC's environment is her home where she is usually positioned in her wheelchair, a high-low chair, and on the floor using bolsters. Her parents make sure she has a variety of experiences such as taking her to the zoo, aquarium, children's museum, and to the park.

AAC Considerations

Preparation for the Evaluation. In preparation for the assessment, several toys were adapted. These included a Dora book with flaps adapted with the use of staggered Velcro dots and ponytail holders to help open the flaps. An Ariel bubble blower was adapted using a single rocking lever switch to assist her in blowing bubbles. A play board was also created using grooming materials and feeding materials for playing with the baby doll. A skidproof material (e.g., shelf liner) was available for her lap tray for when it was time for her snack. RC's parents brought with them yogurt and the spoon she used for feeding.

Three high-tech devices were prepared for the evaluation and were programmed with appropriate core (go, stop, want, that) and fringe vocabulary (blow, pop, brush, spoon, Dora, etc.) to play with bubbles, read the Dora book, and groom the baby. Four different methods of access (direct selection with a keyguard, headpointing, single-switch scanning and eye control) were set up. A formal symbol selection assessment was not conducted, however; the devices selected had a variety of single-meaning icons, SymbolStix (News2You, 2021), Picture Communication Symbols (Tobii Dynavox, 2021b), and multimeaning icons (Minspeak, 2021). Each device was programmed with a different number of locations. Each device was programmed with at least 12 locations with at least 8 locations visible/open for access. Low-tech adapted photo frames were programmed with "more," and "all done/finished" were also made available. A schedule board of photographs of different activities to be used during the assessment was used to assess eye gaze for a low-tech option. Photographs were placed on the four corners of the choice board to allow for observation of accuracy of access.

Rationale for Clinical Decision-Making

Evaluation Process

After a brief interview, the assessment was initiated by presenting RC with a picture schedule including play activities, break time, and feeding. RC's lap tray was covered with the shelf liner to make sure her toys did not slip while she was playing. The two low-tech photo frames were placed on either side of her lap tray. RC's ability to access the switches was confirmed, as she was able to range to them and use them effectively. She was presented with a choice of four activities (bubbles, baby doll, snack, and book). She was encouraged to use eye gaze to choose an activity of her choice. Each activity was presented with the appropriately programmed high-tech device. A laser pointer was used by the assessing clinician to model icon choices on the devices.

While playing with each of the toys, RC's expressive and receptive language and pragmatic skills were assessed using the birth to 3 years' section of the Assessment, Evaluation, and Programming System (AEPS; Bricker & Waddell, 2002). Observation of her ability to interact with her parents, therapists, and student clinicians offered additional information about her language skills. Since RC had difficulty following instructions and completing some of the oral motor movements (tongue elevation and lateralization, lip rounding and spreading), her oral skills were assessed while her mom fed her yogurt.

Results of the Evaluation

Language Skills

Comprehension Language Skills. RC recognized names of actual objects, photographs of objects, and after modeling, she recognized familiar objects represented in colored line drawings (single meaning icons). She understood simple single-step directives and followed conversation when it involved familiar objects and activities.

Expressive Language Skills. RC smiled for affirmation and fussed to express negation. She some-times looked up or nodded for "yes" and shook her head for "no." While using the devices, after modeling, RC expressed her needs and wants using single icons. She did not sequence icons, even when modeled. She vocalized and used head nodding and shaking to confirm her choices.

Pragmatic Skills. RC used eye gaze to make choices and initiate activities by choosing them on the choice board. She used eye gaze to direct her communication partner's attention to objects. She also used her low-tech device after prompting (e.g., tapping on the devices) to indicate recurrence and termination. Turn-taking was difficult; however, it was reported that RC had limited experience participating in taking turns during play activities.

Speech Skills. RC used mainly vowel sounds while vocalizing. Due to her limited vocalizations, voice, fluency, and articulation were not evaluated.

Oral Mechanism Examination. RC presented with an open mouth posture with limited lip retraction and protraction. Although she had adequate tongue protrusion, no lateral tongue movements were observed. During eating yogurt, she demonstrated an immature pattern by sucking on the spoon while taking the food in her mouth. She then demonstrated a prominent tongue thrust while moving the yogurt to the back of her oral cavity. RC ate only four spoonfuls of yogurt. Her hard palate was of adequate height and pink in color; however, velar mobility was not observed.

Fine and Gross Motor Skills. Informal observations confirmed the motor skills listed in the intake form. She used a manual wheelchair, and her positioning was adequate with good head control, trunk support, and lower extremity support. She used a lap tray for hand support. Her occupational therapist (who attended the evaluation) assisted in adjusting her seating and positioning when needed for optimal eye access. These skills were observed informally and with input from the occupational therapist.

Vision and Hearing Skills. RC's hearing skills were adequate for functional use of the device. Her visual acuity was adequate to see locations of size 1.5 × 1.5 inches. She was able to track objects horizontally, vertically, and diagonally using a range of 10 inches. These skills were observed informally and with input from the occupational therapist who attended the evaluation.

AAC Considerations

Low-Tech Assessment. A choice board (cardboard covered with Velcro sensitive material) was used for providing choices as well as presenting the schedule for the assessment. RC easily made selections using the icons on the choice board and selected activities on the schedule.

High-Tech Assessment. Three devices were used in the evaluation. These included the Tobii Dynavox 1-13, ChatFusion 10, and Accent 1400. The Tobii Dynavox was used with Snap+Core First software using 25 locations with 10 locations visible and programmed. The ChatFusion was programmed using WordPower 20 simply software using the 20 locations with 10 locations open and programmed. The Accent 1400 was programmed with 36-location UNITY software with icon sequencing and 10 icons visible and programmed appropriately.

Access Methods. Four different access methods were used. Direct selection on all three devices, head pointing was used on the ChatFusion and the Accent 1400, whereas eye control was used on the Tobii Dynavox I-13 and the Accent 1400. Single-switch scanning was used on all three devices. A wobble switch was mounted near RC's head using a universal mount.

RC had difficulty using direct selection even with the use of a keyguard. She demonstrated limited understanding of the scanning process and some difficulty with accurate and timely access of the switch. Due to her vision issues, RC had difficulty with eye gaze on the Tobii Dynavox I-13 and on the Accent 1400. Last, the ChatFusion with head control was tried. RC understood this access method quickly and immediately accessed icons on the device to make choices, direct actions, and indicate recurrence and termination of activities.

Next Steps

Based on RC's performance, the following recommendations were made:

1. The *ChatFusion* with *Word Power 20 Simply* with head control.
2. A wheelchair mount for access to the device in all environments and safe and easy transportation of the device.
3. Low-tech systems should include a choice board for making choices, and a modified photo frames for indicating recurrence and termination of activities.
4. All systems should be embedded in functional and fun daily activities (e.g., bubble blowing) and routines (e.g., snack time).
5. Speech-language intervention was recommended to work on the following goals and objectives:
   a. Goal 1: Use an SGD device to improve expressive language skills to a functional level.
      i. Objective 1: RC will use an SGD to request items from a variety of communication partners within 3 months.
      ii. Objective 2: RC will sequence two words on an SGD to form phrases/sentences within 6 months.
   b. Goal 2: Use an SGD to develop functional pragmatic skills:
      i. Objective 1: RC will use an SGD to initiate interaction with a variety of communication partners in 3 months.
      ii. Objective 2: RC will use an SGD to take turns with a variety of communication partners within 6 months
      iii. Objective 3: RC will use an AAC device to terminate interaction in 3 months.
   c. Goal 3: Use an AAC device to express medical emergency situations or health-related information independently to an unfamiliar listener within 6 weeks:
      i. Objective 1: RC will use an AAC device to indicate emotions to familiar/unfamiliar listeners in 6 months.

ii. Objective 2: RC will use an AAC device to indicate medical needs to familiar/unfamiliar communication partners within the next 6 months.

References

Beukelman, D., & Light, J. (2020). *Augmentative & alternative communication: Supporting children & adults with complex communication needs* (5th ed.). Paul H. Brookes.

Beukelman, D., & Mirenda, P. (2013). *Augmentative & alternative communication: Supporting children & adults with complex communication needs* (4th ed.). Paul H. Brookes.

Branson, D., & Demchak, M. (2009). The use of augmentative and alternative communication methods with infants and toddlers with disabilities: A research review. *Augmentative and alternative communication, 25*(4), 274–286. https://doi.org/10.3109/07434610903384529

Bricker, D., & Waddell, M. (2002). *Assessment, evaluation, and programming system for infants and children (AEPS®)* (2nd ed.). Paul H. Brookes.

Bristow, D., & Fristoe, M. (1987, November). *Effects of test adaptations on test performance* [Paper presentation]. Annual Convention of the American Speech-Language-Hearing Association, New Orleans, LA.

Bruno, J. (2003). *The Test of Aided-Communication Symbol Performance.* Tobii Dynavox.

CAST, Inc. (2021). *About Universal Design for Learning.* https://www.cast.org/impact/universal-design-for-learning-udl

Dugan, L. M., Campbell, P. H., & Wilcox, M. (2006). Making decisions about assistive technology with infants and toddlers. *Topics in Early Childhood Special Education, 26*(1), 25–32.

Dunn, L. M., & Dunn, L. M. (1981). *Peabody Picture Vocabulary Test–Revised.* American Guidance Service.

Early Steps. (2021). *Early Steps of Louisiana.* https://ldh.la.gov/index.cfm/page/139/n/139

Iacono, T., & Erikson, K. (2016). The role of augmentative and alternative communication for children with autism: Current status and future trends. *Neuropsychiatric Disease and Treatment, 12,* 2349–2361.

Kent-Walsh J., Binger C., & Buchanan C. (2015). Teaching children who use augmentative and alternative communication to ask inverted yes/no questions using aided modeling. *American Journal of Speech-Language Pathology, 24,* 222–236. https://doi.org/10.1044/2015_AJSLP-14-0066

Light, J. C., Drager, K., & Nemser, J. G. (2004). Enhancing the appeal of AAC technologies for young children: Lessons learned from toy manufacturers. *Augmentative and Alternative Communication, 20,* 137–149.

Light, J., Drager, K., & Wilkinson, K. (2010, November). *Designing effective visual scene displays for young children* [Lecture]. Annual Convention of the American Speech-Language-Hearing Association, Philadelphia, PA.

Minspeak, Inc. (2021). *Minspeak symbols.* http://www.minspeak.com/

News2You, LLC. (2021). *SymbolStix Prime.* https://www.n2y.com/symbolstix-prime/

Prentke Romich Company. (2018). *Nu-Eye Tracking System.* https://store.prentrom.com/nueye-tracking-system-br-accent-1400-accent-1200-andaccent-1000

Project Core. (2020). *Universal Core Vocabulary—3D Symbol Format.* https://www.project-core.com/3d-symbols/

Romski, M., Sevcik, R. A., Barton-Hulsey, A., & Whitmore, A. S. (2015). Early intervention and AAC: What a difference 30 years makes. *Augmentative and Alternative Communication, 31,* 181–202.

Rossetti, L. (2006). *The Rossetti Infant-Toddler Language Scale: A measure of communication and interaction.* Super Duper Publications.

Rowland, C. (2011). *Communication Matrix* [Measurement instrument]. https://communicationmatrix.org

Semantic Compaction Systems, Inc. (2018). *Minspeak.* https://minspeak.com

Snyder, P. A., & Hemmeter, M. L. (Eds.). (2018). *Instruction: Effective strategies to support engagement, learning, and outcomes* (DEC Recommended Practices Monograph Series No. 4). Division for Early Childhood.

Tobii Dynavox, Inc. (2021a). *Look to Learn.* https://us.tobiidynavox.com/products/look-to-learn

Tobii Dynavox, Inc. (2021b). *Picture Communication Symbols.* https://us.tobiidynavox.com/products/picture-communication-symbols-pcs

Wetherby, A. M., & Prizant, B. M. (2001). *Communication and Symbolic Behavior Scales™ (CSBS™).* Paul H. Brookes.

Zabala, 2007. Ready, SETT, go! Getting started with the SETT framework. *Closing the Gap, 23,* 5.

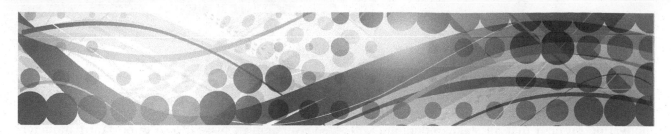

Chapter 9

INTERVENTION AND IMPLEMENTATION FOR TODDLERS AND PRESCHOOLERS USING AAC

Barbara Weber

Fundamentals

When speech-language pathologists (SLPs) work in early intervention, they must be prepared to implement augmentative and alternative communication (AAC) when it can support language growth or serve as the child's primary communication modality. For young children with complex communication needs (CCNs), AAC strategies can be beneficial across multiple stages of language development, both supporting the growth of early language skills (Beukleman & Mirenda, 1992) and augmenting speech and language skills in young children with CCNs (Romski & Sevcik, 2005). Important parameters to consider when developing an implementation plan include consideration of how and when to introduce AAC, building AAC use and communication partner competencies, choosing meaningful and appropriate vocabulary, sensitivity to family issues, and the openness to collaborate with all team members to find the best fit for a child.

Unfortunately, AAC remains underutilized, due to both late identification of AAC needs and misunderstanding of its indications. As mentioned in the previous chapter, many young children with AAC needs are not identified until after the 12 to 24 months of age window, a time when children are learning to understand and say many words. However, prior research has demonstrated that intervening early (prior to 12–24 months) with AAC is ideal (Davidoff, 2017), as early AAC implementation supports the child's development of cognition and receptive and expressive outcomes (Holyfield et al., 2019). AAC supports play and literacy, as well. It is a common misconception that AAC should only be considered when a child is nonverbal. AAC can be utilized for language support in many different ways. Some practitioners may feel reluctant to utilize AAC strategies if they predict that the child will develop verbal skills over time. However, the presence of, or potential for, verbal speech should not deter use of AAC.

There is no one-size-fits-all AAC system, and multiple AAC modalities may be beneficial (e.g., use of gestures, sign language, visual scene displays, communication apps, dedicated devices, such as those discussed in Chapters 2 and 3); each modality may play a role in supporting the child's communication development. The vocabulary chosen for early communicators should support early language development by being developmentally appropriate (Laubscher & Light, 2020), as discussed in Chapter 7. Use of visual scene displays can support capturing, contextualizing, and facilitating engagement with vocabulary targets. One should choose words that are important to the family and child to support participation in family routines.

Early word choices for AAC will also need to be motivating enough that all stakeholders are willing to put in the effort to navigate the complexity of AAC (e.g., the effort to use, practice, program, and/or update an app or device). Additionally, the child must understand the words they are being asked to use. Too often, the focus on expressive outcomes without careful assessment of the child's understanding results in the child being asked to say things he or she does not yet understand. Although focus on core words is an important consideration for generative language and early literacy, a child's early AAC targets may need to capture motivation by first focusing on requests for tangible objects (e.g., bubbles, goldfish crackers, ball, book, video).

Building competency and teaching the child and family to use AAC is an important part of the process. Building in predictability, practice, repetition, use of prompts, and prompt fading are important in effective teaching. For example, after selecting a motivating activity such as blowing bubbles (an activity with a predictable sequence), the child pushes the icon on their AAC device that pictures and says "bubbles" (practice), and continues to do so as long as he or she is motivated to request bubbles (repetition). At first, the adult may demonstrate activating the icon (modeling) or pointing to the icon to indicate the child should point (use of prompts), and as the child learns how to activate the icon for prompts, the adult no longer uses prompts (prompt fading). The child will learn the power of their body to communicate a message when he or she says "bubbles," and the communication partner blows bubbles. These teaching principles can be used with all AAC modalities (e.g., gesture use, sign or picture exchange). It is essential to embed practice into important family routines. Not all families have and/or value playtime routines.

Families need ongoing support for AAC success. Because young children's language is supported by the adults in the child's life, they need to learn how to teach use of AAC to the child (Barker et al., 2019). They are faced with building operational competency to utilize AAC effectively, including positioning and programming the device, deciding when a device is used, choosing vocabulary, building language competence, and

teaching the child, and do so within their already busy, complex lives. These important parameters comprise the initial considerations in planning AAC programming: how and when to introduce AAC, planning for both input and output strategies, generating functional outcomes for the child and the communication partner, and choosing meaningful and appropriate vocabulary reflective of naturally occurring language.

When introducing AAC to very young children, the SLP must be aware that, often, the child's needs are the family's first exposure to AAC, and many of their dreams and expectations may be actively changing. This process can extend across a continuum spanning from a sense of hopelessness and depression that the child may not develop verbal speech to joy and excitement that the child can use a communication modality. Sensitivity, compassion, and understanding are critical skill sets for navigating these feelings. As already reviewed in previous chapters, cultural sensitivity is a vital consideration as well. Variables such as how icons are depicted (e.g., avoiding pictures of foods shown together that a religious practice prohibits, choosing pictured characters that resemble the skin color/dress of the family), who may assume the teaching role in the family, which caregiver typically makes the decisions, and identification of important multiple caregivers or implicit biases must be monitored.

AAC intervention with very young children should focus on speech and language goals, as well as the use of AAC. When focusing on AAC, irrespective of the AAC system being used, vocabulary targets must be motivating, developmentally appropriate, and designed to increase participation in meaningful and relevant routines. The SLP should apply their understanding of the development of concepts, grammar, and so on, so as to choose developmentally appropriate word targets. Embedding AAC practice into motivating, repetitive, and predictable routines will support the child's language learning, and ultimate use of the AAC system; start with one or two routines to first establish success. The use of prompts and prompt fading will support the continuum of learning to independent communication. It is important that the communication partner (whether it be the SLP or a family member) helps the child successfully learn and use the AAC system through prompting (pointing to a target, using a laser to draw attention to it, or providing appropriate guidance to the system), and that their prompting is faded over time to ensure that the child can demonstrate the skill on their own. When AAC has been established within one routine, add one more, continuing to increase participation across the day.

Expert Tips or Practical Advice

1. Attend to the pacing of information, programming, and treatment. The team must follow the family's pace and give information in small pieces when needed. Make a collaborative plan and keep it small. Build intervention in small increments.
2. AAC can support children who are verbal by providing visual support for language learning and increasing intelligibility.
3. Respect the emotional process that may occur when families of young children use alternative modalities for speech.

Case Study: IB

Clinical Profile and Communication Needs

The Individual

I first met IB when he was 23 months of age. IB was referred through early intervention. He has a diagnosis of Pallister-Killian mosaic syndrome, a rare chromosomal disorder that affects many parts of the body. He is not yet ambulatory but can sit with support and hold his head upright, needing support to maintain the head position. He has tracheostomy and gastrostomy tubes. He can vocalize but does not yet say consonants or words. He has a vision impairment that is significantly corrected by wearing glasses, and he has myringotomy tubes for a bilateral conductive hearing loss.

Their Communication Partners and Their Environment

IB lives at home and is cared for by his father. He lives with his father, mother, brother, step-brother, and a 16-year-old cousin. Extended family live nearby and visits often. Family members who do not live nearby call IB using a video application to participate in family routines, such as singing together, or taking part in special occasions, such as birthdays or weekly visits.

AAC Considerations

The AAC evaluation began with a team discussion and the gathering of prior and current assessments of cognition, receptive language, expressive language, vision, hearing, and fine and gross motor skills. Because IB was in early intervention, current assessment and progress monitoring were available. IB did not have much volitional movement of his limbs, head, or fingers, although improvements in movement had been noted. Trunk and head instability made positioning an important variable. The vision specialist, noting how well IB was able to request with gaze, requested an AAC evaluation.

The AAC System

The recommendation for eye-gaze equipment with speech generation was derived from feature matching to IB's presenting physical skills, emerging skills (e.g., making choices with eye gaze), and interprofessional collaboration along with IB's family. IB's family wanted to be sure that the team would also continue to work on using voice and gestures to communicate along with adding AAC strategies.

Rationale for Clinical Decision-Making

Eye-gaze equipment was trialed. IB first demonstrated the ability to sustain gaze to activate and maintain movement of the videos within the device (when IB stopped looking, the video stopped as well) and move his eyes around the screen to play games and choose videos. Next, we identified a highly motivating activity, choosing which music toy to hear, to begin to teach IB that he can use his eyes to choose from pictures of his music items. The repetition and practice across a consistent routine helped IB learn how to effectively and consistently use his eyes to communicate his choice.

Through careful questioning and discussion, we determined that the next step was to add more vocabulary to expand the existing routine or add another routine. This process was not errorless. IB had no interest in indicating "more," "all done," or "stop." He did not seem to have interest in saying "stand" or "sit," as the physical therapist had hypothesized. One of the parents' priorities was that IB would be able to call for his mother and father. Pictures of his mother and father were taken and programmed, but the family did not report much use of these pictures; IB's mother and father were often there, anticipating IB's needs, so there was little need to call for them. At this point, data collection was sparse. We had determined that IB could use his eyes to operate the device. He could choose his music toys. Some of the pre-set screens (e.g., building block towers and knocking them down, core words such as "yes," "no," "all done," and "more") did not seem to meet the family's needs.

After attempts at consistent use, during a discussion about the AAC use, IB's father declared with some consternation, "I want his language to *come alive*!" It was obvious that the device and its settings, despite being appropriately programmed, were not motivating to the family. The family was willing to practice, but something would need to change to make AAC a more functional part of communication.

After many questions and discussions, we determined that, first, seating was an issue. We had IB in a chair specifically positioned to use his eye-gaze equipment. However, IB's father said that he wanted IB to be able to sit on the couch with his family and be able to communicate. The occupational and physical therapist collaborated to support seating on the couch, and this meant we needed a floor stand instead of a table stand for the device. In hindsight, at the time that IB's father

declared he wanted the language to "come alive," the author had gotten a glimpse of the answer for how to help. IB's father had sent meaningful videos to the entire team of IB throughout the day. The family is a happy group who try to engage IB consistently throughout routines. In the videos, one hears IB called many times, as his family attempts to both gain his attention and include him in their activities. When I asked IB's father what would help language come alive during those family routines, he said, "I want IB to be able to *call his siblings like they can call him*." To address this need, we expanded the "mommy/daddy" page to include all family members. The videos also depicted a family gathering time for songs and prayer. When I asked IB's dad if this was a time when he might like IB to be able to fill in a part of a prayer, such as with "amen," or to choose a song to sing, he responded enthusiastically. The family was very excited to try these activities.

Over the following weeks, the family had uploaded the picture to use in these situations but had not yet programmed the device, as, within this time frame, IB required two surgeries, a grandparent experienced a health crisis, and their home Internet connection was spotty. IB's dad explained that he had wanted to program the device, but that there were so many competing priorities and only so many hours in the day. It is important to note that even our best assessment required significant modifications to our programming. Our initial hypotheses, although appropriate, logical, and within typical practice considerations, did not sufficiently motivate the family. Many barriers impacted data collection, and continued discussion helped structure AAC that was exciting for the family. The complexity of life events can also impact the process of AAC. It is paramount that the SLP have realistic goals and provide support every step of the way.

Next Steps

Over time, the SLP and family worked to modify the AAC system in ways that addressed motivation and the family goals. IB had choice-making pages

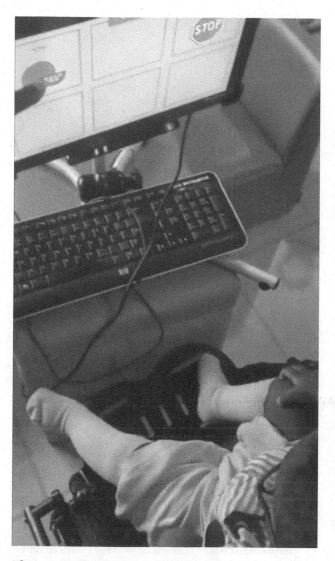

Figure 9–1. Choice-making page.

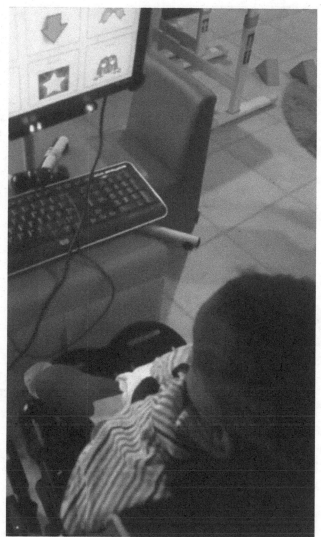

Figure 9–2. Song page.

(like the one shown in Figure 9–1), a page related to singing and song time (shown in Figure 9–2), as well as vocabulary used to engage with his family (like being able to tell them to "clap," like shown in Figure 9–3) programmed into his AAC system.

Now that IB can call family members over and participate in a much-loved family routine, core vocabulary such as "go," "stop," and "more" will naturally become more functional. Some future goals that were proposed included the following: that IB will express his communication intention across multiple functions, express his feelings or state of

being, engage in social communication exchanges with extended family members and friends, and ask and answer questions. For IB and his family, the dynamic journey of early AAC has begun. The family will continue to need ongoing support and programming to meet their changing needs and to gradually increase IB's ability to participate in daily routines that are important to him and his family. His SLP will need to dynamically assess changing family priorities, assess IB's ever-changing receptive and expressive skills, develop functional treatment goals, and plan for generative language growth.

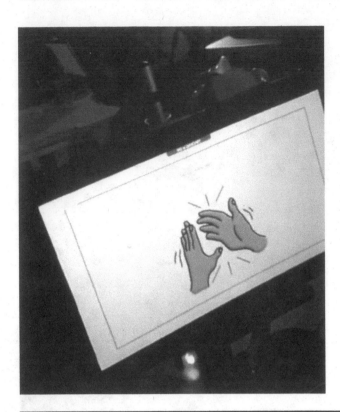

Figure 9–3. Directive page ("clap").

References

Barker, R. M., Romski, M., Sevcik, R. A., Adamson, L. B., Smith, A. L., & Bakeman, R. (2019). Intervention focus moderates the association between initial receptive language and language outcomes for toddlers with developmental delay. *Augmentative and Alternative Communication, 35*(4), 263–273. https://doi.org/10.1080/07434618.2019.1686770

Beukelman, D. R., & Mirenda, P. (1992). *Augmentative and alternative communication: management of severe communication disorders in children and adults.* Paul H. Brookes.

Davidoff, B. E. (2017). AAC with energy—Earlier. *ASHA Leader, 22*(1), 48–53. https://doi.org/10.1044/leader.ftr2.22012017.48

Holyfield, C., Caron, J., & Light, J. (2019). Programing AAC just-in-time for beginning communicators: The process. *Augmentative and Alternative Communication, 35*(4), 309–318. https://doi.org/10.1080/07434618.2019.1686538

Laubscher, E., & Light, J. (2020). Core vocabulary lists for young children and considerations for early language development: A narrative review. *Augmentative and Alternative Communication, 36*(1), 43–53. https://doi.org/10.1080/07434618.2020.1737964

Romski, M., & Sevcik, R. A. (2005). Augmentative communication and early intervention. *Infants & Young Children, 18*(3), 174–185. https://doi.org/10.1097/00001163-200507000-00002

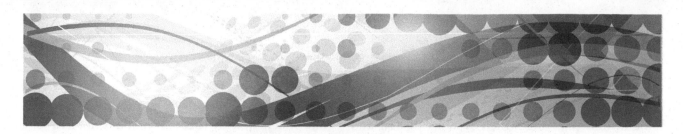

Chapter 10
ASSESSING SCHOOL-AGED INDIVIDUALS

Sarah Gregory

Fundamentals

Before beginning an augmentative and alternative communication (AAC) assessment in any setting, it is important to be aware of some key principles. First, when we consider who would benefit from an AAC evaluation in a school setting, the answer is almost anyone. The candidacy model that was prominent in the 1980s used certain criteria such as age or receptive language skills to determine who would benefit from AAC (Mirenda, 2017). This model required students to prove cognitive or linguistic capabilities before being given an opportunity to use AAC. Instead, Beukelman and Mirenda (1998) suggest using a participation model to provide opportunities to use AAC and support it with evidence-based practice, without asking our student to prove anything first.

There are no prerequisite skills for accessing AAC, and it is never too early nor too late to provide a student with an opportunity to communicate. Many different communicators can benefit from AAC including students who have no speech, intermittent speech, cognitive, and language impairments. It is important to keep an open mind and trial AAC for an extensive period without making an initial judgment on who may or may not benefit from AAC.

Another important consideration before beginning an AAC evaluation is to presume the compe-tence or potential of the person being assessed. We do not know what students are capable of produc-ing with an AAC device until we have a system in place and have taught it extensively. We should not limit a student's ability to communicate before we provide ample teaching and support across envi-ronments to help them become successful.

Presuming competence does not mean that we automatically provide the most complex or robust AAC system to every student. It does not mean that we assume AAC will instantly unlock expressive language skills that are commensurate with same-age peers. Presuming competence means that we do not wait to see specific skills before we begin teaching AAC. It is still important to gain an under-standing of a student's present level of skills and find a system that they can be most successful with in both the present and the future.

In planning for the future communication needs of a student, it is important to select a sys-tem that can evolve with them. We should not put a limit on the vocabulary in an AAC system based on what a student can show us in the snapshot of an evaluation. Consider robust AAC systems that can systematically grow with the student. The defi-nition of robust AAC generally includes a system that has a large vocabulary of at least 3,000 words, has the ability to add personalized vocabulary as needed, supports syntax, embeds principles of motor planning, contains all parts of speech, has a full keyboard, and provides easy access to core vocabulary. These features are important to consider when selecting which systems to trial and which ones to trial first.

In addition to a robust AAC system, start with the largest number of buttons in a grid and the smallest button size that a student can independently navigate. The trial may begin with some of these buttons being hidden, but starting with the largest number of buttons prevents the need to shift button locations as a student's vocabulary grows. Keeping the buttons in the same location over time will support motor planning and automaticity with the device. When button locations move, the person who uses augmentative and alternative communication (PWUAAC) must rely on visual skills, picture recognition, categorization, or literacy skills to relocate the button.

Before beginning an AAC evaluation, consider implementation strategies and supports that can be put in place beforehand. One possible strategy to implement with school-aged students is to provide universal access to AAC in a multitiered approach. This concept has been shared by Karen Erickson and colleagues (2015) and through the work of Project Core with the Center for Literacy and Disability Studies at University of North Carolina, Chapel Hill. Universal access to AAC may include providing a low-tech core board to all students before beginning a trial or evaluation. (Figure 10–1 shows a 36-location Universal Core Communication Board from project-core.com with LessonPix images.) Evaluations can be delayed for many reasons, so it is beneficial to begin supporting symbol-based language as soon as possible. In a school setting, core boards can be integrated into the classroom environment as a tier one support, meaning all students have access to them. This will help identify which students need more intensive or individualized support, which can be provided through an AAC assessment in tier two or three (Erickson et al., 2015).

Similar to a multitiered approach is the Specific Language System First approach to AAC, as described by Chris Bugaj (2019). In this approach, a school district selects one robust AAC system that meets the needs of most of the students. This builds a school culture that strongly supports the

selected AAC system. Providing universal access to one system quickly reveals when it is not a fit for a student, perhaps before a formal evaluation is initiated. The Specific Language System First approach supports staff in being trained across grade levels and strengthens the circle of support, while providing data to guide selection of another system when indicated. Most importantly, this system encourages and helps peers to be meaningful communication partners, despite yearly staff changes (Bugaj, 2019).

Once it is determined that a student requires an AAC evaluation, there continue to be options for how to complete it successfully. It is important to take a team to the fullest extent possible, which means including the student, family/caregivers, SLP, occupational therapist (OT)/physical therapist (PT) if there are motor concerns, Teacher of the Visually Impaired (TVI) if there are vision concerns, classroom teacher, and any other related professionals as needed. Some funding sources, such as Medicaid (state-based, federally regulated insurance), require a licensed SLP to complete the evaluation and sign the report. However, this does not mean that an AAC evaluation should be a solo endeavor, and collaboration with other professionals may be necessary.

Traditional AAC evaluations often consist of an evaluator (e.g., SLP) meeting with a client for one or more sessions, trialing different systems, taking data, and making a team decision about the best AAC system. Another approach can be referred to as "diagnostic therapy," which is similar, but more of an ongoing or trial process in the context of speech and language/AAC intervention sessions. Diagnostic therapy allows clinicians to trial and teach an AAC system and take extensive data on what is working and what changes need to be made. This is a dynamic approach that can also provide insight into future treatment recommendations. Some situations may require a shorter snapshot, due to billing or time constraints, for example. If time allows, diagnostic therapy can provide valuable information and lead to well-informed decision-making. This is because it provides time to assess how the student responds to the system or different intervention strategies. For example, during the first assessment session, a student may

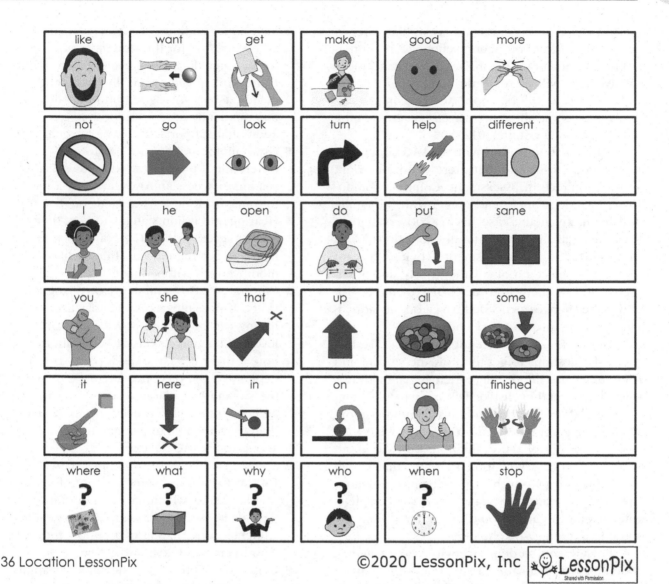

Figure 10–1. Universal Core Communication Board from project-core.com with LessonPix images. Used with permission from LessonPix, Inc.

have used the AAC device only once given modeling and gestural prompts (e.g., pointing to the button on the device). In subsequent sessions, the evaluator has a better understanding of the student's interests, models target words in context with motivating activities, and sees the student independently access these words. The evaluator also notices that the student often hits the button next to the target and brings in a keyguard that increases accuracy of

selections. This more sequential approach characteristic of diagnostic therapy allows evaluators to be responsive to student needs and provides valuable data for the decision-making process.

Teaming is one of the most important aspects of an AAC evaluation. If an evaluator determines an ideal system for a student but does not have support from the whole team, then it may not in fact be the right system. Team members should include the individual being evaluated, as well as caregivers, family members, peers, school team, outpatient clinic, and device representatives. Stakeholder involvement will increase the likelihood that the device selected will be supported by communication partners and therefore increase success of the PWUAAC (Binger et al., 2012).

When getting started with an AAC evaluation, it is important to note that there is not one right way to conduct an assessment. Common components include a "meet and greet" with the family and team, an intake/case history, observation of the individual engaging naturally, selection of AAC tools to trial, direct assessment activities, a team meeting to select a tool collaboratively, and possible diagnostic therapy to teach use of the device and make changes as needed based on the individual's performance and data collected.

During the initial meeting, gather a case history, ask questions to get to know the student and find out what is important to them, what motivates them, and what they dislike. Discuss what the long-term goals are for the student's communication, what their team has tried so far, and what they hope to get out of the evaluation. Be clear about what the process will look like and that it will involve support from the whole team throughout the evaluation and especially after it is complete. Information can and should be gathered from the student and other stakeholders.

Review the student's previous assessments, Individualized Education Plan (IEP)—the plan or program that is developed detailing the individualized instruction needed to support a student with disabilities—and other relevant documents. Determine which other professionals you will need to collaborate with during the evaluation process. For example, if the student may have difficulty physically accessing a device, include a PT or OT. If there are vision concerns, consult a TVI. Collaborating with professionals from other disciplines is always helpful when you have the opportunity because it can provide valuable information for feature matching and implementation of an AAC system.

When generating a report, you will need to mention various domains as they relate to AAC access, customization, and use, such as:

- Fine motor abilities. Determine the best access method for the student (e.g., finger, knuckle, switch, eye gaze, etc.). If the student can physically access the device, assess what size button they can independently access, and if they require additional supports, such as a keyguard.
- Gross motor abilities and posture. Determine if the student requires specific seating to access an AAC device or a mount to transport it on a wheelchair or walker.
- Hearing and vision status and how they impact access to AAC (i.e., can the student hear and see the device? If not, what modifications will be made?).
- Current receptive and expressive language skills. If possible, recent standardized testing can be used to provide present levels of language skills. It is helpful to note if there is a large discrepancy between expressive and receptive language (e.g., if the student has a large receptive vocabulary and can understand much more language than they are able to use due to not having access to an AAC device).
- Spoken/oral language abilities. Many PWUAACs also use some amount of spoken/oral language, which may be intermittent or have decreased intelligibility. Describe the student's current abilities and how they use AAC to augment communication.
- Cognitive abilities (e.g., the student's ability to learn and retain new words on the AAC device) It is important to note that cognitive ability is not a prerequisite for AAC use and should never be used to deny a student access to AAC. Some funding sources require information regarding cognitive status, so this may need to be included in a report.

Data collection, as detailed in Chapter 12, is an important aspect of the trial process and should be clearly outlined before beginning. Be clear about what data need to be obtained (e.g., some funding sources require data to be collected across multiple settings and multiple communication partners).

Consult the team and agree on a method that feels doable to all parties. This may mean that the parents record videos of AAC use in the home, or they fill out a structured form to document utterances, communication attempts, and prompting levels. It is important to find a system that the team is comfortable with, otherwise the trial may conclude with limited data, meaning a funding source does not approve the requested device.

There are many AAC assessments that can be administered at the beginning of the evaluation process to help guide decision-making. A variety of tools (but not an exhaustive list) that can be used for school-aged individuals are detailed in Table 10–1. It is not necessary to use each one of these tools, but familiarity with each of them will help determine which will obtain the most relevant data for the student.

As discussed in Chapter 8, feature-matching is a process that can help guide the selection of an AAC system. This includes determining which features a student requires in a system and then finding a system that matches all of the necessary features. Features include symbols, access method, display and editing features, linguistic features,

portability and positioning, and operational features (as further detailed in Table 10–2). For example, a student with a visual impairment may require high-contrast symbols or the ability to adjust the device settings to provide visual feedback when a button is selected. Consider a student's culture and identity and look for a device that has symbolic, linguistic, and voice features that will accurately represent them. This is an important discussion to have with the student and their family or caregivers to gain their input.

Once the intake and feature-matching across domains of access and language are complete, it is time to select which AAC systems to trial and in what order. It is easy to place a lot of pressure on this decision, but use the information gathered, make a best guess, and proceed confidently while being open to needing to make adjustments to your plan. It is okay if the first system chosen is not the best fit for the student. Be responsive to the student, input from their communication partners, and data gathered, and adjust quickly as needed.

It may be sufficient to trial only one system. If the individual responds positively to the trial device, data from assessments and case history

Table 10–1. AAC Assessment Tools

Assessment Tool	Can Be Accessed At
The SETT framework by Joy Zabala	https://joyzabala.com
The Pragmatic Profile for People who use AAC from AceCentre	https://www.acecentre.org.uk
The Communication Matrix	https://www.communicationmatrix.org
The Assessment for Learning Process for AAC	https://www.alpforaac.com
The QUAD Profile by Russell Cross	https://aaclanguagelab.com/resources
The Functional Communication Profile, Revised by Larry I. Kleiman	Kleiman, L. I. (2003). *Functional communication profile, revised assessing communicative effectiveness in clients with developmental delays.* Pro-Ed.
Augmentative & Alternative Communication Profile by Tracy M. Kovach.	Kovach, T. M. (2009). *Augmentative and alternative communication profile a continuum of learning.* LinguiSystems.

Please note: This is a nonexhaustive list of tools that can help collect assessment data.

Table 10–2. Feature Matching Considerations

Feature	Examples
Symbols	The types of images such as line drawings or photographs
Access method	Such as direct selection with finger, knuckle, or toe, eye gaze, switch access
Display and editing features	Modifications that can be made to the color, size, and shape of buttons
Linguistic features	Parts of speech that are represented, such as pronouns, prepositions, nouns, verbs, adjectives, adverbs, as well as the ability to change grammatical structures such as verb tense or plural nouns
Portability and positioning	The weight of the device and ease of transport, what angles it can be positioned at, ability to be mounted on tables, walkers, or wheelchairs as necessary
Operational features	Tools that can be customized to provide visual or auditory feedback, adjust brightness of the display, adjust volume, change voices, and hold a charge

support the selection, the team agrees, and the AAC device is robust and matches the needed features, there may not be a need to trial a second system. Depending on the funding source, there may be a requirement to trial or at least consider two or three systems. Trialing multiple systems may also be indicated based on professional judgment, school policy, or at the request of the team.

Once you have selected the first system to trial, it is time to begin diagnostic therapy or direct assessment activities (virtually or in person) with the student. Plan to include preferred and novel activities to increase motivation to communicate, as well as nonpreferred activities to provide an opportunity to protest or express displeasure. When evaluating school-aged individuals, it is important to include academic activities, such as answering questions about a text to see how the device may or may not support the student in the classroom. This will also provide data on barriers to accessing academic content, for example, is the student unable to respond to academic questions without access to an AAC system? These barriers are important to include in a final report, as this will help prove the necessity of the device.

During these direct sessions with the student, observe their ability to physically access the device and try different grid sizes (as discussed in Chapter 5). Hide some of the vocabulary and observe if that helps increase accuracy and independence. Provide different levels of prompting to determine if they require less prompting on one system versus another. Provide Aided Language Input, or modeling, and use the device yourself to communicate with the student; observe how often they attend to your use of the device. It is important to observe the student's engagement and interest in the activity, because this will provide the best insight into their ability to use the device. If they are not interested in communicating about something, then we are likely not seeing an accurate representation of their abilities.

After these direct sessions with the student, analyze the data collected from each trial and hold a meeting to make a collective decision about what system to recommend. Carefully consider what system the student prefers and what system the circle of communicative support is most comfortable with implementing and supporting. It is okay to respectfully disagree with team members, be clear about your recommendations, and also be open to the insight of other team members.

In considering final recommendations, let us discuss "the myth of the perfect system." Treating an AAC assessment as a quest for finding the one perfect system for a student may result in a unilateral decision. Often, an AAC assessment will reveal more than one system that will give a student the ability to communicate about anything at any time. The end goal of spontaneous and generative language relies on more than just the perfect system, it relies on buy-in from the student and support from the team. It relies on hours of teaching in fun and motivating environments and hours of device exploration. By searching for the one and only perfect system, one may lose sight of these other important factors and put unnecessary pressure on the evaluation process.

Once a system is selected, it is time to write a compelling report. Be clear about what information is expected so that you can provide relevant data and input from the team. Use resources such as device representatives to help you make the best case for the device you have selected to be funded. Include data across communication partners and settings, focus on what the student can communicate with AAC that cannot be communicated in another way. Data may include vocabulary used by the student, prompting levels used by support people, and how communication changed based on partners and the environment. Many state learning standards have foundations in communication, so include information on how the student cannot access the curriculum without a means to communicate about the curriculum.

One of the biggest factors determining AAC success is evidence-based implementation. When possible, provide training, support, resources, and coaching to the team. Training may include how to model on the device in a way that is manageable at home and school, how to program the device, what level of prompting to provide and when to fade it, how to select vocabulary targets, and how to make AAC support fun and engaging. Seek input from team members about what feels doable and where they need more support. Recommendations for support are only beneficial if they are manageable for the team, otherwise they will not be implemented and can lead to frustration for everyone.

Be creative in providing support and coaching to the team. This could be prerecorded videos on AAC best practices or how to program the device and add vocabulary. Consider taking videos of the student using the selected AAC system to demonstrate prompting levels and wait time. Supporting a student's communication partners can help to avoid device abandonment and increase the student's success with the chosen system.

In a school setting, consider involving peers in AAC teaching to increase the circle of support. Do not involve peers as teachers or helpers but rather as fellow learners of the new system. Provide low-tech versions of the system for all peers to use in meaningful ways. Peer support can have a positive social and academic impact on students with and without disabilities.

AAC assessments with any age group can feel daunting when the end goal is to find the one and only perfect system. A proposed mindset shift is to focus on finding an AAC system that is robust, will meet the student's needs, is preferred by the student, and will be best supported by the whole team across environments. There is rarely one right answer, but we are likely to find success when we involve all stakeholders and focus on teaching and supporting the chosen system.

Case Study: RJ

This is a hypothetical student composed of multiple student profiles from the author's past experiences.

Clinical Profile and Communication Needs

The Individual

RJ is a 5-year-old female. She has a diagnosis of Childhood Apraxia of Speech, a significant expressive language delay, a mild receptive language delay, and a suspected learning disability. Her fine motor skills are moderately delayed; she has difficulty with handwriting and manipulating small objects. Her gross motor skills, vision, and hearing are within normal limits. RJ began receiving early intervention services for speech therapy and occupational therapy at the age of 2.5 years. She recently began attending kindergarten in a public school and continues to receive these services through an IEP.

RJ communicates using vocal approximations, gestures, body language, leading communication partners to desired items, facial expressions, and picture boards. Her speech is less than 20% intelligible. RJ produces one- to three-word spoken phrases that include her family members' names, comments such as "uh oh" and "wow," favorite foods, toys, characters, and carrier phrases such as "I want" and "I see." RJ enjoys playing with her siblings and friends in her neighborhood. She enjoys humor and prefers silly or funny books and TV shows. She is most engaged in back-and-forth communication when humor and laughter are involved.

In preschool, RJ was given communication boards to help her select an item from a category such as food, drink, toys, and classroom activities for the purposes of making choices and to support basic participation. The boards were sent home, but RJ's mom reported that they did not use them because they did not have many of the same items at home and that she can understand RJ better than her teachers. Her SLP provided the choice boards to the classroom and did push-in therapy to help the staff learn how to use them (e.g., during snack time the SLP prompted RJ to use the choice board to pick a snack by pointing to an item on the board and showing it to her, demonstrating this strategy in the moment to staff). RJ did not often seek out the boards but would make a choice if an adult presented a communication board to her. Speech therapy also focused on increasing her speech sound repertoire and verbally producing high-frequency vocabulary words.

Their Communication Partners

RJ's communication partners include her parents, grandma, and two older brothers who live in her home; peers at school and in her neighborhood; teachers; lunchroom workers; therapists; and paraprofessionals in her classroom.

Their Environment

RJ communicates primarily in the home and school environments. Her family frequently socializes with neighbors and attends her brother's basketball games after school. She spends most of her school day in a general education kindergarten classroom with her peers.

The AAC System or Service Considerations

RJ was referred for an AAC assessment by her kindergarten team including her teacher, SLP, and OT. Her team reported that they understand less than 20% of her speech. There is another student in RJ's class who uses AAC (an Accent device with LAMP Words for Life), and every student has access to a core board (which is a paper-based replica of the home screen of the same system). Her teacher uses a large core board replica during circle time and collaborates with the SLP to model core vocabulary for all students. For example, when the words *same* and *different* were targeted, students shared a fact about themselves (e.g., I have one sister), and other students responded if they had the *same* or *different* number of siblings by pointing to the words on the large core replica. The teacher reported that RJ has independently used target core words on the board a few times and that she attends to modeling during circle time. He also reported that she appears interested in her friend's AAC device.

RJ's SLP reported that she has used the core board in therapy and that RJ uses it consistently to request and direct actions, given modeling. Due to RJ's fine motor delay, she was frequently misselecting buttons. Her OT used wax sticks to create a border around target words. This helped RJ visually locate targets and physically access them. Another drawback was the core board being limited to 84 symbols so even though she has access to it throughout her day, it is not robust enough to allow her to fully participate academically or socially.

AAC Considerations

The team met with RJ's family to make a plan for the AAC assessment and to choose a system to trial first. RJ's parents stated that they were in support of her using a voice output device, but they did not have experience with any specific system. RJ's SLP provided a demonstration of three different robust AAC systems. She shared that another student in RJ's class uses LAMP Words for Life (WFL) and that system is widely used in the district, including upper grades that RJ will attend in the future. The school staff (including administrators, teachers, and noninstructional staff) receive general AAC training yearly and have access to online modules to support LAMP WFL. RJ's teacher shared that she is able to point to pictures on the 84-grid board, which is the same size as the buttons on the Accent device. The team also agreed that any system trialed would need to have a full keyboard to support literacy development.

RJ's parents said that they were interested in trialing LAMP WFL but wanted to trial more than one system to see which was the best fit. They also liked how other systems had pages for jokes and preprogrammed phrases, which they felt was important to RJ. The SLP created a folder in LAMP WFL and said she would work with RJ to select jokes to program in during therapy. The SLP has access to LAMP WFL on an iPad, so it was decided to begin using that so that they did not have to wait for a loaner device.

The AAC System or Service

The SLP recommended that she complete diagnostic therapy for approximately 4 to 6 weeks, meaning she would teach RJ to use the device over multiple therapy sessions, collect data, and adjust as needed. This was a possibility because she saw RJ four times per week for speech therapy and felt that this would help the team make the best decision about what device would be best for her.

She did not have room in her schedule to provide training with the staff and family at the moment, but she shared prerecorded videos on how communication partners could model using the device, selecting core vocabulary, and incorporating AAC into daily routines.

RJ's SLP asked that data be collected at home and in the classroom and shared a sample data sheet. RJ's parents said that they were not sure how to use the device at home, and they did not think they would remember to fill out a data sheet every day with their busy lives. They agreed to take videos of RJ using the device at home three times a week so that the SLP could take data from there. RJ's teacher had used the data sheet before and agreed to fill it out daily. RJ's SLP shared that she would also take detailed data in speech sessions and observe her during nonacademic times such as lunch.

RJ's SLP completed the Pragmatic Profile for People who use AAC to take baseline data on how RJ communicated for different pragmatic functions (Martin et al., 2017). She chose the Pragmatic Profile so that she could document RJ's different modes of communication and when she was using AAC versus verbal speech or other nonspeaking methods. This would also allow her to see how her modes of communication change throughout the diagnostic therapy period.

RJ's SLP completed the feature matching process by observing her using the trial device during various therapy activities. She noted that RJ was able to accurately select buttons on a grid of 84 with 50 buttons showing. RJ appeared to be developing motor plans for frequently used words as evidenced by her hand moving toward the second button in a sequence before her eyes moved there. RJ was able to independently carry the iPad. Her teacher reported that in class he had a difficult time hearing the communication device and occasionally missed what she had to say.

During the diagnostic therapy period, the SLP supported the family through tele-AAC (which is discussed in Chapters 35 and 36). She watched the videos RJ's family sent from home and replied with e-mail feedback to help them support device use at home. They participated in one live tele-AAC session so that the SLP could provide feedback in real time. She also met with RJ's classroom teacher twice to co-plan circle time and make sure they were targeting the same vocabulary. RJ's OT observed during one speech session to provide feedback about how her fine motor skills may impact her use of the device and recommended they trial a keyguard.

After 4 weeks, the team met for a second time to review the data and determine next steps. RJ's SLP shared with her family that after reviewing the data they could either write a funding request for a device, continue the trial for 2 more weeks, or choose a second device to trial. She shared that RJ had used 10 words independently across settings and up to 30 words, given a model. She also noted that based on the Pragmatic Profile, RJ used the AAC device for two communicative functions at the beginning of the trial and now had demonstrated use across five communicative functions.

The SLP shared how she had observed RJ learning the motor plans for frequently used words and that she attended to her modeling on her device and less often on the large core board in the classroom. She also described how RJ often produced spoken approximations of words after activating them on the AAC device.

RJ's family reported that she used the device at mealtimes to request food items and that she enjoyed saying people's names on the device and verbally repeating them. They said that the e-mails from her SLP had helped them, but they were still unsure what it looked like when she used the device in school.

RJ's teacher reported that when given a choice, RJ selected to use the SGD over the core board in class. He said that she independently initiated communication using the device approximately twice a day and followed gestural prompts to buttons 70% of the time. He reported that she was using verbal approximations of her peers' names more often. He also shared that it was easier to design lessons knowing that RJ had access to so much language on her device that could be modeled for her.

Based on this information, the team ruled out a low-tech board because it did not provide enough language, RJ chose the SGD over her core board, and she was observed to verbally repeat words

from her device after the speech output was elicited. They ruled out trialing a device with larger buttons as RJ was able to accurately select buttons, which increased when she was given a keyguard. Larger buttons and a smaller grid size would also require more button hits to access language, as there would be less vocabulary displayed on a given page.

RJ's family stated that they were happy with how the device increased her communication skills. They stated that they felt they still needed more training to use it at home but were pleased that her teachers were familiar with the system and already able to incorporate it into academics. They also plan to stay in the district long term and felt comfortable that teachers in higher grades also had experience with this device.

RJ's SLP shared that if they were interested in trialing a second device, the classroom would still do well supporting a different system. They have the foundational skills for supporting AAC, which apply to any device. She explained that they are committed to finding a device that is best for RJ and that everyone is the most comfortable with. RJ's teacher added that he is most familiar with LAMP Words for Life but felt confident that he could support her using any device.

After looking at another similar app together, offering comparable features to LAMP WFL, the team decided to select LAMP WFL for RJ and not trial another system. The team revisited the feature matching they had done at the beginning of the assessment, and the second system did have as many of the required features. In the area of display/editing features, the team felt that consistent button placement and maximum of three button hits on LAMP WFL would make navigation and motor planning easier for RJ. They felt that she had already made great progress and that once her family received more training it would be the easiest system to support throughout her school career.

RJ's teacher brought up his concern that the device was difficult to hear, and the SLP shared that they could pursue funding for a dedicated device that would have a louder external speaker than the iPad but would be heavier. RJ's OT shared that she thought RJ would be able to transport a heavier device. They also discussed that obtaining a dedicated device would give the team and family access to technological support and training on the language system. Since RJ's SLP had limited time, this was a bonus for them. They agreed to request a trial of an Accent device, and if RJ could transport it and liked it they would begin the funding request.

Next Steps

Finally, the team discussed what supports would be needed to support RJ using the AAC device. They decided that RJ's SLP would regularly share videos to a private Google Drive folder so that they could see how she was using the device at school. RJ's teacher would send home word lists that corresponded with lessons, including the button pathways (e.g., a picture of each button that needs to be selected in the sequence to access the target word).

RJ's team would continue to support her language development through multiple modalities including her AAC device and spoken language. Her SLP and classroom teacher planned to meet once a month to co-plan circle time and systematically increase AAC use in the classroom. They would continue to involve classroom peers in AAC learning by using core boards during circle time and academic lessons. The team scheduled quarterly meetings with RJ's family to gain input from home to guide AAC implementation at school. The quarterly meetings would also be used to provide support for RJ's family using the device at home.

RJ's SLP used her present levels on the Pragmatic Profile as well as the Dynamic AAC Goals Grid-2 (DAGG-2) to write IEP goals (Tobii Dynavox, 2015). She wrote one goal for each of the four areas of communicative competence: linguistic, social, operational, and strategic (Light, 1989).

Suggested Treatment Goal Areas

Linguistic: RJ will generate a 2+ word sentence across a variety of communication functions (e.g., protest, comment, gain attention) independently, given modeling throughout the school day.

Social: RJ will use humor with peers and adults by responding to or telling jokes, using

multimodal communication (e.g., nonverbal or programmed on her AAC device).

Operational: RJ will transport her AAC device between classroom activities, given no more than one gestural prompt.

Strategic: RJ will use a different mode of communication (e.g., AAC device, gesture, vocalization) when not understood.

References

Beukelman, D., & Mirenda, P. (1998). Building opportunities and nonsymbolic communication. In D. Beukelman & P. Mirenda (Eds.), *Augmentative and alternative communication* (2nd ed., pp. 265–294). Paul H. Brookes.

Binger, C., Ball, L., Dietz, A., Kent-Walsh, J., Lasker, J., Lund, S., . . . Quach, W. (2012). Personnel roles in the AAC assessment process. *Augmentative and Alternative Communication, 28*(4), 278–288. https://doi.org/10.3109/07434618.2012.716079

Bugaj, C. (2019). *Augmentative and alternative communication spotlight: Addressing challenges to AAC implementation* [Conference presentation]. ATIA 2019, Orlando, FL.

Erickson, K., Hatch, P., Geist, L., & Greer, C. (2015). *Implementation program review for the multi-tiered system for augmenting language* [Conference presentation]. ATIA 2017, Orlando, FL.

LessonPix, Inc. (2021). https://lessonpix.com

Light, J. (1989). Toward a definition of communicative competence for individuals using augmentative and alternative communication systems. *Augmentative and Alternative Communication, 5*(2), 137–144. https://doi.org/10.1080/07434618912331275126

Martin, S., Small, K., & Stevens, R. (2017). *The Pragmatics Profile for People who use AAC*. AceCentre. https://acecentre.org.uk/resources/pragmatics-profile-people-use-aac/

Mirenda, P. (2017). Values, practice, science, and AAC. *Research and Practice for Persons With Severe Disabilities, 42*(1), 33–41. https://doi.org/10.1177/1540796916661163

Tobii Dynavox. (2015). *The Dynamic AAC Goals Grid 2*. TobiiDynavox.com. http://tdvox.web-downloads.s3.amazonaws.com/MyTobiiDynavox/dagg%202%20-%20writable.pdf

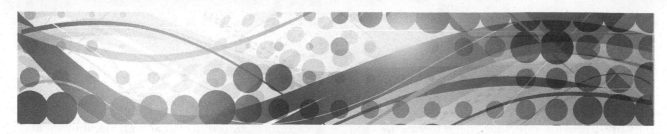

Chapter 11

INTERVENTION AND IMPLEMENTATION FOR SCHOOL-AGED INDIVIDUALS USING AAC

Amanda Soper

Fundamentals

Speech-language intervention for students with complex communication needs (CCNs) who use augmentative and alternative communication (AAC) requires innovators who believe in their students' potential. Speech-language pathologists (SLPs) must acknowledge that AAC is a *means* of communication, and their role is to help students and other educators (e.g., educational assistants, teachers, support staff, etc.) incorporate the use of AAC into the school day. To succeed in the educational environment, students must be able to participate in speaking, listening, reading, writing, and social skills. When data-driven interventions are paired with creative teaching opportunities, students with CCNs can improve their expressive language through AAC and succeed in the school environment.

There is no need to "reinvent the wheel" when it comes to communication and language intervention for school-aged persons who use AAC (PWUAACs). Students with CCNs who use AAC need the same language-based interventions as their peers who do not use AAC. There are many intervention tools available that can be used or adapted to support language acquisition for such learners. However, in addition to these language-based interventions, they also require the use of specific sup-

port strategies (e.g., aided language stimulation, wait time) and training and coaching for communication partners.

In this chapter, we explore the need for AAC intervention to address not only the five domains of language (semantics, syntax, morphology, phonology, and pragmatics) but also the four areas of AAC competence (linguistic, operational, social, and strategic; Light, 1989). Ongoing assessment tools allow SLPs to collect data and probe for new skills to address all of these areas. *While the domains of language overlap with the areas of AAC competence, it is critical to address both to meet the language and access needs for students with CCN.*

In order to meet the language needs of students with CCNs, they must have access to a linguistically robust vocabulary. As discussed in the previous chapter, a linguistically robust AAC system includes a large number of core vocabulary, a range of word classes, the ability to make morphological changes, and access to the alphabet. This provides students with the ability to say anything, at any time, to anyone. This is often referred to as spontaneous novel utterance generation (SNUG; Hill, 2006). Though students who use robust AAC have the ability to achieve SNUG, their expressive language skills are frequently below their receptive language abilities (Binger et al., 2017). This disparity, despite access to an AAC system, must be examined. Having an AAC system is not enough; SLPs must provide direct language instruction and intervention. Given that the domains of language do not occur in a vacuum, AAC intervention should move beyond a focus on semantics and pragmatics to include all domains, including syntax, morphology, and phonology.

Intervention Across the Five Domains of Language

Students with CNNs who use AAC require intervention rooted in established language therapy practices (Van Tatenhove, 2009). As many of these students are still "learning to communicate" rather than "communicating to learn," SLPs should provide educators with the knowledge and tools needed to support **language development** throughout the day. This knowledge can shift instruction from asking students to prove what they know by making choices from a field of answers, to teaching students the vocabulary and language needed to participate in learning opportunities. This "teach, don't test" model can provide students with the foundational language skills they need to succeed in an educational environment and begin to "communicate to learn."

Traditionally, one of the first steps to AAC intervention is introducing vocabulary. An essential part of language intervention for students with CCNs is teaching students how to use core vocabulary, which can be used across contexts. SLPs should remember that in addition to core vocabulary, it is important to teach students to use words of personal importance (e.g., people in their lives, favorite books/shows/characters/songs/foods, etc.) as well as relevant fringe vocabulary (e.g., common toys, places, animals, etc.), as noted in Chapter 7. It is also essential to teach vocabulary in meaningful contexts with consideration to other language domains (e.g., syntax, morphology).

A focus on **semantics**, or the way in which language conveys meaning, is important, but it must not be reduced to simplistic approaches. To teach the meaning of words and word combinations, SLPs often rely on a "Core Word(s) of the Week" strategy. Though it is helpful, especially for

educators, to have target vocabulary, this approach is extremely limiting in teaching vocabulary and meaning to students using AAC. Similar to their peers, students using AAC should be provided with language-rich intervention. One alternate intervention to consider is the Graphic Symbol Utterance and Sentence Development Framework as outlined in Binger and colleagues (2020), a framework of the progression of expressive sentence development using graphic symbols.

Syntax refers to the rules that govern how words can be ordered to form sentences. Syntax typically begins to develop around 18 months of age for typically developing children as their vocabulary begins to expand past 50 words. These utterances are coded by semantic relations (e.g., agent + action, descriptor + object, possessor + entity) and demonstrate how children can use a limited vocabulary to convey a wide range of messages (Binger et al., 2020). When teaching language to PWUAACs, educators should model a variety of syntactic structures while introducing vocabulary to help students narrow the gap between their receptive language abilities and expressive language abilities (e.g., understanding present progressive vs. using present progressive verbs in utterances).

Morphology is the study of morphemes, the smallest unit of meaning (e.g., un, s, es, ly). Similar to syntax, morphology emerges early in spoken language development but is not frequently targeted modeling AAC use for students using AAC. These grammatical markers are important for clarifying messages and should be addressed by educators to improve linguistic competence (Binger et al., 2020).

Pragmatics refers to the rules associated with language in conversation and social settings. When addressing pragmatic skills for PWUAACs, it is helpful to use a variety of assessment tools including but not limited to the Pragmatics Profile for AAC (Dewart & Summers, 1995), the Communication Matrix (Rowland, 2011), and the AAC Profile (Kovach, 2009). Students must learn how to communicate for a variety of functions, establish context, and participate in conversation across contextual variations (e.g., people, setting, topic, etc.). SLPs should consider the social language of typically developing peers when providing intervention and make sure to add age-appropriate and culturally relevant vocabulary to their students' devices (e.g., "uh oh spaghetti-o" for a 2-year-old vs. "ugh" for a 12-year-old).

Phonology, the study of speech sounds (phonemes) and the rules to combine those sounds, is integral in literacy instruction. School-aged students with CCNs must participate in literacy instruction, as literacy is a critical life skill. There are a variety of ways to adapt literacy instruction for nonverbal students including as outlined by Karen Fallon and colleagues (2004) and Erickson and Koppenhaver (2020). Numerous programs and curriculums have been designed with this population in mind, including the ALL Program (Light & McNaughton, 2012) and Readtopia (Don Johnston Inc., 2021), among others. All literacy programs for students with CCNs must include instruction in phonemes and the rules to combine phonemes into words. Many high-tech devices have a phonics keyboard that can be helpful for students to play with sounds and attempt to sound out words. In addition, no high-tech device, no matter how robust, has access to all the words a person could want to say. Therefore, it is imperative that PWUAACs develop an understanding of letters and letter sounds, as it opens a door for them to learn to spell any word they want to say.

Intervention Across AAC Competencies

As part of dynamic AAC intervention that includes assessment, SLPs may use formal tools to measure student progress and needs across AAC competencies—linguistic, operational, social, and strategic (Light, 1989). The AAC Profile (Kovach, 2009) is one such assessment tool that can drive intervention planning.

Linguistic competence should address all five domains of language—semantics, syntax, morphology, phonology, and pragmatics. Using a language sampling tool can help SLPs determine needs in terms of each language domain. There are several ways to collect this data. For early emergent PWUAACs, the Communication Matrix (Rowland, 2011) can help determine semantic and pragmatic

targets. However, as students begin to develop their vocabulary across various functions of language, a tool such as the QUAD Profile (Cross, 2005) can help analyze overall language needs as it has checklists for each language domain. For example, it may reveal that the student's utterances are often unclear because they only talk in first person present tense, do not use possessives, and do not use third person pronouns. This "snapshot" analysis of a language sample(s) should guide the SLP toward intervention strategies aiming to strengthen these areas of weakness. Another tool is a language acquisition monitor (LAM), which can be found on many high-tech devices including several iPad apps (Hill & Romich, 2001). This LAM tool tracks each word that is selected on the AAC device, allowing clinicians to determine areas of need not only in terms of vocabulary and syntax but also times of day that communication partners are struggling to use the device with the PWUAAC.

Operational competence includes the student's ability to fluently access their device and use controls such as volume, power on/off, programming, and so on. These essential functions should be taught by the education team. However, with regard to complex access methods, SLPs must be aware of the needs of their students with CCNs, including changes in physical status and their ability to successfully access the device. Knowing a student's baseline will help clinicians recognize the need for troubleshooting. Difficulties requiring troubleshooting may include but are not limited to inappropriate dwell time, calibration error, unpaired Bluetooth equipment, software glitches requiring an update, hardware errors (e.g., switch no longer works, eye-tracking module not working), and so on. If set incorrectly, access settings can significantly impact a PWUAAC's ability to use their device.

Social competence includes students' ability to participate in conversational exchanges, use socially appropriate language, and form bonds with others. It is an integral part of communication and should consistently be considered and addressed in the school environment, as peer interaction is embedded throughout the school day and often difficult for students with CCNs. This may be addressed through communication circles in which targeted activities are completed with targeted peers to foster social interaction goals and through peer AAC modeling.

Strategic competence refers to a student's ability to repair communication breakdowns, judge which method of communication may be fastest or most appropriate (e.g., gesture vs. saying a sentence), and ultimately be an independent communicator partner who can relay a variety of messages to unfamiliar partners. This area of competency is important to consider when looking at a student's overall skill levels and determining how to help the student become an effective communicator.

These AAC competencies as well as assessment data gleaned from the five domains of language inform AAC intervention and implementation. Through ongoing assessment, SLPs can determine appropriate tools and language interventions to use with their students.

Innovation/Modifications to Existing Language Therapy Tools

There are many tools available for language intervention for school-aged children. Just because they were not marketed for use with AAC does not mean they are not appropriate for students using AAC. Out of the box, these interventions may be difficult to initially implement, but SLPs working with students with CCNs are innovators. Modifications may be made to the intervention tool, or scaffolds and supports might be implemented with the AAC device. For example, a student with limited vocabulary and/or ability to use descriptive language may benefit from a program such as the Expanding Expression Toolkit (EET; Smith, 2015). However, the colors on the EET beads do not necessarily match up to the color-coding system of the student's AAC system and may confuse the student. Therefore, the beads may be modified (e.g., using green instead of blue for "what does it do"/verb) to strengthen the connection between the EET category and AAC system. Another support may be creating masked sets, which involves hiding or "masking" icons on a device and showing only icons relevant to the activity. This may help students to discuss different pictures or topics while minimizing visual clutter and navigation created by nonrelated words. The most important question that therapists should ask is "How can I teach this language skill?"

Descriptive Teaching Method

Students are required to demonstrate understanding of academic topics, typically through referential assessments focused on key content vocabulary (e.g., What is the largest planet? Who invented the light bulb?). However, for PWUAACs, it might not be prudent to add a large amount of content vocabulary to devices that students may have little to no need to access in the future. In such cases, educators should rely on the Descriptive Teaching Method to teach students and help students demonstrate their comprehension of the subject (Van Tatenhove, 2009). With this method, educators use high-frequency vocabulary to discuss content-specific words and key concepts. This highly reusable vocabulary will help students demonstrate understanding of topics. For example, rather than ask, "What is the resistance that occurs when an object moves over another?" educators can ask students, "What happens when these objects move over one another?" Rather than needing the word "friction" on their devices, students can demonstrate understanding of the concept by saying "slow down" or "go slow."

Support and Teaching Strategies

As previously stated, the majority of AAC intervention *is* language intervention. However, there are specific implementation strategies that enable PWUAACs to become successful communicators. These include communication partner training, aided language stimulation (ALS), and wait time.

Communication Partner Training

Knowledgeable communication partners play an integral role in communication and language development for PWUAACs. Many PWUAACs receive classroom support from educational assistants (EAs) such as a paraeducator or instructional assistant (Binger et al., 2010). It is their role to provide students with the learning supports they need to demonstrate their capabilities. For EAs working with PWUAACs, these supports include but are not limited to ALS, wait time, descriptive teaching, hardware/software troubleshooting, and supplemental direct instruction.

Coaching is an effective method to help educators learn how to support their students using AAC (and is fully discussed in Chapters 32, 33, and 34). SLPs should consider providing basic information in a short, informative training, while providing the bulk of their training using a coaching method (Binger et al., 2010). Coaching occurs during real-life scenarios/activities already happening on a daily basis. It generally involves various steps—observation, practice, reflection, feedback, and joint planning. For example, SLPs observe the student with their educators in a naturally occurring activity, and if needed, the SLP may demonstrate a teaching strategy. Educators practice new strategies to help the student. This step is perhaps the most important as it empowers the educators to feel confident using AAC with their students long after the SLP has left the classroom. Reflection and feedback may be used to determine what is and is not working while also generating additional strategies and supports to try. A joint plan allows the SLP and educators to identify a strategy to work on between coaching sessions.

Aided Language Stimulation

ALS (or ALgS) occurs when a communication partner simultaneously talks to a student while selecting key words on their AAC system. It may also be referred to as modeling, aided language input, and a variety of other similar terms. For students whose access method is switch scanning, the model should occur using the scan pattern rather than a direct selection to help the student encode the scan pattern, as ALS teaches students where vocabulary is located on their AAC devices. This means that EAs must know where vocabulary is located on the student's device in order to effectively model. In addition, EAs should model at a language level that is slightly above the student's current language abilities. For example, if the stu-

dent uses one word to communicate, the EA should model two- to three-word phrases during ALS with consideration for syntax and morphology.

Wait Time

Using an AAC device to communicate is typically slower than verbal speech. It is important that communication partners provide adequate wait time so that the PWUAAC can select words and complete thoughts. In the field of special education, many teachers and therapists often refer to a prompting hierarchy (or faded prompting as noted in Chapter 9). It is essential that communication partners pause before using any prompts to allow the student to initiate a response. It is helpful when educators determine a baseline for the needed amount of wait time for their students. For example, some students with Rett syndrome and apraxia may need up to 90 s to initiate a response, whereas a student with autism may initiate a response after 10 s. Knowing the wait time that a student needs will allow them to generate *independent* answers.

Access to AAC allows students with CCNs to more fully participate in school. However, language-based interventions allow students to succeed in school. Using ongoing assessment tools and traditional language interventions, SLPs can implement successful interventions that take students beyond vocabulary and social skills into competent communicators who use more complex language. By addressing phonology through literacy, nonverbal PWUAACs can learn to read and communicate with greater independence. SLPs as coaches ensure that all educators have the tools to help their students communicate to their maximum potential.

Clinical Tips

- AAC therapy is *language* therapy. Consider traditional speech-language interventions and modify them to fit the needs of your student using AAC.
- Ongoing assessment is a critical component of AAC intervention. Use appropriate assessment and measurement

tools to monitor progress and determine areas of need.

■ Coaching and training are a critical piece of AAC intervention as students have limited time with their SLP each week. It is essential that other educators have the tools to support these students throughout their school day.

Case Study: JV

Clinical Profile and Communication Needs

The Individual

JV is a boy who is 9 years, 9 months old. He has a medical diagnosis of cerebral palsy. JV was born at 35 weeks' gestation. Subsequently, he spent several weeks in the neonatal intensive care unit and several additional weeks at a children's hospital. JV began receiving early intervention services when he was approximately 3 months old. During early intervention, JV received physical therapy, occupational therapy, and speech-language therapy. He used a wheelchair as his primary method of mobility until approximately age 6 years; wheelchair use was slowly faded while he improved his ability to walk. He currently walks with handheld assistance or a walker. Though his passive and active range of motion are considered to be within functional limits, JV's fine and gross motor skills are moderately impacted by hypertonia.

Their Communication Partners and Environment

JV lives with his mother and has a support network including extended family and friends. JV uses a combination of verbal approximations and his AAC system, an Accent 1000 with Unity 45 Sequenced, to communicate at home. His family, caregivers, and education team have remarked on how

important his AAC system is, as he is constantly able to show them what he knows, participate in simple conversations, and forms relationships with them. He attends school in a self-contained special education classroom in his district and is in a class with peers who also use AAC systems. He continues to receive speech-language therapy, occupational therapy, and physical therapy. Per his individualized education program, he requires an EA throughout the school day. He has had several over his years in school; however, two have been identified as playing instrumental roles in JV's success. JV loves Mickey Mouse, live-action Disney movies, and cartoon movies. He frequently requests to watch specific movies or to watch songs from movies on YouTube. JV also enjoys reading, playing on the playground, playing with peers, and engaging in social interactions.

AAC System Considerations

JV's AAC journey has led him to trial a variety of systems. Through age 5 years, JV primarily communicated using vocalizations, body movements, facial expressions, and so on. He used low-tech communication boards with pull-off picture symbols, picture symbols presented in a small field, and signs (e.g., more, all done, eat, water, help). Upon arriving at a new school at age 5 years, JV's SLP and educational team recognized that his receptive language skills far exceeded his expressive language skills. His team recognized the need for a robust system and began to consider a high-tech robust AAC system. JV had a raking grasp and an inability to isolate a finger; however, his occupational therapist anticipated that his fine motor skills would improve and requested that the team try direct access first with a keyguard before looking at alternative methods of access.

The team determined that JV needed a large vocabulary that could be used to convey a variety of meanings (semantics). This vocabulary needed to include a large core vocabulary in addition to personal and fringe vocabulary. In order to fully participate in discourse and social situations, his SLP anticipated that he would need to learn rules of sentence construction (syntax) and grammar markers (morphology). As he had behaviors such as tantrums (e.g., crying and body movements) and also struggled to play appropriately with friends, JV needed direct instruction for self-regulation and social skills (pragmatics). Last, in order to fully participate in literacy and communication, it was imperative to determine interventions to teach phonological and phonemic awareness skills (phonology).

For these reasons, his SLP hypothesized that a Minspeak system (Semantic Compaction Systems, 2018) would allow JV to access a large number of words with minimal scanning and navigation. Given an Accent 1000 and Unity 45 1 Hit, a keyguard, and custom activation settings (0.4 s acceptance time, 0.7 s release time), JV moved his whole hand over the keyguard and put his middle finger into the keyguard hole to say his target word (like shown in Figure 11–1). His mother and education team pursued getting JV a device of his own through insurance. JV quickly transitioned to Unity 45 Sequenced upon receiving a device of his own. He

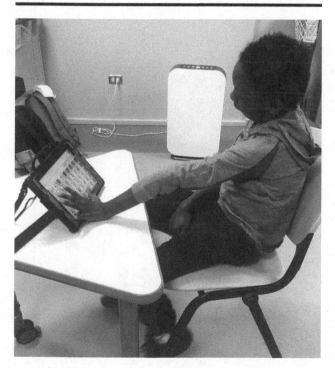

Figure 11–1. JV accessing his Accent device with a keyguard.

continues to use this as his main method of communication with low-tech symbol support boards as needed for participation in academic activities.

Ongoing Assessment

JV's success is largely due to the AAC intervention implemented by his team including his mother, SLP, educators, and JV himself. A variety of assessments have been used over the years to measure JV's progress including the MacArthur Bates Communicative Development Inventories (Fenson et al., 2007), the Communication Matrix (Rowland, 2011), the AAC Profile (Kovach, 2009), and the QUAD Profile (Cross, 2005). All of these assessments have been used to guide intervention planning and to help identify areas of need. Table 11–1 demonstrates JV's progress through four Communication Matrix assessments administered from July 26, 2016, to November 30, 2020, where white rectangles represent skills not seen or used, light gray represent emerging skills, dark gray represent mastered skills, and gray represent skills that are surpassed.

Intervention Strategies and Implementation Supports

Coaching and training have been an essential part of AAC implementation for JV. To support educators, his SLP conducted multiple trainings to help them become more familiar with the vocabulary on his device as well as to become familiar with AAC intervention strategies such as ALS, wait time, and sabotage (a strategy by which a communication partner deliberately creates a problem so the individual must communicate). These trainings followed a similar method to the ImPAACT Program outlined by Binger et al. (2010). Trainings included informative, lecture-style sessions; "silent" breakfasts while using AAC; and coaching sessions. From these trainings and coaching sessions emerged two exceptional EAs who worked with JV at different times. Their dedication has helped JV improve his vocabulary, language (e.g., combining words to convey meaning), social skills, self-regulation, and

Table 11-1. JV's Progress Over Time as Measured by the Communication Matrix

7/26/16

3/1/18

7/17/19

11/30/20

literacy skills, including phonemic awareness and reading comprehension. Both EAs had high expectations for JV and encouraged him to use his device so that they could understand him better. They practiced using his vocabulary system on a loaner device so that they could provide ALS throughout the day. They provided wait time and encouraged others to do so as well to provide him the time needed to formulate simple sentences. These EAs in turn became coaches, helping other educators on JV's team to use implementation strategies and appropriate language-based interventions.

When JV first began to use AAC, his SLP focused intervention on **vocabulary** and **social skills**. His educators were trained using the Hanen It Takes Two to Talk program (Manolson & Hanon Centre, 1992). Using this program, educators engaged JV primarily in play-based activities. They frequently used the "OWL" strategy: observe, wait, listen. Using this method, JV remained more engaged in activities, giving educators the opportunity to model new vocabulary and concepts. Using Hanen-based interventions, JV's vocabulary quickly began to grow, and he spontaneously began to chain utterances into two-word sentences.

JV's SLP introduced an intervention approach based on the Graphic Symbol Utterance and Sentence Developmental Framework (Binger et al., 2020) to target **syntactic structures** and **morphological markers**. Rather than using static AAC boards as recommended in the framework, JV's Accent 1000 with the Unity 45 Sequenced vocabulary was used throughout intervention. Basic semantic structures in first, second, and third person were targeted in speech-language sessions. These included but were not limited to agent-action-object, locatives (e.g., dog in house), possessives (e.g., dog's food), attributes (e.g., big dog), and adverbials (e.g., dog run fast). This intervention took place during play-based activities. The SLP customized materials to include some of JV's favorite Mickey Mouse characters and other interests. This intervention was primarily conducted by JV's SLP; however, his EA attended his therapy sessions and attempted to implement similar strategies throughout his day. Within a 30-min session, the SLP aimed for at least 30 utterances to be modeled, co-constructed, or independently communicated during the session.

The recasting strategy was instrumental in helping JV to expand his mean length of utterance, improve syntax, and begin to use grammar markers (e.g., changing verb tenses, plural s). For example, if JV said, "boy dog fast run," the SLP would recast and model back on his device "the boy's dog runs fast."

Recently, JV was introduced to the Expanding Expression Tool (EET) to help grow his language skills (Smith, 2015). At a basic level, the EET helps students learn to describe objects. However, it also helps students learn to make connections, compare/contrast, make associations, and so on. This tool was modified slightly to more closely resemble the Unity vocabulary color organization system. For example, in the EET, the "group" category is represented by a green bead. However, in Unity, green is used for verbs and category nouns, orange. Therefore, the group bead was changed to orange. This intervention is being introduced in speech-language therapy sessions while his educational team receives training on how to incorporate it into their classroom.

Regarding **phonology**, JV benefited from the Accessible Literacy Learning (ALL) Program to learn letter sounds, segmenting, and blending (Light & McNaughton, 2012). He continues to work on decoding and encoding CVC words. This intervention was provided both by the SLP and his EA who received training from the SLP. Again, JV benefited from customization of materials to engage him. Pictures of favorite shows, toys, and people were used to keep JV interested in the instruction. Typically, instruction in this program follows a discrete trial training method in which the student is given a letter sound and must identify the corresponding letter from a field of four. This was modified for JV to make it more engaging. For example, when learning /l/, JV was provided with 10 pictures of objects or people that began with the /l/ sound like "lion," "lamp," "Ludwig Von Drake," "Lady," "Lilo," "Lightening McQueen," and so on, as shown in Figure 11–2.

He would choose a picture and put it in a book, the clinician would then present him with a field of four letters and name the target sound, /l/, then JV would pull off the correct letter and put it in the book with the picture. As JV has limited verbal speech and is not able to produce most speech sounds accurately, this program has helped him to

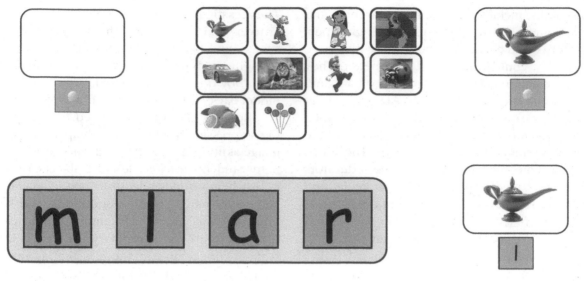

Figure 11–2. Example of a modified phonology lesson.

learn foundational phonemic awareness skills that will help him become a reader and independent communicator.

JV's **self-regulation** and **social skills** have significantly improved over the past 3 years. This is believed to be a result of his increased language and ability to effectively communicate. Many of JV's tantrums were attributed to being denied access to preferred activities or being asked to do "work." JV's educators frequently modeled language such as "I'm frustrated," "I don't want that," "not now," "when can I play," and "when can I go." Though JV does not consistently use full sentences, he did begin to use language to self-regulate and advocate instead. For example, when told he can watch the "hot dog song," he can ask "how many?" to find out how many times he is allowed to watch it. When he does not want to participate in therapy, he will say "I all done, stop goodbye." At this point, educators can review the expectations and let him know when he is all done, circumventing the need for a tantrum. JV also participates in small group play and other activities with peers. His EA helps to

model appropriate language and coach JV in ways that he can participate (e.g., take turns, wait for a friend to finish, use a friend's name instead of grabbing them). This has helped JV to form friendships and relationships.

The combination of these interventions has helped JV to become a more independent and competent communicator. Though many of his utterances are context dependent, he is beginning to use short sentences that allow any communication partner to understand the context and what he is saying (like the one shown in Figure 11–3). It is anticipated that with continued ongoing assessment, his SLP and educational team will choose appropriate interventions to teach and practice a variety of language skills. JV's SLP and educators use intervention tools that have not been marketed toward students who use AAC, but with simple modifications these interventions help students like JV make progress. It is anticipated that he will continue to bridge the gap between his receptive and expressive language skills using AAC as his main method of communication.

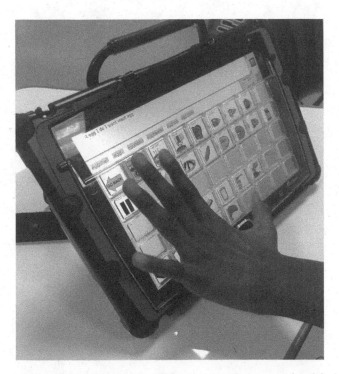

Figure 11–3. JV using his Accent device to build sentences.

References

Binger, C., Kent-Walsh, J., Ewing, C., & Taylor, S. (2010). Teaching educational assistants to facilitate the multi-symbol message productions of young students who require augmentative and alternative communication. *American Journal of Speech-Language Pathology*, *19*(2), 108–120. https://doi.org/10.1044/1058-0360 (2009/09-0015)

Binger, C., Kent-Walsh, J., Harrington, N., & Hollerbach, Q. C. (2020). Tracking early sentence-building progress in graphic symbol communication. *Language, Speech, and Hearing Services in Schools, 51*(2), 317–328. https://doi.org/10.1044/2019_lshss-19-00065

Binger, C., Kent-Walsh, J., King, M., & Mansfield, L. (2017). Early sentence productions of 3- and 4-year-old children who use augmentative and alternative communication. *Journal of Speech, Language, and Hearing Research, 60*(7), 1930–1945. https://doi.org/10.1044/2017_jslhr-l-15-0408

Cross, R. T. (2005). *The QUAD Profile™: A quick and simple language evaluation tool* [Measurement instrument]. https://aaclanguagelab.com/materials/_QUAD_complete.pdf

Dewart, H., & Summers, S. (1995). *The Pragmatics Profile of Everyday Communication Skills in Children* [Measurement instrument]. https://acecentre.org.uk/resources/pragmatics-profile-people-use-aac/

Don Johnston Inc. (2021). *Readtopia™* [Program of studies]. https://learningtools.donjohnston.com/product/readtopia/

Erickson, K. A., & Koppenhaver, D. A. (2020). *Comprehensive literacy for all. Teaching students with significant disabilities to read and write.* Paul H. Brookes.

Fallon, K. A., Light, J., Mcnaughton, D., Drager, K., & Hammer, C. (2004). The effects of direct instruction on the single-word reading skills of children who require augmentative and alternative communication. *Journal of Speech, Language, and Hearing Research, 47*(6), 1424–1439. https://doi.org/10.1044/1092-4388 (2004/106)

Fenson, L., Marchman, V. A., Thal, D. J., Dale, P. S., Reznick, J. S, & Bates, E. (2007). *MacArthur-Bates Communicative Development Inventories* (2nd ed.). Paul H. Brookes.

Hill, K. (2006). Augmentative and alternative communication (AAC) research and development: The challenge of evidence-based practice. *International Journal of Computer Processing of Languages, 19*(04), 249–262. https://doi.org/10.1142/s0219427906001505

Hill, K., & Romich, B. (2001). A language activity monitor for supporting AAC evidence-based clinical practice. *Assistive Technology, 13*, 12–22.

Kovach, T. M. (2009). *The Alternative Augmentative Communication Profile: A Continuum of Learning* [Measurement instrument]. Pro-Ed.

Light, J. (1989). Toward a definition of communicative competence for individuals using augmentative and alternative communication systems. *Augmentative and Alternative Communication, 5*, 137–144.

Light, J., & McNaughton, D. (2012). *The Accessible Literacy Learning™ Reading Program* [Program of studies]. https://www.mytobiidynavox.com/store/ALL

Manolson, H. A., & Hanen Centre. (1992). *It takes two to talk.* Hanen Centre.

Rowland, C. (2011). *Communication Matrix* [Measurement instrument]. https://www.communicationmatrix.org

Semantic Compaction Systems. (2018). *Minspeak.* https://minspeak.com

Smith, S. L. (2015). *Expanding Expression Toolkit* (2nd ed.) [Program of studies]. https://www.expandingexpression.com/

Van Tatenhove, G. M. (2009). Building language competence with students using AAC devices: Six challenges. *Perspectives on Augmentative and Alternative Communication, 18*(2), 38–47. https://doi.org/10.1044/aac18.2.38

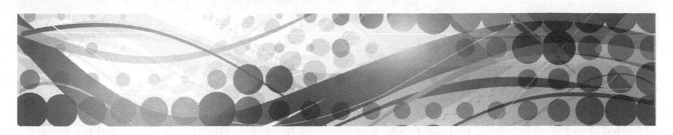

Essay 14

CLINICAL CONSIDERATIONS AND AAC: AAC AND LITERACY

Lesley Quinn

There's a story I tell about entering the field of augmentative and alternative communication (AAC). It starts in my Clinical Fellowship year at a large university hospital in the South, far from the small New England town where I grew up. Here is the gist of it: I was the new speech-language pathologist (SLP), and no one else wanted to do AAC clinic, so they assigned it to me. I expected to hate it, but I loved it.

There is another one I tell: I was a Junior Communication Disorders major, and a faculty member got a grant to train a few students in AAC. She bought one of the first commercially available touch screens, and we met weekly with Dale Gardner-Fox, an AAC/Pragmatic Organization Dynamic Display (PODD) specialist, to learn how to program and implement a system. Dale talked about the importance of "power words," which fundamentally shifted my understanding of communication.

Here is another: Growing up I watched my aunt, who had multiple sclerosis, deteriorate year by year until she was trapped in her body and powerless to communicate. I knew she was listening, wanting to talk to us, and I felt trapped too, because I wanted to talk to her, but I did not know how. When I got to college and learned about AAC, I did not know what to think. Why hadn't anyone who worked with her ever mentioned it?

Each of these stories is true, and they all tell how I got started in the field of AAC. The story I ultimately share depends on which one will help

me connect with a listener. When I am asked to define literacy, I say it is *connecting*. It is an extension of what we do face-to-face, through the air: we connect with others and ourselves using symbols. Literacy allows us to extend face-to-face communication beyond here and now.

Connecting with an author in the distant past through her characters in a novel or with tomorrow's busy version of yourself in a to-do list is going to be harder than connecting face-to-face. The tangible context that is available in person will now be symbolic or inferred, and letter-sound correspondences, number symbols, phonics, and discourse rules will have to be mastered. However, none of this is beyond the reach of persons who use augmentative and alternative communication (PWUAACs). If you told me this when I started in the field (at age 10, 19, or 26 years), I would not have believed you. I could not have imagined I could teach students who were nonverbal, legally blind, motor impaired, and intellectually disabled to do something as complex as read and write. However, the more I connected with learners with complex communication needs (CCNs) and saw their humor, strength, and tenacity, the more I saw how capable they were of learning, and the more I understood it was possible.

Fortunately, I did not need to start from scratch. Pioneers in the field, like Janice Light, Karen Erickson, and David Koppenhaver, have researched, developed curricula, mapped out scope and sequence, written goal hierarchies, and provided frameworks to help us understand what to teach, so students can acquire foundational literacy skills and learn increasingly complex ways of relating to text and through text. Their work is invaluable. Erickson and Koppenhaver recently authored a comprehensive guide to literacy instruction for individuals with disabilities, focusing on learning to read and write (2020).

In my own practice, I found I needed to better understand *how* to teach. In the beginning, out of frustration, I asked myself questions like, "How can you learn to read if you can't focus on a word?" or "How do I help you understand discourse if you don't understand sentences?" I still ask myself these kinds of questions, but it is no longer out of frustration. Now, they are useful frames for establishing where we are and where we need to go. The difficulties are not barriers to learning; they are the skills to be learned. The science of learning is invaluable, too.

If I have gleaned anything in 20 years of working in the field of AAC, it is that humans have an amazing capacity to learn. Even the most "disabled" learners make remarkable gains in understanding, reading, and writing when I teach well. I cannot spell out everything you will need to know to teach literacy, but there are a few key lessons I can share from experience and my own take on the comprehensive literature we now have in human development, learning, language comprehension, word reading, and instructional design:

- Make connecting a cornerstone of your instruction. We evolved to learn complex, socially constructed skills (like language) through social interaction, and we need to be safe and emotionally regulated to do it. Students with severe communication and motor challenges may have never had the experience of connecting and relating to another person, which fundamentally shapes comprehension.
- Attention is key to learning, and social attention is key to social learning. Learners who have difficulty with social attention can develop it with practice and reinforcement.

- Learning requires emotional and cognitive flexibility. Model it, teach it, and reinforce it whenever you see it.
- To learn what something is, we need to see what it is *not*. We need something to compare it to. When introducing letters, numbers, words, and concepts, provide lots of examples of what it is and what it is not.
- Words mean something *to someone*. Understanding involves perspective taking. Learners with semantic and pragmatic challenges can improve their perspective taking skills with instruction, practice, and reinforcement.
- Reading, writing, and math are things we *do*. They are complex processes, and the way we learn a complex process is through deliberate practice with immediate feedback.
- Learners with complex communication needs *can* learn to decode in addition to learning sight words. They need a way to "name" speech sounds along with letters. They also need practice with the component skills involved (see a letter, say a sound; blend sounds; visualize meaning). They may need to break down component skills even further or practice them in less abstract ways first (name parts of a face, discriminate speech from nonspeech sounds), and then practice putting it all together.
- Fluency matters as much as accuracy. Learners can develop it. Start with short (seconds long) sprints to build up speed and endurance.
- Aim high and expect robust progress, because individuals with CCNs can be robust learners with the right instruction. When you get stuck, which you will, take the learner's perspective and ask two questions: *What do I think you know that you don't? What do I think I'm saying that I'm not?* Break down the skill, fill in the gaps, and expect to move forward again.
- Be honest and genuine with praise. Do not say something is easy when it is not, and do not say a student is good at

something if they are not. Learning can be uncomfortable, and it requires significant effort to make gains, but learners with CCNs can handle hard work; they do hard things all the time. They need accurate feedback to progress.

■ Reinforce the process (*I saw how hard you tried*) rather than praising fixed traits (*You're so smart*) and let learners know you have their back. They will work hard when they know you are in it with them.

■ Most important, reach out and connect with the clinicians, educators, and researchers who are at the vanguard of teaching literacy to learners with complex needs. There is great depth of knowledge and skill among them, and we as a discipline are learning more all the time. If it feels daunting, think about Amina and Baxter. Amina is 18 years old and feisty. She had a brain tumor as an infant and has cerebral palsy. She was 14 years old when she used her eye-gaze device to tell me she wanted to learn to read. When I asked her why, she said, "help my mind." Baxter, who is 7 years old, inquisitive, compassionate, and stubborn, has cerebral palsy and cortical visual impairment. He wanted you to know this, which he typed on his iPad with his nose: "[Literacy is] the best way . . . to be the best."

Reference

Erickson, K. A., & Koppenhaver, D. A. (2020). *Comprehensive literacy for all. Teaching students with significant disabilities to read and write*. Paul H. Brookes.

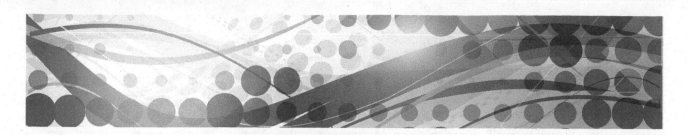

Chapter 12
DATA COLLECTION AND GOAL WRITING IN AAC

Kate Grandbois and Amy Wonkka

Fundamentals

Data collection and goal writing probably seem like two separate processes that are mutually exclusive. We do not often consider them to be related because they tend to happen in a sequential order (goals are usually written first, and the data collection happens second to support that goal). But in practice, data collection and goal writing are intertwined procedures that influence one another and happen in tandem. In fact, data collection and interpretation weave their way through all of our clinical practice. They are equally influenced by outside factors, such as the resources available to you, the environment where you are targeting the skill, the communication partners, and other stakeholders involved with your client. To understand the complex interactions between goal writing and data collection, let's first examine what each process is on its own. We discuss data collection methods first, not because it is a more critical skill, but because we must examine one before the other for purposes of digesting information.

There are many different kinds of data collection, and choosing your data collection system will ultimately depend on the skill you want to measure, the goal you are planning to write (or in some cases, have already written), who is collecting the data, and how many resources are available to do so. It is also important to keep in mind why we col-

lect data in the first place *because collecting data is how we create evidence that our treatment is working* (Olswang & Bain, 1994). We cannot provide evidence-based treatments without data collection. Because of this, good data collection skills are crucial to providing ethical, evidence-based services (Kaderavek & Justice, 2010).

Often in speech and language pathology, we think of data collection as a system of pluses and minuses that we scratch on a piece of paper to count a tally (or the total number of times we have seen a skill). Sometimes, we use that tally to calculate a percentage. The common misconception is that to collect good data, a clinician needs to write down every instance of a communication act. Writing down every occurrence of a target skill is incredibly taxing, since it means we would have to divide our attention between our client and writing down everything we see or hear. As clinicians, our priority is usually being engaged with our clients during therapy (playing games, completing tasks, providing cues and prompting, managing behavior, etc.), which means our data collection suffers. Conversely, if we prioritize taking continuous data, then our clinical work and client interactions suffer. The solution is to *take good data less often*. Design data collection systems that *accurately* measure the skill you are targeting, are a *valid* representation of that skill, and produce *reliable* measurements over time. (Table 12–1 presents definitions and examples of reliable, accurate, and valid data.)

Table 12–1. Accurate, Reliable, and Valid Data

Term	Definition	Example	Nonexample
Accuracy	When the measured value matches the true value	You place potatoes on a scale, and the scale says 2 pounds. This is an accurate measurement if the potatoes actually weigh 2 pounds.	You place potatoes on a scale, and the scale says 2 pounds. This is an inaccurate measurement if the potatoes actually weigh 2.5 pounds.
Reliability	When the measured value is consistent over repeated measurements	You place potatoes on a scale, and the scale says 2 pounds. You come back later in the day and place the potatoes back on the scale. The scale still says 2 pounds. This is a reliable measurement of the potatoes.	You place the potatoes on a scale, and the scale says 2 pounds. You come back later in the day and place the potatoes back on the scale. The scale now says 2.5 pounds. This is not a reliable measurement of the potatoes.
Validity	When the measured value is directly related to the phenomenon in question	You place potatoes on a scale because you want to discover the weight of the potatoes. The scale indicates that the potatoes weigh 2 pounds. This is a valid measurement because it is related to the original question of weight.	You place potatoes on a scale because you want to discover the weight of the potatoes. The scale indicates that the potatoes have a density of 1,380 kg/m^3. This is not a valid measurement because it is not related to the original question of weight.

How exactly do you take good data less often? You need to be familiar with different data collection methods and understand how to use them to measure what you need to measure.

Overall, there are two categories of data that you can take: qualitative and quantitative. Quantitative data are objective, overt, and countable, whereas qualitative data are subjective and require interpretation (Olswang & Bain, 1994). Quantitative data are likely what most people think of when they say "data," but qualitative measures are still "data" and should be considered based on the needs of the task. Sometimes a clinician will choose to only collect quantitative or qualitative data, and sometimes it is more appropriate to collect both. Every data collection method (see Table 12–2 for a list of different kinds of data collection methods) is well purposed for measuring different kinds of skills, depending on the clinical question you are asking. Deciding which kind of data collection system to use will be a reflection of those clinical questions combined with the resources you have available to you. In general, it is in your best interest to choose a data collection system that is doable and yields data that are accurate, reliable, and valid.

Goal Writing

With a general understanding of what quality data collection involves, we can now move onto the goal writing process and take a look at how these two tasks are related. Since data collection and goal writing are intertwined experiences without clear beginnings and ends, it might not be obvious where to start. To approach the task of goal writing, it may be helpful for the reader to sort this process into distinct steps.

Step 1: Create a Skills Inventory

Consider your existing data, from assessments, interviews, and/or observations. To really understand what your client currently does in different environments with different communication partners, you will probably want to use a structured approach to gathering, organizing, and reviewing

Table 12–2. Data Collection Methods

	Definition	Pros	Cons	Example
Quantitative Data Collection Methods				
Frequency	The number of times that a target behavior was observed and counted	Commonly used and understood by others. Gives a total count of a target skill	Can be very time consuming or difficult to capture skills that are frequent or happening in quick succession	Your client produces /th/ for /s/ 57 times during a session.
Rate	The number of times that a target behavior was observed and counted	Well suited for skills that need to occur within a certain time frame	Can be time consuming and/or difficult to accurately capture skills that are frequent or happening in quick succession	Your client produces /th/ for /s/ three times in 10 min
Percentage	The number of times that a target skill occurs out of a total number of opportunities	Commonly used and understood by others. Yields information about how often the target skill occurs in relation to other variables	Requires knowledge of missed opportunity or total number of occurrences	Your client produces /th/ for /s/ 43 times in a session and produces /s/ 32 times. Your client produced /s/ in 42.6%
Duration	The total amount of time that a skill occurs	Well suited for skills that have a clear beginning and ending, or instances where you are interested to know how long a skill or behavior lasts	Requires equipment (stopwatch, clock). Requires consistent visual attention to the client to accurately record when a skill starts or stops	Your client expresses interest in utilizing rate enhancement strategies and asks you to time how long it takes them to compose a message using different access methods
Latency	The amount of time that passes between a stimulus in the environment and a response on the part of the client	Well suited for instances where the question is related to initiation after a cue is given (conversational turn-taking, executing a direction after it is given)	Requires equipment (stopwatch, clock). Requires consistent visual attention to the client to accurately record when an environmental cue is given and when the client responds	Your client begins following a direction 35 s after the direction is given
Probe data[a]	Performance during a subset of trials is measured	When done properly, can efficiently capture valid, accurate, and reliable measurements in a time-efficient manner	When not done properly can yield inaccurate measurements	Your client performs the /r/ sound in isolation 10 consecutive times. You only measure performance on the first three trials

continues

Table 12–2. *continued*

	Definition	Pros	Cons	Example
Momentary time sampling	Total session time is divided into intervals, and you record the occurrence or nonoccurrence of a target communication act at the moment that the interval ends	Well suited for instances where your attention is divided and for communication acts that are continuous, such as communication partner (i.e., providing wait time) or environmental variables (i.e., physical proximity to partners)	In this method, many instances of the target skill may be missed because you are not giving your undivided attention	During a recess observation, at the end of every minute you note whether or not your client(s) was within 5 ft of at least one peer on the playground
Partial interval recording	Session time is divided into intervals. You record whether or not the communication act happened at any point during that interval. If the skill happens multiple times during that interval, you only record it one time. Produces an estimate of the total percentage of time that a communication act occurred	Well suited for instances where your attention is divided	This method overestimates the amount of time that a communication act occurred	During a social skills group, you note if your client initiates communication at any point during the interval
Qualitative Data Collection Methods				
Language samples	A transcription of what an individual communicates, typically in an independent, unprompted format	Ideal for measuring independent language productions, mean length of utterance, grammatical structures, transcription of speech sounds, and comparison of communication between settings	Time consuming, both to transcribe the language sample and to analyze it afterward	You give your client a picture book and ask them to tell you a story. You transcribe each utterance
Interviews	Can be done in both structured and unstructured formats. Collects information related to client performance in different settings as well as values and goals of key stakeholders	Ideal for assessments, new clients, revising goals, and assessing how a skill has been generalized to a nonclinical setting	Can be time consuming, often there is not time allotted within a clinician's schedule to conduct interviews or contact other stakeholders	You are preparing to write new goals for a client. You interview caregivers to determine generalization of skills previously targeted

Table 12–2. *continued*

	Definition	Pros	Cons	Example
Observation	Can be done for both structured and unstructured tasks. Collects information related to performance and current communication status in different environments	Ideal for measuring communication status in different settings. Can be critical for collaboration with other professionals	Time consuming, both to conduct the observation and to analyze it afterward	A new student is assigned to your caseload. You observe the student in the classroom to note specific skills produced in that environment

[a]See the box on p. 195 for more information about probe data.

Note. See *Applied behavior analysis*, by J. O. Cooper, T. E. Heron, and W. L. Heward, 2020. Copyright Pearson; "Data collection," by L. B. Olswang and B. Bain, 1994, *American Journal of Speech-Language Pathology*, *3*(3), pp. 55–66 (https://doi .org/10.1044/1058-0360.0303.55).

information obtained from non-norm-referenced methods such as interviews, observations, and/ or dynamic assessment. This information gathering and organizational process could incorporate commercially available tools such as the Communication Matrix (Communication Matrix, n.d.) and the Augmentative and Alternative Communication Profile (Kovach, 2009), frameworks like the SETT Framework (Zabala, 2005), other resources like the Student Augmentative and Alternative Communication Profile and Portfolio (Van Tatenhove, 2014), or your own customized approach or combination of organizational tools. Regardless of the methods you choose, the inventory should tell the story of what skills your client is able to perform.

Consider analyzing this inventory to identify other important variables, such as communication partners and environmental variables. Communication partners, environmental complexity, and the type of task can all influence a person's performance, and this is particularly true for persons who use augmentative and alternative communication (PWUAAC). By gathering this initial information and considering your client's performance in different contexts (e.g., a testing environment, with you in an office, at home), their skill level with different types of supports, and their performance with different communication partners, you will be better informed when you write goals and objectives addressing these important variables.

Step 2: Identify the Skill(s) to Target

Once you have considered the previous variables and created a skills inventory, it is likely that you have identified a lengthy list of skills and conditions that tell the story of your client as a learner. Typically, we do not write goals and objectives for every single possible skill we have identified for our client. We need to identify which skills are most important and are reasonable and likely to be achieved within our given time frame (e.g., are you writing goals and objectives to be met within a 60-day insurance recertification or to be met within an individualized education program [IEP] school year?).

Step 3: Take Baseline Data

Now that you have created an inventory of skills, environments, and supports that tells the story of your client as a learner and considered the many factors that go into prioritizing skills, you likely have chosen a target skill that meets the needs of the learner and is achievable within your time frame. If you have not done so already, take some data on your student's current performance in this target skill area under the conditions where you would like to see it improve. These data will become your baseline (also called "baseline data") and will guide your clinical decision-making for what criteria you will include in your goal. It will also serve as the jumping-off point against which you measure your client's performance during and after treatment.

Step 4: Consider Variables Related to Client Performance

Considering client and environmental variables is a critical but complex component of goal writing. This step is crucial because you cannot write an appropriate goal without considering the variables that will influence the goal's success. For example, if someone other than you is collecting data for the goal, you will need to account for their availability and training when considering a well-matched data collection system. Considerations will be related to environmental variables (such as "Who is going to take data to measure this goal?" and "Where is the ideal location that this skill will be performed?"), communication partner variables (such as "Is this goal in line with the client's/caregiver's values?" and "Are these skills a priority for other stakeholders?"), and variables related to the client's current status (such as "How does my client learn best?" and "What are the skills that my client isn't demonstrating that would have a positive long-term impact?"). If you consider a variety of client variables before you write your goal, it is much more likely that the goal will be appropriate for your setting, be meaningful for your client, and have a well-matched data collection system.

Step 5: Write Your Goal

Once you have a good understanding of your client's current performance and have considered influencing variables, it is time to write your goal. There is an acronym to help us remember each important component of the goal. Our ideal is to write goals that are SMART: specific, measurable, attainable, realistic, and timely (Swigert, 2014). Knowing that a well-written goal includes these components, it is time to write a goal (or goals) that truly describes the skills you plan to target. As you are drafting your goal(s), we recommend writing it out and going through the mental exercise of how measuring the goal will work.

Step 6: Refine the Goal

Now it is time to ensure you are integrating data collection considerations into your goal writing. Consider gathering some additional information about

- where, when, and how the skills will be targeted and measured
- who will be taking the data to measure the goal (and adjust your goal as needed)

Accounting for these details in advance will help avoid the challenging, frustrating, and sometimes downright impossible task of attempting to collect data using a system that is poorly matched to the task or the demands of the environment. Going through this exercise will increase the likelihood that the goals will be measurable, and the data will also be valid, reliable, and accurate.

Step 7: Follow-Up

Consistently checking in with your data, data collectors, and data collection system is a critical way to make sure that the data remain accurate, valid, and reliable. Data should be analyzed regularly to inform clinical decision-making as your client changes and progresses in response to treatment. Checking in with the individuals who are collecting the data and reviewing the data collection system is also a critical component of a healthy data set. With any data collection system, there is always the risk of observer drift (when the individual using the data collection system begins using it differently over time, resulting in the measurement becoming less accurate). To counterbalance this, consider who will be taking the data and what their level of familiarity is with the data collection system. Consider an initial training and checking in regularly to make sure that the data collection system is being conducted as it was originally intended.

Here are some examples:

- Within an unstructured play-based group activity, given customized visual supports as part of the environment (e.g., a poster on the wall of the classroom), student will use intelligible symbolic communication (e.g., clear speech, his augmentative and alternative communication [AAC] device or a combination of both) to respond to peers a minimum of two times per group session.

■ Student will produce a three-word utterance using intelligible symbol sequences (i.e., sign, dedicated communication device, or both) during structured activities in the absence of verbal and visual cues, a minimum of three times per session.

Being realistic about collecting data that are meaningful and valid is part of drafting a quality goal. Collecting continuous data (or tallying every instance of a response) gives us the actual number of responses, but it is challenging or impossible to do well while providing clinical services simultaneously; we have to balance our data collection with client engagement. One option to consider is probe data (also referred to as discontinuous data). Probe data involves tracking a predetermined subset of responses rather than every instance of a response. Probe data allow for less time-consuming data collection that provides an estimate of the true responses. Variations in probe data collection can increase the accuracy of your data. For example, recording a greater number of probe responses (e.g., tracking data for the first 10 responses in a session rather than only the first response in a session) will result in more accurate data regarding client progress and acquisition of skills (Wonkka & Grandbois, 2020).

Case Study: SB

Clinical Profile and Communication Needs

The Individual

SB is an ambulatory multimodal communicator. Vision and hearing are within functional limits. He is a direct selector who uses his index finger to navigate through multiple levels of a speech-generating device that contains a robust vocabulary and is organized using semantic compaction (Unity 60). This device has up to 60 buttons on a page, allows for spelling/word prediction, and has been customized to include vocabulary that is relevant and important to SB (e.g., family members, pets, important places, etc.). He produces primarily one- to three-word phrases for a variety of pragmatic functions. SB has mild deficits in receptive language, moderate pragmatic deficits, and severe deficits in speech production and expressive language. He is motivated and engaged in therapy and classroom activities and has made steady progress in all targeted areas. In addition to the AAC device, SB also uses oral speech supplemented with gestures, but his intelligibility is poor. Familiar communication partners have improved understanding with context. SB does not yet use interrogatives (question words) to formulate questions, which affects his ability to fully access academic and social experiences. He loves both video games and dinosaurs and enjoys spending time with friends at school and his older brother when he is at home. While his communication skills have improved over the last few years of intervention, communication breakdowns still do occur, and they are frustrating for SB. He is still learning how to optimize his communication modalities across different people and places. He sometimes omits words that would be helpful to enhance his ability to be understood by others.

Their Communication Partners

SB communicates with many different partners across a school day, including familiar and less familiar adults, peers, and students in the broader school community. SB has a small group of close friends at school, several he has known since preschool, and he has a strong connection with his general education classroom assistant. The assistant, Matt, is a college student and knows a lot about both video games and dinosaurs. He is skilled in several communication partner strategies, but most importantly, waiting. SB rarely becomes frustrated when communicating with Matt.

Their Environment

SB is a first grader who receives both individual and small group speech-language therapy services and attends a combination of general education and special education resource classes. In the resource classes, SB receives small group instruction in reading and math along with two to three other first graders. He tends to participate more during small groups, whether in the resource environment or in group activities in his general education classroom. With larger groups, or when time pressure is part of the communication expectation, SB is most likely to be quiet and not participate in the activity unless explicitly told that participation is not optional.

Data Collection Considerations

You reviewed previous speech and language assessments, conducted an observation, and interviewed SB's primary special education teacher, paraprofessionals in the classroom, and SB's parents. Based on these initial qualitative and quantitative data collection strategies, you have created a skills inventory that tells the story of SB's current skill set. During the interview, his team identified asking questions using interrogatives as an area they would like to see improve. He understands questions but does not use question words to ask questions. This can make it hard for partners to understand his intent, as well as for him to take a more active role as a learner. For example, when a substitute teacher covered his small group resource class, SB could not find his red work folder. Instead of using a question such as, "Where folder?" "Where my folder?" "Where my red folder?" SB held up his blue folder and used his AAC device to say, "Red folder," leading to a communication breakdown where the substitute misunderstood and just responded, "No, that folder is blue." Situations like this are one reason SB's team reports that acquisition of this skill is necessary for him to access the academic and social curriculum. They also report concerns with collecting data in the classroom, as there are not resources available to document

every instance of communication. With this information, you determine that formulating questions using interrogatives in a structured setting is an appropriate target skill for your goal. Things you need to consider when designing your goal and data collection include the following:

- In what specific contexts/activities would you like to see this skill increase?
- Who will be responsible for taking data on the goal?
- What supports or environmental modifications, if any, need to be written into the goal to make it attainable/achievable?
- How often does SB need to produce this skill for it to be considered achieved?
- What outcome information tells us the client has achieved the skill?

Prior to writing your goal, you will need to measure SB's current level of performance in this specific area. While communication partners reported that SB does not produce interrogatives, this skill was not directly measured as part of the initial skills inventory. You decide to collect baseline data prior to writing the goal. Due to scheduling restrictions, you are not able to conduct an observation of the general education classroom, so you consult with the classroom teachers to determine their level of comfort with collecting data on this skill. The teachers agree to collect data but express concerns related to measuring missed opportunities for questions. They specifically state they cannot tell when SB intends to ask a question and when he intends to make a statement. Based on this report, you decide that calculating a percentage would not be an accurate measurement, as you would not have an accurate representation of missed opportunities. In discussion with the classroom teacher, you determine that taking frequency data is the most accurate way to measure this skill given the resources available in the setting. Baseline data are collected. The data indicate that during one day of data collection, SB produced zero interrogative forms. This data sample confirms reports from communication partners that SB is not yet producing interrogative forms.

The Data Collection System

Knowing that any goal needs to be SMART (specific, measurable, attainable, realistic, and timely), you consider what fundamental components will need to go into writing a goal that specifically targets the acquisition of interrogatives. Considering the knowledge, skills, and available resources of the classroom staff, you determine that taking percentage data will be difficult, as the current classroom staff do not have a way of accurately tracking all missed opportunities. Additionally, in conversations with the classroom teachers, it became clear that defining an "opportunity" to ask an interrogative is difficult, as his communication partners cannot make assumptions about SB's intentions. You decide that collecting frequency data of SB's production of interrogatives will accurately measure any increases in the skill (notably because the current rate is zero). In the interviews with SB's classroom staff, it was determined that SB has a history of benefiting from visual supports that are systematically faded over time when acquiring a new skill. In your conversations with them, you discuss using visual supports embedded in the environment as cues to produce interrogative forms. His teachers report that initially SB may benefit from gesture prompts to these visual supports, but they feel it is reasonable that these gesture cues could be faded within the year. Given this input combined with SB's learning history, you determine that producing interrogative forms in the presence of a visual cue is achievable within the IEP period. Considering these factors, you write the following SMART goal:

> Within his first-grade classroom environment, given the general visual supports available to all first-grade students (e.g., posters on the wall), and in structured groups of varying sizes, SB will independently use an intelligible symbolic communication (e.g., clear speech, his AAC

device or a combination of both) to ask a minimum of five WH- questions a day.

The Rationale for Clinical Decision-Making

In considering the perspectives of the client, the stakeholders, available resources, and the question you are asking, you rule out other data collection systems, such as percentage of opportunities. You have written a SMART goal that includes specific verbiage related to the setting, the supports required, and the condition in which the skill will be performed. Based on your skills inventory and baseline data collection, you feel this goal is achievable within the given time frame, and you have included a measurement system that will accurately reflect the acquisition of the skill. You have written your goal with your data collection system in mind, choosing a measurement that can be reasonably executed given the resources of the setting without compromising accuracy, validity, and reliability.

Next Steps

You confer with the educational team, and they are comfortable with the goal you have written. You confirm with the classroom staff that frequency data collection is reasonable within the setting. You incorporate their input into the plan for data collection and offer to provide training on the data collection system and intervention strategies. You also plan to check in with the team regularly throughout the year to ensure that the data collection system is being executed reliably. It is likely that Matt will be the primary data collector in the general education classroom, and both he and SB's teacher feel comfortable with the data collection plan. They will write the date on a paper that has been prepopulated with the different WH questions as well as the types of cues they might use, organized by least to most (providing minimal cues at first, such as waiting quietly for up to 15 s, and using more intrusive cues if needed, such as gesturing to the visuals embedded in the classroom). Every time SB uses a question word, they will record the type of word used and what level of prompting was required, if any. You consider your schedule and determine that you will have resources available to you to review the data on a regular basis to make changes to any teaching procedures as needed.

References

Communication Matrix. (n.d.). *About-Communication Matrix*. https://communicationmatrix.org/Matrix/About

Cooper, J. O., Heron, T. E., & Heward, W. L. (2020). *Applied behavior analysis*. Pearson.

Kaderavek, J. N., & Justice, L. M. (2010). Fidelity: An essential component of evidence-based practice in speech-language pathology. *American Journal of Speech-Language Pathology, 19*(4), 369–379. https://doi.org/10.1044/1058-0360(2010/09-0097)

Kovach, T. M. (2009). *Augmentative alternative communication profile: A continuum of learning* [Examiner's manual]. Pro-Ed.

Olswang, L. B., & Bain, B. (1994). Data collection. *American Journal of Speech-Language Pathology, 3*(3), 55–66. https://doi.org/10.1044/1058-0360.0303.55

Swigert, N. (2014). Patient outcomes, NOMS, and goal writing for pediatrics and adults. *Perspectives on Swallowing and Swallowing Disorders (Dysphagia), 23*(2), 65–71. https://doi.org/10.1044/sasd23.2.65

Van Tatenhove, G. (2014). *The Student Augmentative and Alternative Communication Profile and Portfolio*. http://www.vantatenhove.com/files/papers/DataCollection/StudentAACProfilePortfolio.pdf

Wonkka, A. G., & Grandbois, K. B. (2020, December 13). Probe data: The good, the bad, and the ugly (Season 2, No. 14) [Audio podcast episode]. *SLP Nerdcast*. https://www.slpnerdcast.com/episodes/probe-data

Zabala, J. (2005). *Using the SETT framework to level the learning field for students with disabilities*. http://www.joyzabala.com/uploads/Zabala_SETT_Leveling_the_Learning_Field.pdf

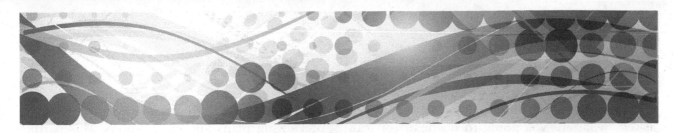

Essay 15

CLINICAL CONSIDERATIONS AND AAC: VISUAL SUPPORT FOR AAC

Amy Wonkka and Kate Grandbois

Students with complex communication needs (CCNs) often benefit not just from augmentative and alternative communication (AAC) but also from visual supports, such as visual schedules, first/then boards, or a token reinforcement system, for example (and like the examples shown in Figure X–1, which shows a first/then board, checklist, and token board setup). Similar to aided AAC, visual supports include the use of something external to a communicator's body and involve the use of symbols ranging from concrete and transparent (e.g., a

spoon to represent snack time on an object-based visual schedule) to abstract and opaque (e.g., a token board with the text, "Snack" indicating that a student must complete five additional work tasks prior to it being their snack time).

While a visual support may use the same symbols as those in the aided AAC system, the purpose of the visual support is different than that of AAC and should not be confused with being an individual's AAC system. Instead of being a tool that is serving as an alternative to or as a means of augmenting communication, the primary purpose of the visual support is related to removing barriers to comprehension, participation, and/or independence.

In general, visual supports are tools designed to help an individual understand and/or demonstrate a desired or expected behavior, and not as a means of communication. These tools are not in lieu of a robust language system for individuals with CCNs. Similarly, AAC systems should not be used as tools to direct the actions of the individual user or to establish their task schedule. Instead, the visual supports and AAC system should be separate but related. The AAC system should have the vocabulary to ask about a schedule ("I did it"), offer a protest ("I don't want to"), or to question ("how many more" before taking a break), for example.

If schedule- or task-related vocabulary is programmed into an AAC system, it is important that the individual is encouraged and shown how to

Figure X–1. Sample first/then board, checklist, and token visual supports.

talk about their schedule or activity (i.e., being asked "what are you going to do next?" or "can you help me choose what you are working for?") rather than the communication partner using the preprogrammed vocabulary on the AAC system as a means of instructing the person who uses augmentative and alternative communication (PWUAAC).

With both visual supports and AAC, aided language stimulation or AAC modeling from the communication partner is necessary. The partner should point to or reference specific words/ icons when talking with the individual and when previewing plans and expectations. This partner strategy is imperative to honoring and demonstrating total communication and can also support an individual's receptive understanding and conceptualization of what is being said. With access to schedule or task-specific vocabulary on an AAC system, it is important to model this language when talking *about* an individual's visual supports, rather than using the AAC as the visual support tool itself.

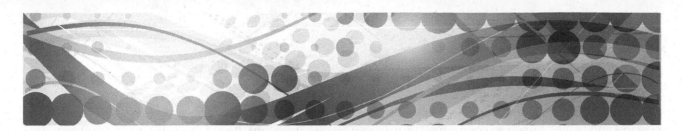

Chapter 13
AAC FOR THE CHILD IN END-OF-LIFE CARE

Rachel Santiago

Fundamentals

The ability to communicate when nearing the end-of-life (EoL) is a critically important facet of care participation, social connection, and preservation of dignity for all people with life-limiting illnesses. For children in end-of-life care and their families, maintaining intimate connections is especially critical. Though many children may not express advance directives or dictate their specific EoL wishes due to age or developmental ability, pediatric patients nearing EoL may require communication access for a wide range of needs. As long as a child is wakeful and cognitively able to participate in even the most basic communicative exchanges, consideration of augmentative and alternative communication (AAC) systems and strategies may be required. Children understand life, death, and illness differently depending on chronological and developmental age; therefore, discussions around illness, medical interventions, and EoL care will inevitably vary for children with life-limiting conditions. However, it is universally important to ensure children can participate in their care, ask questions, express wants and needs, maintain decisional control, summon help, and remain socially connected to caregivers and loved ones through life and, ultimately, until death.

In order to understand how AAC can support children nearing EoL, it is critical to understand the spectrum of care in pediatrics, varying circumstances, and considerations that influence communication. The National Cancer Institute (NCI) offers several definitions for concepts related to EoL care (NCI, n.d.); specifically, EoL care is defined as

> care given to people who are near the end-of-life and have stopped treatment to cure or control their disease. End-of-life care includes physical, emotional, social, and spiritual support for patients and their families. The goal of end-of-life care is to control pain and other symptoms so the patient can be as comfortable as possible. End-of-life care may include palliative care, supportive care, and hospice care. (para. 1)

Palliative care is typically initiated prior to EoL care to prevent, treat, and mitigate symptoms with an overall aim to improve quality of life in patients with life-limiting diagnoses or diseases. Many hospitals and institutions have dedicated palliative care teams, with multidisciplinary providers often including physicians, nurses, nurse practitioners, chaplains, and consulting speech-language pathologists (SLPs). Patients who have stopped curative interventions, may receive "hospice care," a program that provides specific supportive care to ensure comfort and control of symptoms to those nearing end-of-life. Ensuring communication access in the context of palliative care and EoL care is vital to ensuring quality of life and quality of death in children. Although SLPs may not anticipate entering the field with the goal of supporting EoL communication, providers working with children with complex medical care needs and complex communication needs (CCNs) must be prepared to support interactions and autonomy across all situations.

EoL discussions begin at different times in the course of illness depending on a variety of factors. Medical or palliative care teams may prompt EoL discussions in the context of changing or acute medical conditions or known progression of illness. Patients and families may also bring up EoL care needs spontaneously. Discussions may be prompted by changes in a patient's presentation, potentially due to increasing psychological, social, or spiritual distress related to the life-limiting illness, pain, and other symptoms that require higher levels of medication or intervention, increased respiratory distress or cardiac dysfunction, or loss of function in two or more body regions (Fried-Oken & Bardach, 2005). EoL care may also look different for patients depending on their diagnosis and their wishes. For example, some families choose to bring their child into the acute care hospital for EoL support until death, while others may purposefully opt for hospice services in the home setting.

The need for AAC at EoL will be related to the child's baseline communication skills, their abilities, strengths, and needs in the context of their progressive illness, and potentially their prior use of or experience with AAC. Children who use AAC at baseline and are requiring EoL care will continue to require access to communication systems and strategies that best match their needs through the course of illness. Cognitive, linguistic, and physical skills at the child's prior baseline, at the time of assessment, and in relation to illness trajectory, if known, will inform the SLP regarding AAC system selection as part of the feature-matched assessment. Planning ahead for potential changes in skills that will affect communication access should be incorporated, while allowing for integration of

messages to promote a wide range of communicative functions based on the child's evolving abilities, strengths, and needs. Though patient and family readiness for communication planning will vary, it should occur as early as possible to ensure access to needed solutions, potentially before they are required if loss of skills is anticipated.

The Care Team at End-of-Life

SLPs are part of a larger interprofessional team in a child's EoL care. Members of the EoL care team often include the parents and other primary caregivers, nurses, physicians, social workers, child life specialists, psychologists, chaplain or spiritual care practitioners, case managers, physical therapists, occupational therapists, music therapists, home health aides, and hospice resource providers. While the SLP is primed to support assessment, intervention, and access to communication tools and strategies as well as promotion of patient-provider communication (PPC), provision of EoL counseling, guidance, and decision-making should also include input and participation from the interprofessional team. In pediatrics, child-life specialists are specially trained to help children and families navigate difficult conversations and developmentally appropriate coping and normalization. They can also inform clinicians, parents, and patients on helpful topics and vocabulary to integrate into a child's AAC system. The SLP should collaborate with the larger interprofessional team at EoL to provide comprehensive, sensitive, and appropriate care.

Communication Planning

Anticipated Communication Difficulties or Loss of Speech

Certain diagnoses carry an associated expectation that communication difficulties or changes may arise. Examples include, but are not limited to, neurological conditions affecting speech intelligibility, tumors of the brainstem or left hemisphere, degenerative neuromuscular conditions (e.g., muscular dystrophy, juvenile Huntington's disease, and others), certain cancers and oncological diseases, and chronic lung disease. Children with known potential to experience a change in communication skills may be appropriate to participate in communication planning, to strategize how communicative interactions may be supported in the event of anticipated challenges. Depending on the child's age and developmental abilities, this may range from vocabulary selection, symbol selection, Message Banking Process™, creation of low-tech tools, device trial and selection, partner training, and creation of additional visual communication aids. Communication planning may occur over several sessions, especially if fatigue, attention, and illness symptoms warrant breaks. Time for the child and family to familiarize themselves with aided and unaided strategies may also yield the need for subsequent visits to support training, banking of messages if indicated, and the child's ability to practice accessing the recommended system. Disease progression and trajectory will also factor into the planning timeline, with potential for modification and reevaluation as children near EoL due to changing status. Early referral to a SLP to support communication planning and AAC system development is typically advisable, as the course of an illness may change unexpectedly, prompting need sooner than anticipated.

Children who use AAC at baseline may work with known providers, such as SLPs in the school or community setting, to support communication planning when faced with EoL care needs. Some, especially those admitted to the hospital, may work with on-site hospital SLPs. Though a known communication strategy and system may be well established, exploration of modified access strategies in the event of changing physical skills, additional vocabulary (e.g., new terminology related to medical interventions or care needs), or modified field size may be warranted. Depending on each individual's unique needs, new systems and strategies may be explored and recommended. Therefore, ongoing feature-matched assessments will be critical to ensure the most appropriate communication strategies and systems are recommended in context of the child's evolving status.

Acute Communication Difficulties or Loss of Speech

Some children are faced with acute communication deficits and/or loss of speech. When the underlying etiology of these changes is related to a new life-limiting diagnosis, EoL care discussions and the need for an AAC assessment may be prompted. Often, these children and families have little prior experience with AAC which, when coupled with a new and devastating diagnosis or change in skills, may be incredibly overwhelming. For some, the acute change in communication skills may have been unanticipated despite a known terminal diagnosis, for example, due to escalated respiratory support needs or mechanical ventilation. In the context of EoL care, an acute communication deficit may or may not improve over time, prompting the SLP to focus less on restorative strategies and more on compensatory strategies while working carefully with the patient and family to identify the most appropriate, feature-matched, solutions to meet immediate needs and wishes.

Message Banking

Children who use spoken language at the time of diagnosis or prior to advanced illness may wish to participate in message banking. The Message Banking Process is defined as the storing of digital recordings and messages, including words, phrases, sentences, and sounds, using a person's own voice, personality, and inflection (Costello, 2009). Messages can be programmed into a voice-output communication aid or speech-generating device (SGD) for use when the child is no longer able to use natural speech. This strategy may also be appropriate for patients who have difficulty communicating due to a language barrier. These patients may record messages in their primary language and an interpreter may record the translated versions in the language of the medical environment or community. Voice output in both languages ensures that the patient and the communication partner both understand the selected and intended message. When banking messages, children are able to think ahead about their own wants, needs, and preferences in addition to coping strategies and comfort measures. Although every aspect of symptom management, care, and connection cannot be predicted, children and families may embrace the opportunity to participate in conversations about the future and record relevant messages. Those who have experience in the medical setting or who have had a lifelong illness may be very in-tune with their anticipated needs and how they might wish to communicate in times of distress. Children may also be able to build on their legacy by banking messages to loved ones, stories, and memories, or as is often the case for prelinguistic patients, recording the sound of babbling, cooing, and laughter.

Patients who are unable to participate in message banking can still participate in vocabulary selection, which can in turn support future-oriented conversations. Some children may decline banking messages with their own speaking voice, for example, due to perceptions of altered vocal quality or because they believe they lack the endurance and stamina required to participate. Instead, children may choose to use a proxy voice, such as a sibling, friend, or parent, to record the child's selected vocabulary and messages with intended inflection.

Common Needs and Symptoms Children May Experience at End-of-Life

Suttle et al. (2017) describe three primary needs of children at EoL including physical needs, psychosocial needs, and spiritual needs. To mitigate communication breakdowns and misunderstandings while simultaneously optimizing patients' autonomy and control, caregivers and providers should keep these three overarching themes in mind.

Physical Needs

Pain and symptom management are typically at the forefront of direct care provision. However, when a child is unable to effectively communicate their needs, opportunities for symptom management are missed, and unintended suffering may be exacerbated. Children with complex communication and care needs may use nonverbal behaviors to signal discomfort, displeasure, and irritability, but these may be commonly misinterpreted as pain (Schwantes & Wells O'Brien, 2014). In the hospital setting, the inability to communicate effectively may also result in an increased risk of hospital-acquired conditions, which may not have occurred otherwise (Hurtig et al., 2018). Use of visual scenes, for example, a body board, may help young children identify and localize pain or discomfort. Though these concepts are abstract in nature, use of developmentally and cognitively appropriate picture-communication symbols may support a child's ability to distinguish between types of pain (e.g., nausea, aches, burns, tingles, chest pain, headache, constipation, etc.) and other needs. Providing opportunities to describe pain types and levels will help inform caregivers on appropriate symptom management. Rather than reverting to pain medications, which may also be sedating, children need developmentally appropriate ways to identify comfort measures. This might include medical intervention such as pain or nausea relief, or nonpharmaceutical interventions like a cool cloth, hot pack, massage, dimmed lights, favorite stuffed animal, and familial presence or closeness. Depending on their age, children may also wish to ask questions about pain and symptom management to further enhance their ability to participate in their own care and decision-making. Symptoms and physical needs that children may wish to communicate might include pain, nausea, positioning, difficulty breathing, anxiety, seizures, constipation, lethargy, and reduced ability or interest in eating (Polikoff & McCabe, 2013).

Psychosocial Needs

A child's cognitive and developmental understanding of death and how to cope in the context of EoL care will inform how to support those discussions. Some children benefit from open discussions to talk about death and dying as a way to reduce confusion about why certain changes are occurring or why they may be feeling a certain way. Others may not wish to or be able to engage in EoL discussions, and communication opportunities are instead focused on comfort, coping, social connection, and preserving a sense of normalcy. Maintaining intimacy and socialization is often just as important and sanctified for patients and families as pain and symptom management. AAC systems should integrate vocabulary and messages that are personally relevant to the child. Supportive mobile technology may also be provided to promote social connection within and beyond the setting of EoL care. For example, patients using low-tech strategies may still benefit from video calls to loved ones, during which they can see, hear, and engage with others.

In the event of increased sedation, fatigue, and potentially changing cognitive status, some children may not be able to maintain wakefulness or attention for reciprocal interactions as they near EoL. At this stage, even simple but accessible strategies can promote psychosocial support for both the child and their loved ones, for example, activating a single-switch voice-output communication aid to say, "I love you" or "I need you." Partner-assisted scanning may be used to support expression of a range of comfort, emotional, and interpersonal messages in addition to opting in or out of conversations.

Spiritual Needs

Spiritual identification and connection may differ among children and their families. At times, EoL discussions may prompt children, especially older children and teenagers, to think more carefully about their own spiritual beliefs and preferences. For some, this may include programming specific prayers or messages into an SGD or adding vocabulary to express a desire for someone to recite a prayer. For others, preserving spirituality may take form in preservation of intimate connections to loved ones or other meaningful activities. The child's own spiritual preferences and needs should be incorporated, as appropriate, into recommended communication systems and strategies.

AAC Considerations at End-Of-Life

When conducting an AAC assessment to determine the most appropriate communication strat-

egies for a child requiring advanced medical care, whether it is known that the child is nearing EoL or not, a variety of factors should be considered. Like the process described in Chapters 8 and 10, feature-matched assessment should factor in the child's strengths, abilities, and needs across a variety of domains with regard to language skills, vision, sensory needs (e.g., vision and hearing), physical access, environment, communication partners, and cognition to support selection of unaided and aided strategies. When considering aided communication strategies, such as a low- or high-tech system, the feature-matched assessment should support symbol selection, linguistic features, operational considerations, portability, and more with the understanding that the child's abilities and needs may change over time. It should be noted that children in EoL care may also benefit from augmented input to support changes in comprehension and receptive language skills (e.g., visual communication aids, schedules, written text, orientation cues, etc.). Along with input from the patient, family, medical providers, and the palliative care team, the SLP should integrate the following additional factors into the feature-matched assessment.

Age of Child and Understanding of Illness-Related Concepts

Children may be able to participate in EoL discussions and decisions surrounding communication needs and preferences in different ways depending on their chronological and developmental age and abilities. For example, AAC considerations for young children or those with prelinguistic communication skills may focus on expressing immediate wants and needs through aided or unaided strategies, seeking comfort to mitigate symptoms, or gaining attention of loved ones to engage in social connection and physical closeness. Older children may also require access to AAC to participate more fully in conversations and discussions. They may need to ask questions related to their medical care, ask questions about their nonimmediate environment (e.g., "How are my classmates and friends?"), or talk more openly about their illness (e.g., "I'm worried it will hurt").

Children typically develop an early understanding of death around 4 to 5 years old (Panagiotaki et al., 2018) and continue to develop a more mature understanding of death as an irreversible and universal concept until at least 10 years of age (Hunter & Smith, 2008). Despite age-related norms, a child's cognitive skills, past caregiver communication about death, and death experience all contribute to a child's understanding of mortality (Hunter & Smith, 2008). Similarly, the way children understand pain concepts and how pain can be mitigated or treated is related to chronological and developmental age. Each child's unique ability to understand their own illness and experience may inform whether they would benefit from access to more nuanced vocabulary to support these conversations. Additionally, persons who use AAC may require an individualized set of pain-related vocabulary and symbols to support self-reporting of pain symptoms (Johnson et al., 2016). Children with past medical experiences due to chronic illness may have developed their own set of terminology and vocabulary to represent symptoms, interventions, and contexts related to their care. Integration of vocabulary and messages into AAC strategies and AAC options should reflect each child's own understanding and experience. Table 13–1 offers suggested topics and vocabulary to support interactions for pediatric EoL care.

Timing of Consultation and Trajectory of Illness

Though medical teams may be able to anticipate the trajectory and course of illness, timing of death or symptom development cannot be pinpointed consistently. Similarly, each patient and family will inevitably process this information at different rates. Universally, it is critical to gently and sensitively probe about the child's understanding of their own illness as well as the family's willingness to discuss and explore solutions to communication challenges. Simultaneously understanding how the child's condition may change over time will further inform vocabulary selection, methods of access, language organization, and best approaches to repair communication breakdowns.

Cultural and Spiritual Preferences

Every family has their own set of cultural and spiritual practices that will inform EoL discussions, decision-making, and care, and are implicitly integrated into a child and family's interactions. Children may embrace the opportunity to incorporate culturally specific play, traditions, interactions, and needs into their day. Depending on age and familial culture, children may not be expected to participate in EoL discussions, while others are integrated and active in EoL planning. In some cultures, sharing specific information about a child's medical diagnosis and prognosis may be a culturally insensitive practice, and parents may wish to protect their child from such information. Some children may wish to incorporate prayer into their AAC systems along with messages reflecting their personal and/or familial cultural and spiritual values. This may be achieved by recording selected prayers onto an SGD or voice-output communication aid, with the help of a family member, spiritual leader, or hospital chaplain, so the child may actively recite their own prayers. AAC systems should support expression of these needs in a manner that is culturally sensitive and spiritually supported.

System Selection and Maintenance

In determining the most appropriate AAC system and strategies for a patient, with the understanding that skills and needs may change over time, careful consideration should be given to how those strategies will be implemented and maintained. Those providing EoL care and management, including family, loved ones, and care providers, should be trained to support AAC implementation. Some parents and family members appreciate the opportunity to actively engage in vocabulary selection, taking photos or selecting images, and maintaining programming or device setup as a way to contribute to their child's care in a meaningful and tangible way over time. Some caregivers may not be able to take on this aspect of care and will prefer communication system oversight be performed by another family member or clinician. Children who are able to actively design, program, and modify

Table 13–1. Example Messages, Topics, and Considerations to Support AAC and Interactions in Pediatric End-of-Life Care

Message Topics	Possible Considerations	Example Messages
Control and care regulation	Opt in or out of conversations Opt in or out of activities Direct others in care and other contexts	"Please put me back on my BiPap mask" "I don't want to talk about that anymore" "I need 5 minutes" "Push the syringe slowly" "Can we do this later?" "Stop. I need a break"
Legacy building and sanctity of relationships	Message banking Messages specific to loved ones Inside jokes or loving messages Preservation of personality	"I'll love you forever" "Thank you for helping me" "Remember the time when . . ."
Gaining attention	Summoning help Preserving personality	"Mom! Come here!" "I need help please" "Yoo-hoo!! Hurry up!"
Social connection	Participating in conversations Connecting through phone, video, and mobile technology	"Let's call grandma" "How are you today?" "Tell me about my friends"
Emotional expression	Ability to express feelings, humor, anger, statements of comfort, and idiosyncratic expressions	"This sucks!" "It's not fair!" "Knock knock . . ." "Smoooosh!" "@(!*$∧#@*" "Ahhh, that's nice" "Woohoo!"
Participation in care and decision-making	Identifying care needs Describing care preferences Making decisions regarding care needs, medical interventions, and advanced directives as appropriate Deciding who is present at the bedside (home or hospital)	"Please vent my g-tube" "Call my mom before position changes" "I want to try a hot pack first" "I want my sister here" "I need medicine" "When can I eat?" "Am I dying?" "Pray for me"
Comfort and symptom management	Identifying comfort needs Describing comfort preferences Requesting diapering or bathroom needs Identifying and localizing symptoms and needs (e.g., pain, discomfort, nausea, constipation, respiratory needs, temperature control, etc.)	"Blanket" "Get the fuzzy blanket" "I want a hot pack" "Massage my legs" "I have pain. Push my PCA button"

continues

Table 13–1. *continued*

Message Topics	Possible Considerations	Example Messages
Questions	Ability to ask varied questions about varied topics related to, and beyond, medical care	"Will it hurt?" "Where is my [family member]?" "Can I eat or drink?" "Who will help me at home" "Will you stay with me?"
Leisure	Indicate activity preferences Express who to play with and when Participate in play Direct play activities Access to devices	"Sing me a song" "Your turn" "I just want to watch TV now" "Turn on my iPad please" "Call the child life specialist"

their own communication systems may wish to do so, which may provide a degree of control, preservation of self, and opportunity for legacy building.

Medical Interventions at EoL

As children near EoL, certain medical interventions may be warranted to ensure comfort and symptom management. This may include escalated respiratory interventions that can preclude use of natural speech, sedative medications that may alter cognition, attention, and wakefulness, and other interventions that may inhibit baseline skills. It is imperative for the SLP to consider how evolving symptoms and interventions will affect a child's access to their communication strategies and support any modifications to ensure ongoing and meaningful communicative exchanges between the child and their communication partners.

Conclusion

As children transition to end-of-life care and progression of illness or disease evolves, goals shift to support comfort and connection. Communication access must be maintained as an integral foundation of these goals in order to preserve a child's personality, socialization, participation, autonomy, and dignity. AAC recommendations and access methods may require modification over time, but the goal

of maintaining sacred connections with loved ones and autonomy in the face of a changing body and mind remains paramount to EoL communication.

Case Study: GM

Clinical Profile and Communication Needs

GM has been tracheostomy dependent for 5 years due to chronic lung disease and is typically on the ventilator 24 hours a day. During the day, she tolerates cuff deflation to allow for leak speech and is able to converse with age-appropriate language skills despite baseline dysarthria. Though she was prescribed an SGD with eye-tracking technology, GM only accesses her SGD at school to support academics and prefers to use speech to meet all communication needs.

The Individual

GM is a 14-year-old girl with a baseline diagnosis of cerebral palsy. She is a rising sophomore in high school and an active member of her school's drama department and local community. She enjoys going to the movies, listening to show tunes with her younger sister, and served as the stage manager assistant for her high school musical. She has a close relationship with her 12-year-old sister, her parents, and her home nurse who also assists her during the school day.

Their Communication Partners

GM communicates with family members including her parents, her 12-year-old sister, and extended family members who live locally. She also has a close relationship with her daytime nurse, who accompanies her on the bus to school and throughout the day. Other primary communication partners include teachers, therapists (SLP, occupational therapist, physical therapist, and school counselor), other home nurses, school peers, and health care providers.

Their Environment

GM attends her neighborhood high school and is entering the 10th grade. She participates in medical appointments, which occur monthly or with more frequency as needed. GM participates in after-school activities when able, including stage management for the school plays. Given her complex medical needs, GM requires specialized comprehensive care and occasional inpatient admissions at a local pediatric hospital. Over the last year, GM has required multiple hospitalizations to address increased respiratory support needs in the context of repeated aspiration pneumonias. During her third hospitalization in 4 months, GM went into cardiac arrest and she was diagnosed with cardiac failure and secondary end-stage renal disease. Following her cardiac arrest, a magnetic resonance imaging scan revealed a left middle cerebral artery stroke, which resulted in reduced physical strength and coordination bilaterally, right facial weakness, and escalated ventilator settings, which inhibited her from using speech to communicate. In collaboration with the intensive care team, cardiac team, and palliative care team, GM's family made the loving decision to transition to comfort care and remain in the hospital until death, which was soon anticipated due to her progressive and evolving cardiac disease. An AAC assessment was initiated to identify supports and strategies in the context of GM's hospitalization and to support her participation in EoL discussions and care.

AAC Considerations

The AAC assessment by the hospital SLP took place at GM's bedside. A time was arranged with parents and the nurse for a morning visit, when GM was most awake and alert. Though she required some sedative medications, the team was actively weaning them to promote increased time awake to engage in interactions and activities. The goals of the assessment encompassed several factors: establishing consistent and reliable yes/no/I don't know responses, gaining attention, and providing aided strategies to support generative message production. GM identified use of eye and lip movements as her most reliable methods for answering questions. Unaided methods were established, including GM raising her eyebrows to indicate "yes," closing her eyes to indicate "no," and pouting her lip to indicate "I don't know" or "maybe." She demonstrated minimal movement of her head by turning it slightly side to side as well as her right index finger and thumb. To identify an access method for the nurse-call system, several small handheld switches were trialed. Given limited movement, a sensitive switch with a 1-in.-diameter button was ultimately selected and secured to a foam wrap around GM's hand to allow for thumb depression onto the switch, which was plugged into the hospital's nurse-call system.

The AAC System and Rationale for Clinical Decision-Making

Per discussion with the medical team, family, and with GM, it was clear that several strategies to support expressive communication would be beneficial given her evolving status, increased lethargy, and desire for a combination of generative and pre-stored messages. Given her prior experience with an SGD with eye-tracking technology, the SLP supported a bedside trial.

Though GM was able to achieve a successful calibration, she expressed repeated frustration utilizing the system. She was also unable to simultaneously use a switch to access a high-tech system via switch scanning and utilize her call button, which prompted her to endorse her preference to use low-tech strategies. As such, and given the exigency of time, an AEIOU letter board and a text-based communication board with previously stored messages were trialed. GM quickly learned how to use partner-assisted auditory-visual scanning by raising her eyebrows to first indicate the desired row and then her intended letter or message. Thereafter, GM used the letter board via partner-assisted scanning to spell messages she wished to include on her communication boards, which would be organized in a book with pages tabbed by topic.

Once strategies were trialed, recommended, and created, the SLP provided communication partner training to both GM's family and her care team. Signage was posted above her bed along with supportive visuals as a way to inform her care team about communication preferences and instructions on AAC implementation. The SLP was also paged to the bedside to support partner-assisted scanning in the context of bedside discussions with the medical team in which GM wished to be included. Although a high-tech AAC system was available to her, GM indicated her choice to use both partner-assisted scanning to spell messages and her communication boards. The rationale for the clinical decision-making was patient preference in combination with patient's demonstrated ability to use the low-tech options efficiently and with ease.

Next Steps

Over the next month, the SLP worked with GM several times each week with the goal of maintaining communication access and supporting reevaluation and modification of strategies as her clinical and medical status evolved. Communication partner training was provided to new nurses and medical team members who had not previously cared for GM to ensure carryover of all recommendations and strategies.

Over time, GM selected additional messages to include in her communication book that reflected questions about her status, directives to support comfort and pain management, inquiries into the whereabouts of and messages for her family and friends, and desires related to preferred activities. She also requested inclusion of messages to support her participation in video calls from her hospital bed to friends and family in the community. As GM's status continued to progress and she began to experience further escalation in the need for ventilator support and for sedative medications for pain management, as well as increased fatigue, she spent more time using her communication book, usually via auditory scanning, with only intermittent use of the letter board. Her nurse-call switch was modified to support activation of a voice-output communication aid (VOCA) to instead gain parental attention within the room so she could seek their emotional and physical comfort. In the days leading up to her death, GM was in and out of wakefulness and consciousness and unable to participate in the use of her communication book. When awake, she used unaided strategies including eye movements to answer simple yes/no questions and smiles to support communication with her family and care team.

References

Costello, J. (2009). Last words, last connections: How augmentative communication can support children facing end of life. *ASHA Leader, 13*(16).

Fried-Oken, M., & Bardach, L. (2005). End-of-life issues for people who use AAC. *Perspectives on Augmentative and Alternative Communication, 14*(3), 15–19. https://doi.org/10.1044/aac14.3.15

Hunter, S. B., & Smith, D. E. (2008). Predictors of children's understandings of death: Age, cognitive ability, death experience and maternal communicative competence. *Omega (Westport), 57*(2), 143–162. https://doi.org/10.2190/OM.57.2.b

Hurtig, R. R., Alper, R. M., & Berkowitz, B. (2018). The cost of not addressing the communication barriers faced by hospitalized patients. *Perspectives of the ASHA Special Interest Groups, 3*, 99–112. https://doi.org/10.1044/persp3.SIG12.99

Johnson, E., Bornman, J., & Tonsing, K. M. (2016). An exploration of pain-related vocabulary: Implications for AAC use with children. *Augmentative and Alternative Communication, 32*(4), 249–260. https://doi.org/10.1080/07434618.2016.1233998

National Cancer Institute. (n.d.). *End-of-life care.* https://www.cancer.gov/publications/dictionaries/cancer-terms/def/end-of-life-care

Panagiotaki, G., Hopkins, M., Nobes, G., Ward, E., & Griffiths, D. (2018). Children's and adults' understanding of death: Cognitive, parental, and experiential influences. *Journal of Experimental Child Psychology, 166,* 96–115. https://doi.org/10.1016/j.jecp.2017.07.014

Polikoff, L. A., & McCabe, M. E. (2013). End-of-life care in the pediatric ICU. *Current Opinions in Pediatrics, 25*(3), 285–289. https://doi.org/10.1097/MOP.0b013e328360c230

Schwantes, S., & Wells O'Brien, H. (2014). Pediatric palliative care for children with complex chronic medical conditions. *Pediatric Clinics of North America, 61*(4), 797–821. http://doi.org/10.1016/j.pcl.2014.04.011

Suttle, M. L., Jenkins, T. L., & Tamburro, R. F. (2017). End-of-life and bereavement care in pediatric intensive care units. *Pediatric Clinics of North America, 64*(5), 1167–1183. https://doi.org/10.1016/j.pcl.2017.06.012

SECTION IV
AAC Assessment, Intervention, and Implementation for Adults

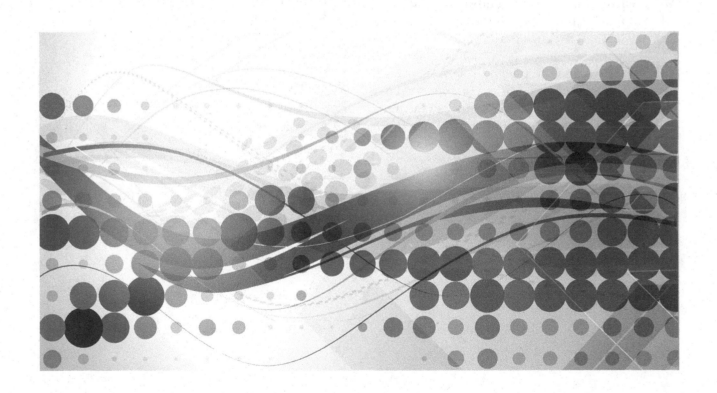

This section is focused on augmentative and alternative communication (AAC) assessment, intervention and implementation of AAC for adults, and started with Chapter 14—a chapter focused on AAC considerations for individuals transitioning into adulthood and into postsecondary environments. Chapter 15 reviews the assessment process for adults, posing the questions practitioners seek to answer in the diagnostic process. Using a custom assessment reporting tool developed for use at Communication Assistance for Youth and Adults (CAYA[1]) as a summative example, the assessment process detailed in Chapters 8 and 10 of Section III is further materialized within this chapter. Essay 16 rounds out the discussion of assessment by reviewing ethical vendor relationships in acquiring AAC systems for individuals needing AAC.

AAC intervention and implementation are discussed in Chapter 16 in the context of supporting adults with neurodegenerative conditions needing AAC, placing emphasis on education and counseling, preservation, augmentation, and adaptation; all essential considerations for supporting adults. Chapter 17 shifts to AAC in the intensive care unit (ICU) and the integral role AAC plays in patient-provider communication. Chapter 18 reiterates the concepts discussed previously in the frame of supporting adults in end-of-life care; and, again, highlights the critical role AAC plays in social connectedness and quality of life.

Key Terms Reviewed in This Section

- Socially valued adult roles
- Transition
- Transition planning
- Transition services

- Multimodal communication
- Participation model
- Social networks

- Communication partner strategies
- Legacy messages
- Neurodegenerative diseases
- Voice amplification

- Acute care
- Intensive care unit
- Patient-provider communication
- Medical decision-making

- Capacity
- Death
- Decision-making
- Dying
- Socialization

---

[1]CAYA. (2021). *What is CAYA?* https://cayabc.net

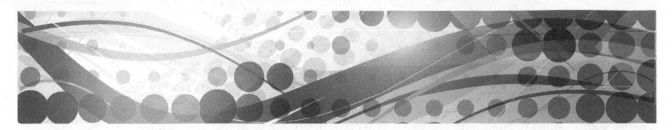

Chapter 14

SERVICES FOR YOUNG ADULTS USING AAC TRANSITIONING TO ADULTHOOD

Diane Nelson Bryen

Fundamentals

Prologue

Years ago, I asked adults with complex communication needs who use AAC technologies the following question:

"How old were you when someone asked you what you wanted to be when you grew up?"

Their answers shocked me. Every one of them indicated that,

"Nobody ever asked me!"

I learned that if this question is never asked, young adults and their families are not likely to begin to think about and start planning for their future. They are not likely to work toward a future that includes doing something meaningful with their lives, having friends and mature relationships, living independently, nor being an active member of their community. As they grow older, they are likely to succumb to having others make decisions about their lives.

With effective transition planning, young adults with complex communication needs (CCNs) and their families can have high expectations for life after school. There are several reasons for this. First, during the past few decades, we have seen documented examples of how augmentative and alternative communication (AAC) devices and services have led to desired outcomes for individuals in college and university settings (Bryen et al., 1995), employment (Carey et al., 2004; McNaughton & Bryen, 2002) and participation in the larger communities where they live (Bryen, 2008).

At the same time, we know that too many individuals who might benefit from specialized and mainstream communication technologies leave school without having access to these devices and the supports needed to effectively use them. Lack of access generally results in the inability to communicate effectively, which severely restricts their participation in traditional adult roles as students, workers, friends and partners, citizens, and parents (Bryen & Moulton, 1998; Light et al., 2003).

New and Emerging Communication Technologies

Higher expectations for life after school are being made possible by access to new and emerging specialized and mainstream communication technologies. In addition to communication boards, specialized speech-generating devices (SGDs) and inclusive mainstream communication technologies for face-to-face communication, new technologies enable young adults to communicate remotely with friends, family, employers, and members of the community at large (Bryen, 2008)

In addition to high-tech AAC devices, topic-specific low-tech communication boards continue to play a role in face-to-face communication. Shown in Figures 14–1 and 14–2 are examples of a few research-based, topic-specific communication boards focusing on communication during times of natural disasters (Bryen & Ravich, 2009), reporting that you have been a victim of crime or abuse (Bryen, 2010), and testifying in court (White et al., 2015). These communication boards are available via free download so that adults with CCNs can live more safely in the community.

Vocabulary needed to support socially valued adult roles, while not always preprogrammed into speech-generating technologies can be downloaded into their communication devices so they can communicate more effectively while engaging in socially valued adult roles (Bryen, 2008), such as

- College Life
- Emergency Preparedness
- Employment
- Sexuality, Intimacy, and Sex
- Reporting Crime and Abuse

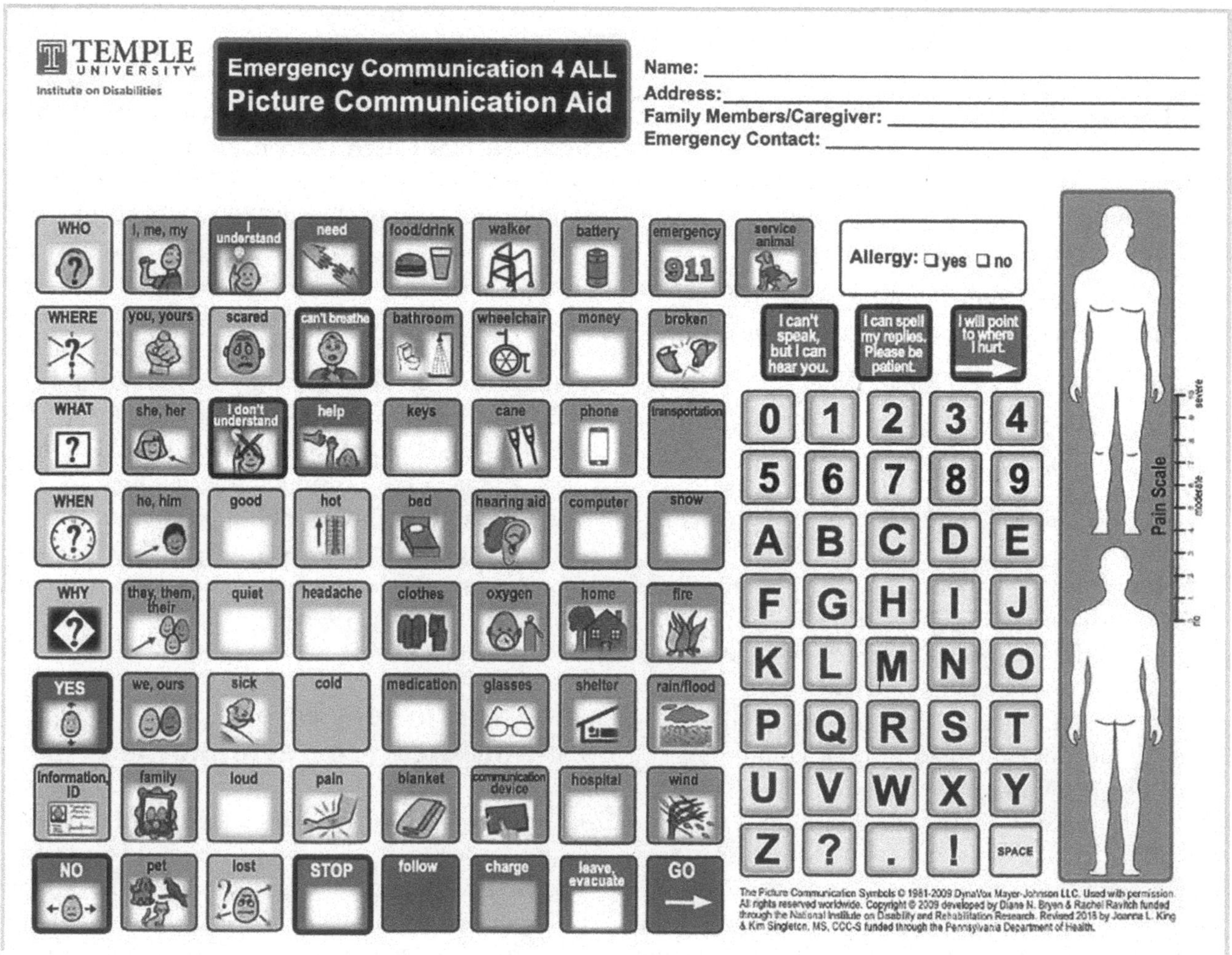

Figure 14–1. Sample communication display for use during emergency situations.

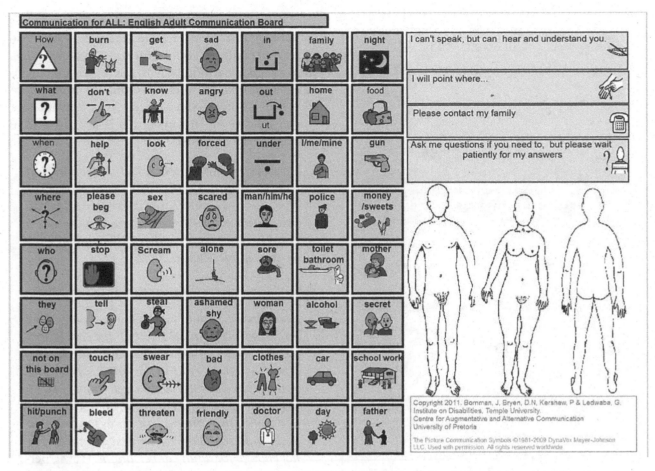

Figure 14–2. Sample communication display for use when testifying in court or reporting on abuse.

- Managing Personal Assistance Services
- Managing Health Care
- Using Transportation[1]

Personal Communication Passports

Personal Communication Passports serve a means of improving face-to-face communication for children, young adults, and adults with the most significant CCNs. Personal Communication Passports are a practical and person-centered way of supporting children, young people, and adults who cannot easily speak for themselves. According to Wilson (2018), a "Communication Passport pulls together complex information about the individual

and presents it in an easy to use format. It is easy to read, informative, useful and fun. Above all, the Communication Passport is in an accessible format, so that the individual can share some or all of the information contained and tries to reflect their personality and interests." They can be paper-made or digital. An example of the first two pages of Ellie's Personal Communication Passport is shown in Figure 14–3.

More recently, SGDs enable young people to communicate remotely via telephones and speakerphones. Mobile phones and smartphones with adaptations for access or built with principles of universal design are enabling many young adults with CCNs to communicate with anyone, anytime,

[1]These research-based vocabulary sets can be downloaded free from https://disabilities.temple.edu/aacvocabulary/

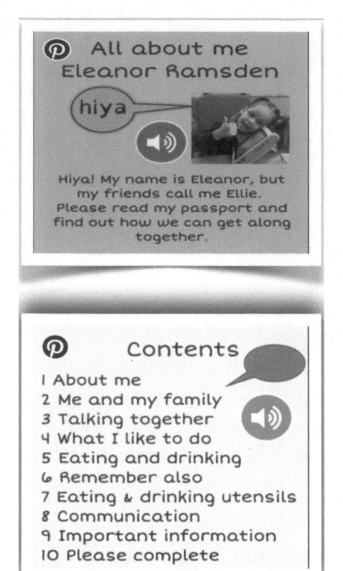

Figure 14–3. First two pages of Ellie's Communication Passport. Used with permission from CALL Scotland.

and from anywhere (Bryen, 2019; Bryen & Moolman, 2015; Bryen et al., 2017). Newer AAC devices enable many young adults to access the Internet for social connection and to obtain the vast body of information via the World Wide Web (Bryen & Chung, 2018) and via intelligent digital assistants such as Alexa or Siri, as shown in Figure 14–4 (Bryen, 2019).

While in K–12, students with CCNs are hopefully being introduced to and learning how to use these specialized communication technologies; they are also learning how to use accessible mainstream information and communication technologies that are being developed using principles of university design. However, this is not always the case, as Sarah laments:

> *Most speech-language pathologists I have worked with want to stay with basic core vocabulary. That was okay until I was 18 years old, which was when I wanted to have some adult words so I could express myself with vocabulary appropriate for my age.* (Lever, 2003, p. 4)

Seven years later, Sarah continues to lament:

> *As adults we want to say anything that we need and want to and we depend on the vocabulary programmed into our devices. Many adult users weren't taught to read in the public schools and to program a device you have to know how to read and spell. So, we depend on our teachers and therapists to program in words that we want to use and the pre-programmed vocabulary is not enough for adult conversations.* (Lever, personal communication, 2010)

AAC and the Importance of Transition

All of us go through many transitions, such as transitioning from preschool to elementary school, from elementary to high school, from K–12 education to college or work, and even transition from work and family to retirement. Each of these transitions can be difficult. However, transition from school to adult living is one of the most critical times in any student's life. In many ways, it is even more difficult for students with CCNs. Students with CCNs will not only have to manage the typical challenges of postsecondary and continuing education, employment, independent living, personal safety, and developing and maintaining social relations, they will have to be prepared to manage their technology, personal assistants, transportation, and

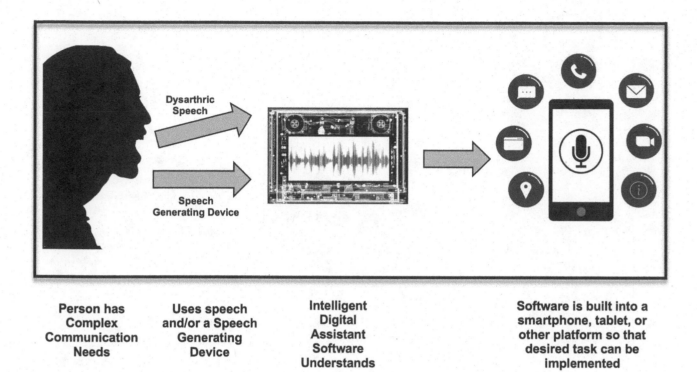

| Person has Complex Communication Needs | Uses speech and/or a Speech Generating Device | Intelligent Digital Assistant Software Understands | Software is built into a smartphone, tablet, or other platform so that desired task can be implemented |

Figure 14–4. AAC Devices plus intelligent digital assistants accessing the Internet.

a host of other challenges, such as communication during times of man-made or natural emergencies (Bryen, 2009, 2010). Many parents worry about this transition, and they have reason to worry.

When the school bus stops at age 21 years, young adults with disabilities are no longer entitled to needed technology, services, and supports guaranteed under the Individuals with Disabilities Education Act (IDEA).[2] As such, careful planning for acquiring AAC and related technologies and services is needed if a young adult with CCNs is to successfully transition to life after school (McNaughton & Bryen, 2007).

When should transition planning begin? It should begin before students with CCNs leave high school, generally at age 14 years. This is the age when typical young adults are already thinking and dreaming about their future. It is the time to begin to dream about jobs and careers; postsecondary, career, and technical training; independent living; community participation; and personal relationships. Thinking about the future can be facilitated by using either person-centered planning processes, such as Making Action Plans (MAPS), or Dare to Dream: Turning your Dreams into Future Realities.

As shown in Figure 14–5, MAPS is a planning process for people with disabilities. It begins with a story—the history—and has a series of empty container questions that ask a person to share some of the milestones on their journey, so the planning circle can get to know them more deeply, dream with them, and begin to build a plan to move in the direction of their dreams. Although MAPS originated in the "disability" sector, its applications cover the full spectrum of life situations.

Similar to MAPS, Dare to Dream: Turning Dreams into Future Realities (Bryen, 2012) is also

---

[2]Congress reauthorized the IDEA in 2004 and most recently amended IDEA through Public Law 114-95, Every Student Succeeds Act, in December 2015.

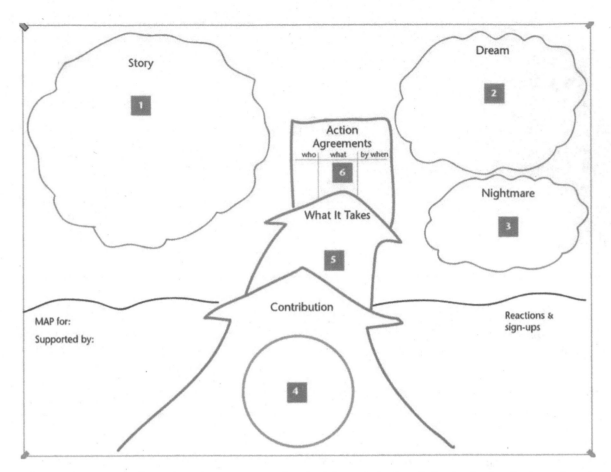

Figure 14–5. MAPS: A Planning Process. Used with permission from Inclusion International.

a planning approach that begins with the person's dream. It is a guided process and is drawn using graphic facilitation.

Case Study: CK

Clinical Profile and Communication Needs

The Individual

Meet CK. He is 18 years old, attends high school in Chicago, and lives with his grandmother. Due to his disability that greatly affects mobility and communication, he uses a variety of assistive technologies including a speech-generating AAC device, an

adapted computer, and a powered wheelchair. CK also relies on personal assistants for most of his daily routines.

As shown in Figure 14–6, CK's dream is to one day live with a buddy in an apartment in Colorado Springs. He wants to be a writer for a national news station. When not working, he wants to be able to communicate with friends.

Their Communication Partners and Environment

CK has been living with his 75-year-old grandmother since the death of his mother 4 years ago. In Chicago, where CK lives, he has many friends both from school and in his neighborhood. He enjoys talking with his friends and working on the high school newspaper. His grandmother came with CK

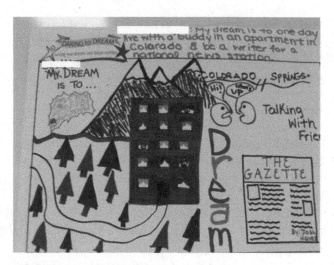

Figure 14–6. CK's dream.

to Temple University to learn how to use his new AAC device and to learn about self-advocacy and independent living. CK is active at his high school where he works on the school newspaper.

Once the student's dream is clearly articulated, it is time to turn their dream into an achievable and measurable action plan. CK's individualized education program (IEP) team is meeting next month to review and revise his IEP and want to start transition planning. CK did not really feel comfortable going to his IEP meetings. He felt like it was just all his teachers and grandmother talking about the stuff he cannot do. His case manager knew how important his input was in a transition plan, so he and CK met and put together a transition plan using the MAPS model. He brought it home and shared it with his grandmother. Once they had time to review it, CK brought it back to his case manager, where they translated the information on the MAPS and wrote measurable postsecondary goals that are required on CK's IEP.

Communication Needs and Goals

CK's dream-driven, measurable goals to accomplish before he graduated included the following that CK will learn:

- How to manage his adaptive technology and his generic technologies

- How to manage personal assistance services (PASs)
- How to manage transportation
- How to manage his health care
- How to apply for a part-time job or internship writing for a school or local newspaper
- How to manage his finances, including his cash and medical benefits
- How to live independently, with personal assistance services (PAS)
- About his interests, employment goals, and/ or postsecondary opportunities
- Sexual and relational roles and responsibilities
- What supports and accommodations he will need
- How to be his own self-advocate
- What services and benefits (cash and other) are available to him?

CK's goals are quite extensive. The transition plan should provide a road map for CK, his grandmother, and his transition team. Where and how will CK and his grandmother learn all of this? It clearly cannot wait until CK is a senior and facing school-leaving. Both MAPS and Dare to Dream: Turning Dreams into Future Realities provide a road map for CK, his grandmother, and his transition team. The content of MAPS, shown in Figure 14–5, is empty. However, when the transition team meets, needed details will be provided. This will include what it takes, and action agreements (i.e., who will do what and by when). If CK has used the Dare to Dream approach, the action plan will be completed using the template illustrated in Figure 14–7. CK's dream will appear in the upper right-hand corner, measurable 1-year goals will be written in the center bullseye. Important people, places, and resources needed to accomplish the 1-year goal or goals will be identified that are both possible and positive. Finally, the first step to be taken by CK is agreed upon. Using either planning approach, annual meetings are important to revisit the original dream, and to celebrate the accomplishment of CK's 1-year goal. The process continues until the dream is achieved or revised.

Fortunately, IDEA provides a realistic time frame for *transition planning*, requiring that it start as early as age 14 years and continue until the

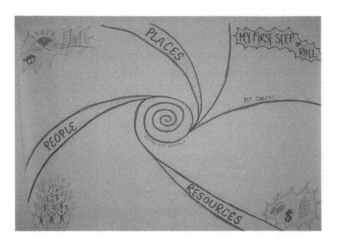

Figure 14–7. Dare to Dream action planning template.

student graduates or reaches age 21 years. Transition planning should prepare students for life after high school, help students plan for and choose high school courses, and help students decide what skills they need to develop to live and work in the community after high school. During this time, students can be given the opportunity to explore work and career options while still in high school. Students and families can also begin to make connections with education and training programs, colleges, agencies, and support services for after high school to continue working toward goals. Students and the entire IEP team learn about student interests and hobbies, what works and does not work in their lifestyles, their skills and talents, and who can help in achieving specific student goals.

AAC Considerations

What is often not considered in transition planning for students with CCNs is the need to have necessary vocabulary programmed into the student's AAC device so that upon graduation they can communicate in socially valued adult roles. Socially valued adult roles include but are not limited to (a) attending college; (b) becoming employed; (c) managing one's personal assistants, health care, and transportation; and (d) engaging in consen-

sual intimate and sexual relationships while at the same time reporting unwanted and often criminal sexual behaviors. Also, since many young adults and adults with CCNs have more limited social networks, during transition planning strategies for increasing social networks are critical to reduce the high rates of unemployment, social isolation, and depression. Finally, transition planning should also focus on increasing personal safety and reducing the risk of being a victim of crime or abuse, since individuals with disabilities, especially those with CCNs, are 4 to 10 times more likely to be the victims of abuse and crime than their peers without disability.

IDEA requires that *transition services* start no later than age 16 years. Transition services are a coordinated set of activities for a child with a disability that is designed to be within a results-oriented process, that is focused on improving the academic and functional achievement of the child with a disability to facilitate the child's movement from school to postschool activities, including postsecondary education, vocational education, integrated employment (including supported employment), continuing and adult education, adult services, independent living, or community participation. It is based on the individual student's needs, taking into account the child's strengths, preferences, and interests. None of this will happen without the IEP.

The AAC System and Transition Planning

Transition planning and transition services must be written into the IEP. Assistive and generic technology devices and services needed for transition must also be written into the IEP. The Colorado Department of Education (2014) has a useful transition checklist, which is provided in Figure 14–8. This checklist is not state specific. Note, however, that this checklist does address how AAC and related assistive technology (AT) are integrated into a transition plan.

It is important to remember that if AT devices and services are not written into the student's transition plan, they will not be provided. Fortunately,

4 to 5 Years Before Leaving School:
Transition activities to consider when preparing transition plans with the IEP team.

- ❑ Identify personal learning styles and the necessary accommodations to be a successful learner and worker.
- ❑ Identify career interests and skills, complete interest and career inventories, and identify additional education or training requirements.
- ❑ Explore options for post- secondary education and admission criteria.
- ❑ Identify interests and options for future living arrangements, including supports.
- ❑ Using your AAC device, learn to communicate effectively your interests, preferences, and needs.
- ❑ Using your AAC device, be able to explain your disability and the accommodations you need.
- ❑ Learn and practice informed decision-making skills.
- ❑ Investigate assistive technology tools that can increase community involvement and employment opportunities.
- ❑ Broaden your experiences with community activities and expand your friendships.
- ❑ Pursue and use local transportation options outside of family.
- ❑ Investigate money management and identify necessary skills.
- ❑ Acquire identification card and the ability to communicate personal information.
- ❑ Identify and begin learning skills necessary for independent living.
- ❑ Learn and practice personal health care.

Two to Three Years Before Leaving the School:
Transition activities to consider when preparing transition plans with the IEP team.

- ❑ Identify community support services and programs (Vocational Rehabilitation, County Services, Centers for Independent Living, etc.)
- ❑ Invite adult service providers, peers, and others to the IEP transition meeting.
- ❑ Match career interests and skills with vocational course work and community work experiences.
- ❑ Gather more information on post-secondary programs and the support services offered; and make arrangements for accommodations to take college entrance exams.
- ❑ Identify health care providers and become informed about sexuality and family planning issues.
- ❑ Determine the need for financial support (Supplemental Security Income, state financial supplemental programs, Medicare).
- ❑ Using your AAC device, learn and practice appropriate interpersonal, communication, and social skills for different settings (employment, school, recreation, with peers, etc.).
- ❑ Explore legal status with regards to decision making prior to age of majority.
- ❑ Begin a resume and update it as needed.
- ❑ Practice independent living skills, e.g., budgeting, shopping, cooking, and housekeeping.
- ❑ Identify needed personal assistant services, and if appropriate, learn to direct and manage these services.

One Year Before Leaving the School:
Transition activities to consider when preparing transition plans with the IEP team.

- ❑ Apply for financial support programs. (Supplemental Security Income, Independent Living Services, Vocational Rehabilitation, and Personal Assistant Services).
- ❑ Using your AAC device, practice effective communication by developing interview skills, asking for help, and identifying necessary accommodations at post-secondary and work environments
- ❑ Specify desired job and obtain paid employment with supports as needed.
- ❑ Take responsibility for arriving on time to work, appointments, and social activities.
- ❑ Assume responsibility for health care needs (making appointments, filling and taking prescriptions etc.).
- ❑ Register to vote and for selective service

Figure 14–8. Transition checklists for the IEP team.

the leadership of the group Quality Indicators for Assistive Technology (QIAT) has developed questions to ask about transition planning for students who use AAC and related ATs.[3] A few of these questions are as follows:

1. Student's transition plans address the AAC and related AT needs of the student, including roles and training needs of team members, subsequent steps in AT use, and follow-up after transition takes place.

   A few questions to consider:

   ■ Does the agency have clearly written guidelines for documenting AAC and related AT transition needs in the IEP, and does the IEP team demonstrate working knowledge of these guidelines?

   ■ How are transition IEPs monitored to make sure that the AAC and related AT needs of students are addressed?

   ■ What supports and services will the team include in the transition planning?

2. Transition planning empowers the student using AAC to participate in the transition planning at a level appropriate to age and ability.

   A few questions to consider:

   ■ How will the student be a participating member of the transition team?

   ■ Does the student use their AAC to support and increase participation in transition planning?

3. Advocacy related to AAC and related AT use is recognized as critical and planned for by the teams involved in transition.

   Some key questions to consider:

   ■ Who will be identified to advocate for the student's use of AAC in the new environment?

   ■ How are self-advocacy skills taught to the student?

   ■ How will the student employ self-advocacy strategies during planning?

4. AAC and related AT requirements in the receiving environment are identified during the transition planning process.

   A few key questions to consider:

   ■ What will the receiving environment need to know about the student's AAC use?

   ■ What changes, if any, are required in the AAC and related technology the student uses to participate and achieve in the new environment?

   ■ What opportunities will the student have to practice needed skills before the transition?

5. Transition plans address specific equipment, training, and funding issues such as transfer or acquisition of AT, manuals, and support documents.

   Some key questions to consider:

   ■ Who is the owner of the AAC device and related AT the student currently uses?

   ■ Will the student be able to use the same AAC device and related AT in the new environment?

   ■ Have funding options for purchase of a new AAC device been identified and accessed?

Next Steps

Transition is the time to dream about careers, postsecondary education, including technical education. It is also the time to think about independent living and what supports may be needed. Many adults with disabilities, especially those who have CCNs and who use a variety of communication technologies are lonely. Therefore, transition planning for life after high school is a key to community inclusion and participation, which can open the door to establishing healthy personal relationships and expanding social networks. Effective use of AAC devices and related AT is important to support a student's dreams by possibly overcoming or reducing functional limitations associated with

---

[3]Based on the QIAT Leadership Team. (2012). http://www.qiat.org

having CCNs. These tools may aid in performing tasks that were difficult or impossible in the past. However, none of this will be possible without planning for future needs.

To help CK's transition become a reality, it would be helpful to develop some sample transition objectives for him. These are based on the socially valued adult roles outlined earlier as well as CK's specific dreams and aspirations. Importantly, these objectives are samples; others may be added, and those that follow may need to be modified, if necessary.

1. Using his AAC device, CK will direct his personal assistance in how to charge his communication device.
2. Using his AAC device, CK will answer selected science questions in order to provide an oral response demonstrating his understanding of the chapter on safe sex.
3. Using his AAC device, CK will preprogram his communication device with responses to commonly asked job interview questions.
4. With the support of his Office of Vocational Rehabilitation counselor, CK will use his AAC device to discuss how much earned income he can make before losing his Medicaid health insurance.

Timely and effective transition planning and services will make a big difference for CK and for many other students with disabilities who have CCNs who will eventually be transitioning from high school to a meaningful adult life.

Expert Tips or Practical Advice

Students should be included in discussion of their AAC, AT, and accommodation needs. Ensure familiarity of which AAC devices, services, and accommodations facilitate completion of class work and higher academic achievement, independent living, and so on. It is easier for the student to express those needs after they leave the K-12 environment, only if they know about needed AT. If tran-

sition services and AT devices *and* services are not written into the IEP, they will not be provided. Students must not be limited by limited knowledge and skills of their educators, related service personnel, or school administrators. The use of AAC and AT is not a goal in itself. When written into a Transition Plan, AAC and AT can be (a) written as part of a goal or objective (e.g., "Using a speech-generating AAC device, student will learn to communicate via telephone with potential employers"); (b) included in Specially Designed Instruction (e.g., "Access to a computer for writing tasks longer than one paragraph"); (c) an accommodation for testing; (d) part of Related Services (e.g., "Student and parents will be trained by an AAC consultant in the use of the student's AAC device"); (e) Supports for School Personnel (e.g., "Teacher of student with CCN will be trained in use and maintenance of the student's AAC approach").

References

Bryen, D. N. (2008). Vocabulary for socially-valued adult roles. *Augmentative and Alternative Communication*, *24*(4), 294–301.

Bryen, D. N. (2009). Communicating during times of natural or man-made emergencies. *Journal of Pediatric Rehabilitation Medicine: An Interdisciplinary Approach*, *2*(2), 123–129.

Bryen, D. N. (2010). Communication during times of natural or man-made emergencies: The potential of speech-generating devices. *International Journal of Emergency Management*, *7*(1). https://doi.org/10.1504/IJEM.2010.032041

Bryen, D. N. (2019). *What people who use AAC say about mainstream mobile technologies*. Interview for the American Association of Occupational Therapists.

Bryen, D. N., Bornman, J., Morris, J., Moolman, E., & Sweatman, M. (2017). Use of mobile technology by adults who use AAC: Voices from two countries. *Assistive Technology Outcomes and Benefits*, *11*, 66–81.

Bryen, D. N., & Chung, Y. (2018). What adults who use AAC say about their use of mainstream mobile technologies. *Assistive Technology Benefits and Outcomes*, *12*, 73–106.

Bryen, D. N., & Moolman, E. (2015). Mobile phone technology for ALL: Reducing the information and communication divide. In Z. Yan (Ed.), *Encyclopedia of mobile phone behavior* (Vols. 1, 2, & 3). IGI Global.

Bryen, D. N., & Moulton, B. (1998). Why "Employment, independence, marriage and sexuality"? *Issues in Special Education and Rehabilitation, 14*(2). Also published in Hebrew in ISAAC-Israel (2001).

Bryen, D. N., & Ravich, R. (2009). *Emergency communication 4ALL—Picture communication aid* (English, Spanish, and Haitian Creole). http://disabilities.temple .edu/aacvocabulary/e4all.shtml

Bryen, D. N., Slesaransky, G., & Baker, D. (1995). Augmentative communication and empowerment supports: A look at outcomes. *Augmentative and Alternative Communication, 11*, 79–88.

Carey, A. C., Potts, B. B., Bryen, D. N., & Shankar, J. A. (2004). Networking towards employment: Experiences of people who use augmentative and alternative communication. *Research and Practice for Persons with Severe Disabilities, 29*(1), 40–52.

Colorado Department of Education, Exceptional Student Services Unit. (2014). *Transition planning* [Downloadable transition checklist]. https://www.cde.state .co.us/cdesped/tk_tab02_planning

Lever. S. (2003). Speaking out: Access to vocabulary. *Alternatively Speaking, 6*(3), 4.

Lever, S. (2010). *Importance of adult vocabulary* [Personal communication].

Light, J., Buekelman, D. R., & Riechle, J. (Eds.) (2003). *Communicative competence for individuals who use AAC.* Brookes Publishing.

McNaughton, D., & Bryen, D. (2002). Enhancing participation in employment though AAC technologies. *Assistive Technology, 14*(1), 58–70.

McNaughton, D., & Bryen, D. (2007). AAC technologies to enhance participant and access to meaningful societal roles for adolescents and adults with developmental disabilities who rely on AAC. *Augmentative and Alternative Communication, 23*(3), 217–229.

White, R., Bornman, J., & Johnson, E. (2015). *Testifying in court.* Centre for Augmentative & Alternative Communication. https://www.up.ac.za/centre-for-augment ative-alternative-communication

Wilson, A. (2018, February 1). Creating personal communication passports. *CALL Scotland.* https://www.call scotland.org.uk/blog/personal-communication-pass ports/

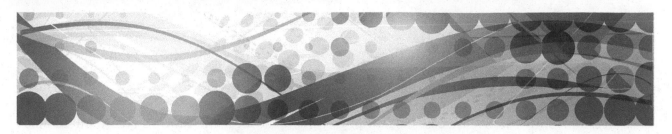

Chapter 15
ASSESSING ADULTS

Jeffrey K. Riley, Lois Turner, and Stacey Harpell

Fundamentals

The reasons that individuals lose their ability to speak or perhaps never acquire the ability to speak are diverse, as are the environments they live in and the people who surround them. Speech-language pathologists (SLPs) as communication specialists have the challenge of teasing apart the many threads of this complexity to determine the best options for communication supports, technology, and practices. The fundamentals of an assessment are observation, measurement, judgment, and decision. The desired outcomes of an assessment are goals and a plan for action. As a skilled professional presented with the challenge of reducing or removing communication barriers for an individual, the SLP will be presented with clients on a wide spectrum of disability and situations. Examples of such situations include an adult who received a devastating diagnosis that will result in the deterioration or complete loss of their speech and/or language, or the parents of a young child with physical and intellectual disabilities that may lead to the child never developing functional speech, or an adolescent who has used a variety of augmentative and alternative communication (AAC) and communication supports for many years and now needs an update, or any individual migrating to new technology or environments and in need of new ways to communicate.

In all of these situations, the challenge for the SLP is to be a keen observer not only of the indi-

vidual and their concomitant physical, intellectual, and behavioral abilities related to communication, but also of the people around the individual and the environments where they live and operate. A sample of observational questions that need to be asked and answered include the following: What does the individual do in their life? Whom do they interact with? What is their home like? Where do they go in the day, or the evening? Who are the people in their lives? Does the individual have aspirations and goals to improve and/or change their communication? How do the people who care, love, and support the individual want their life to change, develop, or be supported? Beyond observation, assessment is also a measurement. It is gauging a person's abilities against standards, norms, or expectations that may predict how successful they will be in communicating with others. This may involve using several standard and/or nonstandard tests to measure and to determine the individual's abilities, strengths, and challenges.

Judgment in the assessment process is informed through the integration of observations and measurements of a host of complex and perhaps atypical individual behaviors, and the complex situations and environments in which they transpire. Some questions to pose include the following: What is consistent? Where is there an opportunity for constructive communication behaviors to grow? What are the possibilities and opportunities to inform or engineer the living and social environments around this individual? How can the people who surround this individual be motivated, inspired, and supported to assume some of the burden of communication for this individual, ease the flow of communication, and build and support autonomy and agency for the individual?

Assessment should lead to decisions and to goals—decisions on what kind of communication system to use, what sort of technology to apply, and what environmental and strategic supports to implement. Decision also involves determining the practicalities and feasibility of selected technologies, systems, and supports in the individual's environment, and identifying resources and limitations of the people, supports, and organizations that surround this person. Decisions must be supported through the articulation of appropriate goals and by the individual, supporters, and the environment to attain desired outcomes. For example, vocabulary customization is a crucial decision to ensure people who are differently abled have access to vital language. People with disabilities are at a high risk for sexual, physical, financial, and emotional abuse and neglect and require access to preferential vocabulary, code-switching, advocacy language, and specific considerations to safeguard them from neglect.

Finally, for the assessment to have lasting impact and value for the participants, it must be compiled into a comprehensive and cohesive report that will document the observations and measurements, substantiate the assessor's judgments, and support collaborative decisions made with the individual, their supporters, and relevant organizations. Effectively, the assessment should synthesize the information and decisions garnered from the assessment and lead to an action plan. In this chapter, we use a custom assessment reporting tool developed for internal use at Communication Assistance for Youth and Adults (CAYA). This tool, the CAYA Communication Assessment and Action Plan (CAAP; Riley & Turner, 2011) will be our touchstone in presenting the many aspects and considerations of a thorough and effective AAC assessment for adults. CAYA is a provincial service program funded by the provincial government of British Columbia (Ministry of Social Development and Poverty Reduction) operating over the past 16 years to serve thousands of adults with complex communication disabilities across a vast geographic area. The CAAP is a customized module of CAYA's digital documentation system. It is not a commercial product. The CAAP assessment framework has been continually developed since the inception of the CAYA program as a means to formalize how staff SLPs conduct and record AAC assessments. It sets the standard for best practice in AAC in British Columbia.

Communication Assessment and Action Plan

The CAAP is the cornerstone document of the CAYA program. This assessment must be completed on each client receiving services from the program. The CAYA CAAP is based on the Participation Model (Beukelman & Mirenda, 2005) that was first published in 1988 and revised numerous times, and it holds that the systematic processes of implementing AAC should be based on the belief of parity between functional participation requirements of peers without disabilities and peers with communication disabilities. In this model, the approach is identifying participation patterns and communication needs, and assessing opportunity and access barriers. The model stipulates planning and intervention for today and tomorrow with postassessment follow-up evaluation of intervention effectiveness on the individual's participation. The CAAP provides a guide for the SLP to consider a client's communication abilities, needs, supports, and the ability of the communication partners and environment to support the chosen communication system. It is embedded within CAYA's proprietary client information system and automatically pulls demographic information from the main client electronic file. The SLP conducts the assessment in conjunction with the client, an SLP assistant, and the rest of the client's team.

SLPs utilize methods of observation, interview, and test administration to gather the information that is entered into the CAAP. A variety of resources are provided to each SLP, and they customize the assessment process according to the situation. This list shown in Table 15–1 does not imply CAYA's endorse-

Table 15–1. Tests and Protocols in Use at CAYA in 2021

Test of Aided-Communication Symbol Performance (TASP)
Peabody Picture Vocab Test (PPVT)
Test for Auditory Comprehension of Language (TACL)
Western Aphasia Battery (WAB)
Boston Diagnostic Aphasia Examination (BDAE)
Test of Language Development (TOLD)
Scales of Cognitive and Communicative Ability for Neurorehabilitation (SCCAN)
The Multimodal Communication Screening Task for Persons With Aphasia (MCST-A)
Social Networks: A Communication Inventory for Individuals With Complex Communication Needs and Their Communication Partners
AAC Genie
Augmentative and Alternative Communication Profile (AACP)
Functional Communication Profile (FCP)
Talking Mats
Communication Matrix

ment of any particular tests and simply reflects the tests that are most frequently used at this time.

SLP assistants contribute to the assessment process under the direction of the SLP and/or other professionals such as an occupational therapist (OT) or vision consultant. They are involved in troubleshooting technology at the initial stages and onward, they produce the nontechnological system(s), and program the technological communication systems. The assessment, trials, decision-making, customizing, and training processes are conducted within a period of 4 to 6 months. Assessment visits range from one to eight sessions depending on the complexity of the individual, geographic realities, and so on. CAYA SLPs have discretion to determine the number of required

visits and whether they are conducted virtually or in person, within oversight limits set by the managers.

An individual's requirement for AAC is generally a lifetime condition. This will bring them into contact with the CAYA team for initial assessment or reassessment as individuals and technology age and change; smaller assessment and technology trials known at CAYA as an "addendum" are related to changes in access, upgrade, or replacement of obsolete technology.

The assessment information is organized into the CAAP. The general format of the CAAP is presented next. Specific content examples from the CAAP regarding goal banks, selection lists, information points, evaluation metrics, and so on, are shared in the context of the case study CAAP evaluation, which follows the case study presentation.

Administrative Information

This information consists of service entry and assessment start dates, the type of CAAP (initial, reassessment, and addendum), the name of the SLP completing it, and links to supporting documents (e.g., reports from other professionals including but not limited to physicians, OTs, physical therapists (PTs), teachers, audiologists, vision specialists, psychologists, behavioral therapists, etc.). Consistent with electronic record systems in use in clinics, hospitals, and schools around the world, the bulk of this information is automatically populated from the CAYA digital client record with additional information optionally added by the SLP. (Of course, if the SLP is operating in a nondigital record environment, this information will need to be manually added.)

Client Information Summary

In the context of a digital record system, individual client information is also automatically populated into the assessment report from the client file; name, date of birth, gender, personal health number, address, languages spoken, communicative function (adapted from Dowden & Cook, 2002) and medical diagnosis. CAYA has adapted

Dowden's communicative independence model by creating four categories: emergent, context dependent, independent, and performance.

The emergent communicator does not have a current, reliable method of expressive communication through symbolic language. They may use nonsymbolic communication strategies such as gestures, body language, and facial expressions, and they require a familiar partner to interpret their messages. This does not necessarily mean that the individual has a cognitive deficit, it simply means that they do not communicate through reliable symbolic language. The context-dependent communicator has symbolic communication that is reliable but limited to particular contexts or partners. They will often use a display with symbols, pictures, and words with support, and may speak, but only familiar communication partners understand them.

The independent communicator has symbolic communication that is reliable and can communicate in most environments and with most partners. They may not have been taught to spell or learned a generative language system, but they are determined to be understood and will use any modality available to them to express themselves. The performance communicator has the ability to communicate anything, on any topic, to any audience. For instance, Glenda Watson Hyatt, a published author, keynote presenter, webmaster, and social media coordinator, is obtaining her master's degree, contributing to shaping public policy and accessibility laws, advocating for herself, expressing her thoughts, and communicating with her husband, family, and friends. Glenda is a multimodal performance communicator.

Communication Status

The SLP considers the client's (a) communication characteristics and issues (e.g., dysarthria, apraxia, aphasia, aphonia, etc.); (b) prognosis (e.g., is functional speech expected to improve, remain the same, or deteriorate); (c) level of intelligibility; and (d) experiences with current and previous communication systems other than speech, all the while considering if the present system is functional for current and future communication needs.

Sensory Abilities

Hearing and vision abilities are screened and referred to an audiologist, optometrist, or other specialist for assessment, if appropriate.

Access

The SLP assesses how the client will access the communication system using a variety of methods, technology, and tools. The SLP evaluates the client's abilities to make direct selections (e.g., pointing with hands, head, or eyes; alternative pointing devices such as mice, joysticks, or trackballs) and indirect selections (e.g., using visual and auditory scanning methods). These evaluations may include the use of styluses, keyguards, and switches. If an indirect selection method is chosen, the type of switch, body site, movement, and movement pattern are documented. The client's body position while using the communication system and wheelchair details, if appropriate, are also documented. Where possible, this portion of the CAAP is completed in consultation with an OT, PT, wheelchair vendor, or other access specialist.

Linguistic Abilities

The SLP considers all aspects of language in this section, including auditory comprehension, verbal expression, pragmatics, symbolic ability, literacy level, written comprehension, composition ability, and stimulability. Within each section, the SLP has the opportunity to indicate whether the assessment was conducted prior to or after receiving a communication system. Additionally, a variety of evaluative observations are available for selection within each category (e.g., "none demonstrated or observed" and "within normal limits"), and each category also has a text box for notes.

The assessment of linguistic abilities is completed using a variety of formal and informal measurements. Standardized scores are not fully tallied and reported in a typical manner (e.g., it is not client focused or respectful of the client's age and social milieu to report vocabulary levels of an infant or child level, when reporting on an adult). Descriptive reporting is more appropriate and will ensure that supporters and family are encouraged to treat the individual as an adult.

Unfortunately, in many regions of the world, scholastic education for students who are nonverbal and have developmental disabilities is not based on the standard curriculum and does not include accommodation for normative developmental or linguistic development. Instead, the level of professional knowledge, skill, and attitudes about AAC in the client's education environment is causal to development of the curriculum. This is also true for rehabilitation medicine. Access to AAC services in inpatient or outpatient rehabilitation settings often depends on the level of knowledge, skill, and attitudes about AAC held by service professionals and organizations. For cognitively intact (or close to intact) clients, linguistic ability is generally directly related to the amount of AAC vocabulary provided and taught either in school or in a rehabilitation setting. The impact of a poorly planned education or rehabilitation process may result in a communication system consisting of a jumble of scattered short phrases, nouns, verbs, adverbs, and fringe vocabulary, regardless of the client's level of cognition or language.

Assessments at CAYA are used to provide a framework for understanding the linguistic skill sets the client is able to access, to find the gaps in developmental abilities and acquired deficits, and to choose appropriate vocabulary for their communication systems.

Cognitive Abilities

SLPs in British Columbia do not conduct formal assessments of cognitive abilities, and this section is clearly documented as an estimation of abilities, including observations of skills of attention, memory, problem-solving and flexible thinking. These skills are observed in context (e.g., ability to independently navigate in familiar and unfamiliar environments, repairing communication breakdowns, navigating the communication system, directing people in the environment, an ability to see another person's perspective). A useful tool for considering cognitive demands on individuals using AAC is a curated online reference library *Thinking About Thinking for AAC* (Mooney et al.,

2019). Again, each section provides an opportunity to choose a variety of observations including "none demonstrated or observed" and "within normal limits," and a text box for notes.

Who Is the Client?

Who is the client (a) as a person (e.g., What are their likes, strengths, dislikes, limitations) and (b) as a learner (e.g., How do they learn most easily and what are their learning challenges)? This is also a place to observe and note the unique details, attributes, and interests of the client.

Communication Partners

This section of the CAAP follows the format of the Social Networks Model (Blackstone & Hunt Berg, 2003) and categorizes partners into four social circles, for example, (a) those who can interpret all of the client's messages and are their intimate communication partners such as an immediate family member or primary care worker; (b) those who can communicate with the client using conventional systems and are familiar, such as family and friends; (c) those who can communicate with the client using conventional systems and are less familiar such as therapists and paid staff; and (d) those who communicate with the client in an unfamiliar manner such as store clerks and bus drivers. In this area, the SLP records the type of communication partner, the social circle, the frequency of interactions, and whether or not they are paid to work with the client.

Daily Communication Needs

The client and the SLP together review the list of daily communication needs in this section, and the client prioritizes them and may, in conversation with the SLP, add individualized needs to the list.

Functional Communication Goals

The goals section of the CAAP follows the format of four functional communication categories: linguistic, operational, strategic, and social (Light & Binger, 1998). Within each category, CAYA has created a bank of specific AAC goals presented in a drop-down menu format and for each AAC goal the SLP also chooses (a) the level of assistance required (e.g., modeling, with assistance, independently); (b) the frequency parameters (e.g., times per day or week); and (c) other parameters (e.g., number of environments, people, instances, and opportunities). The goals are reviewed and revised on an ongoing basis. Goals reflect the client's individual context; some clients may have goals in several or all categories, while others may have as few as one goal in one category. Shown in Figures 15–1 through 15–4 are the communication goal categories and the menus containing the goal banks.

Low-Tech Communication Systems

At CAYA, we believe it is a cardinal rule of AAC assessment that individuals must be provided with a low-tech communication system—technology

Add Functional Goals – Linguistic
- Client will code switch between different communications modalities based on the listener
- Client will demonstrate knowledge of new symbols
- Client will express a linguistic concept using AAC
- Client will combine symbols to express complex messages
- Client will communicate independently
- Caregivers will model use of communication system
- Caregivers will use visual supports with the client

Figure 15–1. Goal Bank Linguistic. Reprinted with permission.

Add Functional Goals – Operational
- Client will demonstrate a skill necessary to purposefully and consistently access a switch/device for cause/effect, participation or communication
- Client will demonstrate a reliable yes/no response through body movement or switch access
- Client will be able to navigate through the communication system
- Client will use row-column scanning or Morse code to access communication system
- Client will use function keys in the communication system appropriately (e.g., speak, home button)
- Client will adjust volume based on environment
- Client will demonstrate the ability to make basic programming changes
- Client will demonstrate use of a partner-assited scanning system
- Client will demonstrate skills necessary to use an eye-gaze system
- Client will use the phone
- Client will use email, social media and other remote communication platforms
- Client will increase speed and accuracy of communication
- Client will use a voice amplifier
- Client will complete voice/message/story banking
- Caregivers will ensure that communication system is available and accessible
- Caregivers will add new content to communication system

Figure 15–2. Goal Bank Operational. Reprinted with permission.

Add Functional Goals – Social

- [ ] Client will gain listener's attention
- [ ] Client will initiate conversation
- [ ] Client will demonstrate turn-taking skills
- [ ] Client will make requests using communication mode appropriate to the situation
- [ ] Client will make choices
- [ ] Client will direct care needs
- [ ] Client will express feelings
- [ ] Client will describe health issues (e.g., pain, discomfort)
- [ ] Client will share information
- [ ] Client will express his/her point of view
- [ ] Client will signal communication breakdowns
- [ ] Client will repair communication breakdowns
- [ ] Client will continue conversation appropriately
- [ ] Client will terminate a conversation appropriately
- [ ] Client will demonstrate an increasing range of communication functions
- [ ] Client will communicate with familiar communication partners
- [ ] Client will communicate with unfamiliar communication partners
- [ ] Caregivers will provide opportunities for interaction
- [ ] Caregivers will respond appropriately to client's communication attempts

Figure 15–3. Goal Bank Social. Reprinted with permission.

Add Functional Goals – Strategic

- [ ] Client will request communication system
- [ ] Client will use an introduction strategy to put partners at ease
- [ ] Client will use stored messages
- [ ] Client will use prediction and other strategies to enhance rate
- [ ] Client will use conversational control strategies to avoid interruptions from partner
- [ ] Client will provide clues and ask listener to 'guess' to bypass vocabulary limitations
- [ ] Client will use mementos/remnants to bypass vocabulary and memory limitations to establish topic of interaction
- [ ] Caregivers will direct conversation back to Client
- [ ] Caregivers will use supported communication strategies with the client

Figure 15–4. Goal Bank Strategic. Reprinted with permission.

notoriously fails, runs out of power, or cannot be used in some environments (e.g., the swimming pool or during a natural disaster). Therefore, it is a requirement that every client in the CAYA program has (or at least is offered) a nontechnological communication system. This can include but is not limited to a communication book or board with any combination of pictures/symbols/words/letters, schedule, partner-assisted display, or tangible symbol system. The SLP records the trials to document what types of low-tech systems were successful and unsuccessful, and the final system is produced and fabricated by the SLP assistant.

AAC Device Trials

In this section, equipment trials are documented, and the final selection, if one is made, is recorded. Specific device trial requirements vary according to local and national regulations and may be dictated by funding rules. The reader is encouraged to apprise themselves of local procedures. At CAYA, the list of equipment that has been lent to the client during the course of service or assessment from the CAYA Technology Loan Bank appears here, and a text box is available to the SLP to compose a trial summary. The trial summary includes a discussion of the relative merits and drawbacks of the different technologies trialed during assessment, and the SLP writes a synthesis statement of the assessment and states the recommended technology, low-tech system, or plan of action. It is important to bear in mind that despite modern advancements in technology, there are individuals who prefer or are better served through nonelectronic solutions.

Mounting

Mounting systems are essential components for the successful use of an AAC system and function in coordination with seating, positioning, and access considerations. SLPs are not formally trained in this aspect of service provision, which highlights the importance of a multidisciplinary team in providing comprehensive AAC services. CAYA provides the funding for mounting systems but due to operational and mandate constraints does not directly employ OTs or other access specialists. In general, OT services are accessed through the British Columbia health system, and private access services are used when and where available. This section allows for input of the name of the professional completing the mounting assessment and a link to their report.

Final Report

At CAYA a system has been designed that automatically aggregates the data and returns a structured professional text document suitable for printing or inclusion in client records, where only the specific chosen items and relevant text appear. Each page is labeled with legally required client demographic information (e.g., name, date of birth, and health number). SLPs working outside of a digital reporting system will need to compile the client assessment information into a formal printed report. The CAAP headings previously discussed in this chapter provide a potential framework for an adult AAC assessment.

Assurances and SLP Signature

CAYA requires the completion of two assurances in this section; the client/family/caregiver/advocate assure they have participated in the assessment; the SLP assures they have no financial relationship with any suppliers of any AAC devices or accessories. The SLP then signs the CAAP and includes their professional designations.

Case Study: GB

This case study is an amalgamation of a variety of cases known to the authors. Personal details and information have been changed and altered to protect privacy.

Clinical Profile and Communication Needs

The Individual

GB is an engaging young man in his mid-20s with cerebral palsy living in the city of Vancouver, British Columbia, Canada. He has a wide and ready smile, an expressive face, and makes excellent use of eye contact in interpersonal interactions. His medical diagnoses include significant physical disability, spastic quadriplegia, intellectual impairment, and developmental delay. Functionally, he is unable to walk but has relatively good control of his arms and hands. GB is able to safely steer a power wheelchair and independently transfer himself for toileting and showering. He is also highly independent in terms of his mobility in the city, traveling significant distances in his power wheelchair, and skillfully navigating the subway system. He does not have functional speech but does have several consistent vocalizations that he uses effectively along with facial expressions and gestures to convey his emotional state.

During his childhood, GB received supports for his communication through the education system. At the time of his graduation from high school at age 18 years, GB was using a Prentke Romich Company (PRC) Vanguard Plus Unity communication device that had been provided through a school support program. Additionally, GB had been provided with light-tech communication supports which mainly consisted of a large binder with printouts of his Minspeak (Baker, 1982) pages with additional picture symbols, organized by topic categories. Upon high school graduation, GB was permitted to keep the communication device and the light-tech communication system, but no further supports were available from the education system in terms of technical support to maintain the communication device or professional support to update either electronic or nonelectronic communication systems. GB used these systems with communication partners in an engaging manner, beckoning them over with his hands and facial expressions to watch and follow as he pointed out his messages using multiple Minspeak and picture symbols in combinations. His communication partners decoded his messages from his light-tech system primarily through word glosses under the picture symbols and additional words that had been added under Minspeak symbols. GB has some limited literacy, he recognizes street and business signage and some sight words, but he is unable to functionally spell. His PRC Vanguard Plus Unity recently stopped working, and friends in his church tried to remedy his loss by providing him with an older donated iPad loaded with scans of

his paper Minspeak pages. A church acquaintance helped him with a referral to a government program that provides specialized SLP services.

GB's Communication Environments

GB is a single child of a single-parent mother and is a member of a visible ethnic minority. GB's mother faced significant financial and psychiatric problems throughout his life, and for extended periods of his childhood he resided in foster care while his mother underwent psychiatric treatment. The family frequently moved about the city, changing neighborhoods and schools. GB now lives in a group home with government assistance. A significant constant in GB's life has been his church and the community associated with it. GB continues to attend church every Sunday and participates in church-led young adult groups. Outside of church, GB participates in a local adapted Bocci sports league, and an adapted music performance group. He is an avid fan of electronic music and is a huge fan of a local synthpop group, attending as many of their local gigs as possible. He also attends a local community college 3 hours per day, 2 days per week in a program designed for young adults with intellectual challenges. In pursuing his interests, he has ventured into new environments, made new friends, and has recently come out as a gay man to his sports, school, and music friends, his group home housemates, and his mother. He has not yet come out to his church, and this step is at present his greatest source of anxiety.

GB's Communication Partners

GB's mother visits him about once a month. Their interactions follow a consistent pattern with Mom talking most of the time, asking few questions, and spending about half the time chatting and visiting with GB's care staff. In his group home, GB communicates mostly with his two primary paid caregivers, two young women from the Philippines, who help him with activities of daily living and planning transportation to his appointments, church, school, and social engagements, and one other housemate, a young man who is close in age and is GB's Bocci buddy. He occasionally interacts with his other three housemates, but they have sensory and intellectual disabilities that make it difficult for them to understand the synthetic speech of his communication device. At church, GB's primary interaction is with a particular family who once hosted him as a foster family in his childhood; they comprise two middle-aged parents and their son and daughter who are close in age to GB. At the adapted music society, GB interacts with the group leader and two other people with disabilities, a young woman near in age to GB, and a man 10 years older than GB who is also gay and shares his interest in the local synthpop group. They usually go to these performances together when the group is performing in town. The community college program is a recent addition to GB's life. In the class,

he interacts mostly with the instructor and assistant, with occasional structured group interactions with the other two students. In addition to these individuals, GB rides transit independently, frequents a bank, a fast-food outlet, and convenience store in his neighborhood where he interacts with service personnel.

The Assessment

The raw data for GB's completed CAAP are presented in the next sections. Sections that are not completed will not appear in the final report. Each item must be assessed using observation (both structured and unstructured), and then supported by both informal and formal assessment.

Communication Status

A. Communication Characteristics and Issue(s):
(select items that apply):

☒ Dysarthria ☐ Dyspraxia/apraxia
☐ Aphasia ☐ Aphonia
☐ Cognition/Executive Functions ☐ Non-Verbal
☐ Others ☐ Speech

B. Prognosis:
Functional Speech is expected to:

☐ Improve
☐ Deteriorate
☒ Remain stable over time
☐ Remain unchanged, no functional speech

C1. Communication Characteristics and Issue(s):
(select items that apply):

☐ Alphabet board ☐ Communication board
☒ Communication book ☐ Book
☐ Schedule ☐ Eyegaze display
☒ VOCA ☐ Computer software
☐ Personal dictionary ☐ Yes/No questions
☐ Emergent Communication Technology ☒ Facial expression
☒ Gesture ☐ Laser pointer
☐ Partner assisted scan display ☐ Limited speech
☒ Other ☐ % intelligible 0

GB has consistent vocalizations that are interpreted by familiar communication partners.

Notes:

Figure 15–5. Ax Communication Characteristics A. B. C.1. Reprinted with permission.

Is it functional for <u>current</u> communication needs? ☐ Yes ☒ No
Is it functional for <u>future</u> communication needs? ☐ Yes ☒ No

C2. Previous Communication System Usage

If the Client has a communication system previously, what does he/she remember about from it? (select items that apply):

☐ Alphabet board ☒ Communication board
☒ Communication book ☐ Book
☒ Schedule ☐ Eyegaze display
☒ VOCA ☒ Computer software
☐ Personal dictionary ☒ Yes/No questions
☐ Emergent Communication Technology ☒ Facial expression
☒ Gesture ☐ Laser pointer
☐ Partner assisted scan display ☐ Client spoke prior to acquired condition

Notes:

Figure 15–6. Ax Current. Future C.2. Reprinted with permission.

Sensory Abilities

GB passed both his auditory and visual screening procedures.

Access

A.	Selection Method		

A. Selection Method
How will the Client access their communication system?
Direct Selection:

☒ Pointing   ☐ Mouse
☐ Joystick   ☐ Trackball
☐ Head Pointing   ☐ Switch – single message
☐ Eye Pointing   ☐ Head Stick

Indirect Selection (Scanning):

☐ Visually
☐ Auditorily

Voice Amplification: ☐

Notes (e.g., scan pattern, processing delay, keyguard, placement of voice amp?):

GB uses an index finger to point, and his accuracy improves when he uses a keyguard.

Figure 15–7. Ax Access A. Selection Method. Reprinted with permission.

B. Body Position
Where will the Client access their communication system?

☐ Ambulatory   ☒ Wheelchair - manual
☒ Wheelchair - power   ☐ Standing frame
☐ Chair   ☐ Couch
☐ Bed   ☐ Floor

Notes:

Figure 15–8. Ax Access B. Body Position. Reprinted with permission.

D. Wheelchair
Make/Model:

Quickie (manual)
Ranger II Storm series (power)

Figure 15–9. Ax Access D. Wheelchair. Reprinted with permission.

Linguistic Abilities

A. Authory Comprehension: ☒ Prior to Device ☐ After Device

- ☐ The client is unable to follow simple directions or responds to yes/no questions.
- ☐ The client is able to follow simple directions and responds to yes/no questions with cueing.
- ☐ The client is able to follow simple directions and yes/no questions without cueing and understands limited conversation about routine events with familiar individuals.
- ☒ The client is able to follow conversation in a structured setting with familiar and unfamiliar individuals. Minor cueing is required form more complex concepts or language structures.
- ☐ The client is able to understand abstract and complex concepts.
- ☐ Within normal limits.

Notes (e.g., how determined or assessed, mitigating factors such as delay?):

This was determined via observation in structured situation, friends and family input, and comparison with subtests of the Western Aphasia Battery.

Figure 15–10. Ax Linguistic A. Auditory Comprehension. Reprinted with permission.

B. Verbal Expression: ☒ Prior to Device ☐ After Device

- ☒ The client is non-verbal.
- ☐ The client uses word approximations.
- ☐ The client uses single word utterances.
- ☐ The client speaks in short phrases and sentences using simple or compound language structures.
- ☐ The client speaks in longer sentences using complex language structures.
- ☐ Within normal limits.

Notes:

GB has consistent vocalizations that are interpreted by familiar communication partners.

Figure 15–11. Ax Linguistic B. Verbal Expression. Reprinted with permission.

C. Pragmatics: ☒ Prior to Device ☐ After Device
(select items that apply)
The Client:

☐ Responds only
☐ Initiates only
☒ Initiates and responds
☒ Maintains eye contact
☒ Uses gesture and facial expression in isolation or to supplement other communication modes
☒ Participates in turn taking
☒ Selects topics appropriate for the environment and conversation partner (e.g., familiar vs. unfamiliar, friend vs. family member)
☒ Maintains the topic of conversation
☒ Signals communication breakdowns
☒ Attempts to repair communication breakdowns
☐ Other

Notes:

GB's pragmatic abilities are a strength.

Figure 15–12. Ax Linguistic C. Pragmatics. Reprinted with permission.

D. Symbolic Ability: ☒ Prior to Device ☐ After Device
Select those levels of symbolic knowledge that apply the majority of the time

☐ None demonstrated or observed
☐ Actual objects
☐ 3D symbols (tangible symbols)
☒ Photos
☒ Line drawings
☒ Symbols
☒ Minspeak
☒ Sign & gestures
☐ Orthography

Notes:

GB is a strong multi-modal communicator. Specific parameters of his dynamic screen display were identified during his participation in the TASP (Test of Aided-Symbol Performance).

Figure 15–13. Ax Linguistic D. Symbolic Ability. Reprinted with permission.

E. Literacy Level: ☒ Prior to Device   ☐ After Device

☐ None demonstrated or observed

☒ *Emergent* (Client recognizes environment print such as road signs and logos, understands that reading proceeds from left to right, "reads" stories based on pictures, demonstrates basic book knowledge)

☐ *Developing* (Client demonstrates letter recognition, grapheme-phoneme correspondence riles, word recognition)

☐ *Acquired-Conventional* (Client can comprehend text and interpret its meaning)

☐ *Recovering* (Attempting to regain previous abilities)

☐ Within normal limits

Notes:

GB recognizes street and business signage, and some sight words, but he is unable to functionally spell.

Figure 15–14. Ax Linguistic E. Literacy Level. Reprinted with permission.

F. Written Composition: ☒ Prior to Device   ☐ After Device
(symbol/letter/word) is primarily...
(select items that apply)

☒ None demonstrated or observed

☐ Practiced but not used functionally (i.e., Client practices spelling and writing at school or home but generally uses a single symbol or word to communicate ideas)

☐ Used in conjunction with another mode of communication (e.g., spells first 2-3 letters of a word to help clarify a spoken message or uses word prediction)

☐ Used as a primary mode of communication (transient – conversational exchange)

☐ Used academically (e.g., essays, poetry)

☐ Used to record personal thoughts and feelings (permanent – lasting record)

☐ Not applicable (please describe below)

Notes:

Figure 15–15. Ax Linguistic F. Written Composition. Reprinted with permission.

G. Composition Ability (using symbols or words):   ☒ Prior to Device   ☐ After Device

☒ None demonstrated or observed
☐ The client can link 2-5 items to form a message with a model
☐ The client can link 2-5 items to form a message with minor assistance/cueing
☐ The client can independently link 2-5 items to form a message
☐ The client can compose grammatically correct simple and compound sentences
☐ The client can compose grammatically correct complex sentences
☐ The client can generate complex, lengthy compositions (e.g., essay)
☐ Within normal limits

Notes:

GB participated in the administration of the Test fir Auditory Comprehension of Language (TACL) using Minspeak

Figure 15–16. Ax Linguistic G. Composition Ability. Reprinted with permission.

H. Stimulability (evidence that the client is learning and retains information taught within a session or over sessions):   ☒ Prior to Device   ☐ After Device

Notes:

GB has an excellent memory and often refers to common activities that happened in another time and place.

Figure 15–17. Ax Linguistic H. Stimulability. Reprinted with permission.

Cognitive Abilities

A. Cognitive Abilities:	☒ Prior to Device ☐ After Device

☒ Within normal limits
☐ Mild impairment
☐ Mild-moderate impairment
☐ Moderate impairment
☐ Moderate-severe impairment
☐ Severe impairment
☐ Unable to determine

Notes:

This is a broad estimation of his cognitive abilities, based on GB's ability to navigate his city and interact with unfamiliar communication partners. Using subtests of the AAC Genie, he is able to identify broad and specific categories.

Figure 15–18. Ax Cognitive A. Cognitive Abilities. Reprinted with permission.

B. Attention Skills:	☒ Prior to Device ☐ After Device

☐ The client is easily distracted by internal and external distracters
☐ The client can attend to a preferred task for a short period of time when distractions are reduced
☐ The client can attend to a non-preferred task for a short period of time when distractions are reduced
☐ The client can attend selectively (i.e., can select and control what he/she pays attention to) regardless of the environment
☐ The client can maintain attention to a preferred task when distractions are reduced
☐ The client can maintain attention to a non-preferred task when distractions are reduced
☒ The client can maintain attention regardless of task or distractions
☐ Within normal limits
☐ None demonstrated or observed

Notes:

GB has given presentations to his peers at a bocci tournament and at church.

Figure 15–19. Ax Cognitive B. Attention Skills. Reprinted with permission.

C. Memory Skills: ☒ Prior to Device   ☐ After Device

☐ Memory for items in isolation (e.g., learned symbols, objects)
☐ Memory for items in association with context or location (e.g., learned and their locations)
☐ Memory for short sequences once learned (e.g., familiar routines, 2 symbol sequences)
☐ Ability to hold and manipulate 2-3 pieces of information (e.g., recalls place in sentence construction, conversation)
☐ Memory for longer sequences (once learned)
☒ Ability to hold and manipulate more than 3 pieces of information at a time
☐ Within normal limits
☐ No reliable memory skills observed

Notes:

GB remembers times and location of meetings and appointments.

Figure 15–20. Ax Cognitive C. Memory Skills. Reprinted with permission.

D. Problem-solving Skills: ☒ Prior to Device   ☐ After Device
(as they relate to communication breakdowns)

☐ The client is unaware of communication breakdowns
☐ The client looks to a caregiver or conversation partner to solve communication breakdowns
☐ The client repeats the intended message when a breakdown occurs
☒ The client rephrases the intended message or supplements with additional information when a breakdown occurs (e.g., adds gesture, key word)
☐ Within normal limits
☐ None demonstrated or observed

Notes:

GB is a multi-modal communicator and is one method does not work he will try another.

Figure 15–21. Ax Cognitive D. Problem-Solving Skills. Reprinted with permission.

E. Flexible Thinking Skills: ☒ Prior to Device   ☐ After Device

☐ The client associates a given symbol with one meaning only
☒ The client is able to use one symbol to represent more than one concept
☐ The client is unable to interpret/use symbols
☐ Within normal limits
☐ None demonstrated or observed

Notes:

GB is a known user of Minspeak.

Figure 15–22. Ax Cognitive E. Flexible Thinking Skills. Reprinted with permission.

Who Is the Client?

As a person?
    Likes, strengths...

GB likes bocci, electronic music, adapted music performance, and going to church.

Figure 15–23. Ax Client Likes Strengths. Reprinted with permission.

    Dislikes, limitations...

he dislikes being undervalued, when people don't give him enough time to talk.

Figure 15–24. Ax Client Dislikes Limitations. Reprinted with permission.

As a learner?
    They learn most easily when...

things are demonstrated to him, opportunities for practice, and he has time.

Figure 15–25. Ax Client Learns Easily. Reprinted with permission.

    They are challenged to learn when...

things are only in writing and there is no one to assist him, and he feels rushed.

Figure 15–26. Ax Client Challenged to Learn. Reprinted with permission.

Communication Partners

THE CLIENT'S COMMUNICATION PARTNERS AND FREQUENCY

Q1: Those few who can interpret all of the client's communication messages (e.g., intimate family members, primary care worker)

Q2: Those who can communicate with the client using more conventional systems and with whom the client shares mutual interests and confides in (e.g., extended family members, friends)

Q3: Those who can communicate with the client using more conventional systems but whom they do not socialize with on a regular based (e.g., rehab professionals, day program and group home staff)

Q4: Those who the client experiences casual interactions with (i.e., unfamiliar communication partners)

Partners	N/A	Q1	Q2	Q3	Q4	Frequency	Paid to work with client
Mom	☐	☐	☒	☐	☐	Once a month	☐

Figure 15–27. Ax Communication Partners 1 of 3. Reprinted with permission.

Partners	N/A	Q1	Q2	Q3	Q4	Frequency	Paid
Group Home Staff	☐	☒	☐	☐	☐	Multiple times a day	☒
Store Clerk	☐	☐	☐	☐	☒	Once a week	☐
Waitstaff	☐	☐	☐	☐	☐	N/A	☐
Bus Driver	☐	☐	☐	☐	☒	Multiple times a week	☐

Figure 15–28. Ax Communication Partners 2 of 3. Reprinted with permission.

Partners	N/A	Q1	Q2	Q3	Q4	Frequency	Paid
Other 1: Church friends	☐	☐	☒	☐	☐	Once a week	☐
Other 2: Bocci ball friends	☐	☐	☒	☐	☐	Once a week	☐
Other 3. Music friends	☐	☐	☒	☐	☐	Once a week	☐

None (no client partners) ☐

Notes:

GB has several groups of friends, depending on the activity that he is participating in.

Figure 15–29. Ax Communication Partners 3 of 3. Reprinted with permission.

Note: the CAAP contains an extensive list of potential communication partners. "N/A" stands for "not applicable" for the particular client being assessed.

Daily Communication Needs

Options	Priority (1=High & 5=Low)				
	#1	#2	#3	#4	#5
☒ Assert control over life	☐	☒	☐	☐	☐
☐ Share information	☐	☐	☐	☐	☐
☒ Communicate with unfamiliar individuals	☒	☐	☐	☐	☐
☐ Initiate and participate in conversation	☐	☐	☐	☐	☐
☐ Communicate using the phone	☐	☐	☐	☐	☐
☐ Direct care needs	☐	☐	☐	☐	☐
☐ Have say in daily activities	☐	☐	☐	☐	☐
☐ Communicate independently	☐	☐	☐	☐	☐
☐ Communicate details to reduce need for questioning	☐	☐	☐	☐	☐
☐ Visual supports	☐	☐	☐	☐	☐
☐ Plan their day	☐	☐	☐	☐	☐
☐ Express negation or opposition within behavior	☐	☐	☐	☐	☐
☐ Closer connection with peer group and/or family	☐	☐	☐	☐	☐
☒ Community volunteering/vocational opportunities	☐	☐	☒	☐	☐
☐ Greet others	☐	☐	☐	☐	☐
☐ Ask questions	☐	☐	☐	☐	☐
☐ Respond to questions	☐	☐	☐	☐	☐
☒ Advocate for themselves	☐	☐	☐	☐	☒
☐ Pursue post-secondary education	☐	☐	☐	☐	☐
☒ Communicate feelings and physical states	☐	☐	☐	☒	☐
☐ Other:	☐	☐	☐	☐	☐

Figure 15–30. Ax Daily Communication Needs. Reprinted with permission.

Functional Communication Goals

Linguistic – the ability to understand and use symbols (text, words, PCS, etc.) to communicate their ideas, thoughts, and feelings to others.							
Client will combine symbols to express complex messages							
Independently	⌄	2021/12/31	*	X	🗓	Times Per Day	⌄	10
GB will combine symbols to express complex messages 10 times per day by the end of the year.							

Figure 15–31. Ax Linguistic Goal. Reprinted with permission.

Operational – the ability to produce messages and operate the AAC system efficiently, minimizing the effects of fatigue.							
Client will use function keys in the communication system appropriately (e.g., speak, home button)							
Independently	⌄	2021/12/31	*	X	🗓	Times Per Day	⌄	10
GB will learn where the new function keys in the Accent are located and operate them appropriately.							

Figure 15–32. Ax Operational Goal. Reprinted with permission.

Social – the ability to interact socially in a way that is deemed pragmatically appropriate.							
Client will communicate with unfamiliar communication partners							
Independently	⌄	2021/12/31	*	X	🗓	Number of People	⌄	25
GB will communicate with 25 unfamiliar people in the coming year.							

Figure 15–33. Ax Social Goal. Reprinted with permission.

Strategic – the ability to use appropriate strategies to bypass linguistic, operational and social domains.							
Client will use prediction and other strategies to enhance rate							
Independently	⌄	2021/12/31	*	X	🗓	Times Per Day	⌄	10
GB will use rate enhancement strategies 10 times per day by the end of the year.							

Figure 15–34. Ax Strategic Goal. Reprinted with permission.

Low-Tech Communication Systems

Used during the assessment
(select items that apply):

☐ Alphabet board   ☐ Communication board
☒ Communication book   ☐ Book
☐ Schedule   ☐ Eye pointing
☐ Yes/No questions   ☐ Tangible symbols
☐ Partner assisted scan display   ☐ Not applicable/appropriate at this time

☐ Other:

Figure 15–35. Ax Non-Tech System during Ax. Reprinted with permission.

Recommended non-tech communication system:
(select items that apply):

☐ Alphabet board   ☐ Communication board
☒ Communication book   ☐ Book
☐ Schedule   ☐ Eye pointing
☐ Yes/No questions   ☐ Tangible symbols
☐ Partner assisted scan display   ☐ Not applicable/appropriate at this time

☒ Other:

SLP-A will create a paper-based visual representation of his Minspeak system.

Figure 15–36. Ax Non-Tech System Recommended. Reprinted with permission.

AAC Device Trials

Recommended Equipment:

Device Name
☒ Accent 1000
☐ Accent 1000 Keyguard

Summary (i.e., provide a rationale for your recommendation, specific detail about use, accessories):

GB was loaned an Accent 1000 with a 45 location keyguard and was able to use it functionally. He previously used his Vanguard as a keyboard to access his desktop computer and it is expected that he will do the same with this device.

Figure 15–37. Ax—Device Recommendation & Summary. Reprinted with permission.

Mounting

Does this person require a mounting system?　☒ Yes　☐ No　☐ N/A

Current mounting system:

GB will use a swing away mount so that he is independent going to the rest room in the community.

Local team member responsible for the mounting of the AAC device:　**Lois Turner**

Mounting quote completed?　☒ Yes　☐ No

If additional support/expertise is required, referral to be made to: _____

Figure 15–38. Ax—Mounting. Reprinted with permission.

Final Report

As discussed previously in the CAAP framework section, at CAYA the digital record system has been designed to automatically aggregate the data and return a structured professional text document where only the specific chosen items and relevant text appear. The printed CAAP can then be shared with relevant professionals and supporters to help GB attain his communication goals.

Next Steps

The CAYA staff will follow through with implementation of the new Accent Plus1000 communication device, for example, (a) programming additional vocabulary, device mounting, training GB on the operational and linguistic differences of the new device (usually completed by the SLP assistant); and (b) regularly and systematically following up on the goals and ensuring his key supporters are provided with training (usually completed by the SLP). GB's formal printed CAAP document will be provided as necessary or as legally required to GB's other care providers. CAYA provides a lifetime service to eligible adults aged 19 years and older in British Columbia. For as long as they live in British Columbia, clients continue to receive support from CAYA and services as required (e.g., repairs, technical support, implementation support, support for aging and disease progression, and upgrade reviews). The CAYA SLP continues to be the case manager for the client, and specific support tasks are determined based on job roles and qualifications.

Please note: CAYA is a provincial service program funded by the provincial government of British Columbia (Ministry of Social Development and Poverty Reduction). They support independent communication through the use of assistive technology.

References

Baker, B. R. (1982). Minspeak: A semantic compaction system that makes self-expression easier for communicatively disabled individuals. *Byte, 7,* 186–202.

Beukelman, D., & Mirenda, P. (2005). *Augmentative and alternative communication: Supporting children and adults with complex communication needs* (3rd ed.). Paul H. Brookes.

Blackstone, S., & Hunt Berg, M. (2003). *Social Networks Inventory: A communication inventory for individuals with complex communication needs and their communication partners.* Augmentative Communication Inc.

Bruno, J. (2010). *Test of Aided-Communication Symbol Performance.* Mayer-Johnson.

Carrow-Woolfolk, E. (1999). *Test of Auditory Comprehension of Language.* Pro-Ed.

CAYA, Communication Assistance for Youth & Adults, 700-655 West Kent Ave N, Vancouver, BC, V6P 6T7, Canada. https://www.cayabc.org

Dowden, P. A., & Cook, A. M. (2002). Selection techniques for individuals with motor impairments. In J. Reichle, D. Beukelman, & J. Light (Eds.), *Implementing an augmentative communication system: Exemplary strategies for beginning communicators* (pp. 395–432). Paul H. Brookes.

Dunn, L. M., & Dunn, D. M. (2007). *Peabody Picture Vocabulary Test* (4th ed.). Pearson.

Goodglass, H., Kaplan, E., & Barresi, B. (2001). *Boston Diagnostic Aphasia Examination.* Lippincott, Williams & Wilkins.

Hamill, D. D., & Newcomer, P. L. (1997). *Test of Language Development-Intermediate* (3rd ed.). Pro-Ed

Hump Software. (2012). *AAC Evaluation Genie* (Version 3.8.5) [Mobile app]. App Store. https://apps.apple.com/us/app/aac-evaluation-genie/id541418407

Kertesz, A. (2006). *Western Aphasia Battery—Revised.* PsychCorp.

Kleiman, L. I. (2003). *Functional Communication Profile—Revised.* LingiSystems.

Kovach, T. M. (2009). *Augmentative and Alternative Communication Profile.* LinguiSystems.

Lasker, J. P., & Garrett, K. L. (2005). *Using the Multimodal Communication Screening Test for Persons with Aphasia (MCST-A).* https://cehs.unl.edu/documents/secd/aac/assessment/picture.pdf

Light, J., & Binger, C. (1998). *Building communicative competence with individuals who use augmentative and alternative communication.* Paul H. Brookes.

Light, J., & McNaughton, D. (2014). Communicative competence for individuals who require augmentative and alternative communication: A new definition for a new era of communication? *Augmentative and Alternative Communication, 30*(1), 1–18.

Milman, L., & Holland, A. L. (2003). *The Scales of Cognitive and Communicative Ability for Neurorehabilitation.* Pro-Ed.

Mooney, A., Kinsella, M., McLaughlin, D. E., & Fried-Oken, M. (2019). *Thinking about thinking for AAC.* http://TAT4AAC.ohsu.edu

Riley, J., & Turner, L. (2011). *Communication Assessment and Action Plan.* Communication Assistance for Youth & Adults, Vancouver, BC, Canada.

Rowland, C., & Fried-Oken, M. (2021, February 23). *Communication Matrix: A clinical and research assessment tool targeting children with severe communication disorders.* https://www.communicationmatrix.org

Talking Mats Limited. (2021). *Talking mats.* https://www.talkingmats.com/

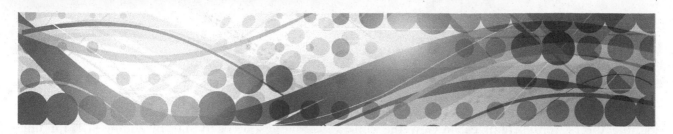

Essay 16

ETHICAL CONSIDERATIONS AND AAC: ETHICAL VENDOR RELATIONSHIPS

Katya Hill

Speech-language pathologists (SLPs) have asked themselves, "What is my relationship with the vendors?" and "How do I ensure that my AAC decisions do not represent a conflict of interest?" ever since the first vendors offered augmentative and alternative communication (AAC) products. The American Speech-Language-Hearing Association (ASHA) provides guiding documents for SLPs to use judiciously when making clinical decisions about AAC technology and to reflect on ethical principles that guide relationships with vendors. Specifically, SLPs need to consider the role an individual vendor plays or played in the AAC evaluation process and selection of AAC technology for an individual.

SLPs conducting AAC clinical services must routinely think about the roles and responsibilities expected of them. Certainly, the ASHA Code of Ethics (2016) and Scope of Practice (2016) are foundational documents to appraise one's professionalism and competencies. SLPs are required to complete financial and nonfinancial disclosures in various professional roles such as presenting at an ASHA continuing education event, submitting an article for publication, or conducting research. Although not every SLP providing AAC services may perform these roles, most SLPs providing AAC services will be in the position of submitting an speech-generating device (SGD) funding request for approval by Medicare, Medicaid, or an insur-

ance provider. Every SGD funding request requires the SLP's signature with an assurance statement verifying that they are not employees of or have a financial relationship with the AAC manufacturer (ASHA, n.d.). However, nonfinancial relationships also may compromise the independent nature of clinical decisions. Let's first look at the role and responsibilities of the AAC manufacturer.

Over 50 years ago, AAC products represented a cottage industry. Today, AAC technology represents a multi-million-dollar industry. The demands of a profit-driven and reimbursement-controlled market create very different business practices from the original "mom-and-pop" companies of past decades (Hill & Hayes-Diges, 2008). AAC manufacturers operate under different business structures that influence their selling and marketing practices and conduct. Paramount to any business is market share and profitability. While businesses value their customers, fiduciary concerns drive a business and have hidden impact on the consumers. For the AAC industry, the consumer is not only the person who uses AAC (PWUAAC), their families, and the SLP, but anyone making purchasing decisions. While SLPs and the clients and families they service want a thriving and growing AAC industry, knowledge of the ownership structure of a durable medical equipment (DME) company like an AAC manufacturer provides insights into the vendor's practices and the role and responsibilities of AAC manufacturers' representatives. Review the contrasting opinions expressed by Woltosz, Bristow, Frumkin, and Romich (1994) about the role of SLPs as manufacturers' representatives in AAC services. The potential conflicts of interest identified in this opinion piece still exist in AAC service delivery. Navroski (2015) attempted to clarify the role of the manufacturer's representative by outlining the types of possible supports. However, SLPs providing AAC clinical services continue to face challenges in coordinating and managing the role of the AAC manufacturers' representative in the assessment, training, and intervention processes.

SLPs may ask whether an AAC business has a code of conduct to compare with a code of ethics. A code of conduct is a set of rules outlining the norms and practices of a company. Hill and Hayes-Diges (2008) found a decline from 20% in 1998 (Hill et al., 1998) to 8% of AAC manufacturers having a code of conduct accessible at their websites. During that time, the market saw major growth in technology options and product lines, acquisition and mergers of companies by larger companies, and the availability of improved SGD funding and billing codes by the Centers for Medicare and Medicaid Services (CMS). With increased Internet accessibility and funding for customers,

AAC manufacturers started to provide additional website resources to SLPs by adding SGD funding request templates and other AAC evaluation and intervention tools to their websites. These are helpful for customers, but to be honest, these resources were created as an economic and marketing solution. However, can you, as a consumer, find an AAC vendor's code of conduct when searching their website for products and resources?

Remember, the vendor's role is not to influence evidence-based clinical practices, decisions, and opinions of interprofessional practitioners.

Whether you are an SLP with years of AAC experience or entering the AAC field as a newly certified SLP, you have resources to monitor your relationship with vendors. You can ask yourself how vendors may directly or indirectly be affecting your clinical AAC practice. Table Y–1 represents five rules that SLPs should follow to ensure independence from vendor influences when conducting an AAC evaluation (Higdon & Hill, 2015).

The knowledge and competence of the SLP influence the communication outcomes of individuals who rely on AAC interventions and their families. SLPs are expected to collect the best clinical and personal evidence (data) to measure the effectiveness of AAC treatment. No one would or should challenge this responsibility. SLPs also are

Table Y–1. Five Speech-Generating Device (SGD) Funding Rules of Commitment

Number	Rule
1	Be committed to following your professional Code of Ethics, Scope of Practice, and American Speech-Language-Hearing Association (ASHA) policy documents.
2	Be committed to conducting a comprehensive augmentative and alternative communication (AAC) evaluation to gather evidence required for SGD funding.
3	Be committed to a fair and unbiased SGD trial process independent of the funding source.
4	Be committed to fully informing the client and family of the comprehensive range of AAC interventions options during the evaluation.
5	Fully disclose potential conflicts of interest regarding financial and nonfinancial relationships.

Note. Created based on "Five SGD Funding Rules of Commitment," by C. W. Higdon and K. Hill, 2015, *Perspective on Augmentative and Alternative Communication, 24*, pp. 129–134.

expected to consider their financial and nonfinancial relationships with vendors to have confidence that clinical decisions are independent of a conflict of interest. No one would or should question this responsibility for consumer protection either.

References

American Speech-Language-Hearing Association. (n.d.). *Medicare speech-generating devices information.* https://www.asha.org/practice/reimbursement/medicare/sgd_policy/

American Speech-Language-Hearing Association. (2016). *Code of ethics* [Ethics]. https://www.asha.org/policy/

American Speech-Language-Hearing Association. (2016). *Scope of practice in speech-language pathology* [Scope of practice]. https://www.asha.org/policy/

Higdon, C. W., & Hill, K. (2015). Five SGD funding rules of commitment. *Perspective on Augmentative and Alternative Communication, 24,* 129–134.

Hill, K., & Hayes-Diges, A. (2008). AAC consumer protection policies in an evidence-based practice, client-centered milieu. In *Proceedings of the RESNA 2008 Annual Conference,* Washington, DC [CD-ROM].

Hill, K., Lytton, R., & Glennen, S. (1998). The role of manufacturers' consultants in delivering AAC services. In *Proceedings of the 8th ISAAC Biennial Conference,* Dublin, Ireland.

Navrotski, D. (2015). Role and responsibilities of AAC manufacturers' consultants in the SGD funding process. *Perspectives on Augmentative and Alternative Communication, 24*(4), 147–154.

Woltosz, W., Bristow, D., Frumkin, J., & Romich, B. (1994). The role of speech-language pathologists as manufacturers' representatives in AAC: Four responses. *American Journal of Speech Language Pathology, 3*(1), 11–18

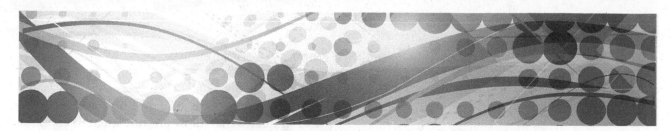

Chapter 16

INTERVENTION AND IMPLEMENTATION FOR ADULTS WITH NEURODEGENERATIVE DISORDERS USING AAC

Catherine Kanter, Emily Kornman, and Annette M. Stone

Fundamentals

The course of augmentative and alternative communication (AAC) intervention for individuals with neurodegenerative conditions involves a focus on current and, perhaps even more critically, anticipated needs and skills of the individual throughout disease progression. Ball, Beukelman, and Bardach (2007) propose the three-phase intervention model in Figure 16–1 to support individuals with neurodegenerative conditions.

This chapter integrates this three-phase intervention model while highlighting the most common and important practical clinical applications of these phases for adults with neurodegenerative conditions needing AAC: education and counsel-

ing, preservation, augmentation, and adaptation. We present these concepts as a cycle in Figure 16–2 because, in clinical practice, SLPs must move between these areas, adjusting interventions based on the changing needs of individuals.

Education and Counseling

Communication difficulties and need for AAC will differ greatly across neurodegenerative diagnoses as a consequence of the different impacts each disease has on the nervous system. For example, each diagnosis results in different types of motor speech disorders, and thus requires different treatment approaches. Progression rate and onset of symptoms within each disease will also vary greatly.

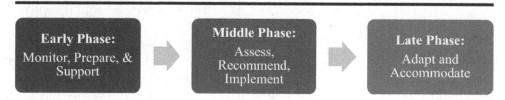

Figure 16–1. Three-phase model for clinical intervention for adults with neurodegenerative conditions.

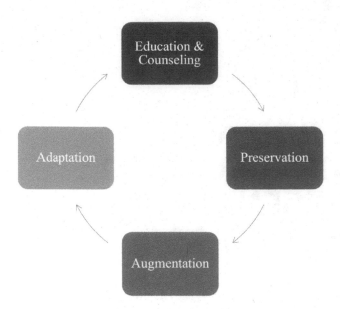

Figure 16–2. Clinical cycle for supporting individuals with neurodegenerative conditions.

Regardless of the disease, counseling should be woven throughout the client-provider relationship as a tool to allow the client to grieve the loss of their previous ways of communicating, while empowering them to preserve the ultimate purpose of communication: human connection (Beukelman & Light, 2020). Counseling should begin with education regarding the progression of the disease and information about potential effects on cognition, communication, language, and social participation. As with any disease, the exact progression cannot be predicted, but as SLPs, it is our role to counsel clients on potential communicative impacts and provide ongoing, evidence-based strategies for continued functional communication. Counseling also helps us identify patient-centered goals, which are more easily accepted and help the client feel heard and see a way forward (Luterman, 2020).

Preservation

Multimodal communication is important to individuals as they experience changes in speech production. Multimodal communication may involve using communication supports or voice preservation strategies that allow an individual to continue using their verbal communication to participate in daily activities. Communication supports, which include strategies, increase participation in communicative interactions (Fried-Oken et al., 2015).

Baseline Measurements

Baseline measurements should be taken during preservation, as early detection of dysarthria, dysphonia, or other cognitive-communicative impairments can lead to timely clinical management. Clinicians should consider using dynamic and criterion-referenced assessments (such as interviews, speech samples, etc.); this combination allows information to be captured in a less direct method (Beukelman & Light, 2020).

- Dysarthria—phonation, respiration, resonance, articulation, and prosody
  - Professional tip: A speech rate of 125 words per minute, or 70% the average speaking rate of 190 words per minute, typically indicates the need for an AAC evaluation (Ball et al., 2020).
- Dysphonia—respiration, rate, vocal quality, loudness, vocal range, and resonance
  - Professional tip: Progression of a neurodegenerative disease may impact the respiratory system, laryngeal mechanism, supraglottic resonatory structure, or coordination between these three systems. Changes could warrant the need for low-tech devices, such as a voice amplifier (see further description later).
- Cognition and Language—cognitive skills, expressive and receptive language skills
  - Professional tip: For neurodegenerative diseases that impact cognition and language, it is important to introduce AAC early on, before this decline, to reduce difficulties with skill

development in this area (Fried-Oken et al., 2015).

■ Contextual Intelligibility—speaker- and listener-related variables that impact communicative effectiveness, such as communication partner familiarity and visual-facial information (Hustad, 2008)

  ■ Professional tip: Assesses functional speech intelligibility across various situations and environments with different communication partners, allowing for the implementation of speech strategies and communication partner training as needed.

■ Additional Considerations—familiarity with technology, current technology use, family member/caregiver motivation and support, communication partners and environments, medications, any current challenges, and the client's interests

  ■ Professional tip: This knowledge will allow for optimal preparation for future AAC use, and client-centered goals.

The ongoing monitoring of deviations from baseline measurements will allow for timely referral to appropriate services and system adaptations during the later stages.

Voice Preservation

Following baseline measurements, voice preservation may be the appropriate next step. Counseling should be heavily embedded into the voice preservation process. One's voice provides an avenue for self-expression and insight into self-concept and identity, conveying information about their personality, humor, emotional well-being, culture, age, and background. Having a voice that one identifies with on their speech-generating device (SGD) is an important factor for continued motivation for use of a device (Creer et al., 2013). Voice preservation refers to the act of saving one's natural voice to later use on a device as either a synthetic voice (voice banking) or with digitized messages (message banking). Voice banking is the process

of recording an individual's voice and turning it into a synthetic voice that can be later used with an SGD. Message banking and legacy messages are complementary to voice banking. Message banking allows for the digital recording and saving of words, messages, phrases, and sounds with emotional tone and other unique qualities of an individual's natural voice (Costello, 2017). Legacy messages are those messages that are unique and meaningful to the individual. They are their ism's or trademark phrases and convey emotion for phrases that express gratitude, pride, love, anger, and frustration (Costello, 2011, 2017). Finally, double dipping is the process used to create a synthetic voice through the use of banked messages. This option allows individuals to focus on banking messages that are important to them, such as phrases to their family members, unique cultural sayings, and so on, and then use these phrases to create their synthetic voice. Through the process of double dipping, the individual in turn has both banked messages, as well as a banked voice, via a single recording process.

The voice preservation process has had significant changes in technology requirements, utterance requirements, and price over the past decade allowing for greater access to individuals seeking these services. Table 16–1 provides a rudimentary overview of the differences in voice preservation options.

Neurodegenerative diseases could take months or years to diagnose. For example, Donaghy, Dick, Hardiman, and Patterson (2008) found a median of 15.6 months from symptom onset to diagnosis of motor neuron disease. Therefore, an individual may not receive speech services until they have already experienced significant changes in their speech intelligibility. There are other options that are now becoming available to individuals who were unable to bank their voice prior to decline in speech intelligibility or loss of speech altogether. These options rely heavily on prior recordings of the individual speaking. Although this is not possible for everyone, every route should be assessed prior to dismissing voice preservation services. The process used for voice preservation is heavily dependent on the client's interests, current speech intelligibility, and future needs. For example, double

Table 16–1. Comparison of Voice Preservation Techniques

	Voice Banking	Message Banking, Legacy Messages	Double-Dipping
Phrase requirement	Between 50 and 1,600 phrases dependent on voice banking platform	No requirement; amount dependent on personal desire	750 or more banked messages[a]
Technology requirement	Most voice banking companies no longer require a soundproof booth. This process can be completed at home with the following technology: ■ Directional microphone, specifications such as noise cancellation, and a frequency range of 80 to 1500 Hz ■ Computer and Internet[b]	■ Recording device that is able to record in .wav format ■ Lightweight, handheld recorder is ideal for recording throughout the day, in the moment ■ Computer to transfer and store the messages ■ Messages could then be stored on a website that would allow for easy transfer to a communication device[c]	■ Recording device that can record in .wav format ■ Lightweight, handheld recorder is ideal for recording throughout the day, in the moment ■ Computer to transfer and store the messages ■ Messages could then be stored on a website that would allow for easy transfer to a communication device[c]
Outcome	Synthetic voice	Digital messages	Synthetic voice and digital messages
Tips	It is important to complete message banking throughout the day, in the moment to capture their most salient emotions and natural sounding prosodic elements. Make sure to capture sounds, such as laughing, crying, and sighs. Encourage the family to participate, and to assist with determining their ism and other phrases to record.[a,c]		

[a]See *Jay S. Fishman ALS Augmentative Communication Program|Double Dipping* by J. M. Costello, 2018 (https://www.childrens hospital.org/centers-and-services/programs/a-_-e/als-augmentative-communication-program/protocol-of-assessment-con siderations/voice-preservation/double-dipping).

[b]From *Frequently Asked Questions*, by My-own-voice team, 2021 (https://mov.acapela-group.com/faq/).

[c]See *Legacy Messages: Message Banking for People With Amyotrophic Lateral Sclerosis and Other Acquired Conditions*, by J. Costello, 2011, American Speech Language Hearing Association.

dipping has a greater time and utterance requirement than some voice banking platforms (Costello, 2018). Therefore, if an individual's voice is deteriorating rapidly, they may be more appropriate for a voice banking platform that requires fewer utterances, and message banking separately. On the contrary, a highly motivated individual whose speech intelligibility is not declining rapidly may be a candidate for double dipping. Regularly scheduled assessments of deviations for an individual's baseline measurements will allow for appropriate determination and provision of services.

Compensatory and Communication Partner Strategies

SLPs should introduce compensatory and communication partner strategies to support individuals with dysarthria and/or dysphonia to continue using speech. It is important for the treating SLP to consider the specific neurodegenerative diagnosis of the individual and address therapy for voice and speech accordingly (Yorkston et al., 1996). Table 16–2 presents common strategies for individuals with neurodegenerative conditions to preserve use of speech.

Table 16–2. Strategies to Support Verbal Speech

Compensatory Strategies	Communication Partner Strategies

• Pacing
• Phrasing
• Speech supplementation
• Alphabet supplemented speech
• Communication breakdown strategies:
  □ Repeat topic
  □ Repeat key words
	• Know the topic of conversation
	• Watch for turn-taking signals
	• Give your undivided attention
	• Avoid communication across long distances (e.g., between rooms)
	• Make sure your hearing is as good as possible
	• Repeat the parts of the individual's phrases that you understood

Note: All strategies adapted from "Comprehensibility of Dysarthric Speech: Implications for Assessment and Treatment Planning," by K. M. Yorkston, E. A. Strand, and M. R. T. Kennedy, 1996, *American Journal of Speech-Language Pathology*, 5(1), pp. 55–66 (https://doi.org/10.1044/1058-0360.0501.55).

Voice Amplification

Voice amplifiers are helpful in extending use of speech and reducing overall fatigue. Amplifying the voice reduces the amount of energy needed at every stage in speech production (e.g., respiration, phonation, resonation, and articulation) (Costello, 2016). Voice amplification has also been shown to increase speech intensity resulting in improved speech intelligibility (Knowles et al., 2020).

Augmentation

As individuals with neurodegenerative diagnoses experience changes in their speech, SLPs must create an individualized communication plan that also explores potential AAC strategies. For each individual with a neurodegenerative condition, it is important that a thorough AAC evaluation includes assessment of four key components: (a) participation patterns and associated communication needs; (b) motor, cognitive, speech and language, visual, and hearing capabilities; (c) constraints and supports affecting AAC decisions; and (d) low- and high-tech AAC options (Ball et al., 2020). Assessment of participation patterns and associated communication needs should include a thorough interview with the individual and key stakeholders discussing communication environments, partners, and modalities. In addition to considering home and community environments, it is important to know the individual's employment goals. Work can influence AAC selection including vocabulary (e.g., preprogrammed, work-specific vocabulary) and access to other features (e.g., e-mail, phone call integration, portability [size and weight], etc.). Emergency preparedness is also a crucial consideration. For example, how will the individual access emergency support across environments, and does the device incorporate features to allow for independence in emergency situations? When identifying the clients' communication partners, it is important to consider those both familiar and unfamiliar with the individual. While some individuals may think they only communicate with familiar listeners, they may encounter unfamiliar people within daily activities (e.g., grocery shopping). Assessment of preferred communication modalities should include both in-person and distance communication such as phone calls, texting, text-to-speech, e-mailing, and use of social media. Caron and Light (2015) reported that use of distance communication leads to greater independence, participation, and overall quality of life among individuals with neurodegenerative conditions. Therefore, discussion of all modalities is crucial to attain and maintain successful communication interactions.

Low-Tech AAC

Low-tech AAC can be used to support or to replace speech for individuals with neurodegenerative conditions. Tools to augment speech include voice amplifiers, low-tech communication books and boards, and speaking valves. Speaking valves may be a temporary option to allow continued verbal communication and potentially improve overall quality of life, increase secretion management, increase swallowing function, and improve taste and smell when an individual requires a tracheostomy tube with or without ventilator assistance. Successful implementation is highly individualized and should be determined through working closely with their multidisciplinary team, such as the pulmonologist and respiratory therapist. A general recommendation for potential candidates is those individuals with ALS in the early to mid-stages (Riley, 2013). Low-tech tools used as an alternative method of communication include writing tools, low-tech partner-assisted scanning grids, low-tech static communication boards with various access options (e.g., head pointer, manual, low-tech eye gaze), and pocket communication cards (revisit Chapter 2 for additional references). Additionally, creating a list of common yes/no questions prioritized by an individual's most common needs, in addition to determining a consistent yes/no signal, can be used in moments of speech fatigue.

High-Tech AAC

Given the different progressions of each diagnosis, AAC assessment and intervention for those with neurodegenerative disorders need to be very individualized. It can be helpful to discuss important feature-matching considerations in the context of disorders with and without accompanying cognitive impairments. The following diagram, Figure 16–3, outlines some of the expected neurobehavioral changes for different diagnoses.

For individuals without accompanying cognitive impairment or decline, motor, communication, and sensory (e.g., vision, hearing) changes should be included in the feature-matching process. For individuals who do have an accompanying cognitive impairment or decline, cognitive changes (e.g., attention, memory, etc.) and accommodations including contextual pictures, reduced clutter on visual displays, and maximized use of previously learned skills should be considered. Table 16–3 highlights additional feature-matching considerations for particular diagnoses.

Given what we know about potential progression of neurological conditions, low- and high-tech AAC supports should be considered during the initial assessment and onset of speech changes. These tools should be used in conjunction with one another to build multimodal communication strategies as the individual's communication deficits change from mild/moderate to severe/profound to continue to maximize participation in communication activities.

Adaptation

Throughout disease progression, SLPs need to include a plan to provide reassessments of the individual's communication function and need to provide necessary interventions such as equipment modifications, communication partner training, and/or introduction of new AAC strategies. For some individuals, this may simply include changing access features on a previous system, while for others this may involve introducing totally new AAC techniques and technologies. Table 16–4 revisits previously discussed neurodegenerative disorders with specific AAC adaptations.

End-of-Life Discussions

For all individuals, one of the most crucial times for communication is at the end-of-life (EoL). Fried-Oken and Bardach (2005) found that the most appropriate time to introduce discussions on EoL care was when individuals or their family members "opened the door" to discussion, when there was a significant increase in pain, and when there is severe psychological, social, or spiritual distress. If possible, it might be most beneficial to discuss EoL care with individuals prior to reaching this stage; however, it will be most crucial to provide access to customized EoL vocabulary and wishes at this phase.

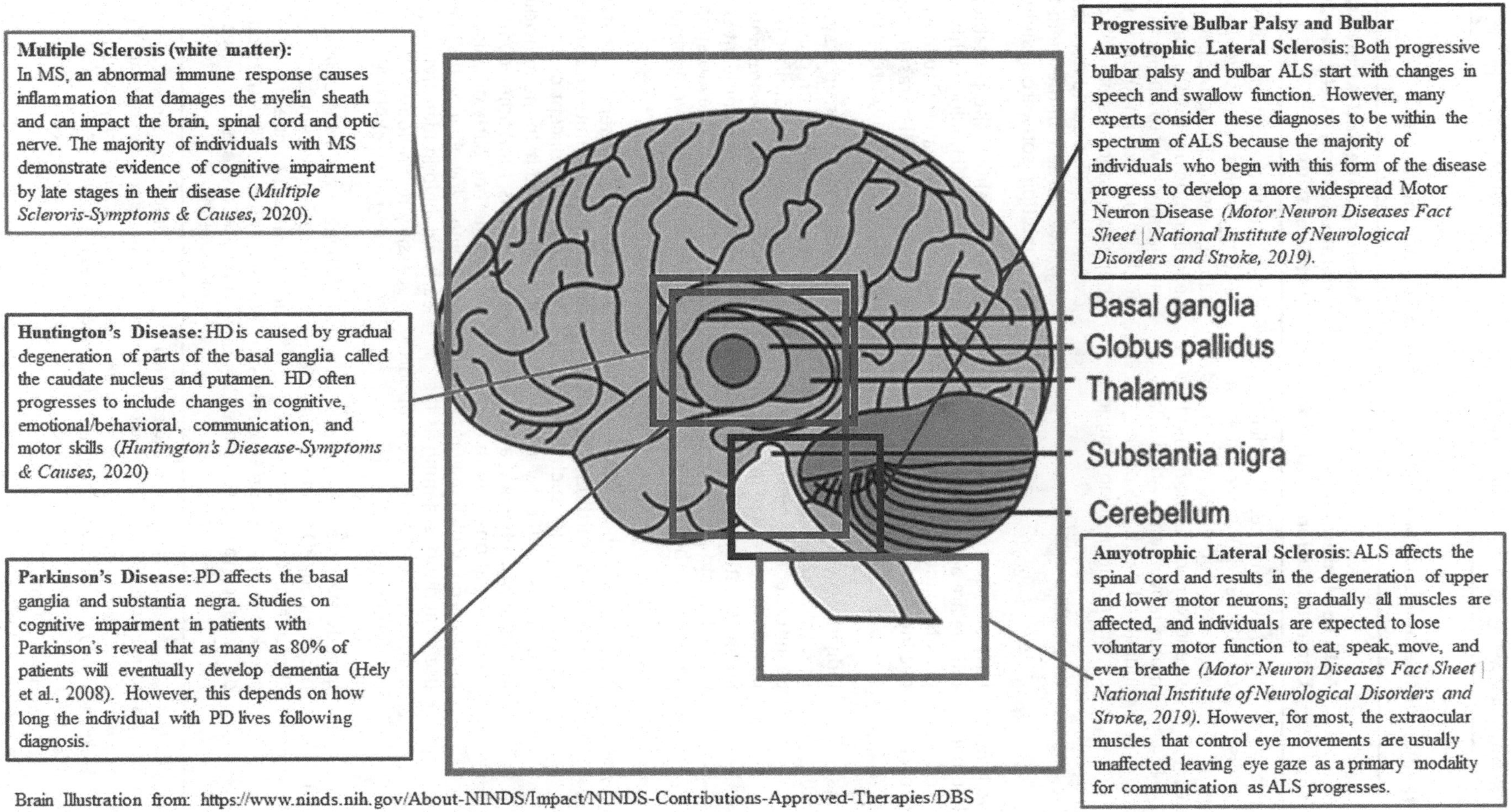

Progressive Bulbar Palsy and Bulbar Amyotrophic Lateral Sclerosis: Both progressive bulbar palsy and bulbar ALS start with changes in speech and swallow function. However, many experts consider these diagnoses to be within the spectrum of ALS because the majority of individuals who begin with this form of the disease progress to develop a more widespread Motor Neuron Disease (*Motor Neuron Diseases Fact Sheet | National Institute of Neurological Disorders and Stroke, 2019*).

Basal ganglia
Globus pallidus
Thalamus
Substantia nigra
Cerebellum

Amyotrophic Lateral Sclerosis: ALS affects the spinal cord and results in the degeneration of upper and lower motor neurons; gradually all muscles are affected, and individuals are expected to lose voluntary motor function to eat, speak, move, and even breathe (*Motor Neuron Diseases Fact Sheet | National Institute of Neurological Disorders and Stroke, 2019*). However, for most, the extraocular muscles that control eye movements are usually unaffected leaving eye gaze as a primary modality for communication as ALS progresses.

Multiple Sclerosis (white matter):
In MS, an abnormal immune response causes inflammation that damages the myelin sheath and can impact the brain, spinal cord and optic nerve. The majority of individuals with MS demonstrate evidence of cognitive impairment by late stages in their disease (*Multiple Sclerosis-Symptoms & Causes, 2020*).

Huntington's Disease: HD is caused by gradual degeneration of parts of the basal ganglia called the caudate nucleus and putamen. HD often progresses to include changes in cognitive, emotional/behavioral, communication, and motor skills (*Huntington's Disecase-Symptoms & Causes, 2020*)

Parkinson's Disease: PD affects the basal ganglia and substantia negra. Studies on cognitive impairment in patients with Parkinson's reveal that as many as 80% of patients will eventually develop dementia (Hely et al., 2008). However, this depends on how long the individual with PD lives following diagnosis.

Brain Illustration from: https://www.ninds.nih.gov/About-NINDS/Impact/NINDS-Contributions-Approved-Therapies/DBS

Figure 16–3. Neurodegenerative disorders' effect on different regions of the nervous system.

Table 16–3. AAC Considerations for Mild-Moderate Communication Limitations

Diagnosis	Mild to Moderate Communication Limitations	Augmentative and Alternative Communication (AAC) Feature Considerations
Amyotrophic lateral sclerosis (ALS)—limb or spinal onset	May have intact direct selection capabilities at initial evaluation with anticipated decline in hand strength, coordination, and fine motor movements. Additionally, individuals with ALS often experience increasing fatigue.[a]	Assess software features, such as compatibility across devices (tablets and dedicated speech-generating device [SGD]), rate enhancement (word and phrase prediction), voice integration into phone calls, and alternative access capabilities. This could decrease the cognitive burden on the client to learn multiple software systems.[b]
Progressive bulbar palsy and bulbar amyotrophic lateral sclerosis (ALS)	Loss of speech and increasing fatigue are anticipated with possible motor and sensory decline.[a]	Consider lightweight, portable, and durable technology with rate enhancement features such as ability to store full-phrase messages and word and phrase prediction.[b]
Huntington's disease (HD)	Individuals with HD motor speech changes (dysarthria) and cognitive-communication decline including decreased initiation of communication, topic maintenance difficulty, and perseverative behavior as the disease progresses.[c]	It is important to consider systems that can rely heavily on previously learned skills (e.g., familiar technology and software). Introduce AAC even before significant speech and cognitive changes to support the greatest skill development prior to decline.[d]
Multiple sclerosis (MS)	Individuals with MS often experience dysarthria, cognitive-linguistic changes such as word-finding difficulty and impaired word fluency, and vision limitations later in their progression, which may require use of auditory scanning as the primary access method to support communication.[e]	Consider AAC systems that allow for auditory prompts and scanning, introduce the concept of auditory scanning, and help the individual practice this sometimes-complex access method early on. Also, including a low-vision specialist early can help in identifying necessary technology and supporting early skill learning.[b]
Parkinson's disease (PD)	In early stages of disease progression, PD is often characterized by decreased speaking volume with progressive dysarthria and voice disorder.[b]	May benefit from use of a voice amplification system, a device worn in the ear to provide simulated noise, which invokes the body's automatic response to increase vocal volume.[b]

[a] *Motor Neuron Diseases Fact Sheet*, by National Institute of Neurological Disorders and Stroke, 2019 (https://www.ninds.nih.gov/disorders/patient-caregiver-education/fact-sheets/motor-neuron-diseases-fact-sheet).

[b] *Augmentative and alternative communication supporting children and adults with complex communication needs* by D. R. Beukelman and J. C. Light, 2020. Copyright Paul H. Brookes Publishing.

[c] Diehl & de Riesthal, 2019

[d] Beukelman, Garrett, & Yorkston, 2007

[e] Yorkston, Baylor, & Amtmann, 2014

Table 16–4. AAC Considerations for Severe Communication Limitations

Diagnosis	Severe Communication Limitations	Augmentative and Alternative Communication (AAC) Feature Adaptations/Modifications
Amyotrophic lateral sclerosis (ALS)—limb or spinal onset, progressive bulbar palsy and bulbar amyotrophic lateral sclerosis (ALS)	At this stage, many individuals will need to consider devices with alternative access as their upper and lower extremities are experiencing increasing fatigue and decreasing voluntary control.[a]	When trialing devices, explore different companies as the eye-tracking cameras vary and often interact with each individual's eyes in unique ways. While one company's device may be a good fit and provide optimal control for one individual, another individual may find this device tedious or not responding to their eyes in an anticipated way. Reach out to your local vendors to trial all the available options.[b]
	While it is rare, some individuals with ALS experience loss of or decrease in range of motion in their extraocular muscles that control eye movements, causing reduced ability to use their device.[c]	Consider adaptations to the display (e.g., larger buttons, clustering buttons in one area, etc.) as well as the eye-gaze interaction settings (e.g., dwell time, calibrating to one eye, etc.) to alleviate some of these barriers; working with vendor support will be helpful in troubleshooting.[b]
Huntington's disease (HD)	For individuals with HD, communication at this stage relies heavily on trained communication partners.[d]	Use of communication partner strategies such as aided language stimulation, giving just a few choices, and repeating key information with gesture and picture supplementation can be most useful at this stage.[d]
Multiple sclerosis (MS)	As individuals with MS may be experiencing more significant cognitive changes at this stage, it may be helpful to reduce the cognitive demand of auditory scanning by switching to partner-assisted auditory scanning.[b]	Simplification of AAC pagesets to include the most highly relevant vocabulary (e.g., medical needs, environmental control, social history) should be considered at this stage to optimize communication.[b]
Parkinson's disease (PD)	For many with PD, in the late stages of disease progression, they may require alphabet supplementation for speech and/or use of a high-tech text-to-speech device. Individuals may also be experiencing more motor involvement (e.g., tremors).[b]	Depending on the motor involvement such as tremors, individuals may also require use of a keyguard or stylus to support more accurate direct selection.[b]

[a]*Motor Neuron Diseases Fact Sheet*, 2019. National Institute of Neurological Disorders and Stroke.

[b]*Augmentative and alternative communication supporting children and adults with complex communication needs*, by D. R. Beukelman and J. C. Light, 2020. Copyright Paul H. Brookes.

[c]Sharma et al., 2011

[d]Beukelman, Garrett, & Yorkston, 2007

Overall, use of AAC at this time supports participation in daily care and EoL discussions (e.g., do not resuscitate orders, hospice), provides instruction to family members following death, and maintains connectedness to say final goodbyes. More information on the role of AAC in EoL for adults can be found in Chapter 18.

Final Thoughts

Individuals with neurodegenerative conditions require ongoing SLP services throughout their disease progression. While this support looks different at each phase, from counseling to implementing high-tech AAC adaptations, the primary role of the SLP is to continue to empower patients to participate in communication activities with their communication partners. Most importantly, it is crucial for individuals with neurodegenerative conditions to know that despite the unpredictable and often frightening changes they face, there is hope in continued and adapted communication.

Case Study: SH

Clinical Profile and Communication Needs

The Individual

SH is a 67-year-old male who was diagnosed with bulbar ALS about 1 year after he began experiencing the symptoms of slurred speech and occasional hand cramping; however, his hands remained largely functional. He did not exhibit any lower extremity symptoms. SH was independent with most activities of daily living (ADLs), such as brushing his teeth, getting dressed, and bathing. SH needed assistance with any ADLs that required communication with unfamiliar partners.

Their Communication Partners

SH's primary communication partner, his wife, reported understanding him approximately 85%

of the time, and frequently translated his speech to other unfamiliar communication partners. SH's difficulty communicating with unfamiliar listeners decreased his social participation in outings, such as trips to the grocery store. SH also stated he depended more heavily on texting as opposed to phone calls due to the listener's difficulty understanding him. In addition to his wife, he frequently communicated with his coworkers, friends, family members, and local church community. He primarily preferred face-to-face communication, as opposed to using social media.

Their Environment

SH mainly communicated at home, at church, in the community, at work, at medical appointments, during medical emergencies, and at family and friend gatherings. SH primarily split his time between work (in retail management) and home. SH and his wife noted a decline in previously enjoyed activities, such as going out to eat, due to his swallowing difficulties. He emphasized concern regarding the use of a device on the go in busy environments, such as at work. His environmental considerations highlighted the importance of multimodal communication strategies. As do most individuals with ALS, SH desired a system that would allow him to maintain independence at work, at home, and in the community.

AAC System or Service Considerations

Education and Counseling

Upon receiving his diagnosis, SH began attending the local multidisciplinary ALS clinic for ongoing monitoring three times per year. At his first visit to the clinic, the SLP engaged SH in an interview to learn about his current communication, communication partners, and experience with technology. The SLP also collected baseline rate of speech (150 wpm) and loudness measurements (60 dB) and provided a brief overview of potential speech changes to expect with disease progression while supporting SH in coping with his new diagnosis. The SLP encouraged SH to continue to reach out with additional questions as he processed the information.

Preservation

At his second visit to the multidisciplinary ALS clinic, his SLP introduced SH to the concepts of voice and message banking. He completed voice banking at home following resources provided by his SLP. He did not complete any further outpatient speech therapy sessions for compensatory strategies, communication partner training, or message or video banking at that time.

At his fourth visit to ALS Clinic, SH's SLP noted that although he still maintained his fine and gross upper and lower extremity skills, his speech intelligibility had declined to 50%, which signified the need for alternative communication. His SLP referred SH back to his local outpatient clinic for an initial AAC evaluation.

Augmentation

SH's local outpatient SLP completed the initial AAC evaluation and determined he needed an SGD. Although SH's fine and gross motor skills were still intact, his SLP was unsure how to get him an SGD without using insurance funding. Therefore, she recommended a device with access via eye-gaze technology given the anticipated disease progression. SH's SLP referred him to a local AAC specialist to seek a second opinion before pursuing insurance funding of an eye-gaze device given his current mobility, environmental, and funding considerations.

At SH's initial evaluation with the AAC specialist, he completed a Communication Needs Questionnaire to determine which communication tasks were most important to him. He indicated that texting, music, and face-to-face communication were most important. The AAC specialist completed a feature-matching evaluation.

SH required a lightweight device that he could carry with him as he moved around his workplace and other environments. He still exhibited gross and fine motor control; therefore, he was able to access the devices via touch. Results of the previous evaluation and informal observation indi-

cated that SH's cognitive skills and receptive and expressive language skills were within normal limits. Therefore, he would benefit from a text-based communication software. He was feature-matched to a text-to-speech (TTS) software with various keyboard sizes and configurations that could accommodate SH if he began to exhibit decreased upper extremity mobility. He also benefited from rate enhancement features such as word and phrase prediction, and the capability to store categories and phrases that SH could use at work or in the community. This would allow for more efficient communication in fast-paced environments. The selected software was compatible with SH's current devices and could also be used on devices compatible with eye gaze in the future; given the progressive nature of the disease, it was important to consider selecting an app that he could become familiar with now. Early modifications and use of this app could build automaticity and require less thinking to navigate through the app, freeing his cognitive resources up to focus on his activities, such as communicating with his friends and family. After the matched application was added to his tablet, SH completed follow-up outpatient therapy sessions to target independent use of the communication device across multiple environments including work, home, and during social gatherings. He attended biweekly 60-min therapy sessions for 3 months.

During follow-up sessions, SH mentioned difficulty using the device in new environments with unfamiliar communication partners, and continued preference for writing and other forms of low-tech communication at work over use of his high-tech system. The importance of multimodal communication was encouraged and expanded on during these sessions. For example, SH was trained to use an alphabet board for word and topic cueing with his wife at home. Given SH's hesitancy to utilize the device in new environments with unfamiliar communication partners, his wife noticed increased dependence on her for ADLs that involved leaving the house, such as going to the dry cleaners. This was addressed through having SH preprogram a page set with phrases typically exchanged during these interactions. SH was provided independent assignments to continue practicing in one new environment with unfamiliar partners per week. SH reported increased independence again with ADLs that involved unfamiliar communication partners, and his spouse reported noticeable improvement in his independence. Sessions were discontinued after six visits as SH exhibited communicative independence across multiple environments when communicating with familiar and unfamiliar communication partners.

Adaptation

Approximately 1 year later, SH returned to the AAC specialist due to changes in mobility. SH was experiencing greater difficulty accessing his tablet via touch due to inability to elevate his arm and hand. He also noted increased head and neck pain due to poor positioning of the tablet and needing to look down at the device, with decreased head and neck control causing difficulty for lifting his head back up after he looked down at the tablet. SH had transitioned to using a power wheelchair, controlled by his wife via attendant control. SH was no longer working and primarily stayed at home. His primary communication partners continued to be his wife, friends, family members, local church community, and a variety of individuals over social media as SH regularly participated in the ALS social media group and attended local ALS support group meetings.

SH continued to use facial gestures for quick yes/no communication. However, he was completely dependent on the TTS software for all other communicative attempts. SH continued to depend heavily on texting as opposed to phone calls and noted complete dependence on his tablet for face-to-face and long-distance communication. SH remained at home while his wife, primary caregiver, went to work for 8 hours. He depended on the tablet to contact her for any medical emergencies. SH did not have a call button or any type of personal alert system in place for any emergencies.

Given his difficulty accessing his prior tablet due to decline in upper extremity motor functioning, his SLP determined at this time that SH required access via eye-gaze technology. This was appropriate for his current motoric status and would accommodate any further upper and lower extremity decline. Device trials were initiated to

determine the most appropriate SGD that would match the features SH required. SH trialed six SGDs with eye-gaze technology across six independent vendors. SH did not exhibit any change in cognitive-linguistic skills, vision, or hearing. The Communication Needs Questionnaire was readministered to evaluate any change in SH's ranking of importance of communication tasks (Bardach, 2017). SH ranked in-person communication, texting, music, and social media as most important, a slight change from his previous preferences. SH also consistently stated the importance of continuing to use his tablet in conjunction with whichever SGD was selected. SH ranked this capability as important as in-person communication, given his comfort level and dependence on the tablet over the past year.

SH no longer needed a lightweight device that he could access via touch as he transitioned from walking to a power wheelchair. He needed a device that could be positioned appropriately on his wheelchair or a rolling floor mount to accommodate his change in environment throughout the day from his power wheelchair to the recliner. SH trialed but ultimately ruled out devices with the same communication software he used on his tablet. Instead, SH indicated a preference for a different text-based system that had features that he required, such as the ability to use all message types, and compatibility with his banked voice. SH was able to easily generalize his knowledge of rate enhancement features such as word prediction and prestored phrases to this new system. SH utilized the eye-gaze accessory to access the TTS keyboard with ease as indicated by the absence of miss-hits or signs of strain. SH's dwell was set at 1 s, with auditory (speaking each letter) and visual feedback (inverting the location). The device also had external computer control features that allowed SH to connect and to access his tablet from the dedicated device.

Next Steps

In addition to initiating the funding process for SH to obtain his SGD through insurance, his immediate difficulty with use of his personal tablet would need to be addressed. The positioning could be adjusted so the tablet would sit right below eye level. Although two-switch scanning would be too fatiguing for SH to be a long-term solution, this could be implemented in the interim while awaiting the arrival of his SGD. The iPad would be able to be controlled by two-switch scanning, which SH could access with both of his knees via hip adduction. This would allow for SH to continue to communicate via the tablet while reducing the poor posturing that was affecting his head and neck. He could utilize the tablet primarily for long-distance communication through social media, texting, and phone calls. Two-switch scanning would be too slow and fatiguing to keep up during in-person conversations.

References

Ball, L., Beukelman, D., & Bardach, L. (2007). AAC intervention for ALS. In D. Beukelman, K. Garrett, & K. Yorkston (Eds.), *Augmentative communication strategies for adults with acute or chronic medical conditions* (pp. 287–316). Paul H. Brookes.

Ball, L. J., Nordness, A. S., & Beukelman, D. (2020). Individuals with acquired physical conditions. In D. R. Beukelman & J. C. Light (Eds.), *Augmentative and alternative communication supporting children and adults with complex communication needs* (pp. 519–552). Paul H. Brookes.

Bardach, L. G. (2017). *Communication Needs Questionnaire.* https://cehs.unl.edu/documents/secd/aac/CommNeedsQuestionnaire.pdf

Beukelman, D. R., Garrett, K. L., & Yorkston, K. M. (2007). *Augmentative communication strategies for adults with acute or chronic medical conditions.* Paul H. Brookes.

Beukelman, D. R., & Light, J. C. (2020). *Augmentative and alternative communication supporting children and adults with complex communication needs.* Paul H. Brookes.

Caron, J., & Light, J. (2015). "My world has expanded even though I'm stuck at home": Experiences of individuals with amyotrophic lateral sclerosis who use augmentative and alternative communication and social media. *American Journal of Speech-Language Pathology, 24*(4), 680–695. https://doi.org/10.1044/2015_ajslp-15-0010

Costello, J. (2011). *Legacy messages: Message banking for people with amyotrophic lateral sclerosis and other acquired conditions.* American Speech Language Hearing Association.

Costello, J. M. (2016, May 8–10). *Augmentative communication supports: A comprehensive and proactive approach for people with ALS* [Conference presentation]. ALS Association Conference, Washington, DC.

Costello, J. M. (2017). *Message banking, voice banking and legacy messages.* Jay S. Fishman ALS Augmentative Communication Program | Message Banking™. https://www.childrenshospital.org/centers-and-services/programs/a-_-e/als-augmentative-communication-program/protocol-of-assessment-considerations/message-banking

Costello, J. M. (2018). *Jay S. Fishman ALS Augmentative Communication Program | Double Dipping.* https://www.childrenshospital.org/centers-and-services/programs/a-_-e/als-augmentative-communication-program/protocol-of-assessment-considerations/voice-preservation/double-dipping

Creer, S., Cunningham, S., Green, P., & Yamagishi, J. (2013). Building personalised synthetic voices for individuals with severe speech impairment. *Computer Speech & Language, 27*, 1178–1193.

Diehl, S. K., & de Riesthal, M. (2019). Augmentative and alternative communication use by individuals with Huntington's disease: Benefits and challenges of implementation. *Perspectives of the ASHA Special Interest Groups, 4*, 456–463.

Donaghy, C., Dick, A., Hardiman, O., & Patterson, V. (2008). Timeliness of diagnosis in motor neurone disease: A population-based study. *Ulster Medical Journal, 77*(1), 18–21.

Fried-Oken, M., & Bardach, L. (2005). End-of-life issues for people who use AAC. *Perspectives on Augmentative and Alternative Communication, 14*(3), 15–19. https://doi.org/10.1044/aac14.3.15

Fried-Oken, M., Mooney, A., & Peters, B. (2015). Supporting communication for patients with neurodegenerative disease. *NeuroRehabilitation, 37*(1), 69–87. https://doi.org/10.3233/NRE-151241

Huntington's disease—Symptoms and causes. (2020, April 14). Mayo Clinic. https://www.mayoclinic.org/diseases-conditions/huntingtons-disease/symptoms-causes/syc-20356117

Hustad, K. C. (2008). The relationship between listener comprehension and intelligibility scores for speakers with dysarthria. *Journal of Speech, Language, and Hearing Research, 51*(3), 562–573. https://doi.org/10.1044/1092-4388(2008/040)

Knowles, T., Adams, S. G., Page, A., Cushnie-Sparrow, D., & Jog, M. (2020). A comparison of speech amplification and personal communication devices for hypophonia. *Journal of Speech, Language, and Hearing Research, 63*(8), 2695–2712. https://doi.org/10.1044/2020_jslhr-20-00085

Luterman, D. (2020). On teaching counseling: Getting beyond informational counseling. *American Journal of Speech-Language Pathology, 29*(2), 903–908. https://doi.org/10.1044/2019_ajslp-19-00013

Motor Neuron Diseases Fact Sheet. (2019, August). National Institute of Neurological Disorders and Stroke. https://www.ninds.nih.gov/disorders/patient-caregiver-education/fact-sheets/motor-neuron-diseases-fact-sheet

Multiple sclerosis—Symptoms and causes. (2020, June 12). Mayo Clinic. https://www.mayoclinic.org/diseases-conditions/multiple-sclerosis/symptoms-causes/syc-20350269

My-own-voice team. (2020, October). *Frequently asked questions.* https://mov.acapela-group.com/faq/

Riley, N. (2013). *Communication and swallowing management for ALS patients with tracheostomy* [PowerPoint slides]. https://ep.passy-muir.com/educationportal/webdashboard.php?mod_1=view&course_id=33&_ga=2.29665206.820540108.1610334800-805001050.1610334800

Sharma, R., Hicks, S., Berna, C. M., Kennard, C., Talbot, K., & Turner, M. R. (2011). Oculomotor dysfunction in amyotrophic lateral sclerosis: A comprehensive review. *Archives of Neurology, 68*(7), 857–861. https://doi.org/10.1001/archneurol.2011.130

Yorkston, K. M., Baylor, C., & Amtmann, D. (2014). Communicative participation restrictions in multiple sclerosis: Associated variables and correlation with social functioning. *Journal of Communication Disorders, 52,* 196–206.

Yorkston, K. M., Strand, E. A., & Kennedy, M. R. T. (1996). Comprehensibility of dysarthric speech: Implications for assessment and treatment planning. *American Journal of Speech-Language Pathology, 5*(1), 55–66. https://doi.org/10.1044/1058-0360.0501.55

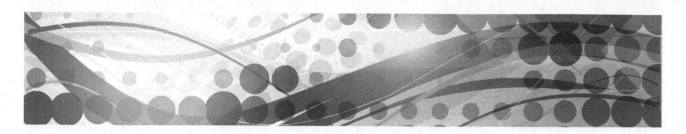

Chapter 17

AAC FOR THE INDIVIDUAL IN THE INTENSIVE CARE UNIT

Richard R. Hurtig and Tami Altschuler

Fundamentals

Introduction: Communication Risks and Barriers Including Health Disparities, Diversity, and Inclusion

Landing in an intensive care unit (ICU) is usually an unexpected event that results from a severe trauma, illness, or postoperative need for intensive care. The ICU is an alien environment for the overwhelming majority of patients. What may seem obvious and straightforward to ICU staff may be foreign to the patient entirely, and especially so for those whose health literacy may be limited. For individuals working in health care, it is quite startling how little many patients, regardless of their educational backgrounds, know about the causes of illness or about the medical interventions needed to treat the illness. The ICU stay can often include a period of time on life support that includes mechanical ventilation. Thus, many patients in the ICU find themselves, for the first time, unable to summon help and make their needs known. The patient's physical state and the medical interventions also make it harder for them to focus and process what they are being told by their caregivers. The typical infection control protocols as well as the heightened protocols that have resulted from the COVID-19 pandemic transform care providers from recog-

nizable individuals into anonymous caregivers in "space suits." All the personal protective equipment (PPE) worn by the ICU staff can significantly impact a patient's comprehension of what they are being told.

Effective patient-provider communication (PPC) is critical to achieving positive outcomes in all medical encounters. Patients who experience a communication barrier are at a heightened risk of experiencing a preventable hospital-acquired condition (HAC) that would extend the length of their hospital stay and, in some cases, lead to a permanent disability or even death (Bartlett et al., 2008; Hurtig et al., 2018). Poor PPC complicates caregivers' assessments of their patients and makes it harder for patients to be active participants in their care. Another factor that can negatively influence patient comprehension is health literacy. It is critical for health care providers to structure the content of their interactions with their patients so that they take the patient's health literacy into consideration.

Poor PPC has also been shown to impact patient satisfaction with their care (Balandin et al., 2007; Hemsley et al., 2007, 2011; Hoffman et al., 2005; Rodriguez et al., 2016) and to increase staff stress (Rodriquez et al., 2015). The human and financial costs associated with poor PPC and the increased incidence of HACs are huge (Hurtig et al., 2018). There is a moral, legal, and financial incentive (Hurtig et al., 2018, 2020) for hospitals to make effective PPC a key component of their "standard of care" for patients across the hospital and in the ICU where communication vulnerabilities are most pronounced.

For a patient to engage in effective PPC, the patient must be able to summon help or attract the attention of caregivers. Many patients in the ICU are too weak to independently summon help using the standard nurse call system pendants that require a patient to generate enough finger movement and force to activate the call button on the pendant. To address this basic need to summon help, it is critical to do a bedside assessment of a patient's ability to produce an intentional gesture. Most hospitals have alternative switches that can allow patients to use other voluntary gestures to activate the call system (e.g., pressure plate, pressure bulb, sip and puff). For patients with even more limited gestures, it is possible to interface assistive technology switches (i.e., mechanical switches, infrared reflectance switches, etc.) with the call system.

When the patient's underlying medical condition or the medical intervention make it difficult or impossible for the patient to use speech to communicate with caregivers, family, and friends, it is important that alternative communication tools be made available. These can range from low-tech strategies, as discussed in Chapter 2, that utilize pen and paper, marker and white board, or printed communication boards, to mid- and high-tech strategies (as in Chapter 3) that utilize tablets with speech-generating software or an electrolarynx for patients who are unable to phonate. How these tools are deployed will also depend on whether the patient has the physical dexterity and strength to independently use a particular tool (i.e., write, point, or use a touch screen). Thus, for patients to be able to use the communication tools, it will be necessary to consider alternative access modalities (as discussed in Chapter 5) ranging from partner-assisted scanning to use of switch access (as with nurse call, above), all of which require the skilled intervention of a speech-language pathologist (SLP) knowledgeable in augmentative and alternative communication (AAC) and comfortable in the medical ICU environment.

Beyond the physical barriers to effective PPC due to the severe trauma, illness, or a postoperative need for intensive care and mechanical ventilation, there are also barriers that can be attributed to cultural and linguistic diversity in the patient population (Bartlett et al., 2008; Hurtig et al., 2015). While hospitals are required to provide interpreter services (The Joint Commission, 2010), there will be bedside interactions that cannot wait for an interpreter (face-to-face, video remote interpreter, or telephone interpreter). The communication strategies employed by the ICU staff may also have to meet the needs of patients with limited English proficiency (LEP) as well as patients with different cultural expectations concerning medical care and patient autonomy.

While many patients in the ICU have not needed any AAC tools/strategies prior to their hospitalization, individuals who use AAC are at a heightened risk of requiring hospitalization. Accommodating the communication needs of these individuals poses additional challenges. If the patient's communication device can be brought into the ICU, there are factors that can negatively influence the patient's ability to access it. Positioning the device to promote optimal access and instructing the ICU staff on how it is used can be challenging. Perhaps equally challenging is making sure the patient's device has appropriate content for communicating in this health setting. Since the communication needs of a patient in the ICU may be unique to that setting, it may not be the case that the relevant messages have been programmed.

Special Considerations for the Intensive Care Unit

Patients admitted to an ICU require a range of intensive care interventions that will make it difficult for them to summon help and communicate. The most frequent of these is mechanical ventilation. Initially, patients may have an endotracheal tube inserted. If they require longer-term ventilatory support, they may undergo a tracheostomy. Many of these patients will be sedated while on mechanical ventilation. More recently, early mobilization protocols have reduced the use of sedation in order to improve patient outcomes and reduce the incidence of post-ICU stress disorders (Corcoran et al.,

2017). These protocols begin with brief withdrawal of sedation to permit nurses to perform assessments and then incrementally extended periods of consciousness. When patients on ventilatory support are conscious, it is critical that their barrier to produce speech be addressed. The early introduction of communication strategies can mitigate the increased stress and anxiety of being unable to communicate and reduce the risk of delirium. For patients on intermittent sedation, it is important to be aware of the potential amnesic side effects of the medications being used. The inability of such a patient to recall how a particular communication tool is used may not necessarily indicate a cognitive decline but rather the side effect of the medication. For that reason, it is important that the bedside staff remind their patients how to summon help and how to communicate with the tools provided. This necessitates that bedside staff are trained in how to use a patient's communication tools so that they can effectively support the patient's use of the tools during care routines and/or when medical decisions need to be made.

A patient's physical weakness or restricted limb use may also contribute to the barriers of access to the use of communication tools. The selection of a communication tool requires a feature-matching process of not only the communication needs but also of the access mode. Ideally the SLP doing the feature-matching assessments will have a working relationship with the ICU staff and be familiar with the unit's treatment protocols. Because of the fragile state of ICU patients, it is also important to continually assess a patient's physical status and to identify alternatives to overcome access barriers that may change as the patient's condition changes.

Under normal circumstances, there may be restrictions to bedside visitation for ICU patients. Thus, the ICU patient will have less support from family, friends, and other nonmedical support personnel (e.g., pastoral care) at a given time. With the heightened restrictions on visitation due to infection control protocols like those imposed by the COVID-19 pandemic, it is also important that the communication tools selected should support communicating with those who cannot be at the bedside. This means that the tools will need to be adaptable to communicating virtually via cell phone or the Internet. For patients who are not fluent in the language being used by the ICU staff, a linguistic barrier further limits PPC. For patients with LEP, this may require use of bilingual communication tools to supplement the use of remote online interpreter services. A further complication may be the need to introduce communication options to a patient who was not familiar with communication technology prior to admission to the ICU. This patient may be faced with the need to acclimate to new technologies or allow strangers to facilitate communication with unfamiliar technology in what can be a frightening environment.

Patient Care Standards

As mentioned in the introduction, patients who face barriers to communication are at a significantly higher risk of experiencing HACs that negatively impact outcomes and lead to extended hospitalization (Hurtig et al., 2018). There are several regulatory and statutory requirements governing PPC that must be addressed in the care of hospitalized patients.

The Joint Commission, the accreditor of U.S. hospitals, recognized the criticality of PPC to patient outcomes and promulgated a set of standards (The Joint Commission [JC], 2010) that mandate that the communication needs of every patient (including those with LEP) must be assessed and addressed from admission to discharge. The JC recognized that AAC strategies should be part of the means by which hospitals addressed their patients' barriers to communication.

Hospitals, along with other places of public accommodation, are bound by the Americans with Disabilities Act (Title III) to address the communication needs of people with disabilities. Thus, hospitals will need to accommodate their standard of care to provide access to communication tools for individuals with preexisting conditions and who may be users of AAC devices prior to their hospitalization.

Further legislation related to communication includes the Convention on the Rights for Persons with Disabilities, which was approved by the United Nations in 2006 (United Nations

Enable, 2007). Among the enumerated rights is to have "the opportunity to be actively involved in decision-making." While President Barack Obama signed the convention, it was not ratified by the U.S. Senate. The National Joint Committee for the Communication Needs of Persons with Severe Disabilities (NJC) has recognized that communication is a fundamental right. The Communication Bill of Rights developed by the NJC (Brady et al., 2016) stipulates that individuals should always have access to a functional AAC solution and any additional assistive technology.

Finally, various forms of Patients' Bill of Rights have been developed that recognize that patients have a right to participate in their care, in medical decision-making, and in end-of-life (EoL) decisions. To ensure these rights to all patients, hospitals must include access to communication tools as part of their standard of care.

Communication Partner Training and Interprofessional Practice

The SLP is the expert in complex communication needs (CCNs) and serves to provide ongoing bedside evaluation and treatment. However, for the hospital to adopt a culture of communication and ensure quality and safety of care, there must be interprofessional collaboration between the SLP and a multitude of other team members including other allied health professionals (e.g., physical therapists, occupational therapists), nurses, physicians, licensed independent practitioners (nurse practitioners, physician assistants), social workers, child life specialists, and respiratory therapists, to name but a few. Communication access becomes standard patient care when all bedside providers integrate communication supports and strategies into their interactions with patients who need them.

To champion a culture of communication, SLPs can offer in-service training or training for new hires during their orientation process and for staff who rotate to units with patients with CCNs. Online modules offer asynchronous learning that may be more efficient for the sharing of information, yet they do not include hands-on learning

and manipulation of communication tools/devices. For example, the SPEACS-2 Communication Skills Training Program (Happ et al., 2014) is a research-based course for nurses designed to teach them how to provide bedside assessment of nonvocal and ventilated patients and to select appropriately matched low-technology communication aids.

It is optimal to provide just-in-time, real-time, "on-the-spot" training to providers at the bedside to demonstrate implementation of communication tools, devices, strategies, and access methods. This offers the greatest likelihood of immediate carryover of a communication system that has been established. The knowledge and skills learned during these training sessions impact the effectiveness of communication supports, service delivery, and patient outcomes. In addition to learning how to utilize communication tools/devices, providers should also understand how to set these up with positioning that ensures access, which may include use of mounting systems to secure a device to the bed or other equipment (e.g., bedside chair or rolling mount for portability) and knowing how to charge devices as needed. It is important to have a troubleshooting plan in place if any difficulties occur. These "on-the-spot" sessions offer the ability to "train the trainer," so providers may in turn train oncoming staff (e.g., nurses during shift changes) on the information learned.

Bedside signage is a valuable way of sharing information specific to the individual patient's communication tools and strategies to ensure continuity and consistency of care (Figure 17–1). This may prevent any confusion with signals used (e.g., "look up for yes") and ensure that all bedside providers are using the same communication strategies when interacting with their patients.

Ideally, health care providers will learn communication enhancement strategies at the preservice education/training level. Some universities offer seminars or courses on this for nursing and medical students with the use of standardized patients or simulations. They may learn how to assess auditory comprehension, manage communication breakdowns, and implement AAC supports for different situations (e.g., alphabet board versus picture board).

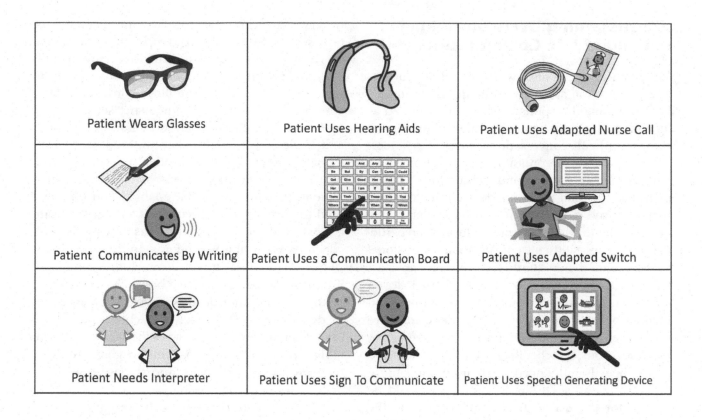

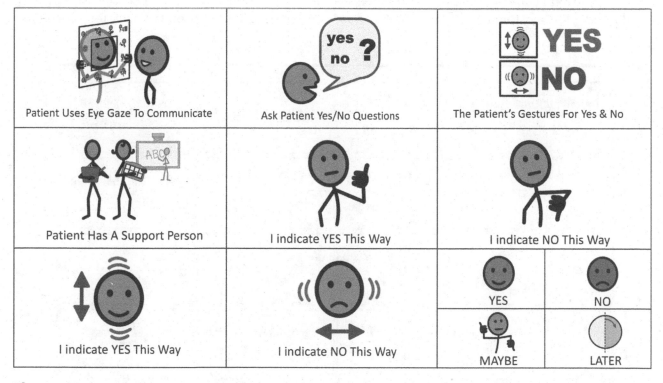

Figure 17–1. Bedside signage. Symbols are courtesy of N2Y SymbolStix. Copyright © 2021 Symbol-Stix, LLC. All rights reserved. Used with Permission, n2y.com.

Life-Sustaining Decision-Making and End-of-Life Communication

When patients encounter worsening illness or disease progression and have difficulty communicating, their limited responses may be interpreted as decisional ambiguity or unwillingness to participate in these difficult conversations. Neuropsychological labels such as depression may be assigned to patients who do not respond. Discussions focused on treatment planning and decision-making are then bypassed to the health care proxy and family members, limiting the patient's inclusion and participation in these difficult conversations. Decisional surrogates are then required to account for any past discussions they may have had with their loved ones regarding their treatment goals, wishes, and religious beliefs surrounding supportive care. There is a burden placed on loved ones to make life or death decisions, which align with these factors and are not heavily influenced by their own emotions.

To mitigate such circumstances, it would be optimal for the SLP to be consulted prior to the need for decision-making discussions with patients to allow ample time for the patient, family, and providers to learn and/or adjust the communication system (Altschuler & Happ, 2019). SLPs can serve an integral role on palliative care teams. Treatment with this population is ongoing with the anticipation that as the illness or disease process progresses, cognitive-linguistic, sensory, and motor abilities may worsen. Communication tools and devices will need to be modified, and treatment planning should consider the current and future communication needs of each individual patient. Patients should be enabled and empowered to participate in discussions so that they can express their wishes, as well as questions and concerns regarding procedures and interventions (Figure 17–2). This should also include augmented input for the patient to have better understanding of the nuances and details of what they agree to or decline (e.g., 3D model of tracheostomy). It is important to move beyond a yes/no dichotomy and allow opportunities for patients to generate their own messages to ask the appropriate questions needed for decision-making.

EoL communication includes more than decision-making. Patients need the opportunity to express their own preferences for procedural

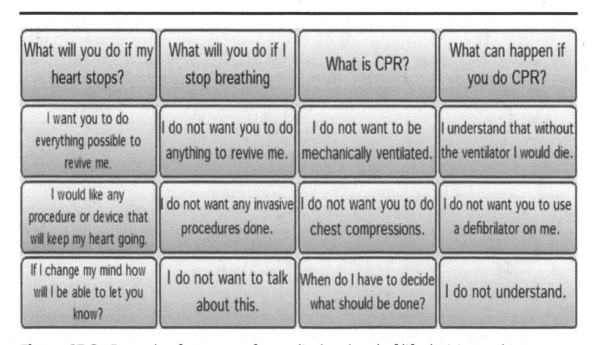

Figure 17–2. Example of messages for medical and end-of-life decision-making.

concerns such as pain management, finances, household instructions, and funeral arrangements. Providing communication support allows opportunities for patients to mend relationships and offer any closure to those who may need to hear affirmations, apologies, or acknowledgments. It is important to remember that effective communication not only benefits the patient but is also critical to care providers and family. Thus, producing voice memos with AAC tools can create individualized digital legacy messages that can last beyond a bedside interaction. If the situation allows, SLPs should consider co-treating with music or art therapy to allow the patient to express themselves through various other mediums in addition to speech and writing; see Chapter 18 for more information about AAC in EoL care for adults.

Best Practices Models

AAC is often underutilized in health care settings due to (a) time constraints, (b) limited staff knowledge and skills in implementing communication interventions, and (c) limited access to AAC resources and equipment (e.g., Blackstone et al., 2015; Gormley & Light, 2019; Hemsley & Balandin, 2014; Hurtig et al., 2015; Santiago et al., 2018). However, there has been an increasing number of SLPs who have led the charge to ensure their patients have access to communication supports in their respective hospitals. The COVID-19 pandemic has strengthened the case for PPC with the surge in patients who are unable to speak due to the respiratory sequelae of the virus and the emergent need for intubation and/or tracheostomy placement (Hurtig et al., 2020).

There has been a shift in the provision of rehabilitation services in the ICU with the development of early mobility programs provided by physical therapists which enable patients to participate in their care early in their recovery process. Patients are ambulating while still on a ventilator and can communicate if provided with the necessary tools and strategies. An interprofessional treatment model involving the collaboration between the physical therapist, occupational therapist, and SLP facilitates mobility, access, and cognitive-linguistic expertise for optimization of AAC evaluation and treatment (Altschuler et al., 2018). AAC may be a part of other hospital initiatives, which may include the SLP as a vital role on interprofessional committees or teams. These may include programs for delirium prevention and treatment, patient safety and quality, and tracheostomy care.

The referral process for AAC evaluations can begin from the first contact patients have with their providers in the emergency department or with a preoperative visit. Screening tools offer an understanding of patients' communication abilities, any existing communication challenges, and any anticipated communication needs. Consultations may stem from order sets or clinical pathways designated for specific diagnoses or procedures that are expected to impact communication abilities (e.g., diagnosis of stroke or recent tracheostomy). It is helpful if the SLP attends unit rounds where each patient on that unit is briefly discussed by the interprofessional team and care needs are identified.

The clinician should put in place a process to ensure meeting all the patient's communication needs (Table 17–1). For each of the individual needs, the SLP should be prepared to provide a communication tool that can be used by the patient. A needs assessment checklist can be used as a guide for clinicians to follow during bedside AAC evaluations and feature-matching assessments (Altschuler et al., 2021). In addition to the patient's communication abilities and potential supports/tools/devices to explore, the clinician should consider the following factors that may impact service delivery:

- *hospital policies* (available communication tools and supports in the hospital, security/safety of equipment brought in from home, infection control)
- *patients' needs and communication strategies* (sensory aids, communication partners, bedside caregivers, positioning and mounting of equipment)
- *provider needs, roles, and responsibilities* (communication partner training and delivery format, designated roles for setting up the communication system, and

Table 17–1. Meeting ICU Communication Needs

Patient Need	Clinician Process
Call for help or gain attention	Evaluate access to standard nurse call pendant and provide alternative switches if needed.
Respond to caregiver questions	Establish easily produced and recognizable gestures that are responsive to questions (yes/no/maybe/later).
Overcome barriers based on limited English proficiency	Provide bilingual communication tools to support bidirectional communication.
Express basic needs/wants	Provide access to communication boards or a speech-generating device that uses pictures, symbols, and/or text.
Ask questions about care, report symptoms, or submit complaint	Provide access to care-specific message content and the opportunity to generate novel messages using an alphabet board or a text-to-speech application.
Participate in decision-making for end-of-life or life-sustaining treatment	Collaborate with the Palliative Care Team and provide access to a medical decision-making communication board.
Engage in conversations with caregivers, family, and friends	Provide access to content to initiate, sustain, and terminate conversations and access to virtual technologies to communicate beyond the ICU.
Maintain personal identity	Provide an opportunity for message and/or voice banking. Start the process preoperatively or before disease progression.
Legacy messages	Provide the means for the patient to write or make digital recordings for family and friends.

monitoring the patient's ability to access and use it)

"Communication Toolkits" offer an array of communication supports from low-tech (e.g., dry-erase boards, alphabet boards) to high-tech (e.g., multimessage speech-generating devices) for providers to access while awaiting an AAC evaluation. Such toolkits do not replace an evaluation; instead, they offer an interprofessional practice partnership to address the communication needs of patients. It is advisable to train all ICU staff on the contents in the Communication Toolkit as well as communication partner strategies. A decision tree or a flowchart may be beneficial for staff to follow as they select the tool that best meets the patient's communication needs at that time.

Conclusion

Effective PPC during an acute care hospitalization is critical to patient outcomes. When patients can make their needs known and participate in medical decision-making, they are at a lower risk of experiencing a HAC and more satisfied with their care (Hurtig et al., 2020). It is essential that patients' ability to communicate be dynamically assessed throughout the hospitalization and that the communication and access strategies be selected to maximize the patients' ability to effectively communicate. To achieve that, it is necessary for the hospital to have developed an institutional "culture of communication" that recognizes each patient's right to effective PPC. The JC accreditation standard identifies the roles that both clinical staff and administrative staff have in addressing each patient's communication needs and preferences (JC, 2010). This requires working to provide adequate staff resources to provide services to patients facing communication and access barriers as well as providing training and support to all bedside care providers. It also requires that adequate funding be available to put together the "communication toolkits" that the SLPs have at their disposal to implement the feature-matched communication strategies for each patient. There are obviously significant costs associated with these efforts. However, the savings that hospitals can achieve by reducing the incidence of HACs and decreased length of stay (LOS), when applicable, more than covers the cost of providing adequate SLP staffing and the communication toolkits (Hurtig et al., 2018, 2020).

Case Study: EG

Clinical Profile and Communication Needs

The Individual

EG was a young adult male with Duchenne muscular dystrophy, a progressive neuromuscular disease with limited life expectancy. He was able to communicate verbally with mild dysarthria, yet his speech was judged to be fully intelligible by his communication partners. With progressive loss of muscle strength, he slowly experienced respiratory insufficiency, and this ultimately developed into respiratory failure requiring an emergent admission to the ICU. He was placed on BIPAP (bilevel positive airway pressure) and was able to speak with a muffled voice and low vocal volume due to airflow noise from the machine. The medical team determined that he needed a tracheostomy for more long-term respiratory support as he was unable to wean from BIPAP support, which is used for more acute versus chronic respiratory conditions. The patient and his family were concerned about his ability to communicate once a tracheostomy was placed. Many people with a tracheostomy can communicate with the use of a one-way speaking valve that redirects

airflow for voice restoration; however, it was anticipated that EG would not be able to tolerate this, and that he would be left nonvocal/nonverbal. He refused to proceed with the tracheostomy until a communication system was established.

Their Communication Partners

EG needed to be able to communicate with his bedside providers (nurses, doctors, physical therapists, occupational therapists, etc.) and his family in the short term. He also wanted to be able to connect with friends virtually through social media and video call platforms. It was his preference to integrate both face-to-face interactions and digital communication within one system versus a setup with multiple devices. Once discharged home, his goal was to reintegrate into his social and religious community, which expanded the number of communication partners exponentially.

Their Environment

EG expressed his desire to be able to communicate immediately after the tracheostomy was placed. There were new medical terms with which he was not familiar but would need to learn to participate in his own care. A Child Life Specialist initiated education/training on this terminology and shared anticipated vocabulary needs for communication. He would return from the operating room to the ICU and need to express novel messages that were new experiences for him (e.g., the need for tracheal suctioning).

AAC Considerations

The SLP was consulted to complete an AAC evaluation and establish a communication system that the patient could utilize postoperatively. Because the patient's respiratory condition was deteriorating, the evaluation and development of the system had to be completed in a week. A feature-matching assessment was conducted, and this provided the information needed to determine an individualized communication system based on his specific abilities in regard to cognition, sensory, and motor functions. He also shared his vocabulary needs, preference for text/picture targets, and organization of pagesets. From the start, EG wanted to lead the development of a communication system and have his preferences, needs, and goals prioritized.

Given the degenerative nature of Duchenne muscular dystrophy, EG had minimal volitional movement of his body, and co-treatment with his occupational therapist revealed that the most reliable point of access for him was his left index finger. He was able to use single-switch scanning via a low-profile and highly sensitive switch. It is anticipated that he will lose his ability to access a communication device with switch scanning with the progression of his disease and that the next or last access method would be via eye gaze; however, this requires an ongoing discussion with counseling for a patient to process the inevitable loss of their abilities. He was briefly educated on eye gaze as an option, yet it was clear that he preferred to maximize his current physical abilities with switch scanning while he had this physical function.

A communication app on a tablet was chosen based on its page layout options, navigation tools, importability of sound files, and ability to back pages up to cloud storage with written consent. It was also important for him to be able to connect with family and friends virtually while he was in the hospital. Social media and video call applications were downloaded and integrated in the communication application for him to access. He was also able to access the hospital Wi-Fi network and learned how to use his personal smartphone as a Wi-Fi hotspot if needed. He practiced single-switch scanning—row/column—and became efficient with this in several days. There were still several days remaining before the tracheostomy, and this allowed for the opportunity to have the patient's voice recorded for message banking. This personalized his messages and preserved the unique characteristics of his voice that a digital output could not convey. He was religious and able to record daily prayers in his own voice, which was meaningful for him and his family to hear. His religious beliefs precluded access to technology during the sabbath. Therefore, a communication binder was made with laminated printouts of all the pagesets on the communication application. Bedside provid-

ers and his family were trained to support use of the communication binder using partner-assisted scanning strategies.

The ICU bedside is filled with medical equipment (e.g., ventilator, intravenous or IV pumps), cables and tubing that cannot be removed from their designated places. The positioning of a communication device required careful consideration so that it was accessible but did not disturb the other medical equipment (Figure 17–3 provides an example of an IV pole-mounted device). It is important to consider the impact of competing noise from medical devices and alarms associated with these devices. The positioning of the speech-generating device (SGD) should ensure that the patient and the communication partners are able to hear the voice output from the device.

A mounting system was set up to allow EG to access his device, placement for the Bluetooth switch interface, and positioning of the switch. EG wanted to be able to use his device in his bed and when he was sitting in the bedside chair. The mounting option selected allowed for easy repositioning of the communication device (Figure 17–4). EG became operationally competent with the ability to navigate the tablet via switch access. He used the accessibility settings to add closed captioning for videos he would view recreationally.

EG is trilingual and fluent in English, Hebrew, and Yiddish. It was important for him to have access to both English and Hebrew keyboards to generate novel messages. He felt it would be most efficient for the text labels of targets to be in both English and Hebrew in order to accommodate the literacy of bedside providers and visitors. When he recorded his voice for message banking, he produced messages in both languages with English first to have immediate care needs met in the ICU.

Although the ICU staff have frequently worked with patients who use AAC, they were unfamiliar with switch scanning and the specific setup of the communication system and its components. Real-time or "on-the-spot" training was provided to EG's care team and family. Bedside signage was posted with instructions for setup, charging the device (both the tablet and Bluetooth switch interface), cleaning, troubleshooting, as well as the contact information for the SLP if any issues arise.

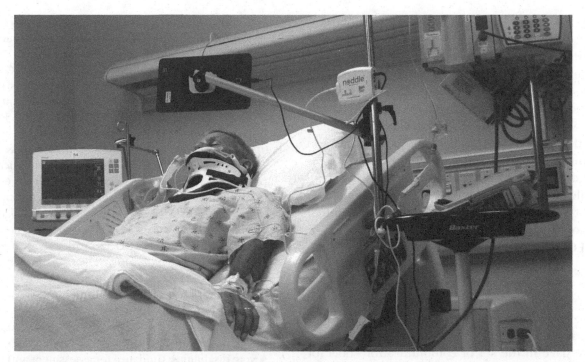

Figure 17–3. Mounting of speech-generating device and switch at the bedside. Reprinted with permission of Richard Hurtig. Image Courtesy of Voxello.

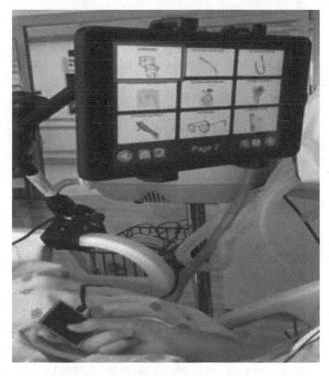

Figure 17–4. EG's initial bedside mounting (pre-operative configuration).

While he was undergoing surgery, the device was mounted to his bed and set up for him to use upon his return to the ICU so that he could immediately express his care needs (e.g., suctioning). From then on, he was able to interact with his care team to express his basic needs/wants, ask questions, share information, and participate in bedside rounds each morning with the medical team. EG independently added vocabulary and pagesets to the device as the need arose. Over the several weeks of his hospitalization, he was able to maintain social relationships virtually and even found a tracheostomy support group on social media. He found it valuable to engage with others who could understand and identify with some of the feelings he was experiencing.

Next Steps

With the abrupt change in his communication abilities due to respiratory distress, EG was provided with all the AAC equipment (tablet and communication application, switch, Bluetooth interface, and mounting) on loan from the SLP department. However, upon discharge, he would not be able to take this equipment home. The possibility of being unable to communicate after he left the hospital was of significant concern to EG. His social worker found funding from local charities that covered the cost of the communication system and would ensure communication access after discharge. The SLP was able to transfer all the files from cloud storage to the new system so as not to disrupt his already established communication system.

EG and his family were advised to pursue an outpatient AAC evaluation to further explore communication options. Since the anticipated progression of his disease will result in EG being limited to eye gaze as his only remaining volitional movement, it was important to consider introducing use of eye gaze in the set of communication tools for EG. It was therefore recommended that EG be introduced to a high-tech eye-gaze speech-generating device and to start learning to use eye gaze before he loses his ability to use switch scanning. EG's family was provided with the acute care SLP's contact information should they have any issues with the communication system once discharged home and awaiting his outpatient visit. The inpatient SLP provided the outpatient SLP and occupational therapist with a detailed report of the communication strategies that had been implemented with EG. Such handoffs are critical for continuity of care.

References

Altschuler, T., & Happ, M. B. (2019). Partnering with speech-language pathologist to facilitate patient decision making during serious illness. *Geriatric Nursing, 40*, 333–335. https://doi.org/10.1016/j.gerinurse.2019.05.002

Altschuler, T., Klein, D., Tesoriero, A., & Scully, A. C. (2018, November 15–17). *Talking early mobility: Get moving with AAC* [Conference session]. American Speech-Language-Hearing Association Conference, Boston, MA.

Altschuler, T., Santiago, R., & Gormley, J. (2021). Ensuring communication access for all during the COVID-19 pandemic and beyond: Supporting patients, provid-

ers, and caregivers in hospitals. *Augmentative and Alternative Communication*. Advance online publication. https://doi.org/10.1080/07434618.2021.1956584

Balandin, S., Hemsley, B., Sigafoos, J., & Green, V. (2007). Communicating with nurses: The experiences of 10 adults with cerebral palsy and complex communication needs. *Applied Nursing Research, 20*(2), 56–62. https://doi.org/10.1016/j.apnr.2006.03.001

Bartlett, G., Blais, R., Tamblyn, R., Clermont, R. J., & MacGibbon, B. (2008). Impact of patient communication problems on the risk of preventable adverse events in acute care settings. *Canadian Medical Association Journal, 178*(2), 1555–1562. https://doi.org/10.1503/cmaj.070690

Blackstone, S., Beukelman, D., & Yorkston, K. (2015). *Patient-provider communication in healthcare settings: Roles for speech-language pathologists and other professionals*. Plural Publishing.

Brady, N. C., Bruce, S., Goldman, A., Erickson, K., Mineo, B., Ogletree, B. T., . . . Wilkinson, K. (2016). Communication services and supports for individuals with severe disabilities: Guidance for assessment and intervention. *American Journal on Intellectual and Developmental Disabilities, 121*(2), 121–138. https://doi.org/10.1352/1944-7558-121.2.121

Corcoran, J., Herbsman, J., Bushnik, T., Van Lew, S., Stolfi, A., Parkin, K., . . . Flanagan, S. R. (2017). Early rehabilitation in the medical and surgical intensive care units for patients with and without mechanical ventilation: An interprofessional performance improvement project. *PM and R, 9*, 113–119. https://doi.org/10.1016/j.pmrj.2016.06.015

Gormley, J., & Light, J. (2019). Providing services to individuals with complex communication needs in the inpatient rehabilitation setting: The experiences and perspectives of speech-language pathologists, *American Journal of Speech-Language Pathology, 28*(2), 456–468.

Happ, M. B., Garrett, K. L., Tate, J. A., DiVirgilio, D., Houze, M. P., Demirci, J. R., . . . Sereika, S. M. (2014). Effect of a multi-level intervention on nurse-patient communication in the intensive care unit: Results of the SPEACS trial. *Heart & Lung, 43*, 89–98. https://doi.org/10.1016/j.hrtlng.2013.11.010

Hemsley, B., & Balandin, S. (2014). A metasynthesis of patient-provider communication in hospital for patients with severe communication disabilities: Informing new translational research. *Augmentative and Alternative Communication, 30*(4), 329–343. https://doi.org/10.3109/07434618.2014.955614

Hemsley, B., Balandin, S., & Togher, L. (2007). Narrative analysis of the hospital experience for older parents of people who cannot speak. *Journal of Aging Studies, 21,* 239–254. https://doi.org/10.1177/1049732311415289

Hemsley, B., Balandin, S., & Worrall, L. (2011). The "Big 5" and beyond: Nurses, paid carers, and adults with developmental disability discuss communication needs in hospital. *Applied Nursing Research, 24*(1), e51–e58. https://doi.org/10.1016/j.apnr.2010.09.001

Hoffman, J. M., Yorkston, K. M., Shumway-Cook, A., Ciol, M. A., Dudgeon, B. J., & Chan, L. (2005). Effect of communication disability on satisfaction with health care: A survey of Medicare beneficiaries. *American Journal of Speech-Language Pathology, 14*(3), 221–228. https://doi.org/10.1044/1058-0360(2005/022)

Hurtig, R. R., Alper, R., Altschuler, T., Gendreau, S., Gormley, J., Marshall, S., . . . Scibilia, S. (2020). Improving outcomes for hospitalized patients pre- and post-COVID-19. *Perspectives of the ASHA Special Interest Groups, 5,* 1577–1586. https://doi.org/10.1044/2020_PERSP-20-00144

Hurtig, R. R., Alper, R. M., & Berkowitz, B. (2018). The cost of not addressing the communication barriers faced by hospitalized patients. *Perspectives of the ASHA Special Interest Groups, 3,* 99–112. https://doi.org/10.1044/persp3.SIG12.99

Hurtig, R., Nilsen, M., Happ, E. B., & Blackstone, S. (2015). Acute care/hospital/ICU adults. In S. W. Blackstone, D. R. Beukelman, & K. M. Yorkston (Eds.), *Patient-provider communication: Roles for speech-language pathologists and other health care professionals.* Plural Publishing.

Rodriguez, C. S., Rowe, M., Thomas, L., Shuster, J., Koeppel, B., & Cairns, P. (2016). Enhancing the communication of suddenly speechless critical care patients. *American Journal of Critical Care, 25*(3), e40–e46. https://doi.org/10.4037/ajcc2016217

Rodriguez, C. S., Spring, H. J., & Rowe, M. (2015). Nurses' experiences of communicating with hospitalized, suddenly speechless patients. *Qualitative Health Research, 25*(2), 168–178. https://doi.org/10.1177/1049732314550206

Santiago, R., Altschuler, T., Howard, M., & Costello, J. (2018, November 15–17). *Bedside AAC service delivery by SLPs in acute care: Current practice and a call to action.* American Speech-Language-Hearing Association Conference, Boston, MA.

The Joint Commission. (2010). *Advancing effective communication, cultural competence, and patient- and family-centered care: A roadmap for hospitals.* https://www.jointcommission.org/-/media/tjc/documents/resources/patient-safety-topics/health-equity/aroadmapforhospitalsfinalversion727pdf.pdf?db=web&hash=AC3AC4BED1D973713C2CA6B2E5ACD01B

United Nations Enable. (2007). *Convention on the Rights of Persons with Disabilities.* http://www.un.org/esa/socdev/enable/rights/convtexte.htm

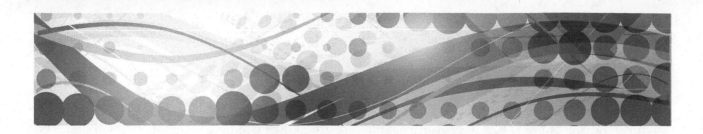

Chapter 18
AAC FOR ADULTS IN END-OF-LIFE CARE

Amanda Stead

Fundamentals

Hospice worker Ann Richardson once remarked, "We cannot change the outcome, but we can affect the journey." This sentiment applies to the intersection of all types of therapeutic professionals with patients nearing the end-of-life (EoL). Due to ever-advancing technologies and the medicalization of death and dying, therapeutic professionals are in closer contact than ever with clients who need support communicating at the EoL (Pollens, 2012). Communication at the EoL is of paramount importance for providing quality end-of-life care (EoLC). Speech-language pathologists (SLPs) can help serve patients near the EoL by facilitating communication for the dual purposes of socializing for quality of life and participating in medical decision-making and symptom management (Pollens, 2020).

Hui and colleagues (2014) sought to define the use of the term "end-of-life" through systematic review. The term "end-of-life" was commonly used to refer to a period of time preceding one's death, which simultaneously implied that the individual's condition was eventually fatal (Hui et al., 2014). Similar terms such as "terminally ill" (a patient's condition), "terminal care" (the actual care received), "hospice care" (benefits received within 6 months of predicted EoL), and "comfort care" (care for EoL focused on comfort) have sometimes been used interchangeably depending on the setting of practice (Hui et al., 2014; Stead et al., 2020).

EoLC often involves an interdisciplinary health team, which can include a diverse range of participants such as primary care physicians, nurse practitioners, physical therapists, occupational therapists, home health aides, social workers, volunteers, and even chaplains. It is the goal of this interdisciplinary team to develop a care plan that meets the patient's needs in terms of pain management, symptom control, and quality of life at the EoL (Stead & McDonnell, 2015). Palliative and hospice care often require referrals to an SLP. The American Speech-Language-Hearing Association (ASHA) has affirmed the role of the SLP in working with patients near the EoL stating: "SLPs are an integral member of the health care team and contribute significantly to the care of patients nearing end-of-life." Describing the role of the SLP at EoL as it relates to the World Health Organization's International Classification of Functioning, Disability, and Health (WHO-ICF) framework can best be described as follows:

- consultation with families and team members about communication and cognition
- development of strategies to support the client in communicating decision-making
- management of swallowing for nourishment
- communicating with members of the hospice team (Pollens, 2004, 2012).

Toner and Shadden (2012) have additionally described the role of the SLP as to provide comfort through communication and swallowing and to counsel clients and family members during EoLC. Through expertise in language, cognition, feeding, and swallowing, SLPs have the ability to provide interventions critical for quality of life for patients and families near the EoL.

Communication Difficulties at End-of-Life

When discussing health-related quality of life (HRQL), Ghoshal et al. (2016) affirmed that physical, emotional, and social well-being are all impacted by one's medical condition or treatment. There are numerous reasons that patients may not be able to communicate well at the EoL, the first of which is their underlying illness. Motor illnesses that affect the nerves, muscles, or structures that control the speech mechanism (e.g., head and neck cancer, motor neuron disease, multiple sclerosis, or Parkinson's disease) can have a direct impact on communication at the EoL. Neurological diseases or disorders that affect cognitive function such as acquired brain injury, stroke, or dementia can also impact a patient's ability to communicate with both family and medical professionals.

Sensory impairment is an additional barrier to effective communication at the EoL. Patients who have a hearing impairment may need additional communication support. For these patients, it is essential to make sure their assistive listening devices or hearing aids are both on and functioning at the correct settings. For patients who are visually impaired, the use of external communication aids and environmental supports may be more limited, but adapting supports through the use of magnifiers, accessible glasses, and lighting may help. It is well documented that sensory issues further compound the effects of other impairments and create additional barriers to participation if left unmitigated.

Emotional distress is common for patients near the EoL. This distress or anxiety can become a barrier to patients communicating what they are feeling or need. Patients may also be concerned they will be judged for their communication wishes or worried they will have an emotional outburst. The impact of the emotional state on communication cannot be understated.

Pain, fatigue, and lethargy all impact patients approaching EoL, with the latter symptoms often increasing throughout the process of dying. Fatigue has been shown to have impacts on physical, emotional, economic, and social aspects of overall quality of life in terminal cancer patients (Ghoshal et al., 2016). The presence of pain has a significant impact on a patient's ability to communicate. Long-lasting pain can impact a patient's ability to attend to tasks and accurately remember information. Furthermore, the presence of pain can impair a patient's ability to communicate, leaving them tired, disengaged, and unfocused. The pharmacological methods used to manage pain can often leave patients tired and "cognitively foggy" as well. These collective symptoms mean that patients with a significant amount of pain associated with their decline can be at a high risk for reduced communication quality and quantity.

The impact EoL has on communication leaves patients and families at risk for having poor quality of life, which is realized through diminished socialization and reduced decisional capacity and medical participation. When patients nearing the EoL are asked what they desire at the end of their lives, the resounding themes are ones of connection. Patients want the opportunity to connect through relationships, say goodbye to those they love, resolve unfinished business, process the reality of death, and consider their legacy (Kuhl et al., 2010). Patients want all of this alongside honest, but hopeful, conversations with their medical providers. Through the use of augmentative and alternative communication (AAC) aids, these goals can be realized.

How AAC Can Support Communication, Socialization, and Decision-Making

Hawksley and colleagues (2017) indicated the predominance of SLP referrals in palliative care were for dysphagia; however, this higher frequency may not reflect the communication needs of patients requiring services. As mentioned, patients near the EoL desire the opportunity to say goodbye to loved ones and have closing conversations with those they care about. It is of the utmost importance that patients and families have the opportunity to meet these goals during this formative moment so as to achieve the "good death." Pollens (2020) described goals for the use of AAC with patients near the EoL or participating in palliative care where a support system was offered to help patients live as actively as possible until death. Another goal of AAC for EoL patients is the integration of psychological and spiritual aspects of care with the final goal of offering a support system to help the family cope during the patient's illness and in their own bereavement (Pollens, 2020).

Fried-Oken and Bardach (2005) used qualitative research to discuss values expressed by individuals who use AAC during their EoL phase. Persons who use AAC (PWUAACs) included those with varying conditions (e.g., amyotrophic lateral sclerosis or ALS, aphasia, developmental disabilities, and other terminal illnesses). With this information, the authors compiled a list of five recurring themes: range of AAC options, techno-connectedness, importance of partners, quality of life, and quality of death. This article offers multiple quotes from different AAC users during EoL, providing a well-rounded discussion of the experiences of individuals during their EoL stage. One quote from a family indicated that despite the advantages of computer-based AAC, the complexity was in fact a disadvantage, and the alphabet board proved to be a more effective tool. Caregivers also mentioned it was essential to train all visitors on how to use the AAC tools. One participant remarked, "I believe having AAC devices for direct communication are not only a medical necessity, but also have a dramatic impact on quality of life and therefore the will to live" (Fried-Oken & Bardach, 2005, p. 17).

In addition to supporting social connection for quality of life, AAC can support individuals in participating in medical decision-making as they approach their EoL. Pollens (2020) explained that written communication, one use of the most basic forms of AAC such as on a pad of paper, mobile tablet, or other electronic device, can help provide individuals relief from pain and other distressing symptoms. In order for patients to be able to make their own medical decisions, they need to have "capacity" defined as the ability to understand the situation, be rational, and appreciate the consequences. Physicians can determine decision-making capacity, and capacity can be supported through the use of external supports (Stone, 2001). Even patients with moderate impairment have the ability to make their own decisions; however, they are often perceived by family members and physicians as being incapable due to their diagnosis. Research has shown through the use of supportive communication tools, individuals can participate in their own care despite the physical or cognitive impact of their disease or disorder. Hurtig and Downey (2008) have shown a positive relationship between client responsiveness and care and how the use of AAC devices improves responsiveness. Further research has illustrated that individuals with dementia can participate in EoL discussions through the use of simple low-tech communication boards (Chang & Bourgeois, 2020). Results indicated that with the use of visual aids, participants demonstrated significantly better overall decision capacity in understanding, reasoning, and appreciation. This suggests that the use of visual aids can not only improve the decision-making capacity for people with dementia (PWD) but can also help clinicians reach a better agreement on their perception of the client's decision-making capacity (Chang & Bourgeois, 2020).

PWUAACs with ALS and other terminal conditions may be better equipped to continue the use of their existing high-tech devices throughout their EoLC. Due to the complex nature of many high-tech AAC devices, previous use and training benefit patients with navigation and ease of use. With more complicated AAC that requires programming, medical staff and families may forgo use entirely (Hurtig & Downey, 2008). All patients who have a high-tech AAC device should have low-tech backup options already in place. Although these may need to be modified to accommodate changes in sensory, physical, and/or cognitive status, PWUAACs should be familiar with low-tech options. When patients are nearing the EoL with new and critical symptoms that impact communication, the use of low-tech AAC or simple communication boards may be more easily implemented. The more universal nature of low-tech communication boards and the ease of training in their use benefit families and patients who are often suddenly in a position of significant and/or accelerating decline. Tools such as alphabet boards or communication charts represent rapidly available options when communication declines (Fried-Oken & Bardach 2005). Whatever the choice of AAC system for a patient and family, it is essential the clinician considers the nature of decline that is associated with the EoL process and implements tools that will have longevity and adaptability across the continuum. These considerations include the decline of sensory systems, mobility, cognition, and energy.

SLPs have a broad role in EoLC to support patients with communication and cognition challenges, and not just in feeding and dysphagia. Low-tech communication boards may be more easily implemented with patients near the EoL due to their ease of use and rapid implementation. Focus should be on participation-based goals to ensure quality of life and involvement in medical decisions and socialization.

Case Study: KM

Clinical Profile and Communication Needs

The Individual

KM is a 64-year-old cis-gendered female currently living at home and under the care of hospice services. Two years prior, KM was diagnosed with breast cancer and underwent chemotherapy treatment and bilateral mastectomy. Despite initial success of treatment, KM experienced a recurrence 6 months ago where her cancer metastasized to her bones and brain. Since the new diagnosis of metastatic breast cancer, KM's symptoms have dramatically changed. Six weeks ago, KM was enrolled in hospice care at the advice of her oncologist when it became clear her condition was terminal. The decision to enroll in hospice care was made to ensure continued symptom management, comfort, and intervention during the dying process for both KM and her family.

Prior to the diagnosis of cancer, KM was a monolingual English speaker with a history of osteoarthritis, farsightedness, and anxiety. KM had a successful career as a financial advisor for the

---

Expert Tips or Practical Advice

For clinicians who work with adults in EoLC, development of a small kit containing a few essential supplies would facilitate provision of some starter low-tech options to individuals whose transition to EoLC was sudden, before a fuller needs assessment can occur.

This kit might contain the following:

- pre-made alphabet displays with different layouts and different font sizes and thicknesses
- nonglare page protectors to hold the low-technology displays
- Sharpie-type markers of various thicknesses to use when creating displays

- cardstock or other thicker paper for creation of sturdy low-technology displays
- prepared (i.e., typed) instructions with screenshots of how to implement partner-assisted scanning (PAS)
- prefabricated communication displays such as the evidence-based Vidatak EZ Communication Boards™ that are available in many languages and formats (e.g., orthographically based options, picture-based options, a combination of the two [i.e., text and pictures] and were designed for use in the ICU and contain a pain scale, etc.; more recently, spiritual care displays were added to the offerings)

past 35 years and had planned to retire at the end of the year. She resides in a townhome with her wife of 13 years and has two adult children and three grandchildren. KM's current primary symptoms include lethargy, pain, reduced strength in extremities, reduced clarity of thought, depression, and anxiety. Objective data are as follows:

- Vision corrected is functional for AAC use.
- When vision is not corrected, patient would benefit from increased symbol and font size, auditory feedback, and familiar photographs.
- Hearing is functional unaided.
- Patient is often positioned in bed in a semireclined position.
- Patient has functional control of extremities, but weakness increases with fatigue.
- Patient is 100% intelligible with familiar and unfamiliar listeners but becomes quiet when fatigued.
- When fatigued or in severe pain, patient prefers not to speak but to write.
- Written language is within functional limits.
- Reading is within functional limits.
- Patient shows signs of comprehension frustration but benefits from repetitions, slower rate, and use of external supports.
- Patient's receptive language abilities are challenged by fatigue and medical management of pain. Patient can follow two-step directions, answer simple questions, and comprehend visual and written information within functional limits.
- Patient is sleeping 14 to 16 hours per day.
- Patient's attention is limited to 20 to 25 min before fatigue impacts performance.
- Patient scored a 24 out of 30 on the Montreal Cognitive Assessment (MoCA), indicating borderline cognitive impairment.
- Quality of Communication Life (QoCL) scores indicated an impact on socialization activities, confidence, and self-concept, as well as role and responsibilities.
- Patient is currently designated as a "specific needs communicator" when not fatigued and requires support to communicate only under certain contexts; however, functional

communication is expected to decline through the end stages of her disease.

Their Communication Partners

KM and her wife MM have been married for the past 13 years. MM is recently retired from a career as a middle school teacher. She is the primary caregiver to KM and is home with her nearly 100% of the time. MM is exhibiting signs of depression and anxiety related to the recent health decline of her wife. She has been attending a support group for spouses of cancer patients monthly for the past 5 months. Recently, she has relocated the couple's bedroom to the main floor of the house in their previous office space. She is very protective of her wife and is struggling with the best way to support her social engagement and her pain status. She frequently declines visits from friends and family stating that "KM needs to rest" or "is not feeling well." She is also struggling with letting KM make her own medical decisions believing she is in "too much pain" to fully understand their ramifications.

KM has two children from a previous marriage. Her son, a 32-year-old cis-gendered male, lives locally and has two children of his own (6 and 10 years old). Her daughter lives in the adjacent state approximately 5 hours away by car, and she has been able to visit monthly for long weekends with her 3-year-old daughter. Each of the grandchildren love to spend time with their grandparents and are excited to tell them about their activities and interests. The youngest grandchild in particular is fond of having stories read to her by her grandmother. KM has developed a deep community surrounding her. She has numerous longtime friends who are interested in visiting with her and spending time with her before she dies. Currently KM has an oncologist whom she sees monthly, a primary care physician she sees as needed, a hired in-home nurse for 2 hours a day, and is also being visited weekly by a hospice nurse and chaplain.

Their Environment

KM and her wife live in a suburban two-story townhome adjacent to a large park and business area. There are several local cafes and restaurants within walking distance that the couple used to frequent. Within the home, the couple's bedroom has been moved to the main floor alongside the main living area and kitchen. KM no longer goes to the second floor of the house due to difficulty with the stairs. KM is currently sleeping in a hospital bed with railings, and her wife has pulled a twin mattress alongside the bed to be near her. There is a mid-sized bathroom adjacent to the kitchen that has a stand-up shower but no accessibility supports.

Communication Needs

KM's primary needs for communication are twofold: to communicate and participate in medical decisions related to symptom management and to socialize with friends and family primarily at home. For communication of medical decisions, it is necessary that KM has multiple modalities of input for information to be sure she is understanding concepts and outcomes, and multiple options for response modes. She has been deemed to have capacity; however, her lethargy and pain often impact information retention. Upcoming medical decisions during her terminal diagnosis of cancer will largely be related to the management of pain symptoms and the relationship with wakefulness and alertness. KM has indicated she would like to have the ability to choose her level of pain medication for as long as she can, knowing that increased dosage often leaves her tired and unable to participate in conversation.

Within KM's EoLC planning, she has indicated she would still like to be able to visit her favorite restaurants as long as she is able and attend her grandson's baseball games. KM would also like to stay at home while she is dying and host visitors and her family there. KM indicated she would like to be able to "review her life" and tell stories from her past and reminisce. This is an important component of saying goodbye to her. She also needs to be able to ask for support to complete activities of daily living (ADLs) due to her extremity weakness and fatigue.

AAC Considerations

KM is farsighted; therefore, she will need to be wearing her glasses as often as possible during points of communication. When this is not possible, it is essential that any communication devices be of sufficient font and picture size to facilitate recognition despite low vision. Fatigue is a major consideration for service implementation. KM's persistent fatigue from her primary condition and from her medication to control symptoms impacts her ability to participate in activities for long periods of time. When KM is fatigued or in pain, she has a difficult time speaking; she would like communication options allowing her to communicate with her caregivers without full exertion or speaking. This is compounded by extremity weakness and pain. Any system selected should reduce needed exertion and limit range of motion in extremities as much as possible. Every tool that is developed must be intuitive and accessed quickly to not accelerate her fatigue.

KM requires support for the input of information due to the myriad of symptoms she currently experiences. Any AAC system chosen should be able to support both caregiver's communication and KM's communication. Shared communication systems are preferable for ease of use and training. One of KM's primary EoL goals is to spend quality time with her family and friends. Because social communication is a primary goal, any system implemented should have a predominance of options for social communication and the review of KM's life. Supportive communication tools should include reference to significant life events and personal stories KM may want to share again or discuss. Tools should also support communication for some limited local exploration so that KM can still enjoy her local communities.

Due to the numerous logistical challenges of KM's terminal condition and the immediacy of the need, low-tech communication boards were chosen as the primary solution for patient and family support in this case. Communication boards are an ideal solution for this client due to the presence of fatigue, the need for cognitive and auditory comprehension support, the ease of communication partner training, and the nature of accelerating functional decline expected as a result of a terminal diagnosis. High-tech AAC solutions have been ruled out as a primary intervention in this case due to the complexity of their construction, the patient's relatively intact ability to use speech when alert, the broad range of communication partners who will need to interact with the supports, and the expected decline in functional status.

The AAC System or Service

Although KM currently has functional speech, reading, and writing, it is unknown if she will retain these abilities throughout the course of her disease decline. Because of this, the development of low-tech communication boards should include a combination of written and visual options. The development of supports will be threefold:

1. development of low-tech communication boards for ADLs
2. development of low-tech communication boards for medical decision-making
3. development of low-tech communication boards for social connection and life review

To support KM's communication of ADL assistance, single-page communication sheets were placed in her kitchen, bathroom, bedroom, and purse. These simple quick referral boards ensure that regardless of where she is in the house, she can rapidly indicate any ADL needs. The communication board lexicon would include words and symbols related to the bathroom, dressing, medication, family, mobility, hunger, and thirst. These boards should also contain simple Yes/No/Maybe response options as well quick responses such as "need help."

For medical decision-making, it is important that a communication board has explicit information regarding the relationship between pain and lethargy. The board should include a seven-point pain scale with both written and visual anchors presented alongside a scale relating to fatigue. This will support medical providers in indicating the relationship between pharmacological pain management and fatigue. The decision-making chart should also include a body diagram so that KM can indicate location of pain. Furthermore, including descriptive words for pain and discomfort (e.g., constant, radiating, throbbing, sharp) and medical

question prompts for her providers (e.g., please explain, what is the plan? how am I doing?) will ensure a two-way conversation and increased clarity of statements when talking with providers.

To support KM's goal of social engagement and life review, the development of a social communication and reminiscence book is warranted. A simple communication board with prompt phrases and social questions should be designed and implemented to uphold this goal. Conversation starters and phrases such as "How is your family?" and "Do you have any interesting plans in the near future?" should be added to support conversational exchange. To support reminiscing and life review, a book should be made with KM's significant life events, formative stories, and experiences, and include pictures of friends and families with some simple text to accompany the pictures. These will allow for a shared context and reminder for storytelling and review. A specific section of this book can also be devoted to interactions with her three grandchildren including kid-friendly symbols of their interests and likes. For example, the oldest grandchild is on a little league baseball team; thus, prompts and pictures can be developed to spur conversation about his current season. A social outing notebook should also be developed consisting of KM's favorite local places for outings, take-out menus, and favorite activities to facilitate choice in social engagement outside of the house.

Next Steps

To implement a therapeutic plan consisting of tool development, patient training, and caregiving training, a short intervention timeline—preferably six to eight visits—should be sufficient. The initial visit would consist of assessment to ensure ability levels and functional declines, establish client preferences and goals, and then determine the appropriate design of the communication boards through trials of different designs, arrangements, and font sizes. Consecutive sessions should be used to design and construct communication boards and external aids for the family with shared input and continued trials for functionality (two to three sessions). Finally, the clinician should focus the training on the use of the boards in a variety of contexts. Once KM seems comfortable with the communication boards and their functions, the next step is to train her caregiver, specifically her wife.

Caregiver training is an essential component of this therapeutic intervention. Once the communication boards and external aids are developed, intervention should focus on shared training with KM and her primary caregiver. Through use of modeling and the teach-back method, the caregiver can be trained to implement the communication boards, build fluency, and troubleshoot problems. Intervention should begin with the clinician modeling the use of conversation starters, presentation of the materials, and solving communication breakdowns. The primary caregiver can then demonstrate use of the boards while the clinician watches and provides real-time feedback and troubleshoots communication breakdowns. Where possible, these procedures should be repeated in a variety of contexts using the full range of materials presented. A medical personnel scenario can also be role-played to ensure both KM and MM fully understand the medical decision-making supports. Some possible goals for intervention are as follows:

- Patient will reduce social isolation risks by using common social messages for greeting, introduction, conversation starters, and turn-taking in four out of five opportunities.
- Patient will use the AAC boards to engage in conversation with a friend/family member five times per week.
- Patient will reduce medical risks and increase medical participation by communicating medical information and physical symptoms with 80% accuracy.

Another option to consider during training is to introduce PAS to both MM and KM. PAS is a technique whereby the communication partner verbally presents the communication options on a person's existing low-technology communication board (e.g., an alphabet display or BB's communication display for ADLs) in an orderly sequence and waits until the communicator indicates "yes" either by head nod, eye blink, thumbs-up gesture, or other preestablished agreed upon signal. Once the communicator has made a selection by indicating "yes," the communication partner can resume the scan, if necessary, or ask the communicator for more detail about their choice. Although this method of communication may initially be slower than pointing directly to a symbol or letter, PAS is both reliable and effective when communication dyads are trained in its use. It decreases the physical demand on the user by eliminating the need for pointing to a symbol on a board. For communication partners who are very familiar with the communication board, the options may be presented auditorily so the user just has to listen rather than look at and/or point at specific options. In this way, the user may have their eyes closed while the communication partner presents choices for communication.

KM's terminal condition means that her functional communication status is likely to decline; thus, she is likely to qualify for additional services should her communication tools cease to serve the family. It is important the family is aware that when there is a change of "prior level of function," they may be eligible for the reinitiation of services. Because the patient's condition is likely to deteriorate, communication boards and environment aids developed for KM may need augmentation or simplification in the future. It is also possible new medical symptoms may emerge or a change in functional cognition may occur, warranting a revision of communication tools. A reinitiation of service could take the form of a short therapeutic plan (three to four visits) to re-create and retrain communication aids and/or address emergent feeding issues. In summary, through the clinician's expertise in communication and cognition, the patient is able to receive critical intervention for their quality of life and their families near her EoL.

References

American Speech-Language-Hearing Association. (n.d.). *End of life issues in speech-language pathology.* http://www.asha.org/SLP/clinical/endoflife/
Chang, W. D., & Bourgeois, M. S. (2020). Effects of visual aids for end-of-life care on decisional capacity of people with dementia. *American Journal of*

Speech-Language Pathology, 29(1), 185–200. https://doi.org/10.1044/2019_AJSLP-19-0028

Fried-Oken, M., & Bardach, L. (2005). End-of-life issues for people who use AAC. *Perspectives on Augmentative and Alternative Communication, 14*(3), 15–19. https://doi.org/10.1044/aac14.3.15

Ghoshal, A., Salins, N., Deodhar, J., Damani, A., & Muckaden, M. A. (2016). Fatigue and quality of life outcomes of palliative care consultation: A prospective, observational study in a tertiary cancer center. *Indian Journal of Palliative Care, 22*(4), 416–426. https://doi.org/10.4103/0973-1075.191766

Hawksley, R., Ludlow, F., Buttimer, H., & Bloch, S. (2017). Communication disorders in palliative care: Investigating the views, attitudes and beliefs of speech and language therapists. *International Journal of Palliative Nursing, 23*(11), 543–551. https://doi.org/10.12968/ijpn.2017.23.11.543

Hui, D., Didwaniya, N., Vidal, M., Shin, S. H., Chisholm, G., Roquemore, J., & Bruera, E. (2014). Quality of end-of-life care in patients with hematologic malignancies: A retrospective cohort study. *Cancer, 120*(10), 1572–1578. https://doi.org/10.1002/cncr.28614

Hurtig, R. R., & Downey, D. A. (2008). *Augmentative and alternative communication in acute and critical care settings.* Plural Publishing.

Kuhl, D., Stanbrook, M. B., & Hébert, P. C. (2010). What people want at the end of life. *Canadian Medical Association Journal, 182*(16), 1707. https://doi.org/10.1503/cmaj.101201

Pollens, R. (2004). Role of the speech-language pathologist in palliative hospice care. *Journal of Palliative Medicine, 7*(5), 694–702. http://doi.org/10.1089/jpm.2004.7.694

Pollens, R. D. (2012). Integrating speech-language pathology services in palliative end-of-life care. *Topics in Language Disorders, 32*, 137–148.

Pollens, R. (2020). Facilitating client ability to communicate in palliative end-of-life care. *Topics in Language Disorders, 40*(3), 264–277. https://doi.org/10.1097/TLD.0000000000000220

Stead, A., Dirks, K., Fryer, M., & Wong, S. (2020). Training future clinicians for work in palliative care. *Topics in Language Disorders, 20*(3), 233–247. https://doi.org/10.1097/TLD.0000000000000219

Stead, A., & McDonnell, C. (2015). End of life care: An opportunity. *Perspectives in Gerontology, 20*(1), 12–15.

Stone, M. J. (2001). Goals of care at the end of life. *Proceedings (Baylor University Medical Center), 14*(2), 134–137. https://doi.org/10.1080/08998280.2001.11927748

Toner, M. A., & Shadden, B. B. (2012). End of life. *Topics in Language Disorders, 32*(2), 111–118. https://doi.org/10.1097/tld.0b013e31825484e0

Vidatak™ Communication Displays. http://www.vidatak.com/

SECTION V
AAC for Persons With Developmental Disabilities

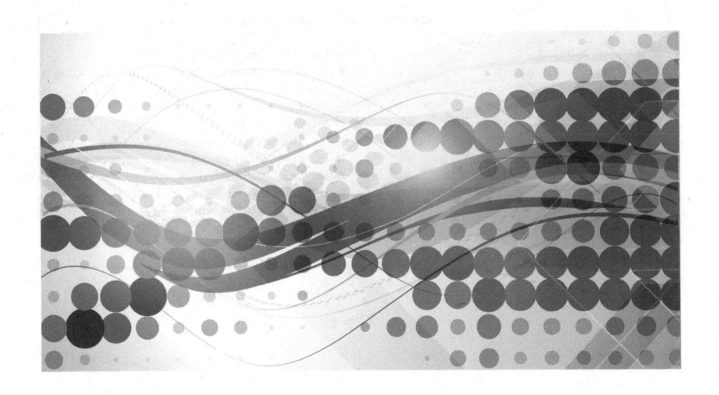

Having established a strong theoretical foundation for augmentative and alternative communication (AAC) fundamentals and service delivery, Section V reiterates these concepts in specific case examples. Section V offers a collection of examples of AAC for persons with developmental disabilities. Before delving into these case examples, Essay 17, *A Parent's Perspective*, reiterates the critical role the speech-language pathologist (SLP) has in not only implementing high-quality services but also involving the family in authentic ways.

AAC for persons with developmental disabilities (Chapter 19), autism spectrum disorder (Chapter 20), and cerebral palsy (Chapter 21) is discussed. Essay 18 revisits the powerful impact AAC can have when serving to augment an individual's existing speech—an important reminder when considering the profiles already discussed in Chapters 19 through 21, as well as those to follow.

Chapter 22 summarizes information about various sensory deficits to offer information about AAC and AAC accommodations for people with auditory and/or visual deficits. Chapter 23 extends this understanding to AAC for individuals with sensory integration challenges and the various ways in which these difficulties can be supported and accommodated. Last, Chapter 24 talks about AAC for individuals with histories of complex trauma. The chapters build upon each other to deepen one's understanding of AAC through examples of individuals with these specific profiles. The ways in which the individual, their partners, and their environment influence the AAC systems and strategies used continue to be displayed within the content of this section.

Key Terms Reviewed in This Section

- AAC intervention
- Accessibility settings
- Arousal
- Attunement
- Autism spectrum disorder
- Buy-in
- Complex trauma
- Cortical visual impairment (CVI)
- Deafblind
- Developmental disability
- Dual sensory impairment
- Dyadic joint attention

- Emotional regulation
- Environmental communication teaching (ECT)
- Gross Motor Function Classification System (GMFCS)
- Intellectual disability
- Investigative intervention
- Language activity monitor (LAM)
- Sensory integration dysfunction
- Sensory processing/integration
- Spontaneous novel utterance generation (SNUG)
- Triadic joint attention

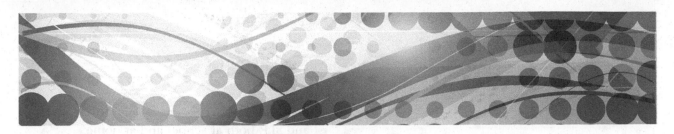

CLINICAL CONSIDERATIONS AND AAC: A PARENT'S PERSPECTIVE

Danielle A. Wagoner

"The most basic of all human needs is to understand and be understood. The best way to understand people is to listen to them."

—Ralph Nichols

Many times, the most important thing you can do for parents is L.I.S.T.E.N.

Language

Think of an augmentative and alternative communication (AAC) system as a language. When I read this analogy for the first time, it was a concept I understood and gave me a new perspective on the bigger picture of AAC. I have always found it very helpful when therapists and professionals use analogies to make new information relatable for that very reason. Our family has a long history with AAC. To sum it all up, we went through roughly five transitions, three different systems, and periods of AAC abandonment over the course of 8 years to end up where we are now. I should explain that we are an active-duty military family and have two children with complex communication needs

(CCNs). The AAC changes were always a result of relocating to a new duty assignment and starting over from scratch with a brand new team.

Now, think about how long it takes to learn a new language (let alone "3"), and how all of the changes and inconsistencies can impact progress. I wish I had known when we started that AAC is less about the device and more about how we use the system to teach language and communication. For example, it was not until about 6 years in and three different communication systems later that I truly understood what modeling was and why it is so important. It is not just about pressing a button to get your needs met. It is about me using the device to immerse my children in what a word means by modeling an action so they can see, hear, and experience what the word on that button means. It is about my responsibility to use the system and model consistently myself without placing any demands or expectations on my children. For my children, using AAC in this way has helped them develop their spoken language and taught them what words mean. Even bigger than that, it has led to the beginning of their ability to advocate for themselves and connect on a different level with the people in their lives.

Include

Include parents in everything. Ask them questions about their child, family life, what they need, what they want, what they hope for. Invite them to observe and participate. Offer consultation and parent training. Educate them on the assessments you use, explain how you arrived at certain answers, and help them understand why you feel what you are proposing is best. Many times I have not been totally on board until I was given information I had not considered that helped me understand why we were doing things a certain way. I would rather have too much information and decide for myself what I think is important as opposed to not receiving enough information. Show parents you value their input. You may be the expert clinician, but they are the expert on their child. They can give you important information and insight about their child that you will not find in their medical or school records, or notice during regular sessions and observations. This information can be helpful when making decisions and considering options for which AAC system might be best for the child. Each family is unique, and there is no one-size-fits-all approach to AAC.

Support

Support the child and family how they need it. It is not just about the child's structured therapeutic sessions with the clinician. It is about using the communication skills learned in those sessions in different environments with different communication partners. One of the most helpful tools and processes for me has been taking videos of myself using the device with my children during certain activities where I could target certain words. I would send them to our AAC specialist and speech-language pathologist (SLP), and they would give me feedback through e-mail, consult notes, and virtual meetings. I was able to go back and watch what I was doing, and eventually started critiquing myself. For our family, I can say with 100% certainty that our success with AAC is a result

of all the support we receive from our AAC specialist and SLP, both at school and at home.

Team

It is important to not only work as a team with families but also consider all consistent communication partners on the child's team beyond the immediate family—teachers, therapists, paraprofessionals, friends, extended family. We are all on the same team, and everyone on the team matters. Be open minded and flexible. Consistency is so important for progress, so it is equally important that everyone on the team is on the same page.

Encourage

Encourage parents no matter how significant or insignificant you think something might be. I will never forget one particular virtual consultation I had with our AAC specialist during the COVID-19 pandemic. I was very motivated and determined to do whatever was necessary so that my childrens' progress would not stall because school was remote. By about 5 to 6 months in, when it was clear there was still no return to normalcy in sight, I began fatiguing. Our AAC specialist had recently taught me how to set up data tracking on the devices, and we arranged a consultation a few weeks later. When it was time for the consultation, I did not want her to see the data tracking since I had lost some steam and felt like a failure. I thought for sure she would be disappointed. Before I could say anything, she got so excited and immediately began applauding how awesome the wordle (word cloud) looked and pointed out all the different words we were using. I was genuinely stunned. Her excitement lifted my spirits and helped me find the motivation I needed to get back on track. Sometimes it is the things you say that you might not even be aware of, or that you may not even remember, that can have a lasting impact on a parent. So, choose encouragement.

Normalize

Normalize nonverbal communication. Normalize what is written in the National Joint Committee for the Communication Needs of Persons with Severe Disabilities (NJC) Communication Bill of Rights.[1] Help give parents the confidence to normalize nonverbal communication and advocate for their child's human right to communicate in the unique way that works for them. There are endless ways of communicating beyond spoken words and listening with your ears. A right is not a privilege. It is an entitlement that belongs to all individuals, regardless of the extent or severity of their disability or difference, that can never be taken away. The more we can normalize nonverbal communication in society, the more individuals with CCNs will have access to their basic human right to communicate.

Always L.I.S.T.E.N.

Language, Include, Support, Team, Encourage, and Normalize. The road to finding what means of communication will work for an individual with CCNs may not always be easy or linear. There is no standard or mainstream way of AAC because we are all unique. However, as long as you stay focused on the goal of communication, you will always be on the right path. And always L.I.S.T.E.N.

"To say that a person feels listened to means a lot more than just their ideas get heard. It's a sign of respect. It makes people feel valued."

—Deborah Tannen, author and professor of linguistics, Georgetown University

---

[1]American Speech-Language-Hearing Association (ASHA). (2021). *Communication Bill of Rights.* https://www.asha.org/njc/communication-bill-of-rights/

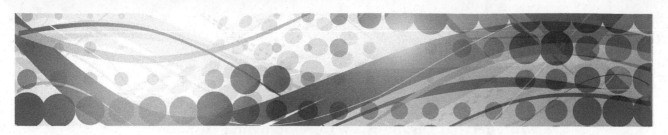

Chapter 19
AAC FOR PERSONS WITH DEVELOPMENTAL DISABILITIES

Jeeva John

The Fundamentals

Augmentative and alternative communication (AAC) tools are commonly recommended intervention strategies for individuals with developmental disabilities and are focused on enhancing communicative competence when speech fails to meet their daily communication needs. Over the years, AAC as an intervention has evolved from being an intervention approach that was considered as an alternative when other speech interventions have failed, to being included and considered early in the intervention process. AAC considerations, especially for individuals with developmental disabilities, need to be seen as a life span intervention approach. This means that the communication tools and AAC strategies identified need to evolve across the individual's life span and its ensuing communication journey.

"Developmental disabilities" is an umbrella term that covers a group of conditions due to impairments in the areas of physical, learning, language, and behavioral development. These disorders may occur anytime from before birth, up until the age of 22 years. Developmental disorders (DDs) would include diagnostic classifications for intellectual disability, autism and pervasive developmental disorders, cerebral palsy, and specific syndromes that exhibit intellectual disabilities and/ or other behavioral manifestations such as Down

syndrome, Prader-Willi syndrome, Williams syndrome, and Rett syndrome, for example (Odom et al., 2007). The National Association of Councils on Developmental Disabilities define developmental disabilities as severe, lifelong disabilities that manifest before the individual turns 22 years and that are likely to be chronic and substantially limit the individual's ability to function in three or more of the following major areas: self-care, receptive-expressive language, learning, mobility, self-direction, capacity for independent living, and economic self-sufficiency.

The Centers for Disease Control and Prevention outline the pre-, peri-, and postnatal causes and risk factors that lead to developmental disorders. They also report an increase in the prevalence of developmental disabilities based on data collected from a survey conducted during 2009 to 2017 of parents of more than 88,000 children, ages 3 to 17 years (American Speech-Language-Hearing Association [ASHA], 2019). The survey completed across the country indicated that the prevalence of autism, intellectual disability, and attention deficit hyperactivity disorder increased during that time, with a concurrent decrease in the percentage of children in the broad category of "other developmental delay." The number of American children with developmental disabilities rose to 17.8% (one in six) in 2017, from 16.2% in 2009 (Zablotsky et al., 2019). Specific increases in prevalence among

---

Intellectual Disability vs. Developmental Disability

The terms "developmental disability" and "intellectual disability" (ID) are often heard being used interchangeably, but they are distinctively different. Intellectual disabilities are included under developmental disabilities, and the title is a term that now replaces the term "mental retardation." An individual with ID presents with below-average cognitive abilities and is further characterized by impairments in both intellectual as well as adaptive functioning. Impairments in intellectual functioning show up as challenges in their ability to learn new information, recall, reason, problem-solve, and so on, while impairments of adaptive behaviors include conceptual skills (related to language, literacy, basic num-

ber concepts), social skills, as well as practical skills that include activities of daily living, safety, understanding and following rules, travel and transportation, money awareness, and telling time, for example. ID can also present itself in varying severities. Interventions around ID have changed significantly as the terminology has evolved to remove focus from intellectual functioning to instead focus on development of functional skills, personal well-being, identifying adequate and appropriate community and family support systems, and using skill development, as well as adaptations of the environment to develop over competences.

---

boys, older children, white and Hispanic children, those living in urban areas, and those with less-educated mothers, among other factors were noted. Variances associated with demographics or socio-economics may likely be due to greater awareness or improved access to health care.

Taking the perspective of the natural variability in the development of language makes it challenging to decipher the presence of a language disorder in the early development of individuals with developmental and intellectual disorders. The population of individuals with developmental and intellectual disabilities is extremely heterogeneous, making it impossible to make generalizations about the language abilities of these individuals. Language delay and language disorder may not be seen as mutually exclusive. There is a prevalence of delayed onset of language development in this population. This presents a notable reduction in the quantity of language produced, looking more like the language abilities of a chronologically younger person (i.e., the expressive language presenting shorter sentences, less sophisticated grammatical structures, and less diverse vocabulary) (Kaderavek, 2010). Only some children with language delays eventually present as having a language disorder. Children with developmental and intellectual disabilities may have significantly impaired speech

intelligibility. They may often present with stronger receptive language abilities than expressive, and these can occur in isolation as well as together. When working with individuals with any developmental disabilities, there are numerous factors that can impact communication development (e.g., delays in development in other domains, such as cognitive, motor, and social domains, can directly influence the individual's language and communication development).

Challenging Behaviors and the Role of Speech-Language Pathologists

A common characteristic of individuals with developmental and/or intellectual disabilities is that they tend to engage in challenging behaviors. These problem behaviors can include noncompliance, tantrums, screaming, hitting, physical aggression, and self-injurious behaviors, as well. These challenging behaviors often have a function to them (e.g., a child with significant intellectual and developmental disabilities may demonstrate an interest to play with someone by hitting them). These socially unaccepted communication acts limit the child's ability to express themselves accurately and engage socially with peers and adults. In some situations, problem behaviors may serve the function of meeting a need, getting attention, and getting social interaction. In other situations, they may result from frustration of not comprehending language, or not being able to express oneself adequately, or both.

Bopp, Brown, and Mirenda (2004) have summarized the research regarding the use of functional communication training and visual schedules as positive behavior support intervention strategies. They also emphasize the importance of SLPs being actively involved in providing AAC supports in a transdisciplinary model, where they need to become familiar with intervention approaches that are implemented by other professionals in order to support the use of AAC and visual supports (the distinction noted in Essay 15) as they support communication-based positive behavior support interventions. SLPs are uniquely positioned between problem behavior and communication, as we have training in verbal, nonverbal, and awareness of using visual support to augment communication (Bopp et al., 2004). Additionally, SLPs are particularly suited in working with professionals across disciplines and environments to determine what the communication function of the behavior is and determining the most appropriate message that can be used to replace that message.

Children with developmental disabilities are also much more than a set of skill deficits and challenging behaviors. They have positive personality traits and social skills that often exceed the stereotypical assumptions and expectations of them. They tend to be loving, affectionate, happy, nurturing toward family, friends, and animals, sociable, friendly, and motivated by social interactions (Colavita et al., 2014). In the author's clinical experience, it has been noted that most often individuals with developmental disabilities have a desire to be seen as competent and active members of their community. They often want to make friends; demonstrate their sense of humor; gain the attention and appreciation of parents, peers, teachers, and other communication partners; and often need to be supported with the language and social skills to execute it effectively. The individual's strengths and motivations to interact socially will vary among the many developmental disabilities but must guide the AAC intervention process.

AAC Evolves Across Their Life Span

Difficulty with communication will affect the individual's ability to communicate effectively across their life span, with varying contexts and their respective demands. In the early ages of an individual, the SLP can develop AAC systems with the family. The SLP might need to coach the family in learning that communication, and hence AAC, plays a crucial role in foundational development, literacy, self-regulation, as well as being able to control one's own environment, and get their needs met at all stages of development. Not being able to control their environment as a result of an inability to communicate can lead to immense frustration, aggression in the individuals, as well as a heightened sense of frustration on part of the communication partners. Exclusively relying on verbal speech or AAC may not be the appropriate fit, especially in situations where problem behaviors exist, or are beginning to emerge, and the individual experiences receptive and expressive language deficits. SLPs are also in a position to motivate the family to avoid the "wait and see" approach with their child.

As these individuals transition into academic environments, the demands related to communicating with unfamiliar communication partners and learning new information call for the SLP and the family to reexamine the appropriateness of the communication system in place. The impacts of language delays or disorders can be seen in the development of literacy skills as well as relationship development with peers. Later, these individuals also transition into adolescence where they will interact with new communication partners in the community as co-workers, supervisors, case managers, roommates, and so on, and will be faced with a different set of communication and social demands.

The use of an effective and efficient AAC system with age- and context-appropriate messages is of critical importance as they will need an effective method of self-expression throughout their life span. Communication partners need to be coached and guided to anticipate numerous changes in the AAC system, either in the form of vocabulary or the tool as a whole, as the system will have to evolve with the individual to meet these dynamic communication demands. Often students may begin their communication journey with one type of dedicated speech-generating device and later transition to a more sophisticated tool, or different platform, that can be identified.

Establish "Buy-in" and Prepare for the Communication Journey

Clinicians and parents often fear that AAC will limit the individual with developmental disabilities from being able to communicate or resort to speech. Research indicates that AAC intervention has significant benefits toward the development of communicative competence and language skills. Over the past 30 years, the advancement in technology and AAC interventions make it imperative that individuals with complex communication needs, regardless of the cause, need access to AAC early in life as a first line of defense in the work of developing communication skills (Romski et al., 2015). Informing and coaching families about these facts and simultaneously demystifying myths about AAC is the beginning of the buy-in process.

The buy-in process is often under-recognized as starting as early as the first interaction the clinicians have with the individual and the family. AAC is typically not the desired outcome for their child, and families may need the clinician to approach them with compassion, patience, and a readiness to meet them where they are at. These early interactions form a foundation for the ongoing buy-in process around AAC, and incorporate AAC tools and strategies not just into the daily activities of the individual with complex communication needs but also those of their numerous communication partners. Family members and other communication partners are likely to have recurring moments of concern, hesitation, and challenges that impact their ability to retain buy-in to the AAC process, especially when problems around communication and the AAC system arise. Creating a routine time to train, coach, and engage in active discussions regarding the myths and facts about AAC, appropriate partner engagement strategies, AAC as it evolves, and facts about the AAC system being used also contributes toward ensuring that families,

other communication partners, and the individuals remain bought-in to the AAC intervention process.

Assessment and Selecting a Tool

The assessment process should highlight the gaps in receptive and expressive abilities, as well as demonstrate the individual's reliance on communication partners to get their needs met. In some situations, the SLP may receive a client with developmental disabilities on whom a comprehensive speech and language assessment has already been completed and AAC intervention with appropriate recommendations were included; in many other situations this is not the case. SLPs need to be mindful to not invalidate another professional's input but also need to emphasize the importance of incorporating AAC early in the intervention.

The SLP will need information on whether these individuals have yet established symbolic communication. Nonsymbolic communication including gestures, vocalizations, facial expressions, proxemics (when an individual uses space between themselves and people/objects/activities to express preferences and interests) and eye gaze may exist in conventional and unconventional means. Symbolic communication including signs, spoken or written words, pictures, and objects may also exist in the same way. Information regarding communicative intent and the functions of their communicative behavior is also important. The framework provided by the Continuum of Communication Independence (Dowden & Cook, 2002) gives the SLP pertinent information to identify individuals as having skills that range from having unreliable use of symbols for communication to competent, consistent, and reliable users of any symbol set to convey messages in varying contexts to various partners (emerging → context-dependent → independent communicators).

Additionally, the Communication Matrix (Rowland, 2011) is an online tool with a series of partner questions designed to identify the kinds of communication behaviors a child is using to communicate and the several functions of that communication behavior. It gives information about which one of seven levels of communication the individual is at and allows a clinician to observe specific strengths and needs in communication for very emergent communicators. Through this tool, clinicians can have a baseline for how a student communicates using their current communication techniques and establish targets moving them along the continuum (with the support of a handy visual matrix), expanding their repertoire of modes and functions to include symbolic communication as soon as they are ready. The matrix also gives results for each student for repeated administrations that can be compared over time, to visually compare progress.

Using the information obtained from early assessment, the selection of the type of tool being used needs careful consideration and trial. Low- and high-tech tools should be considered for all individuals regardless of their age. Recent research indicates that implementation of high-tech AAC can be effective for most individuals with intellectual and developmental disorders of all ages through all school years (Ganz et al., 2017). It also supports the use of high-tech AAC in a natural context to promote generalization of learned skills. It has also been noted that preliterate children with developmental disabilities rely on one of two types of AAC system displays: visual scene displays (VSDs) or grid displays (Light et al., 2019). VSDs can be either low-tech or high-tech and provide important context and meaning for prelowrate individuals.

When selecting AAC tools, a clinician needs to consider a multimodal approach to communication. This approach holds even greater importance, since without its benefits the individual's functional ability to communicate across environments will be compromised. The communicative ability, and eventually the desire to engage socially, of many AAC users with developmental disabilities can be hindered by a number of factors. Factors including fine and gross motor skills, cognitive impairment, social stigma, language, and literacy level can make effective communication and social interaction through a single mode difficult and complicated. "Multimodal communication" is a term used to describe all the different modes we employ with each other, every day, that should be honored and added to the communication toolkit of any AAC

user. This may be via spoken language, texting, e-mailing, handwriting, using photographs and images, social media, body language, gesturing, and pointing.

Investigative Intervention

SLPs need to press forward with an investigative mindset throughout the intervention process. Using the structure provided by the SETT (student, environment, tasks, and tools) framework (Zabala, 1995), SLPs can develop this mindset by recurrently investigating the effectiveness of the tools and strategies set in place and also provide the information needed in designing an effective and meaningful AAC tool. This mindset can be developed by acknowledging that in the beginning phases of intervention, exploration and ongoing analysis are critical. Tools like the SETT framework can be used not just as a formal assessment and report organizational tool, but as a tool to help develop an investigative mindset. It prompts the clinician to consistently focus away from the tool and instead on the student's unique skills, preferences, and motivators, which could evolve with the individual across environments and developmental phases. This also gives the clinician the opportunity to observe how the student learns. SLPs may observe whether the student learns best when introduced to isolated information in a structured, simplified presentation, or if they thrive by learning in context with lots of examples, activities, and models. Information obtained from preference inventories or from surveying communication partners paired with observations are likely to change with maturation (e.g., preferences in food, music, book, media, preferred communication partners, etc.).

SLPs may also repeatedly survey and assess the environment, which includes the communication partners as well as the physical setup of the environment, throughout the intervention process. The resources, materials, and stimuli in the home, school, and work environments can change and will need to be actively observed for change in order to support the communication needs of the individual. Other characteristics, such as how loud, how big or small, or how crowded the environment is might also impact the kind of tool the student is encouraged to use in that environment (e.g., the use of an iPad may be discouraged during a swim class or an active physical education class, but instead a low-tech board with pertinent visuals may be more appropriate). The attitudes, capacities, and communication expectations of all communication partners will need to be observed and respectfully investigated, not only to gauge continued buy-in but also to determine areas in which ongoing coaching and collaboration need to occur. Recurrently assessing the environment also provides the SLP with information regarding meaningful and context-appropriate social messages to be had with these partners.

Surveying the tasks and tools being used is an essential part of the intervention process. Actively observing the nature of the tasks that the individual is engaging in, determining whether they continue to be motivating and supportive of language development is also crucial. When surveying the tool being used, it may become apparent that the individual might benefit from using multiple modes of communication. It is critical that this multimodal approach is openly acknowledged and advocated for. Communication partners at home, school, and other environments will need support through training and coaching to accept the use of gestures, pointing, pantomiming, low-tech pictures, messages on AAC devices, text messages on phones, and photos and pictures on their phones/mobile devices in addition to the newly selected AAC device. It is also essential for the SLP to streamline which modes are most effective in which environments or with particular communication partners. Students may hesitate to use texting or typing at home and prefer pointing and pantomiming, especially if there is a language difference at home.

Designing a Meaningful Communication System

As SLPs, we are practicing in the midst of numerous technological advances that have improved the quality of AAC tools and symbols that we have access to. Low- and high-tech AAC tools are easily customizable with photos, symbols, and 3-D printed objects, for example, that can be adapted to the unique supports that students with developmental disabilities may need as they learn to communicate and navigate the nuances of augmented tools.

High-tech speech-generating devices and communication applications for touch screen tablets now come preloaded with numerous levels of robust vocabulary sets with varying grid sizes. Despite these advances, vocabulary sets may not seem ready to go right out of the box for each individual student. At cursory glance, some may seem overwhelming to the student as well as the communication partner. The challenge becomes knowing how to begin with vocabulary selection while designing meaningful communication tools. SLPs need to note that while most devices are designed with comprehensive vocabulary sets, customization to the individual's interests, preferences, needs, and culture is essential, especially in the early parts of the process. It is also critical that the SLP include the student in the process of customization and design of the AAC system. This approach applies to low- and high-tech systems.

As elaborated upon in Chapter 7, vocabulary sets, regardless of ability and technology level, should consist of a mixture of core, fringe, and personalized vocabulary. These words, specifically fringe and personal vocabulary words, are likely to change rapidly, and the SLP needs to be prepared for this to change, and simultaneously prepare other team members. By way of partner-informed inventories or observations, these words can be surveyed and programmed with the individual using the system. It is important to include familiar and known words in vocabulary sets as well as additional words that the student can learn to use across activities, settings, and with several communication partners. In order to make decisions on adding words with which students are not yet familiar, clinicians are called to presume competence of these individuals to learn new information, expand their repertoire of interests, and be able to express more complex ideas.

In addition to core, fringe, and personal vocabulary, it is vital to incorporate the use of social phrases and quick sentences. Individuals with developmental disabilities repeatedly demonstrate a desire to connect with peers and adults around them. Providing access to social phrases also prompts communication partners and clinicians to mindfully create opportunities for these individuals to use AAC for more than just requesting, rejecting, and answering questions. Directly addressing social interaction with clearly accessible messages is also likely to establish more buy-in through relationship building, peer interactions, sharing of jokes, and telling stories. When incorporating social phrases, it is important to include social messages that help them (a) participate in daily activities across environments (e.g., home, school, grocery store, parks, etc.); (b) express themselves and help them advocate for themselves (e.g., "I have something to say," "that is not on my device," "I don't like that," "I want something different"); and (c) send social messages to support the development of friendships, share information about themselves, and ask questions to curb their curiosity about others? (e.g., "what is your favorite ___?" and "that's cool!" for example).

Consultation Services

When working with AAC and individuals with developmental disabilities, SLPs are encouraged to include time for collaboration and consultation with the team as a whole into their service delivery model. A one-to-one or small group pull-out service delivery model is the traditional route taken when determining how to work within the schools. Ganz, Hong, Leuthold, and Yllades (2019) highlight that these pull-out services should not dominate the services provided to the individuals as those AAC skills learned outside the student's naturalistic environment are less likely to generalize. Through individual or small group pull-out services, the clinician can create opportunities for targeted skill instruction, but those skills will need to quickly generalize in the natural environment to actually make an impact on the student's communication development. Active consultation services are those in which the clinician is able to model on the AAC device to the individual in naturalistic settings, model partner strategies, coach, observe, guide, provide real-time feedback to the individual

using AAC as well as the communication partners all without having to directly design or control the activity or the environment.

Consultation services are powerful when planned thoughtfully after observing and surveying the needs of the teacher, the individual using the AAC system, and the other communication partners (peers and adults). Consultation services should not be reserved for after the individual demonstrates progress in small groups and one-to-one sessions but should be incorporated from the beginning to create more successful communication opportunities for the individual learning to use AAC with novice AAC communication partners. These services are also an optimal opportunity for the SLP to model and teach ways to embed strategies such as asking open-ended questions and using simplistic vocabulary in statements and questions. SLPs may also consider constructing lessons with the teacher as a context for teaching these strategies as well.

Key Takeaways

- Retain communication partner's and the individual's buy-in throughout the intervention process.
- Employ an investigative mindset throughout intervention.
- Encourage the use of multiple modalities for communication.
- Include an active consultation model in addition to traditional service delivery models.

Case Study: KC

Clinical Profile and Communication Needs

The Individual

KC is a 19-year-old young woman with a diagnosis of Down syndrome. She presents with complex communication needs and requires access to AAC to be universally understood given her significantly reduced verbal intelligibility. She is social and enjoys engaging with others. She loves her family and friends. Being able to connect with these important people about their day and her interests brings her joy and is something she looks forward to. She is a vibrant and active member of her community and enjoys anything that is in the realm of performing arts (as seen in Figure 19–1, in her role in a local play). She is a member of a band and partakes in theater classes. Special treats for KC involve musicals and theater productions. She loves to look over playbills and magazines. She has a particular interest in sharing jokes, reciting portions of Shrek the Musical, getting her nails and hair done, and themed birthday parties or get-togethers.

Their Communication Partners

KC spends most of her time with her housemates, mother, father, and their respective families. Text messaging her parents and family is a highly motivating activity, and often her most favorite thing to do. She also receives paraprofessional support from her transition/vocation program, and connects with fellow students, classmates, and educators in the various programs in which she partakes.

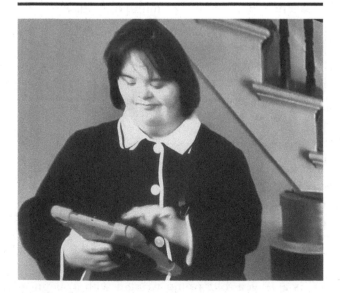

Figure 19–1. KC acting in a local play.

Their Environment

KC, like many young adults her age, desires independence. She currently lives in a shared living environment with one other housemate and a guardian. This is her home. She sees her mother and father every week and will either visit or host them. She participates in daily programs focused on theater, self-advocacy, and other important and enjoyable life skills, where she interacts with a familiar group of students, educators, and mentors. She makes use of what her community has to offer and is often walking into town for lunch (as seen in a local smoothie store in Figure 19–2), some grocery shopping, to get her nails done, or to go to the bank or post office. She has adult support for these tasks and activities.

AAC Considerations

KC demonstrates strong communicative intent. She often seeks out opportunities to connect and engage with her peers and several other individuals in her community. However, her verbal communication is limited, and she uses general gestures intermittently. KC most often uses loose verbal approximations that are hard for unfamiliar (and even familiar) listeners to decipher. She needs access to methods of communication that are understood by all listeners across a number of settings and contexts.

The AAC System or Service

KC has been using AAC across her life span. She has used AAC for a number of years, since the early age of 4 years. However, the specific type and brand of AAC system has changed with her evolving needs as she has transitioned from a school-aged student to a young adult. It is important to note that KC has had access to AAC, signs, and opportunities to develop literacy from a very early age, where her parents advocated strongly for language and literacy exposure. These recurrent and numerous opportunities have enriched and empowered her as an individual with a message to express, as well as allowing her to manipulate words and sounds early

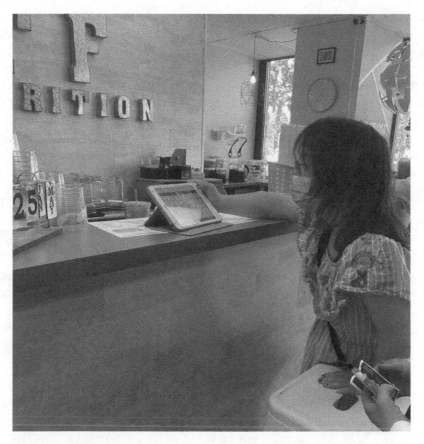

Figure 19–2. KC ordering a smoothie in her community.

on. KC's mother and school team made opportunities for her to engage with literacy even while her prognosis for reading was unpredictable. In KC's early education years, the idea of "literacy for ALL" was just beginning to be discussed and researched extensively. Given the nature and severity of her speech and language deficits, she was fitted with a Prentke Romich Springboard low voice output system with a 36-button grid from the age of 5 years. This system offered her access to a combination of core and fringe vocabulary, with words such as "I," "you," "want," "come," "get," and "help," as well as categories spanning colors, food items, actions, places, and more.

As she progressed in school and intervention, so did her communication system. KC transitioned to Prentke Romich's Vantage low with a 45-button grid, and then onto a 60-button grid. KC continued to work on goals that focused on increasing her ini-

tiation with the device, her utterance combinations and length, and the breadth of her vocabulary. KC has often required encouragement and prompting to use her AAC device, and needed careful implementation of a least-to-most prompting hierarchy to get her to initiate use of high-tech AAC as part of a total communication repertoire.

When KC got a cell phone at the age of 16 years, her AAC needs shifted. She naturally transitioned to texting through iMessage using single typed words, photos, and emojis. This was a very age-appropriate transition that should be anticipated in other young teenage individuals using AAC who have the necessary literacy skills. In an effort to provide KC with a more mobile solution offering programming flexibility, her team moved to Proloquo2Go®. With this system, KC was able to access the AAC app on both a cell phone (larger in size; iPhone 7 Plus) and an iPad. Figure 19–3 shows KC's personalized AAC device and how the team has incorporated core and fringe vocabulary, as well as meaningful short phrases for quick messages to meet KC's social interactions.

Given KC's fine motor dexterity, the overlay on the cell phone needed to have no more than 25 buttons displayed. This represented a significant decrease from the 60-button display of the Vantage low. Because of this, KC's team worked to inventory

her current, future, and anticipated language and communication needs. The team worked collaboratively with various stakeholders in each of the aforementioned environments to ensure that the vocabulary and organization of the overlay were relevant and meaningful for KC.

In discussion with the team, additional elements related to pacing emerged as important features to address in designing an AAC system to

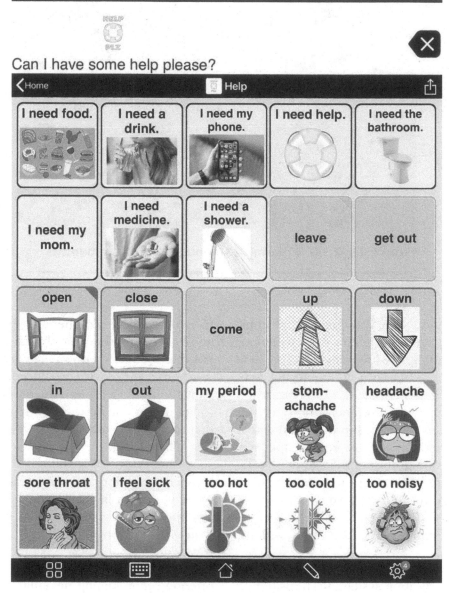

Figure 19–3. AAC overlay with core and fringe vocabulary as well as meaningful short phrases for quick messages. Screenshot from Proloquo2Go® ©AssistiveWare, SymbolStix symbols ©N2Y, LLC.

meet KC's unique needs. More specifically, team members noted that it took too much time for KC to put together a message word-by-word, and by the time she had a message to share, her peers had moved on with the conversation or had appeared to lose interest, despite support in the area. KC's overlay was therefore programmed to offer a wide variety of phrase starters and preprogrammed messages in addition to core and fringe words for novel utterance generation. Figure 19–4 shows KC's personalized phrases and messages that support her in initiating and maintaining social interactions.

KC's AAC consultant worked with KC and stakeholders in each of KC's daily environments (home, programs, and within the community) to modify the overlay as needed, work on establishing opportunities for meaningful engagement and participation, and help stakeholders feel comfortable creating and maintaining opportunities for reciprocal exchanges.

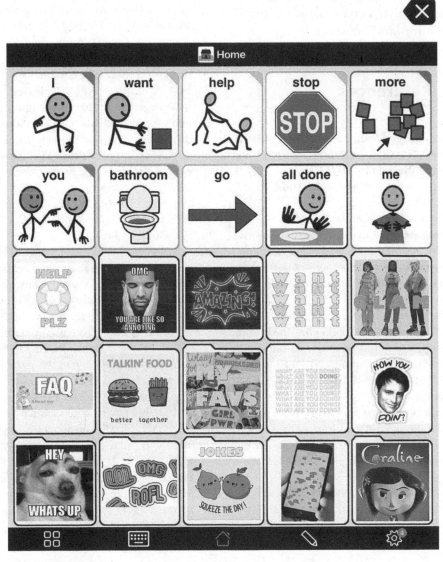

Figure 19–4. An example of personalizing social phrases to match KC's interests. Screenshot from Proloquo2Go® ©AssistiveWare, SymbolStix symbols ©N2Y, LLC.

Next Steps

With the customized AAC overlays established for use on KC's iPhone and iPad, KC's AAC consultant will monitor her success and progress through weekly sessions. Following an active consultation model, the consultant is able to work alongside KC and her communication partners in various environments. The goals focus on increasing independence in using the customized vocabulary in the context of conversational exchanges with multiple communication partners, supporting timely participation in classes, and improving on the viability of text messaging through a combination of Proloquo2Go share features and iMessage.

References

American Speech-Language-Hearing Association (ASHA). (2019, December 24). CDC reports 1 in 6 children has developmental disabilities. *ASHA Leader, 24*(12). https://leader.pubs.asha.org/doi/10.1044/leader.nib1.24122019.12

Bopp, K. D., Brown, K. E., & Mirenda, P. (2004). Speech-language pathologists' roles in the delivery of positive behavior support for individuals with developmental disabilities. *American Journal of Speech-Language Pathology, 13*(1), 5–19. https://doi.org/10.1044/1058-0360(2004/003)

Centers for Disease Control and Prevention. (2020, November 12). *Facts about developmental disabilities.* https://www.cdc.gov/ncbddd/developmentaldisabilities/facts.html#:~:text=Developmental%20disabilities%20are%20a%20group,last%20throughout%20a%20person's%20lifetime

Colavita, V. A., Luthra, N., & Perry, A. (2014). Brief report: Strengths and challenges of children with a developmental disability: A qualitative analysis of parent perceptions. *Journal on Developmental Disabilities, 20*(3), 80–87.

Dowden, P. A., & Cook, A. M. (2002). Selection techniques for individuals with motor impairments. In J. Reichle, D. Beukelman, & J. Light (Eds.), *Implement-ing an augmentative communication system: Exemplary strategies for beginning communicators.* Paul H. Brookes.

Ganz, J. B., Hong, E. R., Leuthold, E., & Yllades, V. (2019). Naturalistic augmentative and alternative communication instruction for practitioners and individuals with autism. *Intervention in School and Clinic, 55*(1), 58–64. https://doi.org/10.1177/1053451219833012

Ganz, J. B., Morin, K. L., Foster, M. J., Vannest, K. J., Genç Tosun, D., Gregori, E. V., & Gerow, S. L. (2017). High-technology augmentative and alternative communication for individuals with intellectual and developmental disabilities and complex communication needs: A meta-analysis. *Augmentative and Alternative Communication, 33*(4), 224–238. https://doi.org/10.1080/07434618.2017.1373855

Kaderavek, J. (2010). *Language disorders in children: Fundamental concepts of assessment and intervention* (pp. 248–250). Pearson.

Light, J., Wilkinson, K. M., Thiessen, A., Beukelman, D. R., & Fager, S. K. (2019). Designing effective AAC displays for individuals with developmental or acquired disabilities: State of the science and future research directions. *Augmentative and Alternative Communication, 35*(1), 42–55. https://doi.org/10.1080/07434618.2018.1558283

Odom, S. L., Horner, R. H., Snell, M. E., & Blacher, J. (Eds.). (2007). *Handbook of developmental disabilities.* Guilford Press.

Romski, M. A., Sevcik, R. A., Barton-Hulsey, A., & Whitmore, A. S. (2015). Early intervention and AAC: What a difference thirty years makes. *Augmentative Alternative Communication, 31*, 181–202.

Rowland, C. (2011). *Communication Matrix* [Measurement instrument]. https://www.communicationmatrix.org

Zabala, J. (1995, March). *The SETT Framework: Critical areas to consider when making informed assistive technology decisions* [Paper presentation]. Florida Assistive Technology Impact Conference and Technology and Medial Division of Council for Exceptional Children, Orlando, FL. https://eric.ed.gov/?id=ED381962

Zablotsky, B., Black, L. I., Maenner, M. J., Schieve, L. A., Danielson, M. L., Bitsko, R. H., . . . Boyle, C. A. (2019). Prevalence and trends of developmental disabilities among children in the United States: 2009–2017. *Pediatrics, 144*(4), e20190811. https://doi.org/10.1542/peds.2019-0811

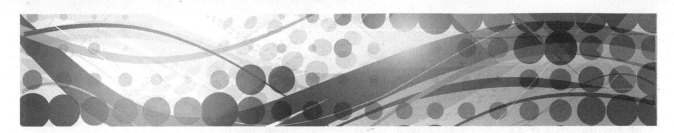

Chapter 20

AAC FOR PERSONS WITH AUTISM SPECTRUM DISORDER

Tanushree Saxena-Chandhok, Deborah Xinyi Yong,
and Sarah Miriam Yong Oi Tsun

Fundamentals

Autism spectrum disorder (ASD) is a pervasive developmental disorder characterized by deficits in social communication and restricted, repetitive patterns of behavior, interests, or activities (American Psychiatric Association, 2013). Individuals with ASD may have significant speech and language skills deficits (Ganz et al., 2011). Recent research studies suggest that 25% to 30% of the children diagnosed with ASD have significant communication needs and remain nonverbal or minimally verbal (Rose et al., 2016; Tager-Flusberg & Kasari, 2013).

When the ability to communicate is severely impaired, the use of an augmentative and alternative communication (AAC) system can become a suitable means for communication (Light, 1989; Light & McNaughton, 2014). AAC can either augment or support an individual's limited or lack of speech abilities, or replace it altogether. AAC refers to the devices, systems, strategies, and tools that assist in communication, apart from use of natural speech. Research has increasingly supported the use of AAC for individuals with ASD to enable effective communication and language development while reducing challenging behaviors. A variety of aided and unaided AAC systems have been used with individuals who have ASD. Unaided systems including manual signs (Total Communication, Makaton signs) and aided systems such as use of visual graphic symbols (including Picture Exchange Communication Systems, PECS), and speech-generating devices (SGDs) have been widely used. Visual supports and social stories have also been identified as effective teaching tools for children with ASD, which present information in the form of photographs, pictures, or illustrations. These supports develop an understanding of a situation or task and its (social) expectations, and manage challenging behaviors while tapping into the individual's strong visual skills.

The selection of a suitable AAC system requires a broad understanding of the individual with ASD. An in-depth AAC assessment and well-planned intervention goals and processes can maximize the possibility of successful and effective communication for the individual using AAC, across contexts and communication partners.

SETT Framework

The assessment process can be guided by several frameworks or models. One such assessment framework is the SETT framework (as introduced in previous chapters), established by Joy Zabala. It is a four-part model that promotes collaborative decision-making in service design and delivery in assistive technology (AT) and is also frequently used in AAC intervention. SETT is an acronym for student, environment, tasks, and tools (Zabala, 2005).

In each part of the model, the assessment team considers questions designed to guide and deepen discussion about the client. In the *student* section, the team considers questions relating to the student's current abilities and special education needs. The *environment* section explores the support given to the student and communication partners, attitudes and expectations of the family and school, along with access issues and the instructional arrangement in his school and home environment. When exploring *tasks*, the specific tasks that occur in the student's natural environments that enable progress toward mastery of goals and objectives and active involvement in his home and school environments are considered. The information gathered about the student, environments, and tasks is used to select the tools during the AAC assessment. *Tools* include devices, services, strategies, training, accommodations, and modifications—everything that is needed to help the student succeed (Zabala, 2005). SETT's holistic framework for AAC prescription and intervention can be a valuable tool for AAC for individuals with ASD, as it focuses on the communication abilities across varied contexts.

Communicative Competence

It is imperative to consider the different communicative competencies that enable an individual with AAC to become an effective and autonomous communicator, across settings and communication partners. In Light (1989), competence is defined as "the state of being functionally adequate in daily communication and of having sufficient knowledge, judgment, and skills to communicate effectively in daily life" (p. 138). Three constructs play an important role in this definition, namely,

■ the functionality of communication (whether communication using the AAC system is functional in nature)
■ adequacy of communication (whether the individual using AAC can adequately convey

information at a desired environment at any given time)
■ sufficiency of knowledge, judgment, and skill (referring to the ability and knowledge of the AAC system by the individual who is learning to use AAC).

The four communicative competencies (operational, linguistic, social, and strategic; Light, 1989) need to be addressed in parallel during goal planning. The ability to attain these competencies can be influenced by specific psychosocial factors, such as motivation, confidence, attitude, and resilience of the individual using AAC (Light & McNaughton, 2014).

A baseline assessment across the competencies provides a good starting point to identify intervention goals. Appropriate tools, such as the AAC Profile (Kovach, 2009) can identify and measure the skill sets under each specific competency. Caregiver's communicative competencies can be measured, and training can further their abilities to support AAC use.

AAC Intervention Strategies

AAC-based interventions support individuals with complex communication needs (CCN) in becoming effective and efficient communicators (Dodd & Gorey, 2014). Communication partners selectively and sequentially apply new communication skills in order to address the challenges of communicating effectively with persons who use AAC (PWUAAC) and to support the communication of these individuals in a wide variety of contexts (Kent-Walsh & McNaughton, 2005).

For the purposes of this chapter, the four AAC strategies highlighted will be as follows:

1. *Aided Language Stimulation (ALS).* ALS is a clinical strategy in which the facilitator points out picture symbols on an individual's communication display in conjunction with ongoing language stimulation (Goossens' et al., 1992). The provision of ALS, also called modeling, promotes communication and comprehension through AAC, enhances

language proficiency, and develops communication competence.

2. *Teaching Core Vocabulary.* A robust vocabulary system of core words (that are used across settings) and fringe words (pertinent to a specific situation) is crucial in developing effective communication. AAC intervention needs to consider the teaching of core vocabulary as these words can generalize across different communication settings (Hammond, 2017).

3. *Expectant Waiting.* Individuals who use AAC need sufficient time to claim their turn, process what they want to say, or compose their sentence. The use of expectant delay, a focus on the child, expectant body posture, and sufficient time should be incorporated into the act of waiting (Light, 2005). Waiting is also more helpful than a question or a command because overuse of those can build prompt dependency or learned helplessness (Zangari, 2014).

4. *Use of Prompts.* Different types of physical, visual, or gestural prompts are sometimes used during AAC instruction with individuals with ASD. Prompts should be used in combination with other AAC intervention strategies. It is important to fade prompts as soon as possible so the individual does not become prompt dependent, or reliant on prompts to perform a new skill (MacDuff et al., 2001).

The Role of the Caregiver in AAC Intervention

The caregiver plays an important role in the AAC intervention. Primary caregiver–implemented interventions promoting generalization of skills to multiple settings have been used effectively with individuals with ASD and their families (Kaiser et al., 2000). We can also extrapolate the effectiveness from existing research related to other developmental disabilities (Ganz & Hong, 2014).

The wider AAC literature supports the important role of the caregiver in the teaching of communication interactions skills and their generalization

as they interact with the PWUAAC in a wider range of communication contexts than educators or clinicians (Kaiser et al., 1998). Caregivers may not initially possess the AAC-specific skills and may require coaching and training to facilitate meaningful exchanges. Kent-Walsh and McNaughton (2005) noted that behaviors of untrained communication partners may result in a PWUAAC that is passive and rarely initiates conversation. They advocate the use of a training model involving observation, demonstration, and self-introspection, and they postulate that the communication partner can learn to use facilitative interaction skills and strategies to better support the individual who uses AAC.

The variability and individuality of an ASD diagnosis make the AAC assessment challenging. An in-depth assessment across skills is necessary, including but not limited to social, communication, sensory, motor, prelanguage skills, and challenging behaviors. The presence of social communication, sensory, and challenging behaviors may impact and limit the communication partners, motivators, and environments of interaction for the individual with ASD. A clear understanding of the individual and their environments is an important part of the assessment, goal setting, and intervention process.

AAC presents information through visual symbols, which is most suited for the visual learning style seen in many individuals with ASD. Successful AAC adoption and use are not dependent only on the appropriate selection of symbols and an AAC device. Other areas that play important roles include AAC instruction and training, the environment, the communication partner's abilities and support, and the communication needs of the individual with ASD.

In the AAC intervention process, careful considerations to individualize the intervention plan can include the following:

■ Individuals with ASD display limited joint attention and reduced observational learning. There is, therefore, a need to provide both explicit instructions and opportunities for learning through trial and error.

■ Skills learned may not easily be generalized to other settings and therefore require explicit training across situations for improved generalization.

- Individuals with ASD generally present with good ambulation abilities and therefore need opportunities to practice and use AAC "on the go."

- Individuals with ASD may possibly display difficulties in eye-hand coordination, subtle fine-motor skills, and motor apraxia. Therefore, AAC training should include opportunities for the development of consistent motor plans that allow for easy access and selection of icons.

- Inherent to the diagnosis of ASD, social communication deviances or deficits exist. The AAC competencies to engage socially and use AAC must be taught explicitly and be addressed across situations to build competency.

- Presence of sensory processing disorders may hinder or interfere with participation and learning of AAC use. Appreciating and providing instruction suitable for sensory needs of the individual and also supporting the individual to manage their own sensory needs is important for AAC success.

Ultimately there must be a recognition of the individual's potential to communicate. The AAC team including the individual with ASD, family members or caregivers, and professionals must work together closely to facilitate and create opportunities for effective communication.

Case Study: EL

Clinical Profile and Communication Needs

The Individual

EL is a young boy living in Singapore. His parents noticed developmental differences in him, and at the age of 5 years a pediatrician diagnosed EL with ASD. Like many Singaporean families, they enrolled him in early intervention programs and intensive one-on-one speech therapy focused on developing language and speech skills. Asian parents typically want their children to speak (Singh et al., 2020; Srinivasan et al., 2010), and this may drive families to focus on improving speech rather than communication. Although EL showed slow speech improvement and was able to produce few speech utterances, he remained ineffective in communicating a variety of needs, wants, or thoughts. Hence, his family started to consider other communication alternatives. As EL's special education school was introducing AAC in the form of PECS, he began to communicate basic requests and exchange picture symbols for concrete objects. Although EL was gaining competence with PECS, by the age of 10 years, his family sought to expand his communication across individuals and environments. EL's parents had also recently purchased an SGD (a tablet with an AAC app), heavily edited to reflect nouns and thus limiting the number of communication functions EL could perform. EL's parents were aware that this high-tech device was not facilitating effective communication, and therefore were keen to explore other solutions.

The family contacted the main Assistive Technology Centre at Singapore for an AAC assessment. The AAC clinical team at the Assistive Technology Centre comprise speech therapists (STs), assistive technology specialists (ATSs), educators, engineers, and occupational therapists (OTs). The team provides interdisciplinary assessments, AAC intervention, caregiver training, and loans of assistive technology (AT) including AAC devices.

An in-person assessment followed, and EL's family were involved to ease him through the interactions and to give the AAC clinical team an opportunity to observe interactions between child and family members. The **SETT framework** was utilized by the therapists during the AAC assessment process. Through observations, direct assessments, and parental reports, the team was able to evaluate the child and determine suitable AAC systems and strategies. Details of the initial assessment follow.

S (Student). EL lives with his Chinese-Singaporean family comprising himself, his parents, and two older siblings. The family speaks English with EL, and some Mandarin Chinese among themselves at home. English is Singapore's common language of communication and the medium of instruction at schools.

He was enrolled at a local special education (SPED) school, where he attended classes to further his activities of daily living, with some instruction on numeracy and literacy. EL was able to recognize alphabets and match words, suggesting emerging literacy skills.

EL had good gross and fine motor skills and could move around easily during interactions, grab his parent's phones or tablet, and select an icon among many to play games and watch videos. His ability to select and navigate to familiar icons was effortless and swift, indicating good visual discrimination skills. He enjoyed these activities and would often rock himself and flap hands (suggesting sensory seeking behaviors) when excited.

In adult-initiated structured activities, EL had fleeting attention, limited eye contact with the communication partner, and poor on-seat behavior. EL's attention span could be prolonged, and he could complete a short task successfully if provided with prompts and motivators. His motivators included strong flavored local snacks and a narrow selection of YouTube videos.

EL had a few challenging behaviors. He had specific ideas of what he wanted, and he persisted in obtaining it, either via vocalizations or grabbing the item. He would throw himself on the floor or become aggressive toward his parents if his wants were not understood. He had thrown a few phones and tablets out the window of his high-rise apartment which led to his parents' wariness about EL's independent handling of devices.

EL could follow simple context-related instructions and was able to locate common items and understand familiar verbs, although his sensory behaviors (such as hand flapping) would interfere with responding to the request or instruction. His parents and teachers relied heavily on the use of motivators to help EL follow instructions. EL was also observed during unstructured environments where he demonstrated greater understanding of his communication partner's intentions as compared to when asked to follow instructions in a structured manner.

EL presented with limited verbal skills. He could produce a few poorly intelligible word approximations for items of high interest (e.g., /bɪʌt/ for biscuit). His utterances were only understood by familiar communication partners in context. EL used gestures (e.g., waving to say goodbye) and natural behaviors (e.g. shouting for refusals) for communication with individuals in his environment.

EL's use of PECS at school and home was limited to exchange of individual symbols for concrete objects for items of interest. As EL was not trained, he did not use syntactic structures in any modality, indicating poor *linguistic competence for AAC*. EL's ability to maintain joint attention and initiate communication were limited to high interest tasks and were often heavily prompted by EL's mother. EL's mother also had difficulty clarifying messages when his AAC system was inadequate. These behaviors indicated poor *strategic competence for AAC*. EL had been introduced to the SGD by his parents, but not in a systematic manner or for varied communicative functions. His mother had occasionally trialed the AAC app with EL during opportune times, for him to make requests of favorite food or to provide reasons for a meltdown by giving choices. EL displayed motor skills to use the low- and high-tech AAC systems but lacked specific skills of *operational competence for AAC* such as the awareness of the purpose or use of the high-tech AAC system. EL's sensory needs interfered with his ability to carry the AAC everywhere. He could not continuously bear the touch and sensation of straps. EL preferred his hands to be free to flap them. EL would rock his body or crouch and hug himself occasionally to eliminate distractions when he felt overwhelmed. He preferred that nothing touch him or was near him at that time.

EL lacked awareness of social rules for communication and was ineffective in initiating or maintaining a conversation with familiar or unfamiliar communication partners displaying inadequate *social competence for AAC*. Communicative functions such as rejection or refusals and directing others for action were expressed through body language or unclear word utterances. His parents would attempt to recognize, interpret, and respond to his behaviors, but often resorted to guessing.

E (Environment). EL's routines and narrowed interests significantly limited his *communication partners* and physical *environments*, as further discussed later.

Their Communication Partners

EL's mother served as his primary communication partner. She was a homemaker and dedicated her time to care for EL's needs. EL's father and older siblings provided care for him whenever possible, but often remained busy with work and school. While it was obvious from their body language that EL and his family had a strong bond, there were very few attempts at interactive communication. They lacked abilities across all communicative competencies (operational, social, and strategic) to support EL's AAC use. At school, he was supported by his supportive and patient teachers and therapy team. He had some interactions with his classmates and school personnel whom he was less familiar with (e.g., the cafeteria operator) but relied heavily on his teachers or therapists to scaffold his communication with them.

The Environment

EL's physical environments included his special education school (where he spent half of his weekdays) and his home (where he spent most of the remainder of his time). The school provided individualized support with a high teacher-to-child ratio. Various materials and supports were used in school, namely, visual supports and PECS. At home, he had one-on-one support from his mother who utilized his motivators in tailoring activities to keep him engaged.

T (Tasks). EL's communication at school and home focused on his needs and wants; pertaining to items of high interest and basic bodily needs such as going to the toilet and eating.

Within school routines, students were involved in social group interactions such as "circle time" or during group "snack time." EL's participation in such tasks was limited, since his preexisting AAC system did not support use of robust language or a variety of communicative functions.

The family hoped that EL would engage meaningfully in more tasks at school, within the community and with unfamiliar communication partners across settings such as mealtime at restaurants or Singaporean Hawker centers (local eateries or food stalls) or with others during his favorite sport (roller skating).

AAC Considerations

Based on information gleaned regarding EL in S, E, and T, the team proceeded to select suitable AAC systems to trial during the in-person assessment.

The AAC System or Service

Tools (T). EL required a systematic-linguistically based AAC system with sufficient core and fringe vocabulary to support his learning, cognitive, and language needs and communication environments. Systems with placement of icons that remain constant and that allow for development of consistent motor plans were also considered. In view of EL's good motor access and visual discrimination skills, the ability to have many symbols on a page was considered for quick and easy access to words. A portable, lightweight system was considered so that he could carry and use it independently.

The AAC clinical team provided ALS throughout the system trials along with sufficient wait time. Both high- and low-tech AAC systems were trialed. Attention was paid to EL's idiosyncratic communicative behaviors including his gestures, body language, and vocalizations.

Using the linguistically robust communication book (30 symbols per page), EL was able to form three- to five-word sentences such as "I want more biscuits" to request for his motivators. He was able to do this independently and accurately most of the time. He had good overall attention during this AAC trial.

An SGD (AAC app loaded on a tablet) with robust vocabulary was also selected, since the voice output would allow for EL to "speak" out loud and gain attention easily at school and home. The dynamic nature of the pages would provide easy access to core and fringe vocabulary; its consistent vocabulary placement would promote motor planning to increase EL's automaticity and efficiency of communication. EL could also imitate three- to five-word combinations modeled by the AAC clinical team member to request for high interest food. He had fairly good physical access but occasionally got distracted by other symbols or apps that caught his interest. EL could tolerate the voice output. However, his occasional and repeated taps of the same symbol created confusion about the purpose and clarity of his message.

The assessment indicated that both systems supported EL's current and future communication needs. The team suggested starting with the low-tech AAC system (a more durable option) as EL had a history of throwing devices out the window. Transitioning to a high-tech system was recommended for the near future.

The SETT framework uses the term "Tools" referring to devices (discussed earlier) and services, strategies, and everything else needed to help the student succeed (described in this chapter in the next section).

Next Steps

Goals and Intervention

Comprehensive treatment goals and intervention plans were developed for EL and his caregivers. The AAC clinical team identified the need to work with the parents and EL's school using a coaching and consultative model to facilitate generalization of skills into the home and other environments in his daily routine.

EL's broad long-term goal was to become a competent and autonomous communicator who uses multimodal communication (including AAC) across settings and communication partners. Achievable short-term goals focused on developing communication skills across competencies and on factors that could impact these competencies, such as caregiver support, motivation, and challenging behaviors.

Over a period of 12 months, two sets of goals were identified for EL and his primary caregivers.

Initial Goals and Intervention. During this stage, the child utilized the low-tech AAC system. EL's goals focused on purposeful use of his AAC system and learning of basic core vocabulary within his daily routines. Through aided language stimulation (ALS), EL was provided with the receptive language input and models of how he could intentionally use his AAC system for communication. The emphasis on core vocabulary taught him the needed words that he could use across situations.

As EL's caregivers lacked the knowledge and communication competencies to apply these strategies effectively in his daily routines, they enrolled in the center's AAC caregiver training program. Through small group discussions based on video snippets of their AAC strategy implementation attempts, they were able to self-introspect on how they could integrate the skills learned within real-life settings. These sessions equipped EL's parents with preliminary skills to support communication in EL's routines. Through engineering of the environment, the family was supported to create suitable opportunities for teaching and modeling of vocabulary (within high interest and motivating situations).

Post caregiver training, EL's mother continued to meet with the AAC clinical team for regular sessions to build specific communication skills that could be embedded in EL's routines. She communicated fortnightly via e-mail communications and met with the team in in-person sessions every 2 months. During the in-person sessions, a coaching model allowed for review of activities and goals (set by the AAC clinical team, together with input from EL's mother and his school). EL's mother reflected with the team on how she had used strategies such as ALS, teaching core words (e.g., "more," "stop"), and expectant waiting during the desired activities across different communicative functions. Within the session, the mother practiced new skills with guidance from the AAC clinical team. Each coaching session ended with discussions for further AAC implementation ideas and repeated practice in his routine environments.

EL's special education team was trained in strategies to support AAC use in the school environment and encouraged to intentionally provide EL with opportunities to participate in group routines.

After 6 months of intervention, EL could use the AAC system with purpose, seeking out the communication book to make requests for highly desired items such as food. He could combine familiar core and fringe words from different pages of the book, within school and home settings. He often continued to use his speech and natural behaviors at first but would clarify himself with the AAC system when individuals around him misinterpreted his verbal message. Such behaviors indicated clear gains in EL's linguistic, operational, and strategic competencies.

At school, EL began exhibiting use of modeled words within tasks of high interest. The teachers reported occasional self-retrieval of the AAC system to indicate a request. He started to see it as a mode of communication when he was not understood.

EL's parents increased in their ability to engineer the environment and provided more opportunities for him to use core words and the AAC systems across planned activities at home. The parents became more adept in using ALS, developing their linguistic and operational competencies. Such strategies were used for modeling requests and comments. With improved skills, EL's parents found the communication board limiting and slow and anticipated moving to the SGD to provide swift access to more vocabulary.

EL's communicative functions, however, remained limited to requests. His communication on the low-tech board was fleeting, and as he lacked joint attention his messages were easily missed by unfamiliar or inattentive communication partners. The family had difficulty in providing EL with sufficient wait time and would immediately react or make assumptions about what he was going to say. The caregivers faced challenges adapting to EL's fast-paced communication interactions as a significant part of their attention was focused on interpreting his idiosyncratic gestures rather than responding to his attempts on the AAC system.

Second Set of Goals and Intervention. The second set of goals focused on transitioning EL to his SGD. The AAC clinical team worked on familiarizing EL with the vocabulary organization of the SGD and the development of EL's motor sequences and planning abilities in order to efficiently access the robust vocabulary on his system. The team taught EL with strategies to use his SGD to initiate communication through the voice output feature across communication partners.

The team worked with EL's parents to expand his communicative functions using ALS. EL's school team identified opportunities to model a variety of communicative functions and to expand communication partners to include peers and school helpers. Caregivers became more mindful of the use of sufficient wait time for EL to initiate or to respond independently on his AAC system.

EL's challenging behaviors and fast-paced motor access of AAC made its community use difficult. He would often press the icons repeatedly, making his message difficult to understand. EL would dart out of sight when he was in public, and his mother found it difficult to manage the use of the AAC system and his behaviors when alone. Given these limitations, EL's home environment was still considered as most suitable for communication intervention.

In light of these challenging behaviors, visual supports (visual schedules, now-then boards, social stories) were used within routines and tasks for EL and his communication partners. The visual supports provided structure, stated expectations of EL's AAC use/behaviors, and reinforced use of AAC.

Six months later, EL and his caregivers showed good improvement and demonstrated further gains across communication competencies. EL was using his SGD within familiar settings, easily navigating to core and fringe words on the system (across several overlays) to request and comment about his wants and the environment (linguistic competence). The voice output on the SGD was a motivating factor as it provided verbal feedback of the selections EL made. His mother recounted how his face would "light up" when he discovered that he could press an icon/message button to ask for a specific item. EL would often use the SGD to augment his speech abilities for clarification of his message (strategic competence). EL's parents began to accept and respond appropriately to such multimodal communication attempts (operational competence).

While EL's repeated selection of icons/message buttons continued to lead to occasional communication breakdowns, EL's mother became more at ease with his behaviors and began to realize that her son was actually "communicating." She also realized that EL's multiple presses indicated the urgency of his message. EL was also receptive to the visual supports resulting in better attention to tasks, instructions, and interactions. EL's mother moved from anticipating EL's behaviors and refraining from using AAC intervention strategies to waiting and letting EL lead a part of an interaction (operational and strategic competencies). As EL's mother was gaining competence and confidence in facilitating use of AAC in structured and familiar contexts, the AAC clinical team began to address generalization of skills across environments in the community. Suitable settings and communication partners were identified, in which the mother would be most comfortable to facilitate AAC use. Within a setting, the team discussed and provided scripts to help loosely structure and plan tasks and use AAC intervention strategies. The mother's anxieties to handle behavioral challenges outside the home environment were overcome by such planning, and she garnered courage to go out in the community with EL.

As a trial, the mother facilitated and preplanned an outing to a neighborhood shop, frequented by the family. The mother prepared and equipped EL with skills and vocabulary (on the SGD). Simultaneously, she sensitized the shopkeeper about the SGD, voice output, and communication style used by EL. During the interaction, EL used preformed sentences to introduce himself to the shopkeeper and initiate the conversation. He then typed a message to request for murukku, an Indian local snack that EL enjoys. The shopkeeper was able to respond appropriately. The mother saw glimpses of success through this exercise. This enabled her to gain confidence in herself and EL to use AAC outside the home setting.

Through the yearlong AAC journey, EL has begun to autonomously express his own opinions, preferences, and choices. EL's parents have gained new insights about their son. They are now equipped to facilitate his AAC use within the community, while respecting his abilities and individual differences. A supportive community of communication partners who can recognize and believe in his potential will provide continued opportunities for self-expression and autonomy, unlocking potential that would otherwise remain hidden. To quote a boy with autism who uses a letterboard for communication,

We all deserve to be challenged and have the opportunity to feel a sense of accomplishment, but that requires people to believe in us and our trapped intelligence and abilities. We can be taught anything if we're blessed with patient mentors who have the ability and desire to look beyond what their eyes can see – past the facade that our uncooperative bodies may present. (Musso, 2019)

References

American Psychiatric Association. (2013). *Diagnostic and statistical manual of mental disorders* (5th ed.).

Dodd, J., & Gorey, M. (2014). AAC intervention as an immersion model. *Communication Disorders Quarterly, 35*(2), 103–107. https://doi.org/10.1177/1525740113504242

Ganz, J. B., Earles-Vollrath, T. L., Mason, R. A., Rispoli, M. J., Heath, A. K., & Parker, R. I. (2011). An aggregate study of single-case research involving aided AAC: Participant characteristics of individuals with autism spectrum disorders. *Research in Autism Spectrum Disorders, 5*, 1500–1509. http://dx.doi.org/10.1016/j.rasd.2011.02.001

Ganz, J. B., & Hong, E. R. (2014). AAC intervention mediated by natural communication partners. In J. B. Ganz (Ed.), *Aided augmentative communication for individuals with autism spectrum disorders*. Autism and Child Psychopathology Series. Springer. https://doi.org/10.1007/978-1-4939-0814-1_6

Goossens', C., Crain, S., & Elder, P. (1992). *Engineering the classroom environment for interactive symbolic communication—An emphasis on the developmental period, 18 months to five years*. Southeast Augmentative Communication Publications.

Hammond, N. (2017). *Generalization of core vocabulary taught to children diagnosed with autism spectrum disorder using an augmentative communication device* (Publication No. 10288058) [Doctoral dissertation, The Chicago School of Professional Psychology]. PQDT Open. https://pqdtopen.proquest.com/doc/1923902143.html?FMT=AI

Kaiser, A. P., Hancock, T. B., & Hester, P. P. (1998). Parents as cointerventionists: Research on applications of naturalistic language teaching procedures. *Infants and Young Children, 10*(4), 46–55.

Kaiser, A. P., Hancock, T. B., & Nietfeld, J. P. (2000). The effects of parent-implemented enhanced milieu teaching on the social communication of children who have autism. *Early Education and Development, 11*(4), 423–446. https://doi.org/10.1207/s15566935eed1104_4

Kent-Walsh, J., & McNaughton, D. (2005). Communication partner instruction in AAC: Present practices and future directions. *Augmentative and Alternative Communication, 21*(3), 195–204. https://doi.org/10.1080/07434610400006646

Kovach, T. M. (2009). *Augmentative and Alternative Communication Profile—A continuum of learning.* LinguiSystems.

Light, J. C. (1989). Toward a definition of communicative competence for individuals using augmentative and alternative communication systems. *Augmentative and Alternative Communication, 5*(2), 137–144. https://doi.org/10.1080/07434618912331275126

Light, J. (2005). *AAC interventions to maximize language development in young children.* http://aac-rerc.psu.edu/index.php/webcasts/show/id/7

Light, J., & McNaughton, D. (2014). Communicative competence for individuals who require augmentative and alternative communication: A new definition for a new era of communication? *Augmentative and Alternative Communication, 30*(1), 1–18. https://doi.org/10.3109/07434618.2014.885080

MacDuff, G. S., Krantz, P. J., & McClannahan, L. E. (2001). Prompts and prompt-fading strategies for people with autism. In C. Maurice, G. Green, & R. M. Foxx (Eds.), *Making a difference: Behavioral intervention for autism* (pp. 37–50). Pro-Ed.

Musso, M. (2019, August 22). *How the letter board changed my life.* https://the-art-of-autism.com/how-the-letterboard-changed-my-life/

Rose, V., Trembath, D., Keen, D., & Paynter, J. (2016). The proportion of minimally verbal children with autism spectrum disorder in a community-based early intervention programme. *Journal of Intellectual Disability Research, 60*(5), 464–477. https://doi.org/10.1111/jir.12284

Singh, S. J., Diong, Z. Z., & Kamal, R. M. (2020). Malaysian teachers' experience using augmentative and alternative communication with students. *Augmentative and Alternative Communication, 36*(2), 107–117. https://doi.org/10.1080/07434618.2020.1785547

Srinivasan, S., Mathew, S. N., & Lloyd, L. L. (2010). Insights into communication intervention and AAC in South India: A mixed methods study. *Communication Disorders Quarterly, 32*(4), 232–246. https://doi.org/10.1177/1525740109354775

Tager-Flusberg, H., & Kasari, C. (2013). Minimally verbal school-aged children with autism spectrum disorder: The neglected end of the spectrum. *Autism Research, 6*(6), 468–478. https://doi.org/10.1002/aur.1329

Zabala, J. (2005). Using the SETT framework to level the learning field for students with disabilities. http://www.joyzabala.com/Handouts_for_Download.html

Zangari, C. (2014, July 29). *On not talking.* https://praacticalaac.org/praactical/on-not-talking/

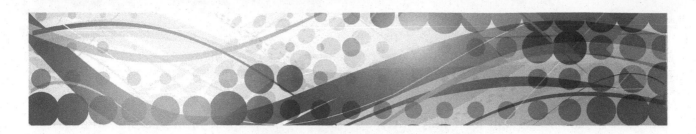

Chapter 21

AAC FOR PERSONS WITH CEREBRAL PALSY

Katya Hill

Fundamentals

Cerebral palsy (CP) is the most common motor disability in childhood (Capute & Accardo, 2008). Recent population-based studies from around the world report prevalence estimates of CP ranging from 1 to nearly 4 per 1,000 live births or per 1,000 children (Sellier et al., 2015). Caused by abnormal brain development or damage to the developing brain, CP is a group of disorders that affect a person's ability to move and maintain balance and posture. The symptoms and severity of CP vary among individuals and last a lifetime. Although the neurological damage of an individual does not worsen, their symptoms may change with growth and aging. While all individuals with CP have movement and posture problems, several related conditions may accompany CP such as spinal problems (scoliosis), joint problems (contractures), seizures, vision, hearing, speech, language, communication, and intellectual disability.

Speech-language pathologists (SLPs) working with individuals with CP should be aware of an individual client's type of movement disorder and type of CP. Through observation of movement, an SLP may be able to identify spasticity (stiff muscles), dyskinesia (uncontrollable movements), and/or ataxia (poor balance and coordination). In addition, medical information should identify whether a physician has classified a person's CP as spastic CP, dyskinetic CP, ataxic CP, or mixed CP. Spastic CP typically is described in terms of the affected body parts: (a) spastic diplegia is muscle stiffness mainly in the legs; (b) spastic hemiplegia indicates that only one side of an individual's body is affected; and (c) spastic quadriplegia affects all four limbs, the trunk, and the face.

The Gross Motor Function Classification System (GMFCS; http://www.cfcs.us) is a useful tool that categorizes CP into five different severity levels for gross motor function on the basis of self-initiated movement abilities (Morris & Bartlett, 2004). The GMFCS does not identify fine motor or functional speech impairments at the different levels. However, the identification of functional abilities for sitting, walking, and wheeled mobility are helpful for an SLP to plan and prepare for an augmentative and alternative communication (AAC) assessment and/or intervention. A child or adult with a GMFCS Level I or II classification may have mild fine motor and speech impairments (dysarthria), whereas an individual with a GMFCS Level III–IV may have moderate impairments affecting functional speech, feeding, and access to assistive technology. An individual at GMFCS Level V will be impaired across all areas of motor function, does not have independent mobility, and would likely require AAC and other types of assistive technology. Note that moderate to severe oral-motor speech and swallowing disorders may occur at any GMFCS level and may indicate the need for AAC.

Once an SLP has reviewed medical records and made initial observations to identify the type, severity, and GMFCS level of an individual identified by a physician, the SLP could use the International Classification of Functioning, Disability and Health (ICF) framework to fill in details specific to a client for each of the appropriate ICF components (World Health Organization [WHO], 2001). Identification of the specific details associated with the ICF components of Body function & structure, Activities, Participation, Environmental factors, and Personal factors assists in targeting variables that may enhance or be barriers to independence and quality of life (National Academies of Sciences, Engineering, and Medicine, 2017). The component of Body function and structure should include the type, severity, and GMFCS level along with any other attendant medical diagnoses such as a seizure disorder, cortical visual impairment, hearing loss, dysarthria, swallowing disorder, and so on. Activities will change over time as children advance across educational settings, engage in community events as adolescents, and mature into adulthood for higher education and employment. Likewise, the type and level of participation will change over time as individuals mature and daily activities require different types of participation. Environmental factors will include use of AAC, any other assistive technology (AT) or durable medical equipment (DME), environmental modifications, accommodations, and support persons. Personal factors to consider include gender identity, cultural/ethnic diversity, socioeconomic status, motivation, beliefs, and values.

AAC Strategies and Technology

Communication is multimodal by nature. Besides speech and vocalizations, we all use facial expressions, gestures, and simple signs when communicating. Unaided multimodal strategies are used together with aided methods that require an external device to achieve effective, interactive communication. Aided AAC strategies may include manual communication boards or notebooks. A variety of speech-output AAC technologies with limited features and memory are available that may be an option as an introductory or trial device. However, for the purpose of this section, we focus on high-performance, computer-based AAC technology as the preferred option for achieving robust spontaneous novel utterance generation (SNUG) or, in other words, communicative competence.

Identification, selection, and manipulation of AAC technology features is a critical step in the assessment process. This matching person with AAC technology (Scherer, 2004) process must ensure that the individual and their family are fully informed of all the possible technology and feature options. Applying a systematic and principled approach to feature selection is achieved when SLPs use a framework based on the primary, secondary, and tertiary AAC components. To optimize the communication performance of an individual who has CP, many features need to be considered, selected, and personalized. Table 21–1 summarizes the features that are available as options on AAC technology and can be manipulated or modified to meet the abilities, needs, and expectations of an individual with CP. The primary features relate to language/linguistic features, including how language is represented and generated, available prestored vocabulary, and methods of utterance generation. The secondary features involve the technology hardware that can be evaluated based on the display software (user interface), the control interface (selection method), and various outputs. The tertiary features include peripheral needs, manufacturer services, and other required or available supports. SLPs need to guide this feature-matching process, since mitigation of an expressive language and communication impairment hinges on the robustness of the language software and ability of the individual to control the selection of display locations.

AAC Assessment

The AAC assessment may be the single most important event in the life of an individual with CP (Hill et al., 2006). For a child with CP, a comprehensive AAC assessment should culminate with a decision about AAC technology and the interventions necessary to build language and communication competence to maximize potential across the life span.

Table 21–1. Primary, Secondary, and Tertiary Features of Augmentative and Alternative Communication (AAC) Technology

PRIMARY FEATURES		
Language Representation	**Vocabulary**	**Method of Utterance Generation**
▪ Alphabet or text ▪ Single-meaning pictures/symbols ▪ Multimeaning icons	▪ Core—high-frequency words ▪ Extended—low-frequency or topic-specific words	▪ Spontaneous novel utterance generation (SNUG) ▪ Prestored sentences
HARDWARE AND SOFTWARE FEATURES		
Display Features (user interface)	**Control and Selection Methods (control interface)**	**Hardware Outputs**
▪ Symbol set (Commercial) ▪ Symbol type (photos, drawings, visual enhancement) ▪ Display type ▪ Display size ▪ Number of grid locations ▪ Number of pages ▪ Color coding	▪ Direct selection—*keyboard, head pointing, eye gaze, brain-computer interfaces (BCIs)* ▪ Scanning—*one or two switches, scanning pattern* ▪ Morse code	▪ Speech—*synthesized, digitized, individually created digital voices* ▪ Other—*display, electronic/infrared/radio frequency, Bluetooth* ▪ *Data logging*
TERTIARY FEATURES		
AAC System Options	**AAC Manufacturer Options and Services**	**Other Clinical Supports (not AAC manufacturer)**
▪ Weight and portability ▪ External computer access ▪ Internet, Wi-Fi ▪ Phone access ▪ Switches ▪ Mounting systems ▪ Carrying cases	▪ Technical support ▪ Repairs ▪ Equipment loans ▪ Warranties ▪ Funding support ▪ Device training	▪ Equipment loan closets ▪ Funding requests, appeals ▪ AAC system training ▪ AAC system programming ▪ Intervention support (speech-language pathologist)

Note. Modified from *The promise of assistive technology to enhance activity and work participation* by National Academies of Sciences, Engineering, and Medicine, Health and Medicine Division, Board and Health Care Services, & Committee on the Use of Selective Assistive Products and Technologies in Eliminating or Reducing the Effects of Impairment, 2017, p. 216 (https://doi.org/10.17226/24740).

For an adult with CP, an evaluation or reevaluation should measure current communication performance and identify unmet needs to maintain or build optimal communication for independence and self-fulfillment. Regardless, the matching person with AAC technology step comes after clinical evidence has been gathered about the individual, compared with the personal and external evidence,

and decisions about how language should be represented and generated are discussed.

As mentioned earlier, details gathered related to the ICF components and the GMFCS level are useful information for making decisions about the tools and instruments to use for gathering clinical evidence. SLPs must conduct formal and informal observations and assessment of an individual's abilities including receptive and expressive language levels (i.e., semantics, morphology, syntax, pragmatic language function, cognition, executive functions, and literacy skills). Gathering and appraising additional related evidence from other team members related to hearing, vision, fine motor (physical) skills, and educational level is also needed. Language sampling is an essential method to evaluate linguistic performance, and a variety of sampling contexts have been described in the literature for use with children, adolescents, and adults including use of play, storybooks and stories, personal narratives, picture descriptions, and interviews. Standardized instruments and informal techniques that are age appropriate may be used to assess the individual's current language levels related to receptive vocabulary and sentence comprehension, expressive use of words and sentences, and reading and spelling skills. In some situations, the use of standardized tests administered in a nonstandardized manner may yield helpful information. For instance, for the individual who cannot point to an item on a page but who can reliably indicate "yes" and "no," administration of a standardized test via partner-assisted scanning may provide valuable information. The SLP must indicate in the report that the test was not administered in the standardized manner.

Once an individual's abilities, needs, and expectations have been documented along with evidence regarding the ICF components, the matching person with technology or feature-match process may start (Scherer, 2004). The SLP and team, ensuring inclusion of the individual and parent(s) if the individual is a child, consider how the primary language components are selected and organized on various displays (user interfaces) of AAC language programs. Equally important is consideration of the individual's most efficient method to select words/messages (control interface) (refer to Table 25–1). An essential principle is not to compromise access to vocabulary and morphosyntactic features for linguistically robust language because fine motor skills compromise direct touch access. Thus, the team may introduce AAC technology by starting with target practice to observe the rate and accuracy with which an individual can select targets from the display without the demand of selecting vocabulary. When observations of direct touch selection observations indicate that the number of locations must be reduced and enlarged to increase accuracy of the individual, then an alternative access method should be considered (Hill, 2006). Chen and O'Leary (2018) provide the basic principles associated with selecting eye gaze as an alternative access method, and Hill and Romich (2002) provide principles on selection rate measurements. Building competence in selecting targets is critical to achieving effective communication. In addition to target selection practice, practice using the various user interfaces across the speech-generating devices (SGDs) under consideration is important. Factors to consider include observation and evaluation of user performance and satisfaction with the symbol set, colors and color-coding features, grid border options, appearance of the target cell when a selection is made, and any display changes that occur with navigation to various targets. These factors all influence user preferences and vary across SGDs. Depending on the SGD, some features may be adjustable (e.g., the background color used on a given display, or the color a device uses when it highlights a selection), whereas others may not be (e.g., grid border options).

Several high-performance AAC systems or SGDs have a data logging feature to support analysis of communication performance. Measures of real-time communication and usage patterns can be used to compare performance among various SGDs trialed or to monitor performance gains provided by the selected SGD once an individual has received appropriate training on the device. Some SGDs may only provide logged data on the number of times a specific location was selected. Other AAC manufacturers have a data logging feature to track how an SGD was used as a loaned device, but the log file is not available to the SLP or client. Other AAC manufacturers have a feature that when activated provides a log file with a time stamp and the event (selected location). In this case, the SLP can collect a language sample allowing for precision performance measurement. The language sample can be analyzed to report standard language measures. The time stamp provides the evidence to report an accurate communication rate (words per minute; wpm) and selection rate (bits per second; bps) that are valuable measures to ensure that progress toward the goal of effective communication is being achieved. In a case study of an adult with CP, data logging was used to compare access methods during an AAC reevaluation to upgrade the individual's SGD (Hill, 2006). The college-aged student was using direct selection with his index finger and thumb on his current SGD and trialing optical head pointing access. His average communication rate on his SGD using direct selection with his fingers was 1.0 wpm and using head pointing was 6.5 wpm. While his peak communication rate (fastest utterances of five or more words) using his fingers was ≤1 wpm, his peak communication rate using head pointing was 21 wpm. Log file analysis provided strong evidence supporting having optical head pointing as an available feature on his new SGD.

Intervention

Quality AAC intervention is quality language intervention. SLPs who have knowledge and skills of the principles of language treatment will be able to identify, plan, and conduct a treatment program to improve communication competence using AAC technology supported by multimodal strategies and learned skill with the technology. AAC treatment starts during the comprehensive AAC evaluation with collection of baseline data during the trial of the selected AAC system, identification of measurable functional communication goals, development of a treatment plan, and confirmation of support persons. While assessment data may indicate that a child needs to improve vocabulary skills using graphic symbols/icons, baseline data to measure growth are essential to determining the effectiveness of treatment. Let's compare two vocabulary objectives: (a) client will increase vocabulary using AAC system by 75% and (b) client will increase expressive vocabulary during play-based activities using graphic symbols on AAC device from a baseline of 5 symbols to 30 symbols in 6 months. The first objective lacks the condition of specificity, is not measurable, and cannot be used to determine the effectiveness of the treatment approaches. The second objective meets the need for specificity and clearly states the what, how, and when of meeting the objective. At the end of 6 months, if the objective is not achieved, the SLP knows that modification to intervention is needed.

An excellent place to start to identify evidence-based intervention approaches for individuals with CP who rely on AAC methods and technology is to review theories on language development and models for adult communication competence. AAC intervention draws from a variety of disciplines including developmental psychology, behavioral psychology, and linguistics to scaffold children and adolescents with CP through the stages of typical language development. Theories and principles related to second language learning have been applied to adolescents and adults using AAC technology, especially for the first time, since use of the AAC system's language has been compared to learning a second language. Again, we need to consider how the ICF framework represents theoretical relationships among the various components as a psychosocial approach to intervention (Clarke et al., 2016). Once an SLP has identified the theory-base to apply to AAC intervention, specific strategies can be selected to complement this foundation.

Direct and indirect modeling has been a typical strategy used to build language competence. Aided language stimulation (direct modeling) has a strong AAC evidentiary base where a communication partner teaches symbol meaning and models language by combining their own verbal output with selection of vocabulary on the AAC system (Binger et al., 2011; Goossens', 1989). Prompting from a partner or clinician is a typical strategy to assist, suggest, or cue someone to use an AAC system. Prompts may be verbal, visual, or physical/tactile with the goal for an individual to be ultimately independent (American Speech-Language-Hearing Association, 2004). Consistency in the prompting hierarchy being used with an individual is important in order to determine when full prompts may be faded to partial prompts or open questions. Ensuring that partners adequately pause when prompting to allow the individual time to process and respond along with providing descriptive feedback when the targeted response is given is also necessary for consistency.

Designing a treatment protocol for an individual with CP who is relying on AAC is a monumental task given that decisions about intervention and its implementation can affect long-term outcomes. Decisions regarding which approach and techniques will result in improvement of functional communication goals are challenging and rest on judicious search procedures to locate and appraise the evidence on the wide range of available intervention approaches and methods. Savvy SLPs will compare the evidence that they have gathered about the client along with their knowledge of the technology features of their client's SGD to arrive at evidence-based intervention decisions.

Case Study: PL

This case study represents a composite of two young adults with CP using the pseudonym PL.

Clinical Profile and Communication Needs

The Individual

At the time of the initial AAC evaluation, PL was a 15-year-old male with severe quadriplegia consistent with GMFCS Level V. PL used a powered wheelchair for mobility with joystick control and customized head and trunk support. Additional ICF Body Function and Structure factors included the diagnosis of cortical visual impairment (CVI) and epilepsy. Speech was nonfunctional and limited to high-pitched vocalizations to request highly motivating activities and to protest. At the time of the assessment, PL relied on a few idiosyncratic hand signs and gestures, enlarged 3-in. picture symbols taped to his wheelchair tray, and a digitized SGD with nine locations of prerecorded messages. These AAC solutions had been introduced over the years in various trial-and-error approaches resulting in

solutions that limited PL's ability to communicate and demonstrate his potential.

Their Communication Partners

PL's functional communication limited his ability to participate with identified communication partners including his parents, teachers, aides, related service practitioners, and fellow students. Personal factors based on the ICF framework indicated that PL was a very social, friendly, and happy adolescent. He was cooperative and engaged in school-related activities but was frustrated by his inability to express himself with his high school peers and at high school events.

Their Communication Environments

PL was enrolled in special education and placed in a high school life skills program. ICF-related activities were identified based on his daily environments of school, home, and the community. Community activities included going shopping, going to the movies, and going to sporting events, especially events that included the high school marching band and music, such as his church. Figure 21–1 represents an example of a completed ICF framework template for PL that identified factors to guide intervention planning once PL received his SGD.

AAC System and Service Considerations

Communication needs were monumental for PL, since he had such limited abilities to express his wants, needs, and thoughts. Review of his individualized education program (IEP), related service progress reports (SLP, occupational therapist [OT], physical therapist [PT]), and multidisciplinary team evaluation records were used to chart his learning trajectory and present levels that included results of standardized testing. The *AAC Profile: A Continuum of Learning* (Kovach, 2009) was used to create a performance profile of his operational, linguistic, social, and strategic skills. Observations of PL's receptive language revealed that he understood

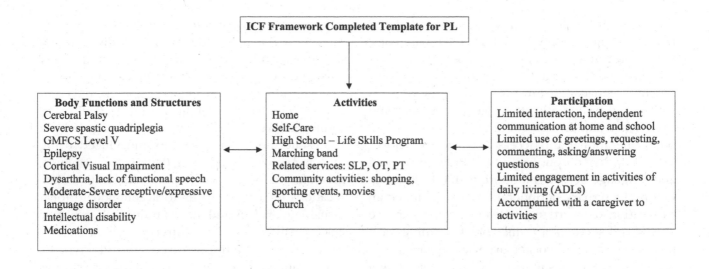

Figure 21–1. School team and parents completed an ICF template with the AAC consultant to guide intervention planning (Copyright Augmentative and alternative communication [AAC] technology by K. Hill, B. Baker, and B. Romich, 2006. In *Introduction to Rehabilitation Engineering* by R. Cooper, H. Ohnabe, and D. Hobson (Eds.), pp. 355–384. Institute of Physics Publishing.

multistep directions, wh- word questions, words out of context, and narratives. He fell within Skill Set Level 4 on receptive language, although his team felt that he demonstrated some skills within Skill Set Level 5 for receptive language (i.e., understanding of narratives and complex sentences, and inferring meaning). His multimodal communication strategies were limited to responses to questions, protests, and requests. He lacked consistent methods of communication to demonstrate spontaneous novel utterance generation (SNUG), his potential linguistic competence or potential for gaining more advanced pragmatic competence. Consequently, he did not score about Skill Set Level 2 for expressive language

since he did not have an AAC system to intentionally select specific words from various grammatical categories and could not construct messages.

The comprehensive AAC evaluation resulted in the prescription of a high-performance SGD for PL, which he received. The team decision was based on the performance data collected at baseline and during the trial, user satisfaction and preferences, and the team and parent preferences and satisfaction. The primary language features included use of all three AAC language representation methods (text-based, single-meaning icons, and multimeaning icons), availability of core and extended vocabulary, and use of SNUG and prerecorded messages.

The secondary user interface features included a language application with 84 locations with icons, letters and numbers, and color coding. The secondary control interface feature for PL was a 14-in. touch screen using direct selection given observation and trials with other access methods and PL's visual impairment (note techniques used to build operational and access competency below). The secondary output features included Bluetooth and language activity monitoring (LAM; data logging). The tertiary peripheral features included an 84-location keyguard to isolate locations to improve access and serve as a framework for hiding locations as access and vocabulary use improved. The AAC manufacturer supports were discussed as a tertiary feature, and clinical supports included training and consultation with an AAC specialist and tele-AAC services. Comparing these identified feature requirements across various SGDs, the interprofessional practice team including PL and his parents selected the Accent 1400 with Unity 84-sequenced (PRC-Saltillo manufacturer).

Critical service considerations, setup, and training included use of strategies to enhance PL's performance given his diagnosis of CVI. Figure 21–2 represents how his SGD was introduced using tape and color-coded piping (yellow for pronouns; green for verbs; purple for prepositions) to isolate locations for target words to accommodate for a visual impairment and access training. Vocabulary chosen was based on high-frequency words associated with motivating activities and PL's type of participation. For example, PL enjoyed music and core words that would be useful for talking about music across environments and activities including the following: want, play, like, stop, turn, on,

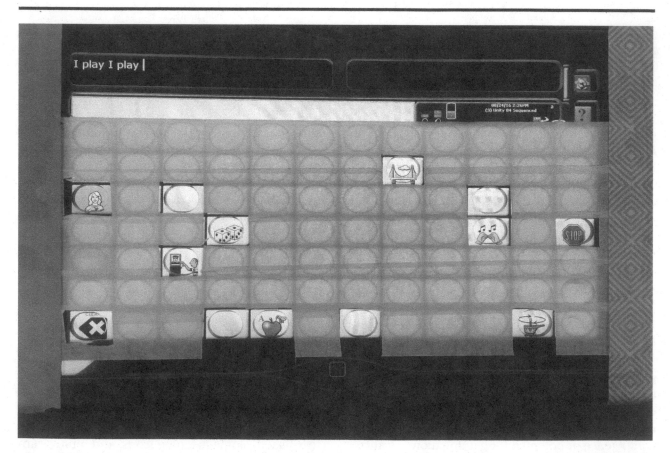

Figure 21–2. AAC system display when introduced to PL. Unity 84 Sequenced is a trademark of PRC-Saltillo. © 2021 PRC-Saltillo.

off, up, down. Social functions that were targeted included requesting, directing, and commenting. Commenting vocabulary was soon introduced to PL to access interjections such as *awesome, yum,* and *sorry.*

A variety of evidence-based intervention strategies were integrated into PL's individualized education program. The three basic principles that were applied involved use of (a) naturalistic teaching strategies that integrated the use of the SGD into daily activities; (b) emphasizing the important role of communicative partners in using the SGD to augment their speech/communication with PL; and (c) providing regular and systematic feedback to PL and his team by monitoring his use of the SGD (Romski & Sevcik, 1996). The team members were trained on how to "talk with" and model language using PL's SGD, apply aided language stimulation techniques (AACtion Points: Aided Language Stimulation, 2014) and to use pause time, using a least-to-more prompting hierarchy during structured and unstructured activities. Consistency in applying this prompting hierarchy was practiced by the team. Especially important was that team members paused for a similar length of time before

the next prompt was given. Table 21–2 shows the steps of the hierarchy used by PL's team and an example prompt at each step (modified from "AACtion Points: AAC & Prompting Strategies" by ICAN Talk Clinic, 2014).

Environmental communication teaching (ECT) activities were created by the team, implemented in school, and shared with parents once PL gained skills to initiate, maintain, and terminate an activity (Karlan, 1989). ECT activities created by the team included highly motivating tasks that required communication to initiate, maintain, and conclude an activity. Examples of ECT activities for PL included listening to music, preparing to go to lunch, and preparing to go to marching band practice. Later ECT activities were created for life skill communication related to providing directions with respect to doing the laundry, preparing food, and playing board games with peers.

By Year 3 of intervention, PL had full access to the 84-location user interface of his touch screen SGD as scaffolding gradually supported moving him to more vocabulary access. Colors were modified from the default vocabulary to provide additional visual supports. His original black keyguard

Table 21–2. Example of the Least-to-More Prompting Hierarchy

Step 1: Pausing	Before initiating an activity, focus your attention on PL and pause. Wait for PL to initiate an interaction using speech-generating device (SGD).
Step 2: Open question	If PL does not respond to the pause, ask a what, who, when, where question, such as "What do you do next?" "Where do you go now?" Then focus your attention on PL and **pause**.
Step 3a: Partial prompt	If PL does not respond to the open question and pause, provide part of the answer, such as "Do you want to listen to music or watch a video?" "Is it time for lunch or band practice?" Then focus your attention on PL and **pause**.
Step 3b: Request for verbalization	If PL does not respond to the partial prompt and pause, request that PL use a proper form of a response, such as "Tell me what you want." "You need to tell me where we go now." Then focus your attention on PL and **pause**.
Step 4: Full model	If PL does not respond to the request to use his SGD and pause, provide the full model for the proper response and **pause**. Use PL's SGD to provide the full model for him to imitate.
End: Descriptive feedback	When PL uses his SGD to give a proper response, provide descriptive feedback and praise: "Great, you want to listen to some music." "Wonderful, you told me it's time for band practice. Let's go!"

was exchanged for a clear keyguard, since he no longer felt the need for the black border grid. Figure 21–3 represents his display.

While LAM data were used to graph overall use of the SGD each week by time periods, these data were used to evaluate consistency in implementing the intervention program to build communication competence and not used for language analysis. Specific observations and/or activities were designed to gather a language sample of at least 100 utterances without partner modeling, and the LAM file was uploaded to a computer for analysis. Although PL's selection rate (2.69 bps) and average communication rate (4.40 wpm) were reduced given PL's visual and motor impairments using direct selection, language sampling data in controlled contexts during the school day showed significant gains in linguistic competence over the five-semester period of intervention. Table 21–3

compares language performance data collected under controlled conditions after the first semester of intervention and at the end of the fifth semester.

It is notable that the majority of PL's utterances could be classified as SNUG. Prerecorded sentences tended to be used for introductions and conversational starters (e.g., "How are you doing?" and "I help manage the marching band."). Over the five semesters of intervention, visual inspection of PL's charted learning trajectory showed a gradual increase in device usage for communication and participation that was confirmed by various communication partners in the activities and environments identified in the completed ICF template.

Gains in the use of social functions were monitored by team members also using the *Augmentative and Alternative Communication Profile: A Continuum of Learning* (Kovach, 2009). After the end of the first semester of intervention, PL

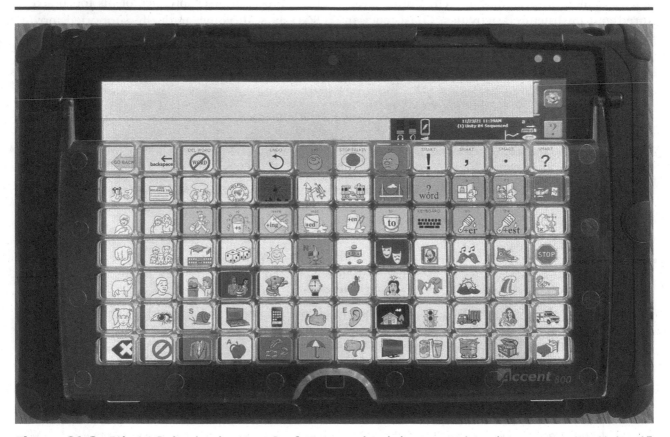

Figure 21–3. PL's AAC display by Year 3 of use at school, home, and in the community. Unity 45 One-Hit and Unity 84 Sequenced are trademarks of PRC-Saltillo. © 2021 PRC-Saltillo. WordPower is a trademark of Inman Innovations, Inc.

Table 21–3. Language Sample Data Comparing Early Performance Using Speech-Generating Device (SGD) With Communication Performance After Five Semesters

Performance Measure	End of Semester 1	End of Semester 5
Total number of utterances	100	100
Mean length utterance (MLU-m)	1.60	3.50
Total number of words	22	248
Different word roots	8	104
Core vocabulary use	25%	47%
Language Representation Method (LRM)		
Multimeaning icons	28%	52%
Single-meaning pictures	72%	48%

fell within the Social Area of Learning and Skill Set Level 3: Practiced Interaction. He demonstrated increased use of and practice with his AAC system and purposefully used his AAC system to participate in social communication more fully. At the end of five semesters, PL fell within the Social Area of Learning and Skill Set Level 4: Social Awareness and Competence. At that point, PL was able to appropriately identify and express opinions and intentions to others, demonstrate increased confidence in using his AAC system for social communication, and interact at appropriate times in conversation. Social validation measures also confirmed the success of the AAC intervention as clinician-made rating scales. PL's teachers, aides, parents, and other stakeholders strongly agreed that PL had made progress; was communicating more frequently, independently, and effectively; and his temper outbursts had declined.

Next Steps

Transition planning is a critical next step for PL who was by then 18 years old. Despite gains in expressive language skills, increased confidence in using his SGD and use of multimodal communication methods, PL's communication has not been optimized, and he had not achieved his potential as a graduating student entering adulthood. Updating the ICF framework template would be a next step to facilitate transition planning and intervention services.

In addition, the team identified objectives related to continued building of PL's expressive language skills which targeted a variety of grammatical parts of speech (e.g., pronouns, verbs, adjectives, prepositions, and articles). In addition, PL would benefit from improvement of morphosyntactic skills—specifically his ability to mark tense as it relates to information being communicated. Improvement in morphosyntax would require use of modeling, recasting, and expansions to increase sentence length and complexity.

These objectives are considered foundational for engaging in daily activities as an adult and building participation skills identified within the ICF framework. The goal of independent living for PL will be to ensure that he has opportunities to make decisions that affect his life, to pursue activities of his choice, and to direct his care. Use of the Communication Bill of Rights (Brady et al., 2016) may facilitate a team's decisions about objectives related to independent communication required for identified ICF activities and participation components. The team and parents completed a Communication Bill of Rights clinician-made inventory based on the published document to identify PL's use of

AAC strategies, including his SGD, and his communication partners' abilities to meet the 15 rights of communication proposed by the National Joint Committee for the Communication Needs of Persons with Severe Disabilities (Brady et al., 2016). Each item was rated on a 0 to 10 scale, with zero reflecting strongly disagree with an ability to fulfill the right to 10 that represented strongly agree to the ability as being independent. Although PL's ability ratings improved from the first use of the inventory for transition planning, the three rights selected to focus on building communication competence included (a) PL using an SGD to interact socially, maintain social closeness, and build relationships; (b) PL using an SGD to refuse or reject undesired objects, actions, events, and people; and (c) PL using an SGD to express personal preferences and feelings. In addition, the team identified objectives related to his ability to express levels of pain, type of pain, and personal care directives as essential communication skills for meeting medical necessity.

After five academic semesters of coordinated interprofessional team intervention with monthly AAC consultant monitoring, PL still had a long way to go in terms of building communicative competence for effective and independent communication during typical adult activities of daily living. PL's progress was attributed to his IEP team (special education teacher, classroom aides, SLP, OT, and PT) being fully trained on his SGD and AAC intervention strategies. All his team members could model target vocabulary and generating messages throughout the day. His parents attended semester trainings provided by the consultant with quarterly reporting of his performance reviewed and discussed with the special education supervisor, team, and parents to make decisions about modifying instructional approaches or suggestions for home and community communication. The principles of evidence-based practice place the individual's benefits first. In PL's case, several AAC solutions were introduced over the years that reflected a trial-and-error approach resulting in solutions that limited his ability to communicate and demonstrate his potential. He was 15 years old before a comprehensive AAC evaluation was conducted that systematically gathered clinical and personal evidence prior to identifying and comparing features on possible SGD solutions. In addition, quantitative performance data were used to monitor progress and guide decision-making. PL's case shows how quality of life can be dramatically enhanced when teams seek the most effective, independent means of communication possible for an individual with severe motor impairments and communication disabilities secondary to CP.

LAM is defined as a language-based theoretical approach to AAC assessment and intervention. It is a data logging feature that allows the recording of a language sample and analysis of an individual's usage patterns of AAC technology for precision measurement. SLPs can check whether the feature is available on an SGD or a communication application. If not, you can contact the AAC manufacturer to request that the feature be added. A variety of resources and publications on LAM and AAC data logging can be found when searching for evidence. Resources on AAC data logging, including some automatic measures of communication performance, are available on various AAC systems including PRC-Saltillo devices, CoughDrop, and Speak for Yourself.

References

American Speech Language Hearing Association (ASHA). (2004). *Preferred practice patterns for the profession of speech language pathology.* https://doi.org/10.1044/policy.PP2004-00191

Binger, C., Maguire-Marshall, M., & Kent-Walsh, J. (2011). Using aided AAC models, recasts, and contrastive targets to teach grammatical morphemes to children who use AAC. *Journal of Speech, Language, and Hearing Research, 54*(1), 160–176.

Brady, N. C., Bruce, S., Goldman, A., Erickson, K., Mineo, B., Ogletree, B. T., . . . Wilkinson, K. (2016). Communication services and supports for individuals with severe disabilities: Guidance for assessment and intervention. *American Journal on Intellectual and Devel-*

opmental Disabilities, 121(2), 121–138. https://doi.org/10.1352/1944-7558-121.2.121

Capute, A. J. & Acardo, P. J. (2008). Neurodevelopmental disabilities in infancy and childhood (3rd ed.). Paul H. Brookes.

Chen, S-H. K., & O'Leary, M. (2018). Eye gaze 101: What speech-language pathologists should know about selecting eye gaze augmentative and alternative communication systems. Perspectives of the ASHA Special Interest Groups, 3, 24–32.

Clarke, M., Price, K., & Griffiths, T. (2016). Augmentative and alternative communication for children with cerebral palsy. Paediatrics and Child Health, 26(9), 373–377. https://doi.org/10.1016/j.paed.2016.04.012

Goosens', C. (1989). Aided communication intervention before assessment: A case study of a child with cerebral palsy. Augmentative and Alternative Communication, 5(1), 14–26. https://doi.org/10.1080/07434618912331274926

Hill, K. (2006). A case study model for augmentative and alternative communication. Assistive Technology Outcomes and Benefits, 3(1), 53–65.

Hill, K., Baker, B., & Romich, B. (2006). Augmentative and alternative communication (AAC) technology. In R. Cooper, H. Ohnabe, & D. Hobson (Eds.), Introduction to rehabilitation engineering (pp. 355–384). Institute of Physics Publishing.

Hill, K., & Romich, B. (2002). A rate index for augmentative and alternative communication. International Journal Speech Technology, 5(1), 57–64. https://doi.org/10.1023/A:1013638916623

ICAN Talk Clinic. (2014, January 14). AACtion point: AAC & prompting strategies. http://www.icantalkclinic.com/aaction-points

ICAN Talk Clinic. (2014, January 21). AACtion point: Aided language stimulation. http://www.icantalkclinic.com/aaction-points

Karlan, G. (1989). The environmental communication teaching training project (Award No. H023C9005). Field-Initiated Research Grant Award from the Office of Special Education, U.S. Department of Education. Purdue University.

Kovach, T. M. (2009). Augmentative and Alternative Communication Profile: A continuum of learning. LinguiSystems.

Morris, C., & Bartlett, D. (2004). Gross motor function classification system: Impact and utility. Developmental Medicine and Child Neurology, 46(1), 60–65. https://doi.org/10.1111/j.1469-8749.2004.tb00436.x

National Academies of Sciences, Engineering, and Medicine, Health and Medicine Division, Board and Health Care Services, & Committee on the Use of Selective Assistive Products and Technologies in Eliminating or Reducing the Effects of Impairment. (2017). The promise of assistive technology to enhance activity and work participation. https://doi.org/10.17226/24740

Romski, M. A., & Sevcik, R. A. (1996). Breaking the speech barrier: Language development through augmented means. Paul H. Brookes.

Scherer, M. J. (2004). The matching person and technology model. In M. J. Scherer (Ed.), Connecting to learn: Educational and assistive technology for people with disabilities (pp. 183–201). American Psychological Association.

Scllier, E., Platt, M. J., Andersen, G. L., Krägeloh-Mann, I., De La Cruz, J., & Cans, C. (2015). Decreasing prevalence in cerebral palsy: A multi-site European population-based study, 1980 to 2003. Developmental Medicine and Child Neurology, 58(1), 85–92. https://doi.org/10.1111/dmcn.12865

World Health Organization (WHO). (2001). International classification of functioning, disability, and health.

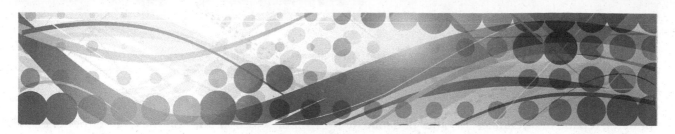

Essay 18

CLINICAL CONSIDERATIONS AND AAC: THE OTHER "A" FOR "AUGMENTATIVE"

Rebecca M. Lavelle

When considering the treatment of motor speech disorders such as dysarthria or apraxia of speech, I often encourage teams to consider what I call "the other A." Throughout my professional career, I have found that most people think of augmentative and alternative communication (AAC) as an alternative to verbal speech. It is easy to understand why this might happen. Low-tech supports such as visual icons are often selected, exchanged, or shown in lieu of verbal output. High-tech speech-generating devices produce utterances that are selected from a dynamic display. It is easy to forget the "other A"—augmentative communication. When we augment verbal speech, we support natural speech using tools to help a speaker communicate with efficiency and efficacy. In essence, we want clients to be able to say what they want to say, when they want to say it, in a way that is understood. There is not only a choice of verbal output or alternative communication to replace natural speech. Augmentative communication can and should be used to support a Total Communication approach.

One of the most important considerations in working with clients who have motor speech disorders is efficiency of communication. In essence, what is the easiest way for a person to communicate what they think, need, feel, or want? When discussing augmentative communication, a primary consideration needs to be ease of use. I often find myself recommending a combination of tools to support natural speech depending on the purpose of communication and the setting. For example, in a classroom setting, a student may benefit from a combination of low-, mid-, and possibly high-tech AAC supports for ease of communication throughout the day. Comment cards with social words or phrases might be made available to reduce pressured speech during social or sharing times. Other low-tech options, such as manual communication boards or individual icons, may be appropriate to clarify utterances or provide specific topic-based vocabulary that may be difficult to produce verbally. Mid-tech switches such as a Step-by-Step Communicator with levels may be programmed in advance of a sharing time to allow for efficient sharing of news and messages.

Efficiency of communication is always the goal, regardless of the modality. In speech-language therapy, traditional interventions for phonotactics and phonology are still employed, but we need to consider the client's functional communication throughout the rest of the day. How can we support a fun, meaningful, connected life experience outside of the clinical setting? The "other A," augmentative communication, can bridge the work between the therapeutic setting and real-world living. Even in therapy, specific intervention targets may be supported with natural aided language stimulation. Clinicians can carefully select carrier phrases, repetitive utterances, or other phonotactic or phonology targets to support with icons, symbols, switches, or high-tech devices. Using natural aided language stimulation with the augmentative supports provides the client immersion into a multimodal communication environment. That can be freeing to those who feel pressured to produce verbal speech. When the focus is on communication and not verbal output, clients can rely on both rote or natural speech as well as augmentative communication tools in a relaxed, natural way. The more we focus on ease of communication, modeling of multimodal strategies, and reducing barriers to communication, the more our clients are able to fully participate in their daily lives.

Another critical consideration when working with clients with motor speech disorders is the efficacy of communication. We should consider not only how easily clients can communicate but also how well they are able to relay a message. At its heart, communication is information exchange. I find that we often overfocus on how someone communicates and forget to consider why they communicate. Humans want to feel heard; they want to belong. Clients with dysarthria or apraxia want to be funny, interesting, creative, reflective, wholly imagined human beings. The most important part of what we do as clinicians is to provide tools for effective communication. That moves well beyond verbal speech. I often ask teams to consider what is being communicated instead of focusing on how it is communicated. If a client communicates via symbol selection and the message is understood, honor that communication the first time. Even if you believe a client can produce that word or utterance verbally, honor the communication exchange. Yes, we have specific phonotactic or phonology targets that we want to reinforce, model, and practice, but that is not why humans communicate. People communicate to be understood. If the communication exchange is supported via low-, mid-, or high-tech augmentative communication, it is still information exchange.

People with motor speech disorders vary greatly as individuals; no two clients are the same. Clients vary in their intelligibility of speech, language competency, motor ability, personality, preferences, and life experience. Each person is unique and important. When treating these clients, short-term efficiency and efficacy of communication are as important, if not more important, than long-term outcomes. Supporting individuals in their daily lives, and what is important to them, is why most speech-language pathologists entered the field. When treating motor speech disorders, one should consider a Total Communication approach, including the "other A"—augmentative communication—to allow clients the most freedom to share their thinking with the world. We need to provide every person with the opportunity to be funny, thoughtful, caring, witty, argumentative, and interesting, because that is what humans do.

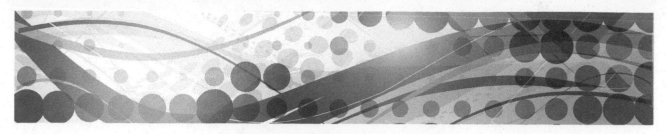

Chapter 22
AAC FOR PERSONS WITH SPECIFIC SENSORY IMPAIRMENTS

Lesley Quinn and Hillary K. Jellison

Fundamentals

Christine Sun Kim is an American sound artist. She was born deaf. Her work has been featured at the Museum of Modern Art, the Hirschhorn, Tate Modern, and the Whitney Museum, among many others. Sound is the subject of her work, and often the medium as well. In her studio she makes boxed nails and brushes dipped in paint bounce around on canvases tied to vibrating loudspeakers. The speakers amplify her voice. The paintings reveal in an instant what Sun Kim knows viscerally—sound is movement; it interacts with things; it is color, shape, and size. Viewers say her work triggers "a radical redistribution of your concept of sense when you understand the idea of sound can be changed in your mind" (Uproxx, 2016).

Growing up, Sun Kim explained in her TED Talk, she was taught to believe sound was not part of her life (Sun Kim, 2015). However, she began to see the influence of sound in her work and has been driven to explore her relationship with it. She realized sound is many things—physical experience, concept, social currency—and rather than being removed from it, she knows it intimately. People are loudspeakers, she says. They amplify sound and transmit it in their responses. Deaf people take this in. Deaf people, she argues, may be more aware of sound than hearing people are.

Cognitive scientists Ghazanfar and Schroeder (2006) shed scientific light on Christine Sun Kim's artistic relationship with sound. They explain that the brain areas we call auditory and visual are not as modular as we thought. "Unimodal" sensory regions process information from other sense organs, and these "lower" cortical areas can contribute to higher-level thought processes. The brain is populated with neurons, whose job is to integrate auditory, visual, and somatosensory input, leading Ghazanfar and Schroeder to wonder if the entire cortex is essentially multisensory. Evidence of cross-modal plasticity is mounting, they say, and pointing to an essential human reality: we do not represent things "in one modality at a time" (p. 284).

We have known about the effect of cross-modal representation on speech perception since McGurk and MacDonald (1976) first showed that /g/ sounds like /d/ when you are watching someone say /b/. Since then, researchers have discovered other ways our auditory, visual, and haptic senses are linked. Newborns recognize what an object looks like based on how it feels (bumpy or smooth) (Meltzoff & Borton, 1979). Four-month-olds recognize the mouth shapes that go with vowel sounds (Kuhl & Meltzoff, 1982). Across languages and cultures, children and adults agree high-pitch sounds go with objects that are small, thin, bright, and up high rather than ones that are big, wide, dark, and down low (Dolscheid et al., 2014; Fernández-Prieto et al., 2015; Haryu & Kajikawa, 2012).

Our symbolic capacity has a concrete foundation, and researchers are increasingly convinced our physical experiences with sensation and our capacity to integrate them are the basis for abstract, metaphorical language. Colors, it seems, can actually be loud, and kindness really is warm (Lobel, 2014). So, what does it mean for individuals who lose their sense of hearing or sight early on? Neurodevelopmental and molecular neurobiologist, Moheb Costandi (2016), explains that early deafness or blindness results in widespread neural reorganization, and it starts at the cellular level, where sensory neurons are prepared to respecialize by turning on or off segments of their genetic code. Reorganization can lead to capacity enhancements, researchers are finding. Bavelier, Dye, and Hauser (2006) convincingly show that deaf adults have better peripheral visual attention. While Pérez-Pereira and Conti-Ramsden (2019), in one of the only comprehensive accounts of blind children's language development, relate specific linguistic advantages, like increased verbal fluency.

By and large, though, research indicates blind children will "arrive at a similar endpoint" as sighted children, as long as they have attuned caregivers, social connection, and no co-occurring disabilities (Pérez-Pereira & Conti-Ramsden, 2019, p. 134). This is true "even for seemingly 'visual' words, such as sparkle, peek and blue," because language "enables people . . . to construct mental models of visual phenomena" even in the absence of visual access to them (Cheng et al., 2020, p. 171).

The same is true auditorily for deaf individuals, who are exposed to a native language from the start. The key to typical language development, says Laura Petitto, who directs the Visual Language & Cognition (VL2) Center at Gallaudet University, is "rhythmic, patterned, maximally contrasting" language input before 10 months old (Petitto et al., 2016). Both natural sign languages and spoken languages have this phonological property, so language development proceeds apace in deaf individuals who have native access to one or more languages, and their skills translate readily to a second signed, spoken, or written language. However,

the picture is very different for individuals who do not have early language access.

Some of the well-documented challenges for deaf children, who learn sign late or only use speech and audition (with hearing aids or cochlear implants), are delays in vocabulary, syntax, theory of mind, and executive functioning (Hall et al., 2018; Lund, 2016; Nicholas & Geers, 2006; Schick et al., 2007). Typically, the longer they go without language access, the more severe their communication challenges are.

In blind children, Pérez-Pereira and Conti-Ramsden (2019) report that communication and language delays occur when adults misinterpret or entirely miss blind children's attempts to engage. They explain that blind infants' "responses to interactions are often less obvious" than sighted infants and may be "idiosyncratic" (p. 45). For example, instead of turning toward a sound, they may drop their head and move it side to side. They may turn their face away from (and their ear closer to) an approaching caregiver. Or they may fail to return a social smile. If these are perceived as signs of rejection or disability and disrupt the cycle of attuned, reciprocal interaction, communication suffers. Adults can learn to recognize interest and engagement in blind children, however. Pérez-Periera and Conti-Ramsden (2019) say that body movements, especially arm and leg movements (excited, active vs. quiet, still), can be highly informative.

Another consideration is the pragmatic behaviors blind children use to recruit attention and keep conversation going. They can look different on the surface but function the same, and they emerge at roughly the same time as sighted children's behaviors. They include offering or showing objects less but requesting them more, using fewer assertions but more protests or rejections, using imitation and verbal routines as a "call and response" strategy to locate caregivers (instead of visually searching), and using personal, internal reports more than externally oriented language.

There do appear to be a few protracted language differences. They involve delays in acquiring deictic terms that convey "shifting spatial reference" (this/that, here/there, I/you); however, they are usually mastered by age 6 years (Pérez-Periera and Conti-Ramsden, 2019, p. 124). There is also a pattern of increased question use with age, while sighted children show gradual decreases. Pérez-Periera and Conti-Ramsden (2019) suggest question formation may be an indicator of additional disabilities in blind children, since those with multiple impairments "seldom" use them (p. 122).

Dual Sensory Impairment

Unlike blind or deaf children, who have language access and whose development proceeds typically, individuals who are both blind and deaf (with at least some degree of vision and hearing loss) experience substantial obstacles to communication (Bruce et al., 2016). Barbra Miles and Marianne Riggio of Perkins School for the Blind stress that the challenges amount to more than a combined sum of the difficulties of being deaf or blind alone. They say, above all, deafblind individuals are challenged by isolation and a lack of information. They explain, hearing and vision are our two "distance senses," and it is through these channels that we develop social relationships, acquire language, and come to understand most concepts about the world. As a result of combined vision and hearing loss, they continue, "the world of a person who is deafblind shrinks. For many it does not go beyond the reach of the fingertips. For others it extends only slightly farther than that." (Miles & Riggio, 1999, p. 72) Deafblind people, they emphasize, are "essentially isolated unless they are in close proximity . . . with another person" (p. 50).

You can experience what an information deficit might be like. Take a piece of paper and poke a pin-sized hole through the middle. Now hold it up to your eye and look around. What do you see? If this were your world from the beginning, how would you make sense of it? What patterns would arise? Would you recognize something if you didn't already know what it was? Miles and Riggio (1999) suggest that in order to learn with such narrowing of the senses, it is essential for deafblind individuals to actively integrate information from the "near senses" of touch, taste, and smell with "whatever remains of vision and hearing," and it is essential

that the people around them be "emotionally and technically equipped" to communicate with them about their experiences (pp. 72–73). They assert that deafblind individuals need learning partners, especially at first, to mediate the process and help them move from isolation toward increasingly active engagement with the larger world.

Lilli Nielsen, researcher, author, and teacher, has worked to encourage active learning in deafblind and other severely impaired individuals. One of her significant contributions was the Little Room, which brings distant sensory experiences to a person with vision or mobility challenges (Nielsen, 1991). Nielsen designed an adjustable, "active learning space" that allowed for small changes in the environment to encourage multiply disabled children to explore. Since her early research in this area, the number of studies looking at "haptic exploration" and spatial learning in individuals with and without disabilities has steadily climbed (McLinden, 2012; Papagno et al., 2016; Peltokorpi et al., 2020; Tivadar et al., 2020).

Cortical Visual Impairment

Christine Roman-Lantzy further contributed to our understanding of the learning needs of nonsighted individuals. She is an authority on cortical visual impairment (CVI), a form of early cortical blindness that leads to difficulty processing visual information. A person with CVI may or may not have an accompanying ocular impairment, which affects visual acuity. CVI is now the leading cause of visual impairment in children in developed countries (Hatton et al., 2007; Kran et al., 2019).

Roman-Lantzy documented a set of common characteristics across individuals with CVI and developed a way to measure it on a continuum from "minimal visual response" to "near typical vision" (Roman-Lantzy, 2019, p. 9). CVI leads to all of the following, to greater or lesser extent: color and visual field preferences, a need for light and movement in order to "see," visual latency (delayed response), difficulty with visual complexity and distance viewing, atypical visual reflexes, and absence of a visually guided reach. She also showed that individuals who receive targeted intervention can increase their functional vision. However, she emphasizes this does not happen "simply with the passage of time" but only when individuals use their eyes during "meaningful, rewarding activities that occur throughout the day" (p. 15).

AAC and Sensory Impairments

Individuals who have vision or hearing loss alone are unlikely to use augmentative and alternative communication (AAC) as a primary mode of communication. They benefit from other assistive technologies to help them access culturally relevant tools and knowledge (closed captions, video relay, refreshable braille display). Some deaf individuals find text-based AAC useful in specific circumstances (a noisy restaurant, with hearing people who do not sign). However, the loss of a single sensory modality does not have an outsized impact on language development if it is accommodated in infancy.

When hearing loss is not accommodated early and an individual has limited language, when a person is deafblind, or when they have a condition that impacts speech and language and they have a sensory loss, AAC becomes integral to communication. Roman-Lantzy (2019) reports that vision loss is both prevalent and underdiagnosed in individuals with developmental disabilities and those with hearing loss. AAC is also more difficult to access for these individuals. Our senses are the admissions ticket for AAC use; without sensory access, successful communication cannot happen. It is therefore critical to assess an individual's sensory needs during an AAC evaluation, to accommodate them when setting up a system, and to address them in intervention.

There are many ways to do this, but it always requires us to consider the ways sensory differences affect an individual's ability to attend to people, language, their environment, and their AAC. Individuals who have peripheral hearing impairments may benefit from hearing aids, cochlear implants, or FM systems to gain access to residual hearing. Individuals who have ocular vision impairments may use special glasses (e.g., prism lenses) to see. However, even with these accommodations, their hearing or vision will remain inefficient, and input will be inconsistent. They will use top-down strategies and frontal lobe executive functions to compensate, and they will tire more easily as a result.

For individuals with CVI, we can anticipate vision will improve with teaching and practice. However, we need to accommodate their changing vision needs at each phase of progress, and we need to plan for inconsistency. Collaborating with a teacher of the visually impaired (TVI) is important, because they can help identify accommodations that will make the AAC system visually accessible. For high-tech systems, this might include adjusting the size of the layout, adjusting the tilt or location of the device, using high-contrast icons, turning off color coding, and increasing the spacing between icons. For low-tech (paper-based) AAC, a TVI might suggest removing lamination, which has a glare, or incorporating reflective material into an image. They might want to integrate movement by taking icons off the board and jiggling them to draw the person's attention. They can also help determine if auditory scanning is needed to access a larger vocabulary.

For deafblind individuals, tactile input and tactile feedback will be important, whether or not they use a system with objects or 3D symbols (Obretenova et al., 2010). Tactile input can include Pro-tactile ASL (PTASL), which is articulated in the hands and on the body. It includes gestures, signed in conventional locations on the person to communicate context, like facial expression or someone coming in the room. Tactile feedback, meanwhile, involves physically "checking in" to let the person know you are there, listening and understanding. The specific input you provide and the ways you connect physically will need to be negotiated with each deafblind person (Bruce & Borders, 2015; Damen et al., 2017; Haakma et al., 2016; Nelson et al., 2016). When we do this, Roman-Lantzy (2019) emphasizes, when our interventions "match their sensory and communication needs," learning "can be robust," even in individuals with the most severe, combined sensory impairments (p. 230).

Clinical Profile and Communication Needs

The Individual

HS is a happy, curious girl who loves music and movement. She is 4 years old and in her second year of preschool in an integrated classroom at her local public school. HS's family speaks English, and they live in a small, rural town with one elementary school. HS and her identical twin were born prematurely weighing just over 3 pounds each. HS required mechanical ventilation to support her breathing, but her sister did not. She spent 2 months in the neonatal intensive care unit, during which time she received high-dose antibiotics for an intestinal infection and developed a cerebral hemorrhage that resulted in damage to the white matter in her brain (leukomalacia). Upon discharge from the hospital, she was referred for an auditory brainstem response hearing test, because she did not pass the newborn hearing screening.

At 3 months old, HS was diagnosed with severe-to-profound bilateral sensorineural hearing loss. She was fitted with hearing aids, and she and her family began early intervention (EI). They worked with a speech language pathologist (SLP) and a developmental specialist to encourage HS's language and cognitive growth. HS and her family were also supported by a deaf mentor, who taught them American Sign Language (ASL).

Over the next several months, HS's parents connected with hearing and deaf families with deaf children. They were motivated to learn as much as they could, and they quickly came to understand the importance of early language exposure. They focused on signing and reading with HS and her sister, and they took advantage of sign language resources online.

During this time, HS and her sister began to roll over, sit up, and push up on their hands and knees. Soon after, HS's sister began to crawl. HS was able to crawl for short distances after weeks of encouragement. At 11 months, HS's sister began to walk, and she signed her first word. Also at 11 months, HS completed the candidacy process for cochlear implantation. She received her first one at 13 months and the second 3 months later. She tolerated activation of both implants well and responded to pure-tone thresholds between 20 and 35 dB in each ear. At 19 months, she began to vocalize and produce different sounding vowels. She began to use furniture to pull herself up and stand. Meanwhile, her sister, who walked around the house, had a vocabulary of 20 to 30 spoken words and a dozen or more signs.

When HS was 20 months old, her EI team referred her for a comprehensive vision evaluation. Her deaf mentor noticed she did not use her eyes in the same way as her sister. HS "looked at things but didn't see them." She noticed movement, but she did not look at faces. She was interested in the flashing lights on her toy, but she did not reach for it when someone held it up. When family members were across the room, HS did not seem to see them.

Upon completing the vision evaluation, HS was diagnosed with cortical visual impairment (CVI). She became eligible for services through the deafblind program in her state. She and her family started to work with a teacher of students who are deafblind (TDB), and they connected with deafblind adults, who encouraged them to learn Pro-tactile ASL (PTASL). Her parents began to use one particular sign with HS and her sister—light scratches on their shoulders—to show when someone was laughing.

HS also began to work with a teacher of the visually impaired (TVI), who was a certified orientation and mobility specialist. He taught the family about the ways vision impacts development and explained that HS's vision would improve with intervention. He helped set up supports to encourage HS to move independently, and he worked with her to "build increasingly stable visual responses" as the first step in developing meaningful, robust representations of her world (Roman-Lantzy, 2019, p. 3).

Now in preschool, HS continues to work with an SLP and a TVI. She participates in an occupational therapy group with students in her class. After school, she does auditory verbal therapy with an outpatient SLP, and she and her family work with a deaf mentor and a teacher of the deafblind at home. HS's team sees that she orients with her hearing more than her vision. She responds to a range of environmental sounds and speech at quiet, conversational levels. She recognizes her father's and sister's voices over the phone and shows she knows them by her smiles and excited vocalizations. She babbles frequently using repeated syllables, like "baba" and "dididi." Whenever her mother says, "Socks and shoes, time to go," she yells, "Baa!" and moves excitedly to the chair next to the door.

Visually, she presents with CVI Range 2–3 skills (Roman-Lantzy, 2019). For HS, this means she orients to toys, people, or animals she likes. She looks at bright lights and moving parts, but she does not get absorbed in them anymore. She looks at shiny or glittery things out of the corner of her eye. If visual "noise" is blocked out with a dark background, she will look at still objects with bright red color. It also means she responds attentively with vision only in environments that are familiar and quiet, and only when objects are close (within 12 in.).

She sometimes blinks in response to a "visual threat," like a hand coming close to her face or a ball that is accidentally thrown at her, but not always. She reaches for objects that interest her, but she turns her eyes away first. Her teachers and family have noticed she sometimes mouths toys or waves them in the air. A main concern for her team is that HS seems to be less purposeful about using her vision and making choices at school than when she is at home. They would like to see her explore her environment, participate actively, learn through play, and demonstrate visual curiosity.

Their Communication Partners

At home, HS spends most of her time with mom, dad, and her sister. She has two dogs she is "learning to like." Her mom said she tolerates their older dog, who is calmer and does not try to lick her; however, they have a smaller, rambunctious dog, Moxie, who will jump up before HS knows it and startle her.

At school, HS has a 1:1 educational support person (ESP), whose job is to orient HS to what is going on around her as she moves through her day. The ESP is learning how to "narrate the scene" for HS, by describing what is happening with words and PTASL signs. She lets HS know in as many ways as she can what others are paying attention to: who is talking, who is not listening to the teacher, and what the group is thinking about. The ESP also works with HS one on one to implement instructional programs.

The students in HS's class were not sure how to interact with her at first and kept their distance, especially when she did not respond to their overtures. However, after 2 years and coaching by their teacher, they now frequently come up and say hi or bring her toys. They are learning to tap her shoulder to get her attention if she does not respond to her name. Instead of, "Look at this," they are learning to give her specific words to show what they are thinking. Several students are getting good at it, and HS seems to know. She will readily turn to face them when they approach and hold out her hand as they say, "Look, it's a stripy pink tiger! Isn't he cute?"

Their Environment

HS's environments undoubtedly do not look, sound, or feel the same to her as they do to her communication partners, but her team tries to understand what it is like for her by putting together what they know about sensory plasticity with the experiences of articulate deafblind adults. Picturing the world from her vantage point is one of the most important tools they have in working with HS. They also know her environments probably feel starkly different, even though they share many of the same features. HS's parents have worked to make their home visually accessible, and HS is mobile and engaged there in ways she is not at school. Because she is calmer and more confident visually, she uses her hearing functionally. She will call out to people who are not in the room. She will hold hands and dance to music, she will babble on FaceTime with her dad, and she will walk across the room to find her parents if they call her.

HS's home has very little visual clutter. The walls are painted a light color, and there are dark wood accents around the doors, ceilings, and floors. There are a few brightly colored decorations on the walls and shelves. The floor is kept clear of toys and furniture that can be tripped over. There is a "HS-height" string that runs from room to room and out to the backyard, which HS can hold onto to guide herself around, but she rarely uses it anymore. The family also leaves up her sensory space that she played in when she was first diagnosed with CVI. She does not use it much anymore, but once in a while, she will go in, lay down, and explore the objects on the sides and ceiling of her little room.

In contrast, her visual experience at school is very likely a "kaleidoscope of meaningless color and pattern where no individual element can be isolated or understood" (Roman-Lantzy, 2019, p. 25). Her classroom is a bustling hub with 11 preschoolers, four full-time adults, and many people who come in and out during the day. Desks, tables, bookshelves, and play centers are packed with brightly colored toys, books, and art materials, and the walls are covered with students' schoolwork, alphabet posters, and reminders about how to be a good citizen. The floors have rugs, and the windows have drapes to dampen reverberation, but there is no dampening the sound of 15 children and adults chattering enthusiastically about their learning.

In order to address this, there is an FM system with sound-field speakers at each station in the room. Teachers and staff wear microphones so the important speech signal stands out from the background noise. HS's school created a learning nook for her in her classroom that is not unlike her little room at home. It is a contained space with extra padding so it is quieter, and HS can do focused listening. It can be made dark for vision work with her light box, iPad, or a spotlight. It is visually uncluttered, and it has some of HS's favorite toys. HS does schoolwork in her "spaceship," but sometimes she invites a student in to hang out. The team also put tactile symbols throughout the school at HS's eye level. They are on the doors to her classroom, bathroom, art room, gym, and cafeteria, and there is a tactile schedule that the preschool students use during morning meeting.

AAC Considerations

HS's team sees she is listening and understanding more this year. However, she is not developing speech or sign as readily, so they have decided to try other AAC modalities. Rather than doing a one-time AAC evaluation, her team has consulted with AAC specialists who are experienced in working with individuals who have vision and hearing differences. They are collaborating with her team and employing dynamic assessment procedures to develop a comprehensive and integrated AAC system that incorporates all modalities available to HS.

HS's central learning task (within and outside of AAC use) is to make meaning of what she sees and hears. Her brain is working hard to determine, out of all the visual and auditory frequencies coming at her, which ones go together. Which colors and shapes make up which objects? Which pitches and rhythms make up which words? Which words go with which objects? And vitally, which of the things she is seeing and hearing are most important to the people around her? It is not easy for her to navigate competing information and focus on what is socially relevant so she can get to know it, remember it, and use it, because both primary learning channels give her inconsistent, inefficient access to information. Therefore, a central AAC consideration is whether she has visual and auditory access to the most salient information: people, words, and their referents. The other main concern is how well her communication partners mediate her attention so she can focus closely for increasing amounts of time on the relevant input she needs to learn.

There is little that has been ruled out for HS in regard to AAC at this point. There is no evidence to suggest she will not be able to develop a robust language system and handle increasing amounts of complexity over time. As Christine Roman-Lantzy (2019) says, "it is important to avoid making assumptions about students' cognitive function when they have experienced a substantial lack of access to . . . information" (p. 12). We also know that HS's visual and auditory skills will improve with intervention. However, at this time she has limited functional use of her vision outside structured, controlled contexts, and she primarily uses her senses of hearing and touch to navigate the world. She is also early on in the process of developing a single-word expressive vocabulary. This means HS will need an AAC system that can grow with her visually, auditorily, cognitively, and linguistically.

Consequently, her AAC system is being designed with flexibility, modularity, and multisensory input in mind. Her team is systematically trialing tactile, low-tech, and high-tech options and working to determine how complex an array can be before she can no longer attend to what she wants to say. They are specifically trialing (a) customized communication boards with 3D tactile symbols (Figure 22–1),

(b) a paper-based communication book with 2D symbols (Figure 22–2), and (c) a speech-generating device (SGD) with a capacitive touch screen and customizable dynamic display (Figure 22–3).

All the displays have been adapted to support visual access. They have a black background with highly saturated or bright, contrasting colors in the foreground. The tactile and paper-based systems have icons that can be removed and manipulated (see Figure 22–1). Figures 22–1, 22–2, and 22–3 highlight similarities and differences between the three systems.

With the tactile and low-tech systems, her team is using partner-assisted scanning, where the communication partner auditorily previews each of

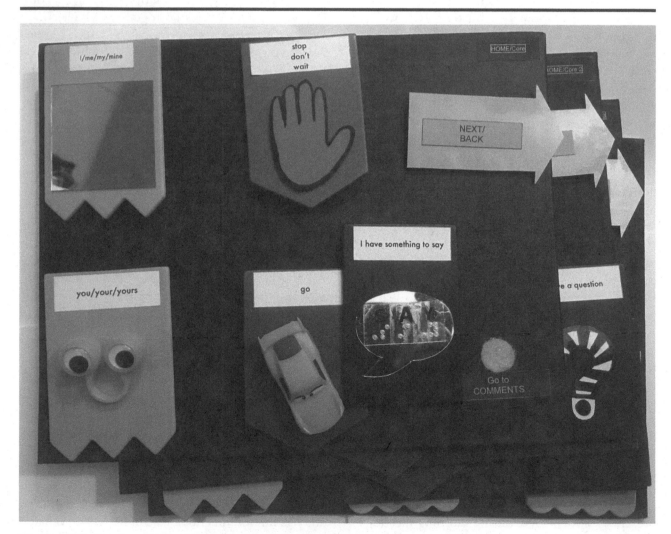

Figure 22–1. Visually accessible 3D tactile AAC display.

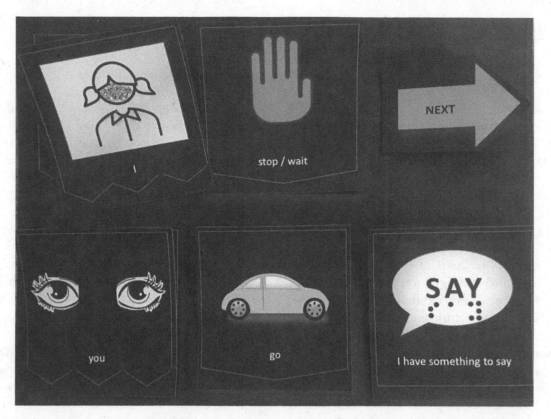

Figure 22–2. Visually accessible 2D low-tech AAC display with manipulable icons.

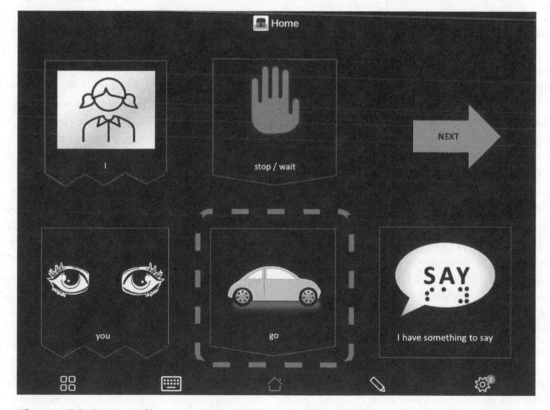

Figure 22–3. Visually accessible, high-tech AAC display with visual highlighting and auditory feedback.

the items on the communication system in a consistent manner, waiting for a response to indicate the intended message. On the SGD, auditory feedback and "visual cue" have been enabled, so HS can run her finger across the screen, hear icons, and see them highlighted before selecting them. The feedback voice is an adult male, while the primary voice is a young girl. HS responds to both.

The AAC System or Service

In customizing an AAC system, the team first needed to identify the signals HS uses to communicate her wants and needs and make sure they have a range of activities and materials to recruit and hold her attention. Team members reported that HS is socially engaging and emotionally expressive, especially when she is relaxed and comfortable. She smiles when she is happy or wants to do something again, and she arches her back or turns her head to the side when she is done. Her parents said she loves to go in the car and visit her cousins or grandparents and will go to the door and turn the knob back and forth to go out. She has also started to go up to family members and hand them a toy, then put her hands on theirs and track while they feel it. She wants to "look with you," her mom said.

She loves people, music, dancing, swinging in a hammock, and gesture songs, like wheels on the bus. Her parents said she smiles and laughs if you can create a sense of anticipation with her, but she did not always do so. They realized early on she was often startled by people kissing or tickling her, because she did not know it was coming. But they came up with games that created a sense of anticipation, so now if you say, "I'm gonna tickle your toes!" and accompany your approach with a rising tone of voice, she smiles and laughs.

Based on this information, the team was able to add a number of activities to HS's repertoire. One she particularly likes is the "sneezing game" (ahh-Ahh-AHH-CHOOOO!), where she elicits each instance of "ahh" from her communication partner using an intentional gesture or action, and the communication partner follows with "CHOO" and a different sensory experience (feather tickling her nose, blanket over her head, gentle poke in the

stomach, a rainstorm of glitter puffs). Another one she likes is the use of "3D model" images within a PowerPoint slide with a dark background. The 3D images incorporate movement and can be manipulated, so she can see them from different angles. She likes to watch "Bebe," the parrot, turn upside-down. Movements are paired with exaggerated vocal sounds (rising pitch for characters looking up, falling pitch for turning down).

With an expanded repertoire of activities and accessible materials, the team has been able to elicit and reinforce an increasing number of communicative gestures and actions from HS, including the signs MORE and EAT (she likes to feed mom and dad, and she will sign EAT to get them to open their mouths). With tactile icons, she has learned to say "GO" when she wants to see one of the 3D images move and when she wants to shift gears and take a walk. She also chooses between a favorite song or a "different" one, using a tactile symbol for one of her favorite songs.

In terms of low-tech versus high-tech AAC, HS has benefited from a gradual, systematic tactile to high-tech transition. First, a tactile symbol is introduced in a highly contrastive pair so HS can get to know what it is and what it is not. She explores them up close, and her team helps her notice salient visual and tactile features to compare the two. She has indicated she knows when an icon is new, because she spends extra time with it, and she puts it to her mouth to feel it with her lips or tongue (she rarely does this after the first or second time). After this, communication partners reinforce her use of the icon communicatively in the context of a motivating activity. HS selects the icon either by pointing or handing it to a communication partner. Eventually, they put the icon back in its place on the communication board within the full tactile array, at which point, HS will search for it with her hands and locate it among six other icons. She will continue to select it with a very low error rate in familiar, motivating activities.

Once HS consistently selects a tactile icon on the board, team members will present her with the corresponding SGD overlay in the context of the same motivating activity and reinforce her use of the high-tech icon. When she started, she alternated between paper-based and high-tech systems, but her team quickly found that HS paid more attention to the high-tech display with backlighting and color highlighting. She was also motivated to select icons on the SGD with auditory feedback. When HS touches a high-tech icon, a thick, red outline pops up and highlights it. When she releases her finger, the highlight goes away, and the device speaks the word.

An activity that reinforced SGD use was for HS to tell her dog, Moxie, to STOP! HS's parents put a bell on Moxie's collar, and HS's dad sat with her at one end of the room, while her mom held Moxie on a long leash at the other end. Mom let Moxie go, and Dad helped HS say, "STOP!" with the volume turned way up. As soon as HS said it, mom grabbed the leash and stopped Moxie. Within a few tries, HS was saying stop on her own, and she has since begun to use stop on the SGD to direct adults' actions at school.

In tracking HS's use of SGD, her team has noticed she starts to tire after 10 minutes of sustained visual attention, and her error rate begins to increase. In the mornings and after naptime, she is highly consistent and highly productive. She also smiles often and is easily directed and engaged. Therefore, when she begins to look away from the device and is less responsive, when she starts to get irritable, when her error rate starts to increase, or when her selection rate starts to decrease, they know she has begun to fatigue. Then they reintroduce tactile AAC. In this way, a dynamic, multimodal approach has helped her become a more active communicator. Similarly, breaking up her day into short periods of "vision on" and "vision off" time has helped her use vision functionally to access AAC for increasing amounts of time.

Her team has been deliberate in devising an assessment system to track her progress, just as they have been in customizing her AAC. Percent correct is not a responsive measure for HS right now, whose performance at any given time is influenced by many variables. We expect she will be inconsistent. A more effective measure of her progress is how much she communicates.

There are no established criteria or norms to guide her team, because there are no "typical" persons who use AAC (PWUAACs), but they can look around and see what HS's peers or fluent PWUAACs do. They can note how many times her classmates volunteer during circle time or how many questions they ask each other during snack time and use these observations to create benchmarks. They can also track what HS does and measure her progress against her own baseline of performance. As they focus on these ecologically based skills, along with her frequency of communication at key times during the day, they are seeing her initiate more and grow as a meaningful communicator.

Next Steps

Over the next year, communication partner training will be an emphasis in HS's program. The team plans to implement an AAC peer training program with HS's sister and a group of students in her class. Her team will encourage her language growth by helping her listen to speech, sign, and nonverbal communication in all the ways she can. They will support her vision and concept development by highlighting the salient visual features of objects and people around her. Thoughtful, purposeful language will help her assign structure and meaning to what she sees and know what to pay attention to.

She and her team will work to build her expressive vocabulary and expand her repertoire of functional communication skills using aided and unaided AAC. They expect she will discriminate between an increasing number of visual and tactile symbols and will encourage her to locate symbols within an increasingly complex array (Bracken & Rohrer, 2014). They also expect she will be able to learn "conceptually referenced" core vocabulary (Snodgrass et al., 2013) and will start to combine words into phrases, given systematic instruction and modeling by her communication partners.

Right now, her AAC system includes a combination of core words and personally relevant, concrete terms, but it is a "proto" system, which is flexible and can transition to any expanded layout. It is possible, because of her vision impairment, that a motor planning approach may facilitate access to larger vocabulary, but for now her team is taking a conservative, bottom-up approach and letting HS's needs and actions guide their next steps.

References

Bavelier, D., Dye, M. W., & Hauser, P. C. (2006). Do deaf individuals see better? *Trends in Cognitive Sciences, 10*(11), 512–518.

Bracken, M., & Rohrer, N. (2014). Using an adapted form of the Picture Exchange Communication System to increase independent requesting in deafblind adults with learning disabilities. *Research in Developmental Disabilities, 35*(2), 269–277.

Bruce, S. M., Nelson, C., Perez, A., Stutzman, B., & Barnhill, B. A. (2016). The state of research on communication and literacy in deafblindness. *American Annals of the Deaf, 161*(4), 424–443.

Bruce, S. M., & Borders, C. (2015). Communication and language in learners who are deaf and hard of hearing with disabilities: Theories, research, and practice. *American Annals of the Deaf, 160*(4), 368–384.

Cheng, Q., Silvano, E., & Bedny, M. (2020). Sensitive periods in cortical specialization for language: Insights from studies with Deaf and blind individuals. *Current Opinion in Behavioral Sciences, 36*, 169–176.

Costandi, M. (2016). *Neuroplasticity.* MIT Press.

Damen, S., Janssen, M. J., Ruijssenaars, W. A., & Schuengel, C. (2017). Scaffolding the communication of people with congenital deafblindness: An analysis of sequential interaction patterns. *American Annals of the Deaf, 162*(1), 24–33.

Dolscheid, S., Hunnius, S., Casasanto, D., & Majid, A. (2014). Prelinguistic infants are sensitive to space-pitch associations found across cultures. *Psychological Science, 25*(6), 1256–1261.

Fernández-Prieto, I., Navarra, J., & Pons, F. (2015). How big is this sound? Crossmodal association between pitch and size in infants. *Infant Behavior & Development, 38*, 77–81.

Ghazanfar, A. A., & Schroeder, C. E. (2006). Is neocortex essentially multisensory? *Trends in Cognitive Sciences, 10*(6), 278–285.

Haakma, I., Janssen, M., & Minnaert, A. (2016). Understanding the relationship between teacher behavior and motivation in students with acquired deafblindness. *American Annals of the Deaf, 161*(3), 314–326.

Hall, M. L., Eigsti, I. M., Bortfeld, H., & Lillo-Martin, D. (2018). Executive function in deaf children: Auditory access and language access. *Journal of Speech, Language, and Hearing Research, 61*(8), 1970–1988.

Haryu, E., & Kajikawa, S. (2012). Are higher-frequency sounds brighter in color and smaller in size? Auditory-visual correspondences in 10-month-old infants. *Infant Behavior & Development, 35*(4), 727–732.

Hatton, D. D., Schwietz, E., Boyer, B., & Rychwalski, P. (2007). Babies count: The National Registry for Children With Visual Impairments, birth to 3 years. *Journal of the American Association for Pediatric Ophthalmology and Strabismus, 11*, 351–355.

Kran, B. S., Lawrence, L., Mayer, D. L., & Heidary, G. (2019). Cerebral/cortical visual impairment: A need to reassess current definitions of visual impairment and blindness. *Seminars in Pediatric Neurology, 31*, 25–29.

Kuhl, P. K., & Meltzoff, A. N. (1982). The bimodal perception of speech in infancy. *Science, 218*, 1138–1141.

Lobel, T. (2014). *Sensation: The New Science of Physical Intelligence.* Simon and Schuster.

Lund, E. (2016). Vocabulary knowledge of children with cochlear implants: A meta-analysis. *Journal of Deaf Studies and Deaf Education, 21*(2), 107–121.

McGurk, H., & MacDonald, J. (1976). Hearing lips and seeing voices. *Nature, 264*, 746–748.

McLinden, M. (2012). Mediating haptic exploratory strategies in children who have visual impairment and intellectual disabilities. *Journal of Intellectual Disability Research, 56*(2), 129–139.

Meltzoff, A. N., & Borton, R. W. (1979). Intermodal matching by human neonates. *Nature, 282*, 403–404.

Miles, B., & Riggio, M. (1999). *Remarkable conversations: A guide to developing meaningful communication with children and young adults who are deafblind.* https://ww2.Ebookit.com

Nelson, C., Hyte, H. A., & Greenfield, R. (2016). Increasing self-regulation and classroom participation of a child who is deafblind. *American Annals of the Deaf, 160*(5), 496–509.

Nicholas, J. G., & Geers, A. E. (2006). Effects of early auditory experience on the spoken language of deaf children at 3 years of age. *Ear and Hearing, 27*(3), 286–298.

Nielsen, L. (1991). Spatial relations in congenitally blind infants: A study. *Journal of Visual Impairment & Blindness, 85*(1), 11–16.

Obretenova, S., Halko, M. A., Plow, E. B., Pascual-Leone, A., & Merabet, L. B. (2010). Neuroplasticity associated with tactile language communication in a deaf-blind subject. *Frontiers in Human Neuroscience, 3*, 60.

Papagno, C., Cecchetto, C., Pisoni, A., & Bolognini, N. (2016). Deaf, blind or deaf-blind: Is touch enhanced? *Experimental Brain Research, 234*(2), 627–636.

Peltokorpi, S., Daelman, M., Salo, S., & Laakso, M. (2020). Effect of tactile imitation guidance on imitation and emotional availability. A case report of a mother and her child with congenital deafblindness. *Frontiers in Psychology, 11*, 540355. https://doi.org/10.3389/fpsyg.2020.540355

Pérez-Pereira, M., & Conti-Ramsden, G. (2019). *Language development and social interaction in blind children*. Routledge.

Petitto, L. A., Langdon, C., Stone, A., Andriola, D., Kartheiser, G., & Cochran, C. (2016). Visual sign phonology: Insights into human reading and language from a natural soundless phonology. *Cognitive Science, 7*(6), 366–381.

Roman-Lantzy, C. (2019). *Cortical visual impairment: Advanced principles*. American Printing House for the Blind.

Schick, B., de Villiers, P., de Villiers, J., & Hoffmeister, R. (2007). Language and theory of mind: A study of deaf children. *Child Development, 78*(2), 376–396.

Snodgrass, M. R., Stoner, J. B., & Angell, M. E. (2013). Teaching conceptually referenced core vocabulary for initial augmentative and alternative communication. *Augmentative and Alternative Communication, 29*(4), 322–333.

Sun Kim, C. (2015). *The enchanting music of sign language*. TED Fellows Retreat. https://www.ted.com/talks/christine_sun_kim_the_enchanting_music_of_sign_language?language=en

Tivadar, R. I., Chappaz, C., Anaflous, F., Roche, J., & Murray, M. M. (2020). Mental rotation of digitally-rendered haptic objects by the visually-impaired. *Frontiers in Neuroscience, 14*, 197.

Uproxx. (2016). *Exploring the sound of silence with Christine Sun Kim: HUMAN* [Video]. YouTube. https://www.youtube.com/watch?v=6FI5Z_aw3Fc

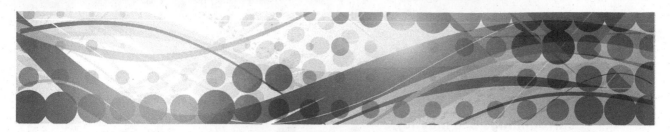

Chapter 23
AAC FOR INDIVIDUALS WITH SENSORY INTEGRATION CHALLENGES

Sarah Gregory and Elisa Wern

Fundamentals

Individuals with communication difficulties do not exist in a vacuum. They are living within bodies that must perceive, process, integrate, and make meaning of the information from their senses as they navigate the world. Each of us must take in information from the world around us and determine whether to act or not based on that information. This is known as sensory processing. Sensory processing broadly describes the way the information a person gains from the environment is received, transferred, and transmitted through the nervous system. At any point during the detection, movement, and processing of a sensation, there could be an error or issue. You might also hear the term *sensory integration* (SI). Ayres used the evaluation measures she developed in research with both typically developing children and children with learning and behavioral difficulties in order to identify key SI ideals and to gain insight into how these functions are related to occupational performance. Sensory processing is defined as the neurological process that organizes sensation from one's own body and from the environment and makes it possible to use the body effectively with the environment (Ayres, 1971). The sensory system is composed of the more common senses of tactile, auditory, visual, olfactory, and gustatory, along with vestibular, proprioceptive, and interoception.

The vestibular system is from the information in one's inner ear as it moves forward, back, tilts, rotates, or goes side to side. Proprioception tells us where our joints and other body parts are in space. Recent work on interoception that has been done by Mahler (2017) defines interoception as the awareness of one's internal body states, such as pain, body temperature, itch, heart rate, hunger, sleepiness, and when one needs to use the restroom. Figure 23–1 defines the different sensory processing areas.

Many therapy professionals prefer not to use the term *sensory processing disorder*, because it is not a formally recognized diagnosis in the current *Diagnostic and Statistical Manual of Mental Disorders, Fifth Edition* (*DSM-5*; American Psychiatric Association, 2013), there is not clear diagnostic criteria, and occupational therapists (OTs) are not able to diagnose per their framework (Occupational Therapy Practice Framework [OTPF], 2020). Instead, therapy professionals tend to talk about an individual's pattern of sensory processing and how there is a mismatch between their sensory processing and the environment or task they are engaged in. This mismatch is what causes the sensory processing difficulty and can also be referred to as sensory processing dysfunction, sensory integration disorder, or simply sensory processing delays.

In the autism spectrum disorder (ASD) population, prevalence estimates of sensory difficulties range from about 40% to more than 90% (Baranek

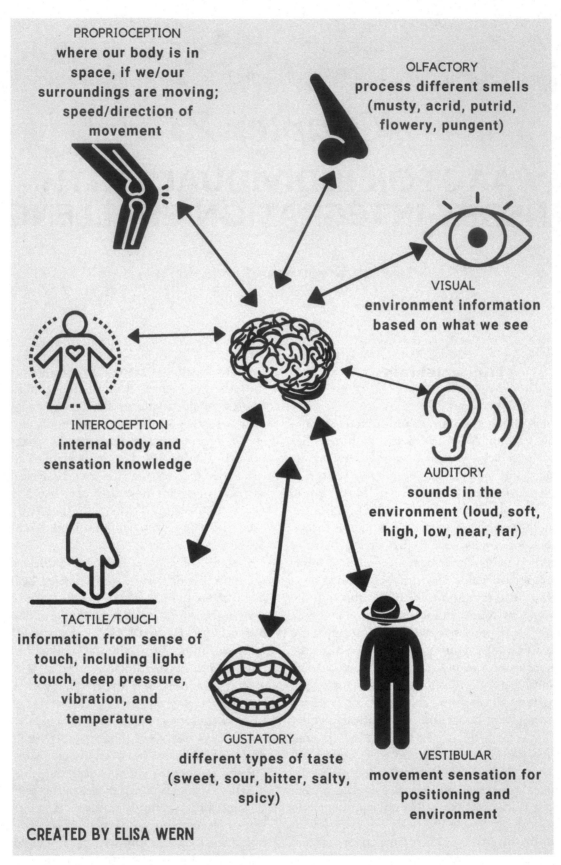

Figure 23–1. Sensory processing differences defined. Image created by Elisa Wern. Graphics freely available via Canva program.

et al., 2014). Miller (2006) estimated that 40% of children with sensory processing difficulties also demonstrate symptoms of attention deficit hyperactivity disorder (ADHD), based on data from a national sample of 2,410 typically developing children. Each area of sensory processing, as well as comorbid diagnoses, should be considered as communication-related interventions are implemented.

When determining how best to implement augmentative and alternative communication (AAC), it is important to consider skills within the four domains of communicative competence as outlined by Janice Light (1989)—linguistic, operational, social, and strategic. They also include communication functions such as gaining attention, initiating, and maintaining conversation (Light, 1989). As previously discussed, these four areas of communicative competence help to frame how AAC and sensory integration disorders interact. When an individual has difficulty processing sensory information, it is important to consider the linguistic aspect; does the individual have the language needed to understand and describe what they are experiencing? Some of the less visible areas of sensory integration (such as olfactory) may not impact an individual's physical use of an AAC device, but they will need the language to be able to explain what they are experiencing and strategies to seek support.

In addition to linguistic competence, it is important to consider skills that fall under social competence. How will an individual express a need for support with sensory processing? Who will they tell and when? Should they ask for the nurse? All of these questions must be navigated within the context of different social situations. For example, at home a student may be able to adjust the lights as needed, but at school may need to talk to a teacher first. The linguistic and social areas of communication also overlap as we support self-advocacy. Students must have the language to describe their sensory needs/accommodations and also navigate social complexities when expressing these needs.

Strategic competence may be targeted in helping an individual express their sensory needs beyond the AAC device. This could be a low-tech paper-based visual support, a gesture, or finding another way to gain attention when someone is not listening. Another strategy is preprogramming phrases on the AAC system so that the individual can be quickly and easily understood when their sensory system is already overwhelmed.

Finally, operational competence must be supported when looking at some of the more common or "easy to see" areas of sensory integration—tactile, auditory, and visual. Unlike olfactory processing, these areas may directly impact one's use of AAC. Fortunately, there are many device settings that can be adjusted to support sensory integration needs, such as auditory feedback or changing the buttons visually. The area of operational competence is sometimes overlooked in therapy but can greatly support individuals with sensory integration needs as outlined next.

Competencies Versus Sensory Integration Areas

Sensory processing difficulties can be supported through a variety of solutions depending on the area of need. Some competency areas can be supported by the solutions generated during consideration or feature matching, while others are addressed through explicit instruction in language and vocabulary. As with all communication supports, the consideration of needs must be based on individual needs with input from the AAC user first and foremost.

Tactile processing, the difficulty of being defensive or hyposensitive to the feel of items, can limit a device user's desire to interact with and use a touch screen device. This can affect the operational and strategic competences and should be included in any intervention plan. Some AAC users might be hesitant to touch the screen of a device. This access can be accommodated by the use of a stylus to make their choices. It might be a commercially available stylus or one that was fabricated through low-tech materials or by 3D printing. The important thing to remember about any stylus is that it must enable better access to communication. Settings within most dedicated devices also allow for adjustment in how buttons or areas are selected. For example, settings can be changed for whether buttons are selected when pressed or when released, as well as how often repeated selections are allowed. Figure 23–2 depicts different AAC application settings for selection.

[Authors' note: Screenshots were selected from a variety of vendors; however, it is important to note that these do not showcase every feature from every AAC program available but are meant to serve as a highlight of features available across vendors. Please check with your specific AAC application or program to determine where these settings may be if available.]

> Decreasing the use of hand-over-hand support for all persons who use AAC (PWUAACs) is a distinct means to support communicators' autonomy and has the added benefit of supporting those with tactile-based sensory processing needs.
>
> Other strategies for tactile defensiveness are as follows:
>
> - use of tactile overlays
> - use of keyguards or touch guards for guidance without being forced upon them
> - adjusting the touch sensitivity in device/language system preferences to necessitate more or less "touch time" before button activation
> - use of a stylus
> - for combined tactile input needs, use of a textured bath glove with fingers removed (can simultaneously give increased tactile information to the user as well as encourage finger isolation for more accurate selection)
>
> A small group study analysis of AAC evaluations for 181 cases, most of whom were children under the age of 8 years, revealed that 50% had some visual abnormality, and 59% had other sensory or self-regulation deficits (Del Monte et al., 2019). These prevalences show the importance of addressing these sensory and self-regulation deficits when considering and implementing AAC.

Those who struggle with auditory processing can be impacted by the sounds and voice chosen on the device. It is important to involve the PWUAAC in selecting a voice and customizing other sounds to assist them in processing the information from the environment. This might mean that a student prefers to use auditory feedback, where the PWUAAC hears the message on a button before it is spoken out to aid in their correct selection of their intended message. Adults using AAC have reported that they prefer to have button selection feedback turned on, which serves as confirmation that they have selected a button when they operate primarily based on motor planning. From an operational competence point of view, it is important that each PWUAAC knows how to adjust the volume on their device and can do so as independently as possible. This might mean that an adult could help program a page with function buttons for power, volume, speech adjustment, and so on, within the capability of each device or AAC application. Most devices also have the ability to compose word by word with voice output as well as waiting and only speaking sentence by sentence. For many individuals with auditory processing issues, hearing each word as it is spoken can be confusing and make composing a full message more difficult. As with all things, this should be a person-by-person, individual-led decision. Figure 23–3 shows adjustments that can be made to speech settings in different current applications for AAC.

Visual processing may also affect access to an individual's device. The number one factor affecting a user, especially of an app-based device, is screen glare. When a device is placed flat and the included stands or kickstands are not utilized properly, the overhead lights create a glare that can make accurate selection difficult. Matte screen protectors can also be applied to assist in decreasing glare. Color sensitivities might also impact a PWUAAC. This can be assisted by changing the backgrounds or the screen display intensity/brightness within the device settings. Figure 23–4 shows different settings in AAC programs that can be adjusted for visual processing difficulties. If the PWUAAC also has tactile processing needs and uses a keyguard, they should be able to trial a few different colors of them so the contrast between it and the device screen is not an issue.

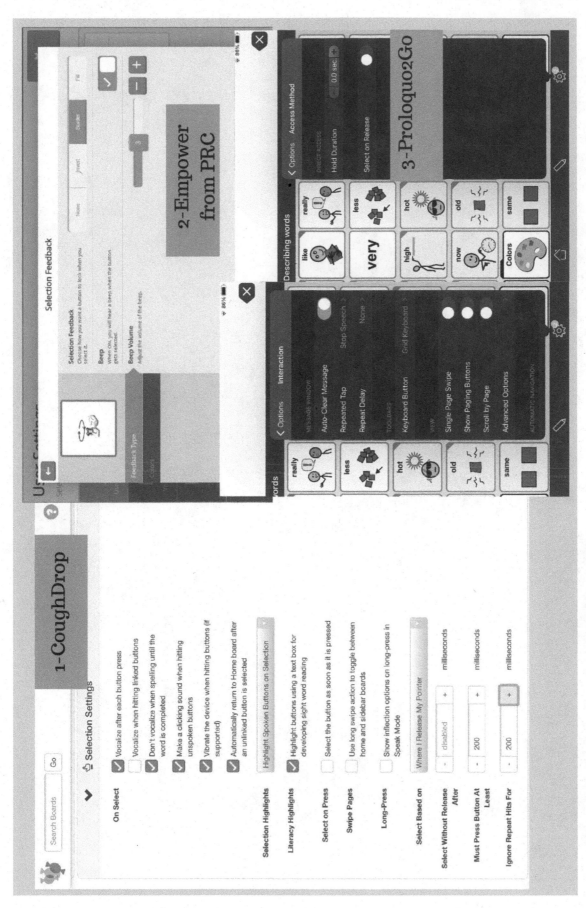

Figure 23–2. Selection settings from CoughDrop (CoughDrop AAC), Proloquo2Go (Assistiveware), TouchChat HD with WordPower (Prentke-Romich), Speak for Yourself (Speak For Yourself AAC), Snap Core First (Tobii Dynavox). TouchChat, and Empower are trademarks of PRC-Saltillo. © 2021 PRC-Saltillo. Minspeak® symbols used under exclusive license from Semantic Compaction Systems, Inc. WordPower is a trademark of Inman Innovations, Inc. *continues*

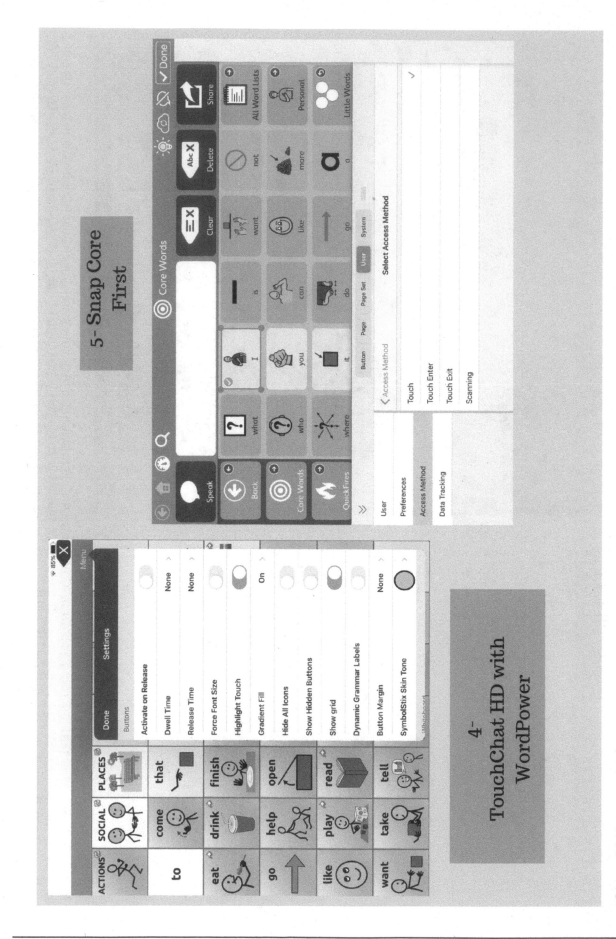

Figure 23–2. *continued*

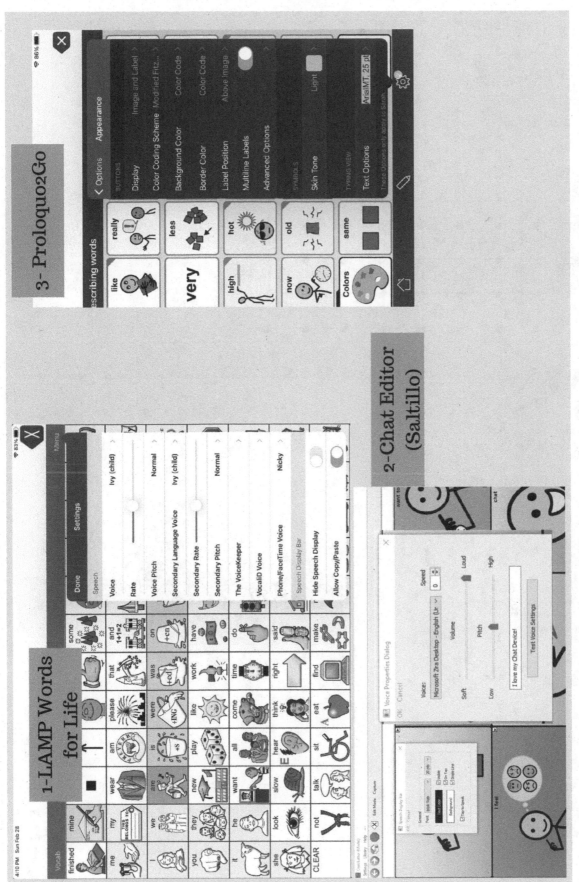

Figure 23–3. Voice and speech settings from LAMP Words for Life (Center for AAC and Autism), Chat Editor (Saltillo), Proloquo2Go (Assistiveware), TouchChat HD with WordPower (Prentke-Romich), and Speak for Yourself (Speak For Yourself AAC). ChatEditor, LAMP Words for Life, TouchChat, and Empower are trademarks of PRC-Saltillo. © 2021 PRC-Saltillo. Minspeak® symbols used under exclusive license from Semantic Compaction Systems, Inc. WordPower is a trademark of Inman Innovations, Inc. *continues*

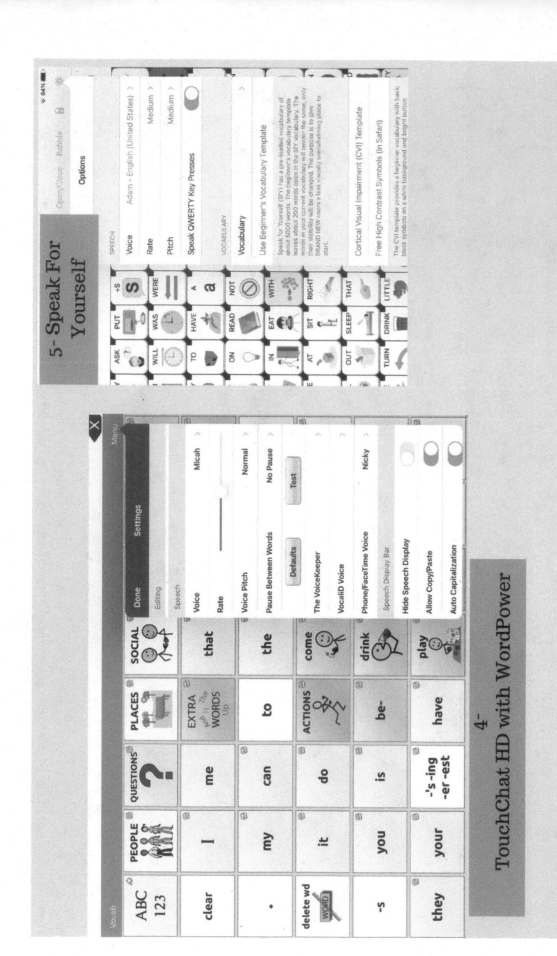

Figure 23–3. *continued*

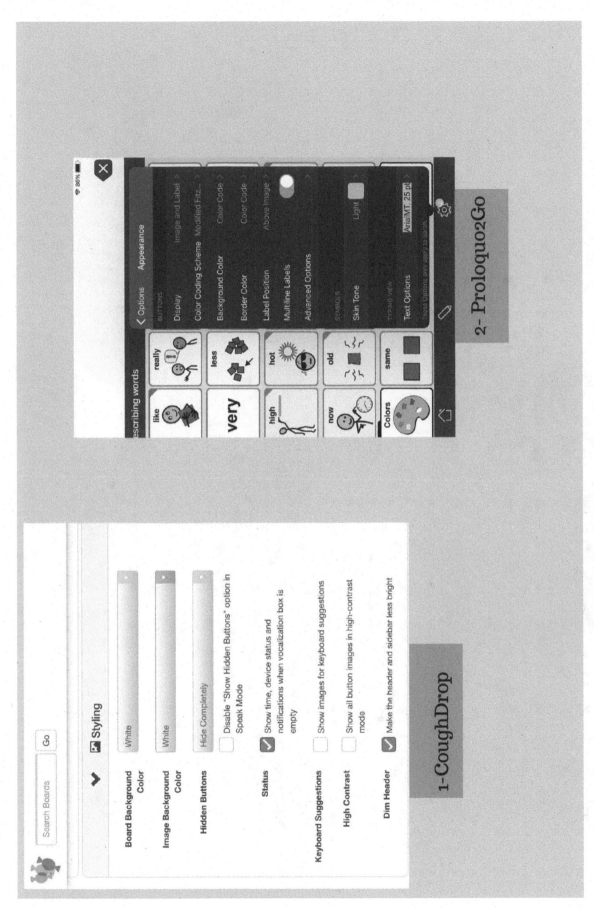

Figure 23–4. Visual processing settings from CoughDrop (CoughDrop AAC), Proloquo2Go (Assistiveware), TouchChat HD with WordPower (Prentke-Romich) and Snap Core First (Tobii Dynavox). ChatEditor, LAMP Words for Life, TouchChat, and Empower are trademarks of PRC-Saltillo. © 2021 PRC-Saltillo. Minspeak® symbols used under exclusive license from Semantic Compaction Systems, Inc. WordPower is a trademark of Inman Innovations, Inc. *continues*

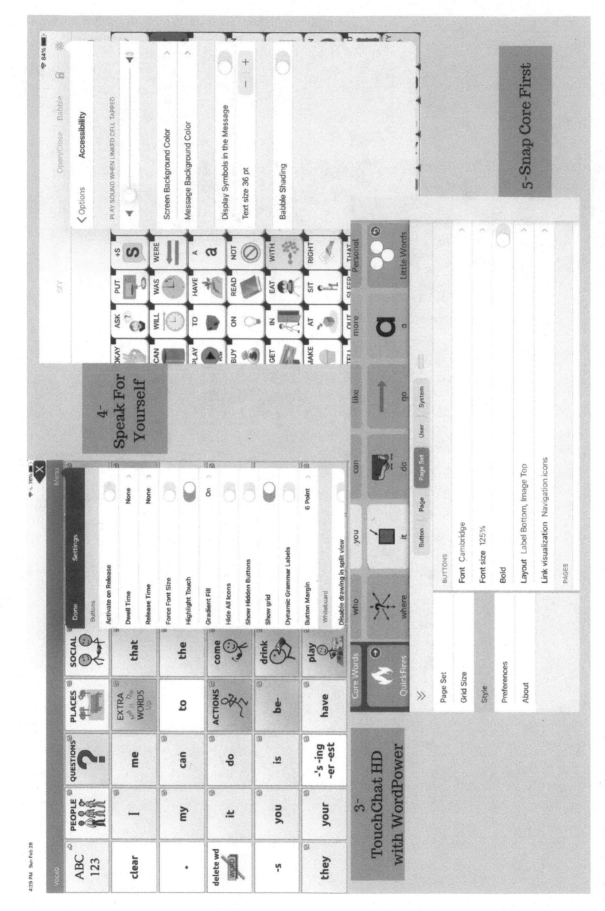

Figure 23–4. *continued*

For supporting other sensory processing difficulties, accommodations tend to be less about physical changes to the device. For these areas of gustatory, vestibular, proprioception, olfactory, and interoception, the need shifts more toward ensuring that the PWUAAC has appropriate vocabulary to speak to their needs. When planning for those with challenges in these areas, having words available and accessible such as those in Table 23–1 will assist the PWUAAC in communicating about and advocating for their specific needs. All PWUAACs need access to language they can use to self-advocate. These vocabulary words are often the areas where decreased language skills occur when they are frustrated or overwhelmed.

Considerations for the Trial Process

It is critical for a successful communicator that those assisting with making device and language system selections take into account an individual's sensory needs. During the trial process, one might have to continually adjust based on an individual's changing needs. Be sure to involve the individual and value their input and preferences first and foremost. Those familiar with the SETT Framework (Zabala, n.d.) will know that student/society member is the place to begin, and this holds true for sensory processing concerns as well.

If the PWUAAC has limited awareness of their sensory needs or language to describe what they need, this information should be gathered through clinical observations and caregiver interviews. One might also elicit feedback using low or no language-based strategies such as visual supports or imagery to support "I like that" or "I don't like that." It is also important to show the PWUAAC all possible options on how to customize device settings to meet their sensory needs.

Instructional Strategies

When a student is struggling with an area of sensory integration, their needs may present differently in different settings (e.g., home, school, vocational). All environments should be considered in a multi-disciplinary evaluation. Therefore, it is important to support the PWUAAC in not only recognizing when a change needs to be made to their AAC device, but to build the operational competence to make changes when needed.

When targeting operational competence, it is beneficial for the SLP and OT to collaborate and problem-solve together. It is important to identify what an individual's sensory needs are and how to make accommodations to the environment and communication device. Involve the PWUAAC as changes are made to the system so that they have agency over the process.

Table 23–1. Commonly Needed Key Vocabulary for Sensory Integration Needs

Sensory Processing Area	Commonly Used Key Vocabulary
Gustatory	Tastes sweet/sour/bland; need to spit it out; I like that/don't like that
Vestibular	Dizzy/headache/spinning; I need to sit down
Proprioception	I need to move around; I am afraid of falling; device is too heavy
Olfactory	Smells bad; I'm allergic to that scent/perfume
Interoception	Hungry/tired; need to use the bathroom; stomach hurts; body parts for pain

Ideas for targeting operational competence in therapy:

- Use natural opportunities, for example, when the device has low battery demonstrate how and where to plug it in.
- Help the PWUAAC test out different voices and give them agency to select their own voice.
- Adjust the volume in different settings, and discuss when to use a quiet versus louder voice.
- Demonstrate how to adjust screen brightness and practice using the setting in different environments with different lighting.
- Turn on auditory feedback (e.g., a beep every time a button is activated) and ask the PWUAAC if it is helpful.
- Adjust visual feedback settings such as a boarder highlight when a button is selected.
- Demonstrate different access methods such as direct selection or a stylus.

Teach how to add new vocabulary and create quick access phrases to help describe sensory processing needs (e.g., "my stomach hurts").

After the settings are adjusted, provide support to help the individual become independent with changing settings, such as volume and brightness of the device. Provide intervention across settings to work through realistic challenges to the sensory system. For example, go outside and demonstrate how the device reflects light differently depending on where it is placed in relation to the sun. Discuss what makes it easier or more difficult to use the device depending on the glare. Another important instructional strategy is to teach language that will help the individual understand and describe their sensory needs. Teaching individuals to express preferences can also help with sensory integration (e.g., "I like it," "I don't like it," "change it," "I want a different voice"). Also, collaborate with the PWUAAC to create phrases, in their own words, that can be programmed into the device for quick access (e.g., "please turn down the lights").

Case Study: ES

Clinical Profile and Communication Needs

The Individual

This is a hypothetical student composed of a few different students from the authors' past experiences.

ES is a 7-year-old male. He has a medical diagnosis of autism, as well as a vision impairment of convergence insufficiency, affecting his ability to track and read fluently. ES attends a public elementary school and spends most of his school day in a general education classroom. He receives services through his individualized education plan (IEP), including speech/language therapy (SLP), occupational therapy (OT), and special education services.

Based on standardized assessments, ES's receptive and expressive language fall within the below average range. He communicates through multiple modalities including gesture, facial expression, and echolalia. ES has had a communication device (iPad with a communication app) for 1 year but does not often choose to use it. ES also has a moderate learning disability that impacts his reading, writing, and executive functioning skills. Outside of school, ES enjoys spending time with his older brother, having dinner at his grandparents' house each week, going to swim classes, and participating in 4-H.

Their Communication Partners

ES's communication partners include his peers at school, swimming, and 4-H, teachers and instructors, parents, grandparents, cousins, lunchroom workers, therapists, and paraprofessionals in his classroom.

Their Environment

ES communicates in many different environments each week, including his public school campus, special education classroom, swimming class, 4-H, private therapy center, and his grandparents' house. He spends most of his school day in a first-grade classroom with his peers.

AAC Considerations

ES's school team was concerned that he does not like to use his current AAC device but still needs communication support. His school team and family both reported that he does not like to touch or be touched and appears to have tactile defensiveness. Bright lights and glare appear to be aversive to him and affect his vision significantly as well as his medical diagnosis of convergence insufficiency. They requested an updated AAC evaluation as well as an updated OT evaluation to gain more information about his sensory integration needs.

The team agreed to begin with the OT evaluation to determine how sensory processing would impact ES's use of AAC. The evaluation revealed that ES demonstrated difficulty with visual processing secondary to his convergence insufficiency, as well as tactile defensiveness with most surfaces, including that of his tablet device.

After the OT evaluation was completed, ES's school team and family met to complete the SETT framework (Zabala, n.d.). First, they discussed the **student**, ES, his current diagnoses, and IEP services. They listed his strengths and areas where he needed more support. Specifically, he has difficulty with communication, sensory integration, and literacy activities.

Next, they discussed the **environment** and described different places where ES has to perform the activities that are difficult for him. This included the general education classroom, special education classroom, hallways, lunchroom, special classes, home, and the community. They also listed the accommodations that were already in place including adapted seating, visual schedule, and iPad with an AAC app.

They discussed the **tasks** that ES needed assistance with. These included writing, reading, com-

munication, accessing the curriculum, and sensory integration. Once they had gathered information for the first three areas (student, environment, and tasks), they were ready to discuss the **tools**. They started with communication and began by outlining the necessary features, rather than naming specific tools.

The team discussed the continued need for a voice output device. Low-tech communication systems were ruled out as they would limit ES's communication partners to people who can read. He would also need a variety of accessibility features that could be adjusted to accommodate his sensory integration difficulties. Needed features included options for visual, auditory, and tactile feedback. It was also important to trial different icon colors such as high-contrast icons to support his diagnosis of convergence insufficiency. A dedicated SGD would provide more of these accessibility features than an iPad.

They ruled out systems with more than four button hits to access vocabulary; due to his vision challenges, they wanted to provide more language with fewer button hits to support motor planning. Another reason to rule out low-tech AAC systems was because the voice output or auditory feedback would help ES know that he hit the right button if he was not looking directly at the device.

The team decided to trial devices that had voice output, a full keyboard, few button hits to access language, a system with the ability to adjust settings such as brightness, color contrast, dwell time, visual/auditory feedback, and a device that would accommodate a keyguard. Once the trial started, data were collected by his SLP, OT, and special education teacher at school as well as his parents at home and in the community. They collected data across all settings outlined in the SETT meeting.

The AAC System or Service

Fortunately, the AAC app that ES had been using for a year was available on a dedicated SGD, so the team decided to trial that first since he was familiar with it. They hoped that by accommodating his sensory integration needs, he may be more interested in using the device. Based on the SETT meeting, and feature-matching process, they decided to trial a keyguard with a stylus to help with ES's tactile defensiveness. The current system required no more than three button hits to access any word and supported principles of motor planning. They decreased the brightness of the screen, added auditory feedback for each button hit as well as visual feedback (button highlight on touch). Consistent motor plans and auditory feedback may make it possible for ES to access language without always needing to look directly at the device.

ES's SLP and OT collaborated to find the best accessibility settings for the device and observed how his needs changed in different environments. They actively involved him in problem-solving and taught him the operational skills to independently change settings as needed. These skills will help him have more ownership of the device and help him independently support his sensory needs.

Next Steps

Based on the trial of ES's current language system on a dedicated SGD, changes to access and accessibility, he greatly increased his use of the system. He used a stylus to activate buttons and looked at the device more often given the decreased brightness and high contrast symbols. As motor planning became more automatic, he was able to look away from the device and continue to produce short messages accurately. The team decided to complete a funding request to obtain an SGD.

Once a device has been secured, the SLP and OT will provide training to ES's teachers and family. They will focus on what to look for when ES is having difficulty with sensory processing (e.g., not touching or looking at his device) and how they can support him, such as giving him a stylus or adjusting the angle of the device. They will make visual directions for how to change specific device settings so that ES or one of his teachers can make adjustments as needed. The OT and SLP will also create a short video about ES's sensory needs to share with his family and instructors in the community. In addition, they will check in monthly to see if any new challenges arise.

They added one session a month where the OT and SLP can co-treat in order to best support ES in using his device. Again, they will actively include ES and give him agency over the settings, such as auditory and visual feedback, and help him select a voice that he likes.

ES's SLP completed the Dynamic AAC Goals Grid 2 (DAGG-2) in collaboration with the team (Tobii Dynavox, 2015). This provided information to select goals in all four areas of communicative competence (Light, 1989). His OT will also target operational skills to help ES independently change settings on his device.

To support linguistic competency, ES and his SLP will target creating longer utterances across multiple pragmatic functions. They will use a core word of the week approach so that language can be consistently supported across related services, special education, and general education. For each core word, the SLP will provide sample two-word phrases across multiple pragmatic functions, for example, requesting, protesting, greeting, commenting, asking/answering questions, and directing.

Operational competency will be supported by both the SLP and OT. They collaborated to write a goal to support ES in adjusting settings to help his vision needs, such as changing the brightness and moving the device away from light. They also wrote a goal for ES to make adjustments based on his level of tactile defensiveness, such as using the stylus. Therapy activities will include helping ES select a voice and add preferred vocabulary that is not preprogrammed into the device.

Social competency support will include helping ES identify when he has a sensory need that he cannot independently navigate and seek help from a teacher. This will include initiating communication and preprogramming quick phrases such as "it's too bright in here." ES's SLP will support him to create the phrases in his own words and then program them.

Finally, strategic competency skills will include gaining attention before communicating a message. They will also work on using multimodal communication and choosing a different modality when not understood.

References

American Psychiatric Association. (2013). *Diagnostic and statistical manual of mental disorders* (5th ed.).

Ayres, A. J. (1971). Characteristics of types of sensory integrative dysfunction. *American Journal of Occupational Therapy, 25,* 329–334.

Baranek, G. T., Little, L. M., Parham, L. D., Ausderau, K., & Sabatos-Devito, M. (2014). Sensory features in autism spectrum disorders. In F. Volkmar, R. Paul, K. Pelphrey, & S. Rogers (Eds.), *Handbook of autism* (4th ed., pp. 378–408). Wiley.

Del Monte, B., Trujillo, C., Conaster, M., & Norris, G. (2019). *Complicated sensorimotor systems accessing AAC: A data driven approach.* Assistive Technology Industry Association 2019 Conference, Florida: ATIA.

Light, J. (1989). Toward a definition of communicative competence for individuals using augmentative and alternative communication systems. *Augmentative and Alternative Communication, 5*(2), 137–144. https://doi.org/10.1080/07434618912331275126

Mahler, K. (2017). *Interoception: The eighth sensory system.* AAPC Publishing.

Miller, L. J. (2006). *Sensational kids.* Putnam.

Occupational Therapy Practice Framework: Domain and process—fourth edition. (2020). *American Journal of Occupational Therapy, 74*(Suppl. 2), 7412410010. https://doi.org/10.5014/ajot.2020.74S2001

Tobii Dynavox. (2015). *The Dynamic AAC Goals Grid 2 (DAGG-2).* TobiiDynavox.com. http://tdvox.webdownloads.s3.amazonaws.com/MyTobiiDynavox/dagg%202%20-%20writable.pdf

Zabala, J. (n.d.). *SETT framework documents.* http://joyzabala.com/Documents.html

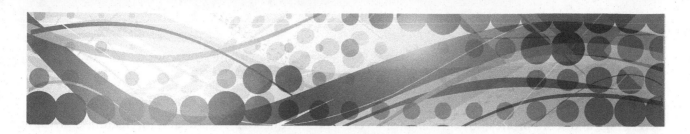

Chapter 24

AAC FOR PERSONS WITH COMPLEX TRAUMA

Lesley Quinn

Fundamentals

Abuse and neglect in early childhood impact every major system in the human brain from the brainstem to the cortex, from the sense of balance to the sense of self (Fisher, 2018).

There is growing consensus that maltreatment is harmful to children. That might seem like a surprising statement, but prior to 1998, it was not conventionally accepted that trauma, abuse, and neglect affect children's development. The Adverse Childhood Events (ACE) study shifted our thinking. For the first time, the medical community was presented with clear evidence that early adverse experiences are linked to later physical, mental, and economic well-being (Felitti et al., 1998). The ACE study is now an ongoing, nationally funded, multistate project, and data indicate that one in seven children experiences neglect or abuse (Centers for Disease Control and Prevention [CDC], 2020). Children with disabilities are at even greater risk for maltreatment than nondisabled children for a number of reasons (Hibbard & Desch, 2007).

It is not an overdramatization to say abuse and neglect cause brain cells to die. Researchers continue to look for the mechanism of action, but many studies have shown that gray matter decreases as severity of maltreatment increases (there are no differences in brain volume in mal-

treated children to start with) (Lim et al., 2014). There are also functional connectivity problems within and between cortical and subcortical brain regions (Teicher et al., 2003). While there is variability among individuals, certain brain regions are consistently affected: the somatosensory cortex, the right orbitofrontal-temporo-limbic area, and the left inferior frontal gyrus, which together are involved in sensory perception, attention, inhibition, emotion, and reward processing (Lim et al., 2014). In regard to sensory perception, Lim, Radua, and Rubia (2014) note that there is thinner cortex specifically in areas that correspond to body parts that were abused. They suggest developing brains adapt by "sensory gating" overwhelming experiences as a protective mechanism (p. 860).

Downstream, these neurological changes are associated with a host of sensory, motor, attention, learning, memory, language, social, emotional, and behavioral problems, which physicians try to capture with multiple diagnoses, like attention deficit hyperactivity disorder (ADHD), post-traumatic stress disorder (PTSD), reactive attachment disorder, oppositional defiance disorder, bipolar disorder, conduct disorder, developmental language disorder, and developmental coordination disorder, because no one diagnosis fits (van der Kolk, 2014).

In the area of language, maltreatment seems to have its own effects above and beyond low socioeconomic status (SES), IQ, or other developmental disorders (Lum et al., 2015). Children with histories of maltreatment can sometimes pass language screenings and score proficiently on sentence-level tests; however, as a group they have greater difficulty with receptive and expressive language, and invariably, with pragmatics, narrative language, and autobiographical memory (Brien et al., 2020; Ciolino et al., 2020; Sylvestre et al., 2016). Bessel van der Kolk, a leading trauma researcher, explains that verbal fluency is also affected. He says, while a nontraumatized person may be able to generate 15 words a minute, one with PTSD may only be able to name four. "The effects of trauma are not necessarily different from—and can overlap with—the effects of physical lesions like strokes," van der Kolk adds (2014, p. 43). With brain scans he shows that Broca's area goes offline in trauma survivors when they are experiencing strong emotions, so they literally "cannot put their thoughts and feelings into words" (p. 43).

For persons who experience pain, abuse, bullying, or neglect, it is essential to be able to communicate about sensitive issues (Johnson et al., 2017, p. 276).

Studies have not specifically addressed trauma, abuse, or neglect in children who use augmentative and alternative communication (AAC) or explored AAC use in children with histories of maltreatment. A few studies have addressed abuse and victimization in adults with complex communication needs (CCNs; Bornman, 2017; Bryen et al., 2003; Collier et al., 2006; Johnson et al., 2017). The studies pay particular attention to the vocabulary and environmental supports persons who use AAC (PWUAACs) need to self-advocate, protect themselves, report maltreatment, and access the legal system.

For PWUAACs, it is of particular concern whether they have access to the words they need to talk about traumatic experiences. Collier et al. (2006) found that only three of the 26 adults in their study had vocabulary they needed. Johnson, Bornman, and Tönsig (2017) explain that published vocabulary sets are often limited because they are based on observations of typical peers doing "fun things" or daily activities (p. 276).

When Collier and colleagues asked individuals using AAC and their communication partners

what words they needed to discuss maltreatment, they requested vocabulary for feelings, privacy, and bodily functions most often. Bornman (2017) found that verbs ranked most important (scream, hit), and that five words came up repeatedly when participants were asked to generate vocabulary lists: man, woman, hit, sore, sad. Johnson, Bornman, and Tönsig (2017) propose an iterative process for customizing AAC tools to discuss sensitive topics. They say preestablished lists will "rarely suffice," and in order to create personalized supports, implementers should use hypothetical scenarios to generate word lists (rather than asking about personal experiences), seek out the different perspectives of the PWUAAC and familiar others, and ask literate adults using AAC to socially validate the tools (p. 282).

Another concern Collier and colleagues address is that individuals in the study did not necessarily recognize maltreatment as abusive or neglectful, because they did not have a schema for thinking about it. However, given the opportunity to talk safely in groups with other individuals using AAC and counselors, they came to identify and organize their experiences differently. Some then wanted to report caregivers for abuses, like withholding or destroying their equipment, inappropriately administering medication, providing services while intoxicated, threatening them with the withdrawal of services, talking about the "dirty pictures" in their devices, making degrading comments, giving them the "silent treatment," or not allowing them to communicate. However, many others were hesitant to report out of fear of reprisal. It was not a hypothetical concern. Bryen et al. (2003) found that in 97% of instances individuals knew their abusers, and in 22% of participants the abuse was ongoing. Regardless of whether or not they wanted to report incidents, participants were keen to discuss an "overall lack of respect from people in their lives, a sense of condescension, and being treated less than equal to non-disabled people" (Collier et al., 2006, p. 68). Many participants requested help accessing mental health services to deal with past and current maltreatment, as they felt services were limited due to counselors' lack of training around their communication needs.

Trauma changes not only how we think and what we think about, but also our very capacity to think (van der Kolk, 2014, p. 21).

The experiences the adults using AAC reported to Barbara Collier and her colleagues of being degraded, threatened, and seen as less than by people on whom they depended are the ones that are most traumatic, according to van der Kolk. Beyond any objective measure of damage, he says a few characteristics determine whether incidents will have lasting traumatic impact and how severe it will be, namely, if they are unpredictable, inescapable, and isolating (van der Kolk, 2014). These subjective experiences make abuse and neglect deeply stressful, and when children—and by extension, adults with disabilities, who are dependent on others for care—experience prolonged or recurrent loss of safety, agency, and connection, which is inherent in abuse or neglect, it is traumatizing. Over time, at very basic levels, traumatic experiences reshape the way a person attends to and perceives the world. Early abuse and neglect are "complex trauma," precisely because traumatic interpersonal experiences are interwoven in complex ways with children's development in all areas.

Pamela Snow, a registered psychologist, researcher, and former speech-language pathologist (SLP), is "inviting speech-language pathology to the prevention table" when it comes to maltreated children (Snow, 2009). She has drawn the link between abuse and neglect and complex communication needs. She says the discipline of speech pathology "is an untapped resource" and has much to offer, given the depth and breadth of SLP's knowledge about language, which seems to be both a mitigating factor in the development of complex trauma and a key to its resolution. However, she emphasizes, "This expertise must be contextualized within the broader milieu of mental health." She continues, "Language competence is acquired through the relational milieu of parent-child interactions. Where these are positive and secure, both language and mental health develop synchronously and in ways that promote intra and inter personal skills in the child." (p. 100)

Where a safe, attuned relationship is lacking, Snow and van der Kolk agree, it must be a focus

of treatment. In addition, van der Kolk (2014) says successful intervention for children with complex trauma must address core features of the disorder that lead to language challenges: pervasive emotional dysregulation, problems with attention and concentration, and social challenges, "getting along with themselves and others" (p. 157). Light and McNaughton (2014) advocate for something similar to improve outcomes for individuals with CCNs. They say it is important to expand our focus and address "personal psychosocial factors," like motivation, attitude, confidence, and resilience alongside AAC competencies, so that AAC use is not the end goal but the means by which individuals with CCNs relate to others and engage in meaningful learning and work.

AAC assessment and treatment plans that take into account relationship and psychosocial needs are more likely to lead to successful outcomes for individuals with CCNs who experience abuse or neglect. They are also more likely to lead to success for individuals who have medical trauma related to their conditions. At the same time, as the language needs of individuals with severe complex trauma are spotlighted, SLPs will be asked to play an increasing role in their treatment. This may include AAC supports for those whose communication is significantly impaired due to speech or mental health challenges. In this group, addressing core relationships and psychosocial needs will be critical.

Case Study: PW

Clinical Profile and Communication Needs

The Individual

PW is 10 years old and in fourth grade. She likes curly fries, watching *Kratts' Creatures*, playing on the iPad, and riding her purple EzyRoller. She also likes to watch baseball with her uncle and bake with her cousin. She is from a Caucasian, English-speaking family. She has many diagnoses, including PTSD, Mood Disorder—NOS, Reactive

Attachment Disorder, and Developmental Speech and Language Disorder. She takes several different medications to help with her behavior, impulse control, and sleeping.

PW and her younger brother, who is 9 years old, were removed from their biological mother's care when PW was 6 years old. They have been living with their uncle since PW was 7 years old. He is now their legal guardian. Although not much is known about PW's early years, she experienced abuse and neglect. Her team suspects she was exposed to drugs, weapons, and prostitution. PW's brother has a diagnosis of intellectual impairment.

PW has received speech and occupational therapy since preschool. Her speech is difficult to understand. She repeated kindergarten and was soon placed in a self-contained classroom with increased staff support. Her behavior became increasingly aggressive (toward adults, peers, animals, and herself) in first grade, and she was placed in a partial hospitalization program. Since then, she has been in three different residential treatment programs and is currently in one near her home. She has missed many days of school as a result of the many transitions.

PW has difficulty participating in testing, but she has been able to complete some. Her IQ test scores vary from low average to very low, but team members do not believe they accurately reflect her potential. Her literacy and numeracy skills and her knowledge of basic concepts are estimated to be at prekindergarten levels. Her most recent CELF-5 Core Language score was 61, with scaled scores ranging from 1 to 6. When she speaks, she uses single words or short phrases. She does not have any alveolar or palatal consonants in her speech-sound repertoire. She also does not have consonant blends, and she only produces /m/, /n/, and /ng/ in syllable-final position. Her primary SLP at school observed that her production varies even with words she can articulate, and she has "reduced precision." Often, she will not speak for long periods of time at school and home.

PW's occupational therapist (OT) explained that she has difficulty planning and executing fine-motor movements. Her hands shake at rest and when she is pointing at something, which may be a side effect of medication. Her counselor said OT has been "monumental" in helping her identify strategies to calm her body.

In regard to communication, PW's uncle expressed the following frustration:

She loves languages. It is puzzling. She has a severe communication deficiency, but she is not confused by other languages. She knows a bit of Spanish. She can name body parts in German. She is obsessed with people, but she is unable to have the simplest appropriate interaction. She asks everyone she sees in public, 'What's your name?' They answer, and they ask her what her name is, but she never answers. She cannot have a "normal" conversation with us, where she tells us about her day, or anything personal, like what she likes, what she would like to do, what her thoughts are. I know her favorite fruit is watermelon, but she cannot tell me if I ask. When she is asked things at school that we don't provide information about she never tells "the truth." If I ask about things that I know did not happen, like it was raining and I ask if she played at the park, she says yes.

PW's team experienced these challenges when working with her:

"She has low frustration tolerance and resistance to completing tasks."

"She gets irritable quickly and can't maintain self-control when faced with adversity. She has weak resiliency, and she struggles to overcome stress."

"She is unable to play by herself, except for a minute or two."

"She doesn't respond to positive reinforcement. She's food motivated—she'll only work for McDonald's hash browns."

Their Communication Partners

At home, PW lives with her uncle and brother. Her uncle, now in his 60s, became the children's legal guardian when PW was 8 years old. PW's mother is his niece. Her uncle has two adult children, who live nearby. His wife died when his daughter and son were young, and he and his children are close as a result. His daughter is helping him raise PW and her brother. His daughter, her partner, and her partner's two children, who are PW's age, come over often. PW's uncle confirmed that her mother is not in contact with her or her brother. The family spends time with neighbors, friends, and many of his late wife's relatives.

At her local public school, PW was reported to interact most with her special education teacher and the educational service providers (ESPs) in the classroom. She sought out one ESP in particular, who was described as "calm, deliberate, and respectful." PW sometimes initiated interaction with other students but did not often respond, and she needed "a great deal of support" to play a game or have a conversation. She is expected to return to this school after she has completed her residential treatment program.

In her residential placement, PW goes to school on campus with the seven other students from her house. She spends a full day at school with the special education teacher, support staff, and peers. She sees her counselor individually once a week, but the counselor is a daily presence in the program. After school, she spends afternoons and evenings with her "house parents," her staff mentor, and other students in the program. When she is discharged from the program, she will have an in-home therapy team, with a counselor, mentor, and OT to support her transition, help her maintain skills, and work with her family to build new ones.

Their Environment

In her current placement, PW's day is highly structured and supportive. There is one adult for every three students. The program offers students trauma-informed care and integrates OT and dialectical behavioral therapy. Social-emotional learning is emphasized throughout the day. PW participates in weekly counseling with her family, and she sees them on weekends at the program or for home visits.

At school, PW receives individualized instruction. Academic work is designed to be high-interest, interactive, and thematic, and to support the development of creativity and responsibility. There are extracurricular activities, like wood-shop, an

organic vegetable garden, and an exercise gym with a climbing wall and a sensory space.

Evenings and weekends, PW and the other students do homework, personal care, cooking, and chores. Students go on frequent outings with staff, and there are opportunities to watch TV and play video games. Students participate in equine-assisted therapy, and they have regular visits from a therapy dog named Mars, who is trained to provide support to individuals with PTSD. They also have daily group meetings, where students and staff discuss concerns and engage in collaborative problem-solving and relationship repair.

AAC Considerations

The mental health and allied health communities widely cite therapeutic alliance as integral to successful intervention (Malhotra & Chauhan, 2020; Ormhaug, 2014). The key elements of a therapeutic alliance are said to include the personal bond that develops between client and therapist and the mutually agreed-upon goals and tasks involved in the process. Where AAC is concerned, it includes the AAC device and other tools. This means it is essential to consider an individual's AAC preferences, especially since it is becoming clear that even young children with significant disabilities have preferences for the AAC they use (van der Meer et al., 2011). For individuals with complex trauma, no other AAC consideration may be as important as preference.

Since there were no major physical, sensory, or cognitive access needs to consider for PW, the main considerations were what she preferred to use and what best supported her ability to connect and relate, although it was clear these were not going to be easy or quick decisions to make. During the first few sessions, PW showed overt fear. Her eyes were wide, her posture was rigid, she stood behind staff members, and retreated backward if we approached. She entered a therapy room only when staff promised hash browns, and she kept her head down on the table between folded arms. She refused to look at us or the AAC. On two occasions, she lay down on the floor, fell asleep, and could not be roused.

Over the course of a 3-month extended evaluation, which allowed PW time to adjust and move at a comfortable pace, she began to connect, show interest in materials, and take up to three turns in an activity. She began to use AAC to inform or request, and she did this while coordinating her attention for up to 15 min. Ultimately, she began to relate, and she showed us which AAC system she preferred. However, it required us to carefully consider her needs in the areas of (a) safe and positive relationships, (b) emotional regulation, (c) attention, and (d) social attunement, and to use an assessment procedure that provided immediate feedback about meaningful behavior change in areas where there are no established group norms and a great deal of individual variability.

The system she chose was an iPad mini with a communication app that used "word tree" organization. She preferred an iPad mini over a dedicated device, a standard-size tablet, a plus-size smartphone, or a paper-based communication book, and she preferred word tree organization over pragmatic, environment, and core word/semantic compaction layouts. Figures 24–1, 24–2, and 24–3 show her progression with three AAC systems over the course of assessment. For PW, the learning picture with word tree organization was one of increasing joint attention and meaningful communication week by week, with decreasing noncommunicative intent.

The AAC System or Service

The following are steps PW's team took to help her begin to relate with AAC. They are not an exhaustive or prescriptive list of what to do for an individual with complex trauma, but they provide a framework for making decisions and developing a responsive assessment or treatment plan. The steps could broadly be described as (a) laying the foundation for a positive relationship with PW by fostering positive, collaborative relationships within the team; (b) keeping PW's level of arousal within the "learning bandwidth"; (c) helping PW and her communication partners think about the same thing at the same time; and (d) activating attunement to encourage back-and-forth communication.

Positive, Supportive Relationships. In order to lay the foundation for a positive relationship with an individual with complex trauma, it is important for the people in their circle to support one another and collaborate, both to model positive relationships and to address very challenging behaviors

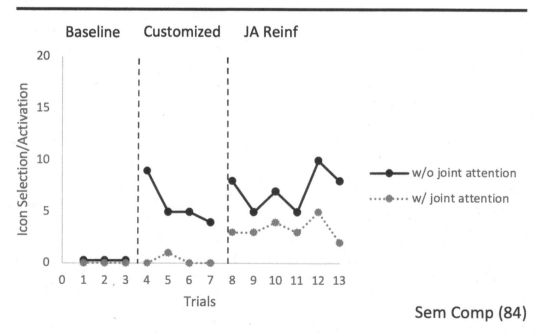

Figure 24–1. PW's learning picture with AAC system 1.

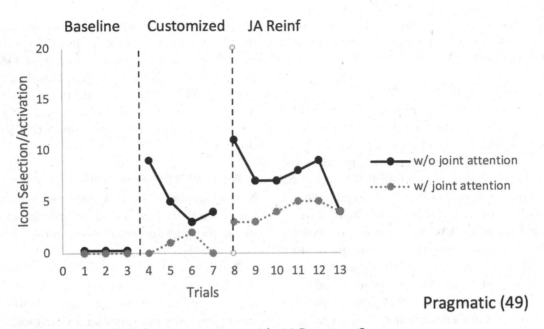

Figure 24–2. PW's learning picture with AAC system 2.

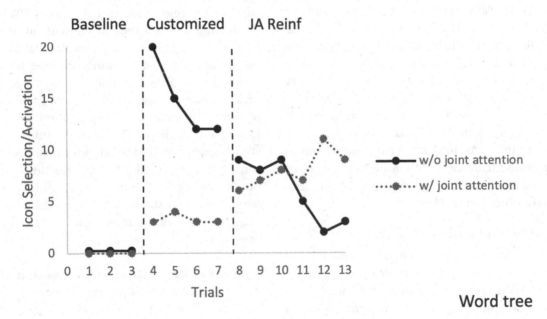

Figure 24–3. PW's learning picture with AAC system 3.

that come up. The steps team members took to do this for PW were as follows:

- Define the shared narrative.

Narratives can highlight problems and suggest common themes, which, if addressed, can move communication in a more meaningful direction. We asked, "What was the most enjoyable time you've had with PW?" and "What was the hardest time you've had with her?" PW's team members voiced similar frustrations that she initiated but did not respond, and she could not or would not share personal information. They suggested it was hard to get to know her and hard to connect. She was "there but not really there."

■ Clarify expectations for AAC use.

Miscommunication and unmet expectations can lead to frustration for the PWUAAC and their communication partners, so it is good practice to discuss expectations up front. Several team members said PW did not need AAC, while PW's uncle said he would like to have a conversation and have her tell him what she did at school. We made sure to discuss PW's use of AAC to express her feelings when she was dysregulated. Team members often suggest this as a goal. We concluded it would not be a reasonable goal at first, because she would need extensive support and skill building to do this, just as she would if she were communicating orally.

■ Clarify roles.

Language, especially narrative language, is integral to trauma treatment. The SLP/AAC specialist's role is not to discuss specific traumatic experiences but to help individuals develop the language skills they need to do trauma work. This includes vocabulary for feelings, mental state words, and autobiographical memory for positive personal events, which can be used as a template for discussing negative experiences in counseling. It was also important to clarify with the team how to handle disclosures of abuse or neglect and how to support PW in identifying safe others to disclose to.

■ Identify professional resources.

PW's team had access to many professional resources, with OT being a critical one. For an individual with complex trauma, it is often beneficial to have the support of a trauma-informed behavior analyst (TIBA). PW's team consulted with a board-certified behavior analyst (BCBA), who identified behavioral strategies that were contraindicated, given her history of neglect and abuse, and ones that would support her growth. She provided an in-service to the team about the risks of using procedures that mimicked past neglect or abuse. Attention-related extinction (ignoring bad behavior) and contingent praise to establish compliance

(praising obedient behavior) were two procedures that were deemed risky until adults were conditioned as "neutral" stimuli and had established a history of safe, consistent, helpful interactions with PW. The TIBA identified noncontingent reinforcement on a fixed schedule (something positive coming at a set time) as one important strategy to do this.

■ Confirm the safety plan.

New team members were provided with a written list of unsafe behaviors and instructions for whom to call for help and what to do in each instance.

■ Identify triggers and calming strategies.

Residential staff had extensive knowledge of PW's triggers, and they were starting to identify calming strategies. They put together a visual reminder and gave a copy to each team member. It had five feelings (happy, sad, mad, scared, disgusted) with PW's triggers on one side, and the ways PW showed the feeling on the other, along with strategies that helped her regulate. For example, fear at low levels looked like fast blinking, looking to the side, or hand-wringing. At higher levels, it became skin picking, hairpulling, rocking, pacing, or vasovagal response (dizziness, ringing in the ears, fainting). It was a useful tool, because it indicated which strategies worked best at which times. For PW, sensory strategies like finger brushing or walking outside worked when she was mildly dysregulated, but when she was so scared that she became aggressive or dissociated, she needed others to leave the room.

Emotional Regulation and Attention. Level of arousal and attention interact in ways that impact learning. If a task is easy or automatic, higher arousal helps us perform; however, if it is new or complex (which almost all AAC learning is) lower arousal is better (Teigen, 1994). Past a certain level, both under- and overarousal become incapacitating. A central difficulty for individuals with complex trauma is that they are frequently understimulated or overstimulated, so they cannot attend. Sometimes they are both at the same time. They also find it very difficult to emotionally regulate or adjust.

Arousal also drives attention—it guides us to see and do things that engage us if we are under-aroused and calm us if we are overstimulated. Because of this, we see things differently in different states of arousal. If you are hot and thirsty, a glass of water looks like a drink. If you are not, it could just as easily be a science experiment, a percussion instrument, or a diving opportunity for your action figure. The value we assign something, how close or far removed it feels, and whether we see the whole or its parts are influenced by arousal. Individuals with complex trauma, for example, tend to focus on eyes and view neutral expressions as angry or threatening. In these ways, arousal and attention influence learning and creativity. For PW, severe dysregulation meant we could not know what she was seeing. It also meant that telling her to "look" or "pay attention" did not ensure she was looking at or thinking about something in the same way as we were.

To address regulation, PW's team took steps to help her achieve a calm, alert state in order to learn complex, new things. We worked to do the following:

- Frame emotional regulation as an underdeveloped skill that could be improved and see small gains in this area as big successes.
- Avoid taking anything personally, even when it seemed targeted.
- Find something we genuinely liked about PW and let others know.
- Do something prior to each session to help ourselves maintain a calm, confident presence.
- Communicate pleasure in seeing PW at the beginning of each session, especially if the last session was difficult, and make sure PW perceived we were happy to see her.
- Establish predictable routines and introduce novelty within them.
- Minimize bright lights, noise, and fast movements to avoid PW's hyperstartle reflex.
- Implement a sensory strategy at the beginning of each session: holding

something warm, feeling something soft, or tasting something sweet.
- Avoid communicating shame verbally or with body language.
- Use a calm, even tone of voice.
- Show we are on the same side by using "we" ("We'll practice together." "Let's figure it out." "What should we do?").
- Ask PW her thoughts and ideas ("How can I help?" "What do you think?" "What would work here?").
- Go first, show how it works, and let PW direct our actions.
- Model making mistakes and trying again.
- Identify early signs PW was becoming dysregulated and intervene quickly.
- Keep sessions brief, end on success, and work to increase endurance each time.
- Avoid reasoning, rationalizing, or problem-solving with PW when she was dysregulated.
- Negotiate in advance with PW when she was regulated, how to handle difficult situations when they arose ("What should we do when __?").
- Focus on opportunities to do better next time.
- Ask PW how long she could tolerate doing a nonpreferred task and set a timer ("We can do hard things when we know they're going to end").
- Practice playing and having fun during each session.

In addition, team members took steps to establish joint attention with PW so she and her communication partners were "thinking together." We worked to do the following:

- Reinforce hand tracking.

Joint attention is as much about referencing a speaker's hands as it is their eyes. Eye contact was a trigger for PW, so we started by reinforcing dyadic joint attention, or hand tracking and orienting to a point. When PW was emotionally regulated, saying "thank you for looking" with a genuine tone of voice was highly reinforcing. Meanwhile, noncontingent reinforcement on a fixed schedule helped her stay regulated.

■ Shape communicative intent and "thinking together" by reinforcing eye behavior.

PW would not make eye contact or respond volitionally, either verbally or nonverbally, so we focused on how she engaged with the nonsocial world in automatic ways with her eyes. Psychologist Daniel Kahneman (2011) explains that working memory and pupil dilation are linked. He notes that our pupils start to dilate when we engage working memory and keep dilating up until the moment we find an answer or give up. With nonverbal, severely motorically impaired individuals, pupil response might be the only reliable behavior we have to work with, but we can also reinforce eye behavior with individuals like PW, who struggle to communicate for social-emotional reasons.

When we asked PW a question, gave her a direction, or showed her an item and her eyes dilated, we responded, "Thank you for thinking about it" or "I see you thinking." When she was tolerating these exchanges, we became more direct. We asked, "Are you thinking about this part?" or "What do you see?" Within several sessions, PW began to respond by nodding or pointing. We expanded on these interactions with comments like, "Me too; we're thinking about the same thing" or "I see that too. And I can see this." Once we had a sequence of three contingent exchanges, where she attended to the speaker, responded with her eyes or a gesture, and responded to a follow-up, we began to focus on AAC use.

What is important to notice is that we did not reinforce eye contact. Direct eye contact can be highly triggering. But more than that, sustained, unbroken eye contact is not what happens during natural exchanges. Eye behavior is fluid, as communication partners check in with each other to make sure they are, literally, on the same page. The goal with PW was to reinforce shared looking, and then establish triadic joint attention by reinforcing a sequence of looks, first to an item (materials or AAC), then the speaker's face, then back to the item, or vice versa. It took time and practice for PW to do this consistently, and it had to be reinforced

with each new communication partner, but starting with the kinds of experiences very young children have with attention helped PW build her capacity. Shifting attention is the basis for "back-and-forth" conversation, and we have increasing evidence that early differences in attention predict later language skills in children with disabilities, with a growing call to address attention and other executive functions (Amso & Scerif, 2015; Atkinson & Braddick, 2011; D'Souza et al., 2020; Hsu et al., 2014; Scerif & Steele, 2011; Schuymer et al., 2011).

Social Attunement and Reciprocity. While we addressed emotional regulation and attention, we also worked to activate PW's system of social attunement. Van der Kolk (2014) describes early social interaction as "the dance of attunement." (p. 111). He explains that the back and forth of conversation has its roots in physical rhythms and attuned movements between infants and caregivers, and is the reason rocking, singing, hand games, and rhymes are part of caregiving routines across cultures. These rhythmic experiences are the early basis for conversation, and disruptions in these attuned rhythms are consequential for brain development. One of the most striking consequences is its effect on the "self-sensing system," otherwise known as the default mode network (DMN). The DMN runs down the midline of the brain and connects frontal and parietal areas with parts of the brain that process internal sensations. These areas, he says, work together to integrate body sensations with conscious perceptions and create a sense of self. It is also involved in many later developing, higher-level skills, like social cognition and narrative language. The network is so important to humans it is the default brain state. In other words, when we are not actively doing something else, we are thinking about our social selves. Van der Kolk takes care to explain that there can be near complete inactivation in the DMN for individuals with complex trauma, and that "the lack of self-awareness. . . is sometimes so profound that they cannot recognize themselves in a mirror" (p. 92).

To address rhythm and attunement with PW, we aimed to do the following:

■ Start each session with a nonverbal, attuned, rhythmic activity and transfer the rhythm to a communication task.

PW was able to establish a rhythm nonverbally with a communication partner relatively quickly. Within several sessions, she could bounce on a yoga ball, rock on a balance board, blow a tissue, volley a balloon, trace lines in a sand tray, fill a cup with cotton puffs, or color a picture with a bingo dabber in the context of "at the same time" or "I go, you go" exchanges. One activity that worked well was taking turns adding shapes to create a picture in a tangram app on the iPad. Initially, the tempo that engaged her was slow, with 15- to 20 s pauses; however, it increased with time. Since the goal was not to do rhythmic activities per se, but to establish attunement, once we activated it, we switched to communication tasks with AAC. In addition, as we were better able to modulate her level of arousal, rhythm and reciprocity were established more quickly.

A final social need we began to address was the language of self. We worked to do the following:

■ Attend to and recognize faces.

We used the "selfie" view on an iPad instead of a mirror. PW would not come into view of the camera at first, but she would watch a communication partner and sometimes direct them by pointing. Later she was willing to look at herself with a communication partner in view at the same time.

■ Establish her understanding of I/you.

We practiced *What do I see?/What do you see?* with cards that had different pictures on the front and back. This was challenging, and she consistently matched her answer to what she saw on the front of the card, even when asked by her communication partner, "What do *I* see?"

■ Create a concrete representation of PW.

We used a customization feature on an AAC app to take "selfies" and decorate them. PW created a messy image of herself, unrecognizable and full of scribbles, but it became the *I* symbol on the AAC devices. PW began to select *I* with increasing frequency after this activity, even though she did not use it self-referentially in phrases. Going forward, team members will take photos of her as she is comfortable and see which one she wants to use to represent *I*.

Next Steps

PW's team decided to pursue AAC with her. Some were very surprised at her responsiveness to it and the clinicians who did the AAC evaluation. Her team is optimistic about what she will be able to communicate over the next year, having seen her growth with AAC/language therapy. Her communication partners are also excited about word trees. They have created a number of lite-tech supports, as word tree organization seems to be a useful scaffold for her. Her OT and counselor have taken screenshots and created lite-tech supports to help her identify emotions and sensory experiences in therapy. Her teacher has made word tree activities for students to practice categorizing. PW's family is using a word tree to help her identify her likes and dislikes. Every time she tries something new, they give her an icon to go with it, and she puts it on either the *I like it* or *I don't like it* tree posted in the kitchen. As Figure 24–4 shows, they have also made it a shared experience by drawing or embellishing icons.

Her team is now thinking about the language foundations PW needs to engage in trauma work in the coming years. Understanding others' intentions, making predictions about their behavior, and having a coherent narrative about herself and her past are long-term mental health goals. To lay the foundations for that work, team members will continue to address vocabulary for self and others, perspective taking, and early skills in autobiographical memory, like identifying present versus past experiences ("What do you see now?" "What did you see before that?"). It will be months before PW is discharged from her residential treatment center, but her team believes she is making progress, and they are eager to see it continue.

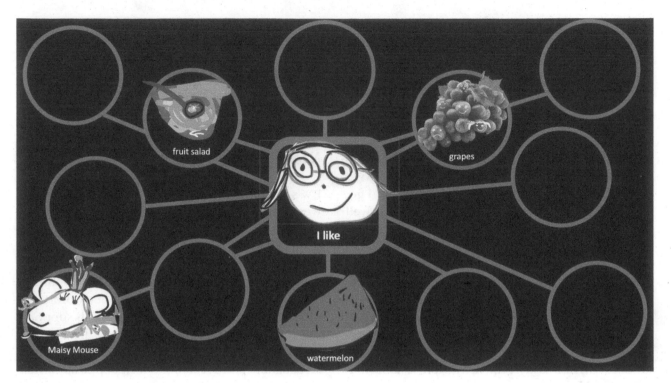

Figure 24–4. PW's paper-based word tree for likes.

References

Amso, D., & Scerif, G. (2015). The attentive brain: Insights from developmental cognitive neuroscience. *Nature Reviews. Neuroscience, 16*(10), 606–619.

Atkinson, J., & Braddick, O. (2011). From genes to brain development to phenotypic behavior: "Dorsal-stream vulnerability" in relation to spatial cognition, attention, and planning of actions in Williams syndrome (WS) and other developmental disorders. *Progress in Brain Research, 189*, 261–283.

Bornman, J. (2017). Preventing abuse and providing access to justice for individuals with complex communication needs: The role of augmentative and alternative communication. *Seminars in Speech and Language, 38*(4), 321–331.

Brien, A., Hutchins, T. L., & Westby, C. (2020, November). Autobiographical memory in autism spectrum disorder, attention-deficit/hyperactivity disorder, hearing loss, and childhood trauma: Implications for social communication intervention. *Language Speech and Hearing Services in the Schools, 30*, 1–21.

Bryen, D. N., Carey, A., & Frantz, B. (2003, June). Ending the silence: Adults who use augmentative communication and their experiences as victims of crimes. *Augmentative and Alternative Communication, 19*(2), 125–134.

Centers for Disease Control and Prevention (CDC). (2020). *Preventing child abuse and neglect. How big is the problem?* https://www.cdc.gov/violenceprevention/pdf/can/CAN-factsheet_2020.pdf

Ciolino, C., Hyter, Y., Suarez, M., & Bedrosian, J. (2020). Narrative and other pragmatic language abilities of children with a history of maltreatment. *Perspectives of the ASHA Special Interest Groups, 6*(2), 230–241. https://doi.org/10.1044/2020_PERSP-20-00136

Collier, B., Mcghie-Richmond, D., Odette, F., & Pyne, J. (2006, March). Reducing the risk of sexual abuse for people who use augmentative and alternative communication. *Augmentative and Alternative Communication, 22*(1), 62–75.

D'Souza, D., D'Souza, H., Jones, E., & Karmiloff-Smith, A. (2020). Attentional abilities constrain language development: A cross-syndrome infant/toddler study. *Developmental Science, 23*(6), 129–161.

Felitti, V. J., Anda, R. F., Nordenberg, D., Williamson, D. F., Spitz, A. M., Edwards, V., . . . Marks, J. S. (1998). Relationship of childhood abuse and household dysfunction to many of the leading causes of death in adults: The adverse childhood experiences (ACE) study. *American Journal of Preventive Medicine, 14*(4), 245–258.

Fisher, S. (2018). *Developmental trauma: New thinking, new treatment, new challenges* [Event]. Sebern F. Fisher. https://www.sebernfisher.com/upcoming-webinar-developmental-trauma-new-thinking-new-treatment-new-challenges/

Hibbard, R. A., & Desch, L. W. (2007). Maltreatment of children with disabilities. *Pediatrics, 119*(5), 1018–1025.

Hsu, N. S., Novick, J. M., & Jaeggi, S. M. (2014). The development and malleability of executive control abilities. *Frontiers in Behavioral Neuroscience, 8*, 221.

Johnson, E., Bornman, J., & Tönsig, K. (2017). Model for vocabulary selection of sensitive topics: An example from pain-related vocabulary. *Seminars in Speech and Language, 38*(4), 276–285.

Kahneman, D. (2011). *Thinking, fast and slow*. Farrar, Straus and Giroux.

Light, J., & McNaughton, D. (2014). Communicative competence for individuals who require augmentative and alternative communication: A new definition for a new era of communication? *Augmentative and Alternative Communication, 30*, 1–18. https://doi.org/10.3109/07434618.2014.885080

Lim, L., Radua, J., & Rubia, K. (2014). Gray matter abnormalities in childhood maltreatment: A voxel-wise meta-analysis. *American Journal of Psychiatry, 171*(8), 854–863.

Lum, J. A., Powell, M., Timms, L., & Snow, P. (2015). A meta-analysis of cross-sectional studies investigating language in maltreated children. *Journal of Speech Language and Hearing Research, 58*(3), 961–976.

Malhotra, S., & Chauhan, N. (2020). The therapeutic alliance between the child, parents, and health professionals. *Handbook of Clinical Neurology, 174*, 323–332.

Ormhaug, S. M., Jensen, T. K., Wentzel-Larsen, T., & Shirk, S. R. (2014). The therapeutic alliance in treatment of traumatized youths: Relation to outcome in a randomized clinical trial. *Journal of Consultation and Clinical Psychology, 82*(1), 52–64.

Scerif, G., & Steele, A. (2011). Neurocognitive development of attention across genetic syndromes: Inspecting a disorder's dynamics through the lens of another. *Progress in Brain Research, 189*, 285–301.

Schuymer, L. D., Groote, I. D., Striano, T., Stahl, D., & Roeyers, H. (2011). Dyadic and triadic skills in preterm and full-term infants: A longitudinal study in the first year. *Infant Behavior and Development, 34*(1), 179–188.

Snow, P. (2009). Child maltreatment, mental health and oral language competence: Inviting speech-language pathology to the prevention table. *International Journal of Speech-Language Pathology, 11*(2), 95–103.

Sylvestre, A., Bussières, È. L., & Bouchard, C. (2016). Language problems among abused and neglected children: A meta-analytic review. *Child Maltreatment, 21*(1), 47–58.

Teicher, M. H., Andersen, S. L., Polcari, A., Anderson, C. M., Navalta, C. P., & Kim, D. M. (2003). The neurobiological consequences of early stress and childhood maltreatment. *Neuroscience and Biobehavioral Reviews, 27*, 33–44.

Teigen, K. H. (1994). Yerkes-Dodson: A law for all seasons. *Theory and Psychology, 4*(4), 525–547.

van der Kolk, B. (2014). *The body keeps the score: Brain, mind and body in healing trauma*. Viking Press.

van der Meer, L., Sigafoos, J., O'Reilly, M. F., & Lancioni, G. E. (2011). Assessing preferences for AAC options in communication interventions for individuals with developmental disabilities: A review of the literature. *Research in Developmental Disabilities, 32*(5), 1422–1431.

SECTION VI
AAC for Persons With Acquired Disabilities

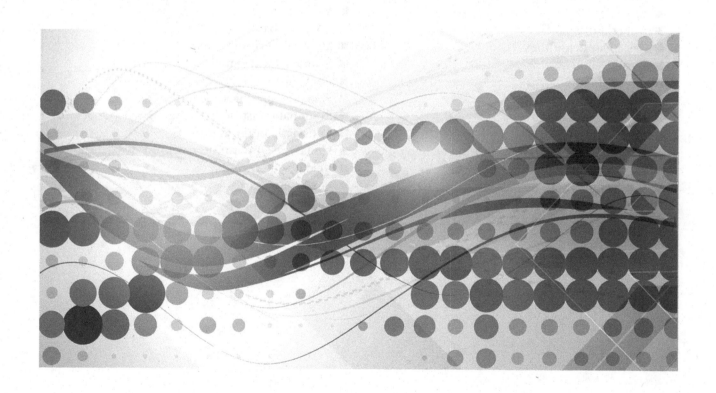

Section VI provides the theoretical foundation and case study examples of augmentative and alternative communication (AAC) for persons with acquired disabilities. The section is headed by Essay 19, which centers on decision-making and how AAC serves to ensure understanding and participation in this critical process.

Chapter 25 is about AAC for persons having sustained a traumatic brain injury, and the distinction between AAC, assistive technology, and information and communication technology is made in the context of understanding how to support the functional outcomes for these individuals. Motor speech disorders and the various resulting presentations with respect to speech abilities are detailed in Chapter 26 to help understand how AAC can serve to augment an individual's existing speech or be an alternative (or both).

Chapter 27 discusses AAC for individuals with amyotrophic lateral sclerosis (ALS), illustrating the flexibility of the systems to accommodate the evolving health care needs of individuals carrying this diagnosis. Chapter 28 provides suggestions for AAC for persons with aphasia, and Chapter 29 covers the various ways individuals with dementia are supported using AAC. The last chapter of this section, Chapter 30, details AAC for individuals who are medically complex in their profiles, warranting creative programming and support.

Key Terms Reviewed in This Section

- AAC facilitator
- Aphasia
- Apraxia of speech
- Assistive technology
- Chronic illness
- Counseling
- Declarative memory
- Dysarthria
- Flaccid dysarthria
- Information and communication technologies
- Intervention phases
- Intervention staging
- Interprofessional practice
- Medically complex
- Memory book
- Message banking
- Motor speech disorders
- Nondeclarative memory
- Reminder cards
- Social communication
- Systematic instruction
- Traumatic brain injury
- Unilateral upper motor neuron dysarthria
- Visual sequencing aids
- Voice banking
- Working memory

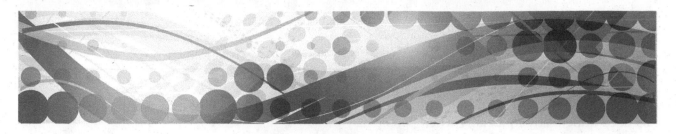

Essay 19

ETHICAL CONSIDERATIONS AND AAC: CRITICAL HEALTH SITUATIONS, INFORMED CONSENT, AND THE IMPORTANCE OF APPROPRIATE AAC

Paula Leslie

Following on from optimizing communication to enable autonomous decision-making in general, we must address critical health situations. This applies for the person at the center of our care and for surrogate decision-makers. Such decisions typically bring increased stress and therefore decreased communicative ability (Pochard et al., 2005). People often presume that decisions regarding end-of-life (EoL) situations create greater burden, but the evidence does not support this (Dekel et al., 2005). What is true is that as we age, or have increased disease and comorbidities, each decision we make narrows the paths ahead of us (Altschuler & Happ, 2019). Advance care planning is for *every* one, at *every* time-point, and thus having the vocabulary and subtlety of sentence construction and comprehension becomes ever more crucial.

In recent years, there has been an avalanche of studies, policies, and protocols regarding the importance of good communication and shared decision-making; but rarely do we see consideration of persons who use augmentative and alternative communication (PWUAAC). Comprehensive and excellent policy statements guide many details *but* the mode of communication (Kon et al., 2016). Reference to AAC is rare and usually in disease-specific guidance (National Institute for Health and

Care Excellence, 2017). Interestingly, where we see the use of AAC being progressively acknowledged is in the support of people with cognitive impairments such as dementia. Here the concept of the *supportive toolbox* has been built on a range of professionals' common techniques and more specialized approaches such as AAC (Sinclair et al., 2019).

Thirty years ago in describing the undoubted *magic* of AAC, David Beukelman cautioned us to look at broad and sometimes hidden costs that will be part of the package of increased communication options (Beukelman, 1991). These include the facilitators who support those using AAC approaches. These are the same people who may be the surrogate decision-makers, or those involved in best interest decisions in critical health care scenarios. As noted in other essays and chapters of this text, exercising the right to autonomous decision-making relies on an individual being able to understand the information shared with them, consider the costs, benefits, and implications, and *communicate that decision to others*. This requires a proactive approach to building AAC competence in all those who support the person at the center of the decisional process (McNaughton et al., 2019).

Predicting who feels the greater burden and what classes as a critical situation is somewhat in the eye of the beholder. We as health care professionals need to be ready to identify when people may be under greater emotional and cognitive burden than usual. For the caregivers and surrogate decision makers we know there is increased pressure (Pochard et al., 2005). This may be compounded further with having to deal with AAC whether used by themselves or with the patient. We as health care professionals need to be addressing the possible use of AAC earlier in the disease progression so that patients, families, and others are primed for its use, if and when a critical time arrives. Alongside the AAC consideration, we should all be taking responsibility for engaging in advance care planning decisions earlier. This will help to avoid such issues springing up without notice and allows us to be prepared in a culturally sensitive manner (Friend & Alden, 2020).

A final thought regarding regret and guilt: as health care professionals we have a responsibility to our patients' families to ensure that guilt is minimized even where regret is experienced (Cox, 2009). Regret is that sense of missing a loved one, of being sad that they have died. Guilt is the feeling that as a person involved in their care, in any decision-making process, or simply knowing them but not spotting something, you are somehow to blame for poor outcomes or even the death. We have a duty to try to reduce the blame a person might put upon themselves, that is almost a default position. Recent work shows that regret is associated with factors in three areas: decision antecedents (characteristics of the patient or caregiver), decision-making processes, and decision outcomes. Of particular interest in the world of AAC might be the most significant predictor of regret in decision antecedents: caregiver desire to avoid making a surrogate decision (Elidor et al., 2020). Of course, many factors contribute to this, but we need to be mindful of the unfamiliarity and perceived complexity of doing such a task via AAC. We can address that, if not the outcomes of the disease process, and reduce guilt. Death itself is not a bad outcome—it is a natural part of life, and associated regret does not indicate pathological grief. Minimizing the burden of the communicative process is within our realm and where we can make a real contribution in critical health situations.

References

Altschuler, T., & Happ, M. B. (2019). Partnering with speech language pathologist to facilitate patient decision making during serious illness. *Geriatric Nursing, 40*(3), 333–335. https://doi.org/10.1016/j.gerinurse.2019.05.002

Beukelman, D. (1991). Magic and cost of communicative competence. *Augmentative and Alternative Communication, 7*(1), 2–10. https://doi.org/10.1080/07434619112331275633

Cox, J. (2009). Making the healing difference: Guilt and regret. *American Journal of Hospice & Palliative Medicine, 26*(1), 64–65.

Dekel, R., Solomon, Z., & Bleich, A. (2005). Emotional distress and marital adjustment of caregivers: Contribution of level of impairment and appraised burden. *Anxiety, Stress, & Coping, 18*(1), 71–82. https://doi.org/10.1080/10615800412336427

Elidor, H., Adekpedjou, R., Zomahoun, H. T. V., Ben Charif, A., Agbadje, T. T., Rheault, N., & Legare, F. (2020). Extent and predictors of decision regret among informal caregivers making decisions for a loved one. A systematic review. *Medical Decision Making, 40*(8), 946–958. https://doi.org/10.1177/0272989X20963038

Friend, J. M., & Alden, D. L. (2020). Improving patient preparedness and confidence in discussing advance directives for end-of-life care with health care providers in the United States and Japan. *Medical Decision Making.* https://doi.org/10.1177/0272989X20969683

Kon, A. A., Davidson, J. E., Morrison, W., Danis, M., & White, D. B. (2016). Shared decision making in ICUs: An American College of Critical Care Medicine and American Thoracic Society Policy Statement. *Critical Care Medicine, 44*(1), 188–201. https://doi.org/10.1097/CCM.0000000000001396

McNaughton, D., Light, J., Beukelman, D. R., Klein, C., Nieder, D., & Nazareth, G. (2019). Building capacity in AAC: A person-centred approach to supporting participation by people with complex communication needs. *Augmentative and Alternative Communication, 35*(1), 56–68. https://doi.org/10.1080/07434618.2018.1556731

National Institute for Health and Care Excellence. (2017). *Parkinson's disease in adults: Diagnosis and management* (NICE Guidance NG71). https://www.nice.org.uk/guidance/ng71/evidence/full-guideline-pdf-4538466253

Pochard, F., Darmon, M., Fassier, T., Bollaert, P-E., Cheval, C., Coloigner, M., . . . Azoulay, É; French FAMIREA Study Group. (2005). Symptoms of anxiety and depression in family members of intensive care unit patients before discharge or death. A prospective multicenter study. *Journal of Critical Care, 20*(1), 90–96. https://doi.org/10.1016/j.jcrc.2004.11.004

Sinclair, C., Bajic-Smith, J., Gresham, M., Blake, M., Bucks, R. S., Field, S., . . . Kurrle, S. (2019). Professionals' views and experiences in supporting decision-making involvement for people living with dementia. *Dementia (London)*, 1471301219864849. https://doi.org/10.1177/1471301219864849

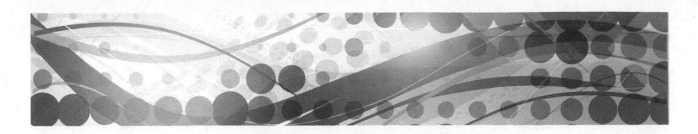

Chapter 25
AAC FOR PERSONS WITH TRAUMATIC BRAIN INJURY

Lindsay R. James Riegler and Laura P. Klug

Fundamentals

Traumatic brain injury (TBI) is a form of nondegenerative acquired brain injury that occurs when a sudden trauma causes damage to the brain (American Speech-Language-Hearing Association [ASHA], 2021; National Institute of Neurological Disorders and Stroke, 2021). TBI can lead to various communication deficits including but not limited to, aphasia, dysarthria, and apraxia. In this chapter, the authors outline cognitive communication deficits common to TBI and methods to aid in improving verbal output using various technology-focused modalities while accounting for the cognitive sequelae often associated. The cognitive communication deficits associated with moderate to severe TBI often have lifelong effects that evolve over time and, as such, should be evaluated at regular intervals to ensure individual communication needs continue to be met.

It is important to understand the similarities and differences between augmentative and alternative communication (AAC) devices, assistive technology (AT), and information and communication technologies (ICT) and how one device may be appropriate for multiple deficits. Rapid advancements in technology have yielded numerous improvements in communication. Technology-based applications now afford the person with a brain injury the ability to communicate with conversational partners using speech-to-text– and text-to-speech–based modalities. There are many factors to account for when recommending technology for the purposes of communication among persons with brain injury. Understanding the unique communication needs of each patient and leveraging their personal goals will assist with proper selection of devices and generalization of skill across settings.

Review of Cognitive-Communication Deficits in TBI

TBI can result in a range of communication impairments including language and motor speech disorders. TBI-related cognitive disorders can negatively impact functional communication. The use of an AAC system may aid in facilitating improved communicative outcomes. Cognitive-communication impairments are different from motor speech or primary language disorders in that the cognitive impairment is the catalyst of the communication deficit. Underlying attention, memory, executive function, and processing difficulties can hinder one's communicative abilities in the areas of comprehension, expression, and social communication. Cognitive-communication deficits include tangential topics, extraneous conversational utterances, egocentrism, and difficulty with the quality and quantity of language produced (Bond & Godfrey, 1997; Elsass & Kinsella, 1987; Tran et al., 2018). A wide array of social communication breakdowns can occur due to difficulty initiating and maintaining conversational topics and misinterpreting verbal and nonverbal cues. Due to the variability of deficits that can occur following a TBI, a broad spectrum of cognitive-communication impairments may present. Persisting cognitive-communication deficits can have a significant impact on a person's quality of life by negatively impacting community engagement, academics, vocation, and social involvement. Therefore, individualized care planning, which may include a tailored AT, AAC, or ICT selection, is essential and is ideally delivered in a therapeutic milieu.

Comprehensive evaluation and treatment of neurocognitive functioning, including cognitive-communication disorders, in individuals with TBI remain the standard of care. The use of telehealth assessment and treatment (as substantiated in Section VII) versus an in-person environment has been demonstrated to be an acceptable and often preferred delivery modality for TBI care (Turkstra et al., 2012). Cognitive-communication abilities post-TBI can change dramatically over the course of recovery, necessitating ongoing AAC reevaluation. In addition, professionals should consider multimodal communication, message representation, and navigation when evaluating AAC needs for individuals with TBI (Wallace, 2010). In proceeding with rehabilitation for cognitive-communication disorders, modification of therapeutic strategies needs to be gauged, dependent on cognitive ability and the AAC demands. The literature supports cognitive rehabilitation for remediation of cognitive deficits following a TBI. Cicerone et al. (2019) conducted a systematic review of clinical literature to derive evidence-based, domain-specific, clinical recommendations. Recommendations, including those for cognitive-communication deficits, were classified into Practice Standards, Practice Guidelines, or Practice Options based on the level of evidential support. The Practice Standard for social-communication skills post-TBI incorporates pragmatic conversational skill training and recognition of emotions from facial expressions into clinical interventions. Cognitive interventions for specific language impairments such as reading comprehension and language formulation following TBI are recommended as a Practice Guideline.

Practice Options include group-based interventions for social-communication deficits after TBI and computer-based interventions as an adjunct to clinician-guided treatment for cognitive linguistic deficits after TBI (Bjorkdahl et al., 2013; Cicerone et al., 2009, 2019; Griffiths et al., 2016; Neumann et al., 2015; Radice-Neumann et al., 2009; Vallat-Azouvi et al., 2009).

Motor speech, traditional language, and cognitive-communication disorders post-TBI should be evaluated at regular intervals by a speech-language pathologist (SLP). Individuals with moderate to severe communication disabilities following TBI need to be assessed for, provided with, and trained in the use of appropriate AAC aids (Campbell et al., 2002; Doyle et al., 2000; Powell et al., 2012; Togher et al., 2014; Wilson, 2000). Assistive technology for cognition (ATC) or utilizing ICT can be a better approach for those with mild cognitive-communication deficits (Brunner et al., 2017). Both informal and standardized assessments are recommended when evaluating individuals with TBI. However, the evaluating professional must be cognizant that communication barriers and/or use of AAC systems can negatively and inaccurately impact standardized neurocognitive test results.

AAC Versus Assistive Technology Versus Information and Communication Technologies

Utilizing technology as an aide for individuals with complex communication needs can help reduce negative TBI outcomes in academia, vocation, and social settings. Brunner et al. (2017) identified three technology categories that have been widely examined for use in cognitive rehabilitation that include: (a) AAC tools, systems, or strategies; (b) AT; and (c) ICT. However, additional investigation is required to clarify the use of technologies in cognitive-communication rehabilitation among persons with TBI. While technology categories will overlap in clinical practice, it is important to know the distinct differences each option offers. Refer to Table 25–1 for classification of communication technologies in TBI research.

Table 25–1. Selection of Assistive Technology (AT), Augmentative and Alternative Communication (AAC), and Information and Communication Technologies (ICT) to Support Communication Based on Traumatic Brain Injury (TBI) Severity

Technology	Technology			TBI Severity		
	AT	**AAC**	**ICT**	**Mild**	**Moderate**	**Severe**
AAC speech-generating devices (high-tech)	YES	YES	YES (on Internet)	NO	YES	YES
AAC mobile devices (phones, tablets, smart pen)	YES	YES	YES	YES	YES	YES
Alphabet/picture/writing board (low-tech)	YES	YES	NO	NO	YES	YES
Unaided AAC (gestures, mime, facial expression, keyword sign)	NO	YES	NO	YES	YES	YES
Adapted keyboards/mouse	YES	YES	NO	YES	YES	YES
Switch access for computer or speech-generating device	YES	YES	NO	NO	YES	YES
Eye-gaze access for computer or speech-generating device	YES	YES	NO	NO	YES	YES
Computer programs	YES	YES	YES (on Internet)	YES	YES	YES
Internet hardware and software	NO	YES	YES	YES	YES	YES
Video-teleconferencing	NO	NO	YES	YES	YES	YES
Online learning	NO	NO	YES	YES	YES	NO
Social media	NO	YES	YES	YES	YES	YES

Note. See *Communications report 2012–13*, by Australian Communications and Media Authority, Commonwealth of Australia, 2013; "Review of the Literature on the Use of Social Media by People With Traumatic Brain Injury (TBI)," by M. Brunner, B. Hemsley, S. Palmer, S. Dann, and L. Togher, 2015, *Disability Rehabilitation, 37*(17), pp. 1511–1521; "Evidence-Based Cognitive Rehabilitation: Updated Review of the Literature From 2003 Through 2008," by K. D. Cicerone, D. M. Langenbahn, C. Braden, J. F. Malec, K. Kalmar, M. Fraas, T. Felicetti, L. Laatsch, J. P. Harley, T. Bergquist, J. Azulay, J. Cantor, and T. Ashman, 2011, *Archives of Physical Medicine and Rehabilitation, 92*(4), 519–530; "Traumatic Brain Injury and AAC: Supporting Communication Through Recovery," by M. Doyle and S. Fager, 2011, *The ASHA Leader, 16*(2) (https://doi.org/10.1044/leader.FTR8.16022011. np); "Language Representation for the Augmentative and Alternative Communication of Adults with Traumatic Brain Injury," by M. Fried-Oken and M. Doyle, 1992, *Journal of Head Trauma Rehabilitation, 7*(3), 59–69; *Augmentative and alternative communication clinical guideline*, by Speech Pathology Australia, 2012; "INCOG Recommendations for Management of Cognition Following Traumatic Brain Injury, Part IV: Cognitive Communication," by L. Togher, C. Wiseman-Hakes, J. Douglas, M. Stergiou-Kita, R. Teasell, M. Bayley, and L. S. Turkstra, 2014, *Journal of Head Trauma Rehabilitation, 29*(4), 353–368 (https://doi.org/10.1097/HTR.0000000000000071).

Augmentative and Alternative Communication

Communication boards, speech-generating devices, signs, gestures, drawings, and tangible objects are all examples of AAC systems used with individuals with TBI. The need for AAC may be temporary for those with developmental or acute communication needs; however, some persons who use AAC have permanent communication disabilities and require AAC for use over a lifetime. Doyle and Fager (2011) proposed an assessment and intervention framework for persons with TBI who can benefit from an AAC system that includes three communicator types: emergent, transitional, and long-term augmentative. Individuals are assessed by level of cognitive function, recovery stage, and purpose of rehabilitation; based on their communicator type, specific AAC methods and goals are targeted. The dynamic recovery process for TBI often means these individuals will move through the various communicator types while the professionals support their changing needs with appropriate methods and goals (Doyle & Fager, 2011).

Technology Displays

Computerized communication books and devices may serve as aided AAC systems for communication-impaired persons secondary to brain injury. Thoughtful consideration regarding the modality of message representation is importation for optimal patient utilization (Thiessen et al., 2017). Clinicians should remain mindful of the patient's current and anticipated strengths and needs. The identified needs are then paired to match features offered by available AAC hardware/software, often referred to as "feature matching" (Costello et al., 2013). The intended outcome of the conversational exchange is of equal importance. Communicative intent refers to the underlying action desired by the conversational initiator, for example, sharing or requesting information. The way in which the information is displayed within the AAC/computerized system, text versus images, is referred to as message representation (Beukelman & Mirenda, 2013). Grid and visual scene displays are the most common methods of message representation. When designing the AAC display, clinicians must attend to the cognitive effort required to understand the displayed content (Brown et al., 2015, 2019), as little empirical evidence exists outlining the way in which persons with TBI interpret AAC displays (Thiessen et al., 2019).

Grid Displays. As previously reviewed, grid displays use decontextualized content, line-drawn icons/pictures, or text depicted on plain backgrounds into rows or columns of individual cells, each item representing a different word or concept (Thiessen et al., 2019). Special consideration should be made when utilizing grid-based displays. Persons with brain injury may lack the ability to understand the intended message from a static image due to the lack of movement-based cueing (Adolphs et al., 2003; Brown et al., 2016; Collignon et al., 2008; McDonald & Saunders, 2005; Schultz & Pilz, 2009; Turkstra, 2008). Successful utilization of grid-based displays requires the individual to identify then select a sequence of words/cells and combine for the intended message. Tangible space on the communication device often forces the user to navigate between pages which may contribute to additional user difficulty if working memory, attention, and cognitive flexibility deficits are present.

Visual Displays. Additionally, visual displays may prove a successful alternative to grid displays for message representation in persons with brain injury given the contextualized nature of the images. Visual scenes display objects and people in their natural environment and are intended to mimic specific situations/events or experiences (Dietz et al., 2006). Research using visual display for message representation in persons with brain injury demonstrated increased processing time and slower navigation compared to decontextualized images. However, the literature reports increased accuracy navigating displays containing scenes (Visual Display) than those containing decontextualized photos (Grid Display) (Thiessen et al., 2019).

Assistive Technology

AT was first defined in 1987 as part of the *Individuals with Disabilities Education Act* as a mechanism to protect against discrimination for individuals with disabilities like the protection provided on the basis of race, gender, age, nationality, and religion. An AT device is referred to as "any item, piece of equipment, or product system, whether acquired commercially off the shelf, modified, or customized, that is used to increase, maintain, or improve the functional capabilities of a child with a disability. The term does not include a medical device that is surgically implanted, or the replacement of that device" (Individuals With Disabilities Education Act, 20 U.S.C. § 300.5, 2004). Individuals with TBI can have motor, sensory, behavioral, and cognitive deficits requiring an interdisciplinary team approach to AT evaluation and implementation. SLPs play an important role in facilitating communication between the caregivers, interdisciplinary team members, and the individual with cognitive-communication deficits. AT for TBI rehabilitation can include but is not limited to mobility aids, adaptive switches and tools, physical modifications to the environment, hearing aids, computer software and hardware, and cognitive aids (Eunice Kennedy Shriver National Institute of Child Health and Human Development, https://www.nichd.nih.gov/health/topics/rehabtech).

Research supports the efficacy and effectiveness of utilizing AT to improve independence and life participation for people with cognitive deficits (Sohlberg, 2011). Smart devices (phones, tablets, watches, pens, etc.) are examples of AT devices commonly used with the TBI population to help compensate for cognitive impairments. A further illustration of utilizing a smartphone as an AT device would be to program reoccurring phone alarms for an individual with memory impairment as a reminder to take medications at specific times. AT has had a notable impact in the field of cognitive rehabilitation for brain injury, affording individuals with TBI greater independence. AT devices can be utilized for AAC when they are used explicitly to assist or support communication (Brunner et al., 2017). For example, an iPad programmed with a specific speech-generating application can be used as an AAC device (like discussed in Chapter 4). Numerous tablet/phone applications can be downloaded and used to assist with speech-to-text and text-to-speech needs. Functional implementation of technology in TBI rehabilitation often requires use of technologies from multiple categories (AAC, AT, ICT) to optimize communication across individualized settings.

Information and Communication Technologies

ICT refers to any device or application used for communications. E-mail, computer programs, Internet, smartphones, and social media are all examples of ICT because these tools allow individuals to access, store, transmit, and manipulate information (Australian Communications and Media Authority, 2013; Brunner et al., 2017; Davies & Riley, 2012). Given the wide range of cognitive-communication disorders following TBI, applying ICT in rehabilitation as an adjunct to more traditional forms of rehabilitation can assist an individual in meeting their communication goals. For example, given the portable, socially acceptable, and accessible nature of texting, an ICT strategy that may be beneficial is to text oneself key points for conversations to engage in more meaningful communication (Brunner et al., 2017; Newby & Coetzer, 2013).

Social Media and Apps

Social media platforms have become a standard form of functional daily communication and should not be overlooked in TBI rehabilitation. There are advantages and disadvantages to using social media with individuals with TBI. Creating a therapeutic environment safe for the utilization of social media platforms to support communication delivery and access to information is recommended and can be difficult to implement. Risks when using social media, including stalking, cyberbullying, trolling, scams, and identity theft (Brunner et al., 2019; Jenaro et al., 2018), are often heightened for individuals with TBI due to lack of insight or poor judgment. Age of the person with the brain injury must also be considered, as oversight into appropriate use of social platforms must be considered and discussed if caregiving needs are necessary. There are several benefits to using social media in the field of communication disorders and sciences. Social media communication allows for a greater response time, is tolerant of spelling and grammar errors, and provides messages in both text-based and multimedia forms, which can be beneficial for people with disordered communication (Brunner et al., 2019; Hemsley et al., 2017). Social networking groups/platforms may also offer persons with brain injury a sense of community and engagement alleviating some feelings of social isolation. Despite many challenges individuals with TBI may experience when utilizing social media, research suggests that most individuals with TBI do utilize social media (Baker-Sparr et al., 2018; Flynn et al.,

2019; Tsaousides et al., 2011; Wong et al., 2017). Therefore, structuring social media communication to optimize the benefits and minimize the risks can be a functional target in TBI rehabilitation.

Due to a multitude of applications (apps) that are appropriate for use in TBI rehabilitation for organization, time management, communication, and so on, in addition to the rapid release of updated and new apps, a comprehensive review of apps will not be provided in this publication. Building app-based technology strategies into TBI rehabilitation may be beneficial; however, the lack of regulation and high variability of applications should be noted (Brunner et al., 2017). Like all aspects of TBI rehabilitation, app-based treatment needs to be individualized regarding patient skills. Visual cuts and deficits are an additional consideration when introducing devices and applications to individuals post TBI.

Special Considerations

The environment in which rehabilitation personnel successfully train and utilize AAC devices warrants additional discussion. Although not the primary focus of this chapter, clinicians must be aware of known limitations to AAC implementation. It may be surprising that the use of AAC within the acute care/hospital, despite access via trained SLPs, remains poor (Stans et al., 2017). There are several factors that contribute to reduced access including cost of device, insurance reimbursement, and acuity of health needs while the individual remains inpatient. Of particular concern is the lack of knowledge regarding persons with brain injury's communication vulnerability among health care personnel (Stans et al., 2017). Health professionals are often unaware of strategies to use to increase communication between persons with brain injury and lack confirmation of intended message. This can lead to both the health professional and person with brain injury lacking the necessary information to make informed medical decisions. The role of the SLP in any health care setting is to advocate on behalf of the person with brain injury; to educate staff on the modalities of AAC and train all invested parties on the use to maximize communication and improve

quality of life. Finally, in an age where technology is supported on a large scale, health professionals must be aware of their own biases and stigmas attached to recommending/utilizing or training persons on AAC devices for the purposes of increased communication and comprehension (Stans et al., 2017).

> ### Case Study: TH

Clinical Profile and Communication Needs

The Individual

TH is a 25-year-old college graduate working on her master's degree in nutrition. She sustained a moderate TBI, Glasgow Coma Scale 10 (Teasdale & Jennett, 1974), when she was impacted by an automobile while walking home from the gym. TH spent 11 days in the hospital, four of which were in the neuro–intensive care unit (ICU). Once transitioned out of the neuro-ICU and to the medicine floor, she received intensive inpatient rehab services including physical therapy for gait instability due to left-sided weakness, occupational therapy (OT) for assistance with feeding/writing/bathing/visual inattention, and speech therapy for mild spastic dysarthria, moderate attention deficits, and impaired executive functioning.

TH's visual inattention complicated her ability to "see" text, despite 20/20 vision. She had poor frustration tolerance and was impulsive with her decisions. Constant fatigue limited her ability to actively engage in treatment with all disciplines. As a result, rehab disciplines decided to rotate co-treatment groups to maximize therapeutic gains. TH's awareness of her deficits was limited at first. With assistance, she was able to recognize the need to slow her rate of speech and overarticulate to improve functional verbal communication at the word level.

Their Communication Partners

TH's primary support system includes her parents, her sister who lives out of town, and a handful of close friends. While TH's friends made efforts to provide empathy and support, they too were busy with school and work-related responsibilities making consistent interactions challenging. TH endorsed feelings of loneliness and isolation.

Their Environment

TH was discharged from the hospital and resided in her second-story apartment with her parents who split their time between TH and their full-time jobs 3 hours north of her location. Alternating every other week, TH's mom and dad drove her three times per week to outpatient rehab appointments for continued speech, physical, and occupational therapies. Her prolonged impulsive behavior, reduced insight into deficit, and poor judgement precluded her from living independently when discharged from the hospital. As TH continued to make progress in her therapies, she gained independence.

AAC Considerations

TH's condition was assessed routinely as she gained strength, insight, and awareness. Her AAC needs changed throughout the course of her recovery, ranging from no tech, low tech, to high tech. Regular considerations for AAC selection included attention, and executive function abilities and visual considerations for screen size/grid displays to reduce confusion and improve expression of intended message. Fatigue was monitored during AAC training, and frequent breaks were implemented. Establishing attainable goals prior to AAC training improved frustration tolerance.

The AAC System or Service

While in the neuro-ICU, TH's new medication to prevent seizures left her extremely fatigued rendering her verbal output limited. To ensure her wants and needs were met, the inpatient SLP trained nursing staff and family how to utilize a low-tech laminated visual display to improve communication of basic needs and single yes/no questions (see toolbox for resource). TH's visual inattention to her left side and constant fatigue made use of this AAC aid challenging at first. With education provided to hospital staff and family to stand on

TH's right side and cues for TH to attend to the left side of the page, she was successful in making her wants and needs known by pointing to pictures on the low-tech board with 80% accuracy across four sessions and nursing reported reduced frustration as evidence by limited use of calming medication during the daytime hours.

TH demonstrated rapid improvement in her level of alertness; however, she continued to struggle with thought formulation, fluidity of speech, and poor topic maintenance. Once transitioned to the medicine floor, TH benefited from the use of pen and paper and was encouraged to use mind mapping to assist with interactions with her medical providers. TH was encouraged to map out her thoughts/questions and used her personal smartphone to record the conversations, with permission, using voice recorder software. Cognitive demand was reduced through visual representation of her thoughts and served as a written reminder for questions when interacting with medical personnel. Becoming an active participant in her own medical decisions increased TH's motivation to adhere to therapy recommendations and improved mood. As TH demonstrated increased awareness and motivation, different software applications/functions on a tablet were gradually introduced. Tablet training replaced paper-based activities given her preference for technology and need to minimize the number of strategies in use to reduce confusion.

As TH's cognitive-communication status continued to improve, her treatment focused on improving speech rate and breath support using a metronome app on her tablet. TH was assigned independent homework using strategies trained during her therapy sessions to increase generalization. The data were recorded on the app and reviewed by the SLP each session to track progress. With the successful use of the metronome app on her tablet, the SLP downloaded and trained TH how to use a deep-breathing application to assist with poor frustration tolerance. TH enjoyed the new app and downloaded a mindfulness and relaxation app to help her fall asleep.

The SLP continued to reinforce the use of her tablet as an AAC device to improve conversational fluency and topic maintenance across all functional tasks including at home, in therapy sessions, and in the community. TH's sister assisted with generalization of topics learned using social media apps downloaded on her tablet. TH used popular social media application(s) to practice topic maintenance and conversational vigilance with friends and family members. The use of these applications also improved TH's feelings of isolation.

Four months after her injury, TH discussed returning to graduate school. In preparation for the next semester, both OT and SLP worked on strategies to set TH up for a successful transition back to school. OT targeted residual visual inattention while reading/studying through use of reminders on her cellphone. The team, including TH, mutually agreed that TH should enroll part-time upon her return to graduate school. Classroom and testing accommodations were developed based on the results of her performance on neuropsychological tests completed approximately 1 month prior to the start of the semester and input from her physiatrist, OT, SLP, and the college's Office of Disability Services. The SLP trained TH on a smartpen to aid in note taking and facilitated classroom and testing accommodations through collaborations with TH, her neurologist, and the college's Office of Disability Services. TH used folders on her tablet to assist with coursework organization and memos to remind her what questions to ask her professor while studying at home. TH was trained to set a timer when studying to allow for numerous breaks to reduce fatigue and improve sustained attention.

Next Steps

Long-term treatment goals include sustainment of tablet use as an AAC device to improve functional cognitive communication.

Expert Tips or Practical Advice

Understanding the unique needs and motivating factors of each patient will help ensure adequate buy-in. Identifying patient goals and using AAC training to target those goals will help in generalization of skills learned.

References

Adolphs, R., Tranel, D., & Damasio, A. R. (2003). Dissociable neural systems for recognizing emotions. *Brain and Cognition, 52*(1), 61–69.

American Speech-Language-Hearing Association (ASHA). (2021). *Traumatic brain injury in adults*. https://www.asha.org/practice-portal/clinical-topics/traumatic-brain-injury-in-adults/#collapse_8

Australian Communications and Media Authority. (2013). *Communications report 2012–13*. Commonwealth of Australia.

Baker-Sparr, C., Hart, T., Bergquist, T., Bogner, J., Dreer, L., Juengst, S., . . . Whiteneck, G. G. (2018). Internet and social media use after traumatic brain injury: A traumatic brain injury model systems study. *Journal of Head Trauma Rehabilitation, 33*(1), E9–E17. https://doi.org/10.1097/HTR.0000000000000305

Beukelman, D. R., & Mirenda, P. (2013). *Augmentative and alternative communication: Supporting children and adults with complex communication needs* (4th ed.). Paul H. Brookes.

Bjorkdahl, A., Akerlund, E., Svensson, S., & Esbjornsson, E. (2013). A randomized study of computerized working memory training and effects on functioning in everyday life for patients with brain injury. *Brain Injury, 27*, 1658–1665.

Bond, F., & Godfrey, H. P. (1997). Conversation with traumatically brain injured individuals: A controlled study of behavioural changes and their impact. *Brain Injury, 11*(5), 319–330.

Brown, J. A., Hux, K., Knollman-Porter, K., & Wallace, S. (2016). Use of visual cues by adults with traumatic brain injuries to interpret explicit and inferential information, *Journal of Head Trauma Rehabilitation, 31*(3), E32–E41. https://doi.org/10.1097/HTR.0000000000000148

Brown, J., Thiessen, A., Beukelman, D., & Hux, K. (2015). Noun representation in AAC grid displays: Visual attention patterns of people with traumatic brain injury. *Augmentative and Alternative Communication, 31*, 15–26. https://doi.org/10.3109/07434618.2014.995224

Brown, J., Thiessen, A., Freeland, T., & Brewer, C. H. (2019). Visual processing patterns of adults with traumatic brain injury when viewing image-based grids and visual scenes. *Augmentative and Alternative Communication, 35*(3), 229–239. https://doi.org/10.1080/07434618.2019.1609578

Brunner, M., Hemsley, B., Palmer, S., Dann, S., & Togher, L. (2015). Review of the literature on the use of social media by people with traumatic brain injury (TBI). *Disability Rehabilitation, 37*(17), 1511–1521.

Brunner, M., Hemsley, B., Togher, L., & Palmer, S. (2017). Technology and its role in rehabilitation for people with cognitive-communication disability following a traumatic brain injury (TBI). *Brain Injury, 31*(8), 1028–1043. https://doi.org/10.1080/02699052.2017.1292429

Brunner, M., Palmer, S., Togher, L., & Hemsley, B. (2019). "I kind of figured it out": The views and experiences of people with traumatic brain injury (TBI) in using social media—Self-determination for participation and inclusion online, *International Journal of Language & Communication Disorders, 54*(2), 221–233. https://doi.org/10.1111/1460-6984.12405

Campbell, L., Balandin, S., & Togher, L. (2002). AAC use by people with traumatic brain injury: Issues and solutions. *Advances in Speech-Language Pathology, 4*(2), 89–94.

Cicerone, K. D., Azulay, J., & Trott, C. (2009). Methodological quality of research on cognitive rehabilitation after traumatic brain injury. *Archives of Physical Medicine and Rehabilitation, 90,* S52–S59.

Cicerone, K. D., Goldin, Y., Ganci, K., Rosenbaum, A., Wethe, J. V., Langenbahn, D. M., . . . Harley, J. P. (2019). Evidence-based cognitive rehabilitation: Systematic review of the literature from 2009 through 2014, *Archives of Physical Medicine and Rehabilitation, 100*(8), 1515–1533. https://doi.org/10.1016/j.apmr.2019.02.011

Cicerone, K. D., Langenbahn, D. M., Braden, C., Malec, J. F., Kalmar, K., Fraas, M., . . . Ashman, T. (2011). Evidence-based cognitive rehabilitation: Updated review of the literature from 2003 through 2008. *Archives of Physical Medicine and Rehabilitation, 92*(4), 519–530.

Collignon, O., Girard, S., Gosselin, F., Roy, S., Saint-Amour, D., Lassonde, M., & Lepore, F. (2008). Audio-visual integration of emotion expression, *Brain Research, 1242,* 126–135.

Costello, J., Shane, H., & Caron, J. (2013). *AAC mobile devices and apps: Growing pains with evidence based practice.* https://www.childrenshospital.org/centers-and-services/programs/a-_-e/augmentative-communication-program/downloads/app-and-clinical-feature-matching-handouts

Davies, G., & Riley, F. (2012). Glossary of ICT terminology. In *Information and communications technology for language teachers (ICT4LT).* Slough, Thames Valley University. http://www.ict4lt.org/en/en_glossary.htm#GlossI

Dietz, A., McKelvey, M., & Beukelman, D. (2006). Visual scene displays (VSD): New AAC interfaces for persons with aphasia. *Perspectives on Augmentative and Alternative Communication, 15*(1), 13–17. https://doi.org/10.1044/aac15.1.13

Doyle, M., & Fager, S. (2011). Traumatic brain injury and AAC: Supporting communication through recovery. *The ASHA Leader, 16*(2). https://doi.org/10.1044/leader.FTR8.16022011.np

Doyle, M., Kennedy, M., Jausalaitis, G., & Phillips, B. (2000). AAC and traumatic brain injury. In D. R. Beukelman, K. M. Yorkston, & J. Reichle (Eds.), *Augmentative and alternative communication for adults with acquired neurological disorders* (pp. 271–304). Paul H. Brookes.

Elsass, L., & Kinsella, G. (1987). Social interaction following severe closed head injury. *Psychological Medicine, 17*(1), 67–78.

Flynn, M. A., Rigon, A., Kornfield, R., Mutlu, B., Duff, M. C., & Turkstra, L. S. (2019). Characterizing computer-mediated communication, friendship, and social participation in adults with traumatic brain injury. *Brain Injury, 33*(8), 1097–1104. https://doi.org/10.1080/02699052.2019.1616112

Fried-Oken, M., & Doyle, M. (1992). Language representation for the augmentative and alternative communication of adults with traumatic brain injury. *Journal of Head Trauma Rehabilitation, 7*(3), 59–69.

Griffiths, G. G., Sohlberg, M. M., Kirk, C., Fickas, S., & Biancarosa, G. (2016). Evaluation of use of reading comprehension strategies to improve reading comprehension of adult college students with acquired brain injury. *Neuropsychological Rehabilitation, 26,* 161–190.

Hemsley, B., Palmer, S., Goonan, W., & Dann, S. (2017). *Motor neurone disease (MND) and amyotrophic lateral sclerosis (ALS): Social media communication on selected #MND and #ALS tagged tweets.* Paper presented at the 50th Hawaii International Conference on System Sciences, pp. 41–47.

Individuals With Disabilities Education Act, 20 U.S.C. § 300.5. (2004). https://sites.ed.gov/idea/regs/b/a/300.5

Jenaro, C., Flores, N., & Frías, C. (2018). Systematic review of empirical studies on cyberbullying in adults: What we know and what we should investigate. *Aggression and Violent Behavior, 38,* 113–122.

McDonald, S., & Saunders, J.C. (2005). Differential impairment in recognition of emotion across different media in people with severe traumatic brain injury. *Journal of the International Neuropsychological Society, 11,* 392–399.

National Institute of Neurological Disorders and Stroke. (2021). *Traumatic brain injury information page.* https://www.ninds.nih.gov/Disorders/All-Disorders/Traumatic-Brain-Injury-Information-Page

Neumann, D., Babbage, D. R., Zupan, B., & Willer, B. (2015). A randomized controlled trial of emotion recognition training after traumatic brain injury. *Journal of Head Trauma Rehabilitation, 30,* E12–E23.

Newby, G., & Coetzer, R. (2013). The use of emails and texts in psychological therapy after acquired brain injury. In G. Newby, R. Coetzer, A. Daisley, & S. Weatherhead (Eds.), *Practical neuropsychological rehabilitation in acquired brain injury: A guide for working clinicians* (pp. 255–270). Karnac Books.

Powell, L. E., Glang, A., Ettel, D., Todis, B., Sohlberg, M. M., & Albin, R. (2012). Systematic instruction for individuals with acquired brain injury: Results of a randomised controlled trial. *Neuropsychological Rehabilitation, 22*(1), 85–112.

Radice-Neumann, D., Zupan, B., Tomita, M., & Willer B. (2009). Training emotional processing in persons with brain injury. *Journal of Head Trauma Rehabilitation, 24,* 313–323.

Schultz, J., & Pilz, K. S. (2009). Natural facial motion enhances cortical responses to faces. *Experimental Brain Research, 194*(3), 465–475.

Sohlberg, M. M. (2011). Assistive technology for cognition. *The ASHA Leader, 16*(2). https://doi.org/10.1044/leader.FTR3.16022011.14

Speech Pathology Australia. (2012). *Augmentative and alternative communication clinical guideline.*

Stans, S. E. A., Dalemans, R. J. P., de Witte, L. P., Smeets, H. W. H., & Beurskens, A. J. (2017). The role of the physical environment in conversations between people who are communication vulnerable and healthcare professionals: A scoping review. *Disability and Rehabilitation, 39*(25), 2594–2605. https://doi.org/10.1080/09638288.2016.1239769

Teasdale, G., & Jennett, B. (1974). Assessment of coma and impaired consciousness: A practical scale. *The Lancet, 304*(7872), 81–84. https://doi.org/10.1016/s0140-6736(74)91639-0

Thiessen, A., Brown, J., Beukelman, D., & Hux, K. (2017). The effect of human engagement depicted in contextual photographs on the visual attention patterns of adults with traumatic brain injury. *Journal of Communication Disorders, 69,* 58–71. https://doi.org/10.1016/j.jcomdis.2017.07.001

Thiessen, A., Brown, J., Freeland, T., & Brewer, C. H. (2019) Identification and expression of themes depicted in visual scene and grid displays by adults with traumatic brain injury. *American Journal of Speech-Language Pathology, 28,* 664–675. https://doi.org/10.1044/2018_AJSLP-18-0086

Togher, L., Wiseman-Hakes, C., Douglas, J., Stergiou-Kita, M., Teasell, R., Bayley, M., & Turkstra, L. S. (2014). INCOG Recommendations for management of cognition following traumatic brain injury, Part IV: Cognitive communication. *Journal of Head Trauma Rehabilitation, 29*(4), 353–368. https://doi.org/10.1097/HTR.0000000000000071

Tran, S., Kenny, B., Power, E., Tate, R., McDonald, S., Heard, R., & Togher, L. (2018). Cognitive-communication and psychosocial functioning 12 months after severe traumatic brain injury. *Brain Injury, 32*(13–14), 1700–1711. https://doi.org/10.1080/02699052.2018.1537006

Tsaousides, T., Matsuzawa, Y., & Lebowitz, M. (2011). Familiarity and prevalence of Facebook use for social networking among individuals with traumatic brain injury. *Brain Injury, 25*(12), 1155–1162. https://doi.org/10.3109/02699052.2011.613086

Turkstra, L. (2008). Conversation-based assessment of social cognition in adults with traumatic brain injury. *Brain Injury, 22*(5), 397–409.

Turkstra, L. S., Quinn-Padron, M., Johnson, J. E., Workinger, M. S., & Antoniotti, N. (2012). In-person versus telehealth assessment of discourse ability in adults with traumatic brain injury. *Journal of Head Trauma Rehabilitation, 27*(6), 424–432. https://doi.org/10.1097/HTR.0b013e31823346fc

Vallat-Azouvi, C., Pradat-Diehl, P., & Azouvi, P. (2009). Rehabilitation of the central executive of working memory after severe traumatic brain injury: Two single-case studies. *Brain Injury, 23,* 585–594. https://doi.org/10.1080/02699050902970711

Wallace, S. E. (2010). AAC use by people with TBI: Effects of cognitive impairments. *Perspectives on Augmentative and Alternative Communication, 19*(3), 79–86.

Wilson, B. A. (2000). Compensating for cognitive deficits following brain injury. *Neuropsychology Review, 10*(4), 233–243.

Wong, D., Sinclair, K., Seabrook, E., McKay, A., & Ponsford, J. (2017). Smartphones as assistive technology following traumatic brain injury: A preliminary study of what helps and what hinders. *Disability and Rehabilitation, 39*(23), 2387–2394. https://doi.org/10.1080/09638288.2016.1226434

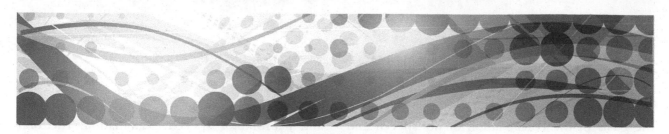

Chapter 26
AAC FOR PERSONS WITH MOTOR SPEECH DISORDERS

Mary Andrianopoulos

Fundamentals

Speech is a complex process that involves the integration of cognitive, linguistic, resonatory, articulatory, phonatory, and respiratory processes. The neurological substrates and integrity of the central nervous system (CNS), peripheral nervous system (PNS), and associated sensorimotor neural networks must be intact for humans to communicate with intelligible speech. When the CNS, PNS, and neural networks are injured or affected by neurological diseases, speech production is inevitably compromised. Motor speech disorders (MSDs) are neurological in origin due to breakdowns within the CNS and/or PNS and associated sensorimotor systems. MSDs can be classified into two primary types: problems with motor execution (dysarthria) and problems with motor programming and planning (apraxia of speech [AOS]). Although MSDs affect both adults and children due to acquired or congenital etiologies, respectively, the presentation of symptoms typically varies in children due to the beneficial effects of neurodevelopment and neuroplasticity. MSDs in children are referred to as Childhood Dysarthria and Childhood Apraxia of Speech. In addition to the differential diagnosis of MSDs in children and adults, it is important to consider the severity, prognosis, client candidacy for intervention, and appropriate selection of interventions that are evidence based. Since MSDs are neurological in origin and affect motor execution and/or motor programming and planning, the focus of intervention should be on movement, incorporating principles of motor learning in therapy to facilitate neuroplasticity, acquisition of skill and retention (generalization), and restoring communication. Most importantly, it is vital to identify and help to alleviate the impact of the MSDs on the individual's ability to communicate and quality of life. In the sections that follow, MSDs will be briefly reviewed with respect to the neurosubstrates, neuropathologies, speech, and acoustic-perceptual features consistent with dysarthria and AOS. This chapter and case study focus on an adult with an acquired MSD.

Dysarthria. Dysarthria is an umbrella term that refers to MSDs that disrupt movement and motor execution of the neuromuscular and neuroskeletal systems. Depending on the location of neurological involvement, dysarthria affects the precision (accuracy), timing (speed), strength, steadiness, range of movement, muscle tone, and coordination of speech processes (Strand et al., 2014). Speech production is compromised due to the side effects of the neurological disorder or condition on respiration, phonation, articulation, resonation, and prosody. The dysarthrias can be classified on the basis of the constellation of nonspeech and speech symptoms, acoustic perceptual properties, and underlying neuroanatomical or neuropathologies associated with each dysarthria (Darley et al., 1975). The etiology of dysarthria ranges from vascular, degenerative, and neuromuscular diseases; to surgical or nonsurgical trauma; to neoplasms (e.g., tumors); to toxic, metabolic, and infectious diseases; to congenital or developmental malformations; to multiple system involvement; and to indeterminate causes. The onset of dysarthria can include developmental or congenital conditions (e.g., genetic or chromosomal causes); and acute (e.g., cerebral vascular accidents, physical or surgical trauma), subacute (e.g., transient ischemic attack), chronic and progressive (e.g., muscular dystrophy, amyotrophic lateral sclerosis, multiple sclerosis, myasthenia gravis, etc.), and multifactorial causes. Tables 26–1, 26–2, and 26–3 provide overviews of each type of dysarthria by location, speech, and other symptoms.

Assessment of Dysarthria. Differential diagnosis of dysarthria requires that one assesses the structural and functional integrity of the motor speech mechanism. A basic examination of the speech mechanism consists of an oral peripheral and neuromotor speech examination. The oral peripheral examination is necessary to determine if there are any inadequacies to the speech mechanism and its articulators. It is important to determine if the skeletal structures and/or soft tissues of the teeth, hard palate, soft palate, tongue, jaw, pharynx, face, mouth, nose, laryngeal skeleton, and so on, are present, intact, and adequate for communication purposes. It is of the utmost importance to assess the functional integrity of the speech mechanism to determine if the CNS and PNS and their neural networks are intact, not impaired, malfunctioning, or suboptimal for the innervation of the speech mechanism. The neuromotor speech examination allows one to assess the interconnectivity and integrity of the pyramidal tract and extrapyramidal tracts (CNS), the control circuits (e.g., basal ganglia and cerebellum and their interconnectivity to other neuroanatomical regions and sensorimotor networks), and the lower motor neuron (LMN) system or PNS (e.g., cranial and spinal nerves and their neuromuscular innervation) for speech production. The neuromuscular structures are examined at rest, during voluntary oral motor movement, sustained movement, and spontaneous production of speech.

Table 26–1. Classification of Dysarthria Due to Supratentorial Lesions

Dysarthria	Localization of Neuropathology	Speech Symptoms	Other Symptoms
Spastic	Bilateral upper motor neuron (UMN)	■ Slow speech rate ■ Imprecise articulation ■ Distorted vowels ■ Strained-strangled phonation ■ Harsh vocal quality ■ Monopitch, monoloudness ■ Hypernasality	■ Spasticity
Unilateral upper motor neuron	One cerebral hemisphere	■ Imprecise articulation ■ Irregular articulatory breakdowns ■ Slow rate of speech ■ Slow and/or irregular alternate motion rates (AMRs) ■ Harsh voice or hoarse voice	■ Affects mostly contralateral lower face, tongue ■ Weakness ■ Spasticity ■ Incoordination

Table 26–2. Classification of Dysarthria Due to Subcortical Lesions

Dysarthria	Localization of Neuropathology	Speech Symptoms	Other Symptoms
Hypokinetic	Basal ganglia	• Breathiness • Reduced loudness • Monopitch, monoloudness • Short, fast rushes of speech • Long pauses between sentences	• Slow initiation of movement • Movement reduced in range • Rigidity
Hyperkinetic	Basal ganglia	• Specific to type of movement disorder superimposed on speech production • Dyskinesia, dystonia • Chorea, athetosis • Myoclonus, tremor, spasm	• Involuntary movement • Fast versus slow • Rhythmic • Arrhythmic • Mixed symptoms

Table 26–3. Classification of Dysarthria Due to Infratentorial and/or Supratentorial Lesions

Dysarthria	Localization of Neuropathology	Speech Symptoms	Other Symptoms
Flaccid	Lower motor neuron (LMN) Cranial + spinal nerves Neuromuscular junction	• Cranial nerve specific and impact on speech production • V, VII, IX, X, XI, XII • Resonation, articulation • Phonation, respiration	• Weakness • Atrophy
Ataxic	Cerebellum	• Breakdowns in articulation • Imprecise consonants • Distorted vowels • Monopitch, monoloudness • Atypical stress and intonation • Incoordination	• Incoordination • Ataxic gait
Mixed dysarthria	More than one neurological region	Varies on location of neuropathologies	Varies

The examiner observes the neuromuscular structures of the face, tongue, soft palate, jaw movement, pharynx, larynx, shoulders, and abdominal diaphragmatic structures for symmetry, weakness or paralysis (hypotonia), spasticity or rigidity (hypertonia), atrophy, involuntary movements, breathing, and coordination of systems.

As previously stated, speech and nonspeech movements are examined and observed for precision (accuracy), timing (speed), strength, steadiness, range of movement, muscle tone, coordination of speech processes, and the impact of these salient features on speech (Duffy, 2013). During speech tasks, reading aloud and connected speech, the examiner observes for the presence of deviant speech characteristics, such as imprecise articulation, articulatory breakdowns, distorted vowels, slow initiation or voice onset problems, long pauses between words or phrases, dysfluent-like repetitions (e.g., palilalia), nasal emission, precision and coordination of speech processes, speech rate or variability, duration of syllables and utterances, and the presence of involuntary movements. The acoustic perceptual qualities of phonation and resonation are assessed for deviant vocal characteristics, such as hyper- or hyponasality, nasal snorting, monopitch, monoloudness, excessive or reduced loudness, voice decay, excess or equal stress, atypical prosody, pitch and pitch range, pitch breaks, strained-strangled phonation, hoarseness, harshness, diplophonia, and tremor. Speech is assessed for severity, variability of symptoms, and consistency or inconsistency. Examination of neuropathological (e.g., suck reflex, jaw jerk reflex, palmomental reflex) and vegetative reflexes (e.g., gag) are assessed for their presence, absence, and degree of briskness (e.g., hyporeflexia vs. hyperreflexia). Evidence of atrophy and the presence of fasciculations are confirmatory signs and can assist the examiner in the differential diagnosis of the dysarthria type with respect to the location of the neurological involvement (e.g., LMNs, cranial and spinal nerves, or neuromuscular junction).

The type of dysarthria, etiology, projected course, prognosis, and management of the MSDs once the individual is stable should be addressed in a timely manner and are influenced by a number of factors. However, not all individuals are good candidates for speech therapy. Treatment for dysarthria can include behavioral (speech-oriented), medical, prosthetic, compensatory techniques, and environmental adjustments (Duffy, 2013). In cases with severe dysarthria or anarthria, the use of assistive technologies (ATs) and alternative and augmentative communication (AAC) can be implemented to augment or substitute oral communication. AT and AAC can also be used in conjunction with behavioral treatment approaches to improve verbal communication, increase speech intelligibility, and provide the individual opportunities to practice, improve performance, and learn. Empiri-

cal research has demonstrated that using AAC does not hinder an individual who uses AAC from learning to speak (Millar et al., 2006). Research also supports that AAC interventions do not inhibit, but instead increase speech production (Schlosser & Wendt, 2008).

Apraxia of Speech. The classic theoretical model of apraxia of speech (AOS) is attributed to a breakdown in the motor speech programmer (MSP) that selectively impairs (a) articulator-specific plans of movement (motor planning), and (b) muscle-specific biomechanical programming that controls the speed, timing, and force of voluntary movement during spontaneous speech (Darley et al., 1975). Hence, AOS impairs an individual's ability to program and plan sensorimotor signals necessary to produce spontaneous, voluntary speech despite intact and functional linguistic and motor systems. AOS occurs in the absence of weakness or problems with motor execution (e.g., spasticity, rigidity, etc.). An acquired AOS can occur in either adults or children due to a lesion in the language-dominant hemisphere involving the frontal lobe and other subjacent cortical or subcortical regions. Children who fail or are slow to acquire speech due to a congenital or neurodevelopmental problem affecting motor programming and planning of speech exhibit a childhood apraxia of speech (CAS). The neurological underpinnings of CAS are typically indeterminate in origin; however, CAS is attributed to involvement of the language-dominant hemisphere since a coexisting language impairment may be present. The etiology of an acquired AOS ranges from degenerative conditions (e.g., primary progressive aphasia or AOS), vascular lesions (e.g., stroke), neoplasms, and trauma (e.g., physical or surgical trauma), as well as other indeterminate causes involving the CNS in the language-dominant hemisphere. The onset of an acquired AOS ranges from acute, subacute, chronic, to progressive. An acquired AOS often coexists with a nonfluent and/or fluent aphasia and unilateral UMN dysarthria, and frequently, a nonverbal oral motor apraxia and limb apraxia. Speech characteristics and symptoms of AOS (e.g., sound substitutions) frequently resemble those that occur with other neurolinguistic problems like aphasia (e.g., phonemic paraphasias). It is important to remember that sound errors in AOS are motoric in nature, yet phonemic paraphasias in aphasia are linguistic (Duffy, 2013). If swallowing, chewing, and drooling are present, one should suspect the presence of neuromuscular issues (e.g., weakness). Table 26–4 provides an overview of the clinical symptomatology attributed to an acquired AOS.

Assessment of Apraxia of Speech. Since motor speech abilities are intertwined with cognitive-linguistic processes and may coexist with fluent and nonfluent aphasias and/or dysarthria, differential diagnosis of an acquired AOS frequently presents a challenge to clinicians and researchers. In the past decade, greater emphasis has been placed on using more objective operational metrics and assessment protocols to differentially diagnose an AOS and identify the clinical symptoms most supportive of an AOS as compared to other neurolinguistic and neuromotor problems (Basilakos et al., 2015; Haley et al., 2012; Strand et al., 2014). The Apraxia of Speech Rating Scale (ASRS) is a structured assessment protocol developed by Strand et al. (2014) that uses operational metrics to assess an AOS in individuals with other comorbid neurological conditions (e.g., nonfluent and fluent aphasia, dysarthria). This ASRS assesses the presence or absence of approximately 16 distinguishing

Table 26–4. Clinical Symptoms Associated With Acquired Apraxia of Speech

Apraxia of Speech Symptoms			
Articulation	**Contextual Influences**	**Speech Rate Prosody**	**Fluency**
Distorted consonants, vowels, sound substitutions	Increased number of distorted sounds with increase in complexity of syllables, words, phrases	Segmentation of syllables within words and multisyllabic words	Difficulty initiating articulation
Overshooting and undershooting articulatory targets in place and manner	Increased number of sound substitutions with increase in complexity of syllables, words, phrases	Segmentation of syllables in phrases, sentences	Repetition of sounds and syllables
Articulation errors similar for imitation and spontaneous speech	Increased number of sound substitutions and distortions with increase rate of speech	Prolonged or lengthened duration of vowel segments	Attempts to self-correct speech errors
Distorted voicing	Slow overall speech rate	Prolonged or lengthened duration between consonants, syllables	Starting and restarting attempts to voluntarily articulate or speak
Greater number of consonant cluster errors than single consonants	Slow speech alternate motion rates (AMRs)	Prolonged or lengthened duration between words, phrases	Visual and audible effortful trial and error articulation and/or groping
Increased variability and abnormal distribution of voice onset time for voiced, voiceless fricatives and stops	Difficulty sequencing speech sequential motor rates (SMRs)		Fewer words produced on one breath compared to vowel prolongation

clinical features (operational metrics) that are most frequently observed in individuals with an acquired AOS with and without a coexisting aphasia and/or dysarthria. The ASRS' 16 clinical features or variables fall into four discrete categories: (a) six primary distinguishing features of AOS with no overlap with dysarthria or aphasia for which one of more of the six variables must be present for diagnosis of AOS; (b) six distinguishing features unless dysarthria is present; (c) two distinguishing features unless aphasia is present; and (d) two distinguishing features unless dysarthria, aphasia, or both are present (Strand et al., 2014). Many of the 16 distinguishing features or clinical symptoms that are inventoried using the ASRS rating scale are included in Table 26–4. The ASRS evaluates severity using a 5-point ordinal scale ranging from 0 to 4 as follows: 0 = not present, 1 = detectable but infrequent, 2 = frequent but not pervasive, 3 = nearly always evident but not marked in severity, and 4 = nearly always evident and marked in severity. The ASRS' normative data show that the ASRS rating scale has strong inter-rater reliability ranging from .91 to .98.

Treatment for AOS should focus on improving speech production, increasing speech intelligibility, and introducing alternative modes for communicating when indicated, such as AT and/or AAC, sign language or manually signing, context-specific communication boards, and electronic speech output devices. It is important to note that AOS is a disorder of speech production, yet a coexisting language problem may be present. Treatment approaches fall into the following categories: articulatory-kinematic, rate and rhythm control, facilitation/reorganization, scripted training, sensory or tactile cueing, restructuring oral muscular phonetic targets, a variety of instrumentation, including some that use ultrasound, and AAC (Duffy, 2013). Principles of motor learning should be incorporated into intervention to facilitate performance, skill acquisition, and retention. For moderate to severe nonfluent AOS, AAC is very beneficial to augment or provide a means for the individual to communicate. The use of AAC with nonfluent individuals also facilitates reorganization (neuroplasticity) of the CNS and associated neural networks.

Case Study: RL

Clinical Profile and Communication Needs

The Individual

RL is a 50-year-old, right-handed, monolingual English-speaking male with 23 years of education. His past medical history is unremarkable with the exception of hypertension, mild-to-moderate obesity, and a coronary artery bypass graft (CABG) which he underwent 1 year ago. In addition, he is 1 year post onset of a single left middle cerebral artery (MCA) embolic cerebrovascular accident (CVA) that occurred during or immediately following the CABG surgery. A T1-weighted magnetic resonance imaging (MRI) study following surgery showed a lesion in the left cerebral cortex and subjacent white matter involving the left posterior inferior frontal lobe and insula. Neurology reported mild weakness involving his right upper extremity (RUE), a positive Babinski reflex of the right lower extremity (RLE), and right-sided facial droop. The RLE, left upper extremity (LUE), and left lower extremity (LLE) are intact.

Immediately following the stroke, he was found positive for a unilateral left vocal fold weakness involving the left recurrent laryngeal nerve (L-RLN) due to complications during the CABG surgery. He underwent laryngeal electromyography (L-EMG) that confirmed a mildly weak left vocal fold. He underwent a series of assessments to evaluate his swallowing ability and risk for aspiration, including modified barium swallow (MBS) evaluations for dysphagia. He transitioned from a nasogastric tube (NGT) feeding to soft and pureed diets, including oral nutritional supplements (ONSs). He was evaluated and treated by Otolaryngology for the unilateral left vocal fold weakness and was referred for voice therapy to Speech-Language Pathology for glottal insufficiency. The speech-language pathologist (SLP) diagnosed him with a flaccid dysarthria due to LMN weakness to the left vocal fold affecting the vagus (Cranial X) nerve. He was also found positive for a mild unilateral UMN dysarthria affecting the lower face on the right side and right side of the tongue. Three months post-CABG and stroke and following voice therapy for his dysphonia, he received bulk injections from an Otolaryngologist to manage the mild weakness of his left vocal fold.

Postoperatively, RL was classified as having moderate-to-severe nonfluent transcortical motor aphasia as indicated by his performance on subtests of the Boston Diagnostic Aphasia Examination, Third Edition (BDAE–3; Goodglass et al., 2001). His performance on the BDAE fell in the 80th percentile based on the mean of three auditory comprehension tasks and 32/60 on the Boston Naming Test Second Edition (BNT–2; Kaplan et al., 2001). A comprehensive neuromotor speech evaluation was performed (Darley et al., 1975; Duffy, 2013), including assessment of his ability to volitionally program and plan speech for communication purposes using the ASRS (Strand et al., 2014). The Consensus Auditory–Perceptual Evaluation of Voice (CAPE–V, Kempster et al., 2009) was also administered at that time to assess vocal quality. Although RL is nonfluent due to the embolic stroke to his left hemisphere, he exhibited mild to moderate breathiness, hoarseness, reduced loudness, mild shortness of breath, and diplophonia when trying to phonate due to the flaccid dysarthria affecting the left vocal fold.

The comprehensive neuromotor speech evaluation revealed a marked to severe AOS based on the results of the ASRS (Strand et al., 2014). RL's communication is generally limited to one- to two-word responses, often ending with "I can't say" or "May." The latter is a reference to his wife, Megan, on whom he generally relies when speaking with others, although he occasionally produces what sounds like grammatically accurate but distorted propositional phrases. The ASRS identified the following most notable features consistent with an acquired AOS: marked difficulty initiating speech; significant deterioration of repetitive speech on trials with increasing word length and complexity; schwa vowel inclusion; abnormal prosody; self-awareness of his speech errors; groping and frustration with visible and audible searching; numerous and varied off-target word attempts on volition; and phonemic transposition errors. RL

was slightly more fluent on automatic tasks (counting 1 to 30) and markedly to severely nonfluent on volitional tasks, such as describing a picture and trying to read aloud.

In summary, RL was diagnosed with the following complex communication problems that severely hinder his ability to communicate verbally:

- flaccid dysarthria due to LMN weakness involving the left vocal fold
- unilateral UMN dysarthria due to central weakness affecting the right lower face and right tongue
- AOS due to embolic stroke and marked to severe programming and planning of volitional speech
- transcortical motor aphasia affecting expressive more than receptive language problem due to L-MCA embolic stroke
- dysphagia, mild in severity due to mild left vocal fold weakness

Current Communication Status: The flaccid and unilateral UMN dysarthrias have improved and are stable, and residual side effects are negligible. Swallowing is stable and functional, and RL is deemed to be low risk for aspiration. Receptive language abilities have improved and are stable. Auditory comprehension is functional and mildly compromised at most. His AOS is stable and not expected to improve. It is difficult to tease out the impact of the transcortical motor aphasia since he is severely nonfluent. RL does not show evidence of agrammatism or word-finding difficulties, but it is difficult to determine the extent of his nonfluent aphasia since his speech is limited to one- to two-word utterances. Nonfluent speech is deemed to be secondary to the AOS. Oral-verbal communication is limited to very short utterances that are very unintelligible.

Mini-Mental State Examination and screening of cognitive abilities revealed he was oriented to time, place, and year. He exhibits functional cognitive and receptive language abilities. RL does not wear glasses or a hearing aid to correct vision or hearing abilities, respectively. Hearing and vision are intact. RL has full use of his left hand, RLE, and LLE. Physical function is only mildly compromised due to mild RUE weakness. RL walks independently without the assistance of a cane or wheelchair. RL and his family are significantly frustrated.

His current communication is highly inefficient at expressing his needs, detailed and complex information at work, and himself at social interactions with family and communication partners. RL is no longer social due to his limited verbal communication and frustration when trying to speak. His nonfluent speech is often unintelligible to unfamiliar and familiar communication partners, and he cannot respond effectively to simple questions and conversational speech.

Their Communication Partners

RL is unable to communicate independently without the assistance of his wife. RL has two adult children who live out of state and with whom he speaks less frequently since his stroke. In the past, he used FaceTime, videoconferencing, and his cell phone to communicate with his children, colleagues, and friends. RL and his wife were very social prior to the stroke. RL's wife heard about a university speech clinic that has a Stroke Support Group, and she wanted RL to attend so he could practice speaking with a communication partner. RL and his wife attended the Stroke Support Group, but he exhibited groping and frustration trying to communicate with others at the support group. RL and his wife noticed that some of the individuals with compromised communication abilities at the support group communicated effectively with the help of ATs, AAC, and speech-generating devices (SGDs). RL and his wife inquired with the SLP staff running the support group about the process for obtaining a referral and workup for an AT, AAC, or SGD. The staff recommended that he speak to his primary care physician and/or neurologist about a referral and provided him a list of SLP specialists in the region who can assess his candidacy for a low-technical (tech) or high-tech device to augment his communication.

RL and his wife identified his communication needs in the following contexts:

Occupation and Professional Role: RL returned back to work part-time 4 months ago to assist preparing legal cases for trial; however, he is no longer trying cases in court due to his inability to communicate. His contributions at work are significantly limited, and he and his wife are concerned since he is the wage earner in the family. RL would like to resume interacting with colleagues, staff, clients, family members, and friends.

Psycho-Social-Emotional Well-Being: Since his stroke, RL has been less engaged with family, friends, colleagues, staff, and former clients. RL would like to resume his old lifestyle and be able to interact and communicate more independently. He would like to contribute in a more meaningful manner at work and at the Stroke Support Group that he recently joined and enjoys attending for emotional support and interacting with a communication partner. RL would like to communicate with familiar and unfamiliar people in his community.

Routine Medical and Emergency Needs: RL would like to be able to schedule appointments and communicate with his physicians and other professional personnel (SLP, PT, etc.) independently. In the event of a car and other medical emergencies, he would like to be able to call and communicate more effectively.

Their Environment

RL lives with his wife of 30 years on whom he relies when trying to communicate with others. He lives in a suburb just north of a relatively large city. He is able to walk and drive without assistance. Prior to his stroke, RL prepared and tried cases in court. He is able to walk and perform activities of daily living (ADLs) independently and has good use of his arms and hands. Although his RUE has mild residual weakness, it is functional to perform ADLs.

AAC Considerations

Past Treatment: RL participated in both inpatient and outpatient services once weekly for PT therapy and two to three times weekly for SLP therapy for approximately 1 year following his stroke. SLP therapy initially consisted of regaining glottal sufficiency for phonation and swallowing. Speech and language therapy was focused on articulatory-kinematic speech therapy and constraint-induced language therapy to improve articulation and his speech intelligibility, oral-motor skills, accuracy and intelligibility of verbal productions for single-syllable and multisyllabic words, and receptive and expressive language. Although cognitive-linguistic abilities improved and stabilized, RL's verbal productions did not improve significantly. RL is 1-year post-onset of his stroke, and given his current severity of AOS, his prognosis for improving functional speech is poor. Despite being able to use pantomime, hand gestures, and writing, he is not able to effectively express his ideas and function. Since RL is very social and employed as an attorney, he requires a more efficient and effective method for communicating. Cost is not a factor when considering an appropriate AAC device for him.

The AAC System or Service

RL can use direct selection to access a device with both his left and right hands when he places the device on a table or lap. As previously stated, his hearing and vision are within normal limits and adequate for SGD use. A low-tech device is not appropriate for RL given his level of education, demands of his work, social needs, and current cognitive linguistic function. An SGD is the most appropriate option for RL. The following SGDs were considered and introduced to RL: Tobii Dynavox Indi7 and I-110, MessageMate, and a Lingraphica AAC device. The SLP specialist engaged RL to try out several of the SGDs to determine which one best suited his current communication needs and level of intellectual function.

RL was able to quickly learn and navigate each device to form messages, stringing words together for short sentences and longer complex phrases with little to no training. Among the selection introduced to RL, the Lingraphica AllTalk and MiniTalk SGD devices were best suited for him as they provided a number of options with which he could express himself by combining text, images, pictures, and speech with the use of one finger to touch icons that activated speech for simple, frequently used words, phrases, and sentences. The Lingraphica SGD also enabled him to organize icons into pages on specific topics, which is ideal for the type of work he does as a criminal lawyer and social person. Since he has use of both hands, he was able to use the white board on the SGD to write and draw and the keyboard to type out words and sentences that provided voice output. The built-in videos, activities, and treatment applications will also enable him to practice speaking words and phrases since he is no longer actively working with a SLP. He would like to be able to connect to advanced therapy online provided through Lingraphica.

Next Steps

RL would like to work with the SLP specialist to learn how to use the Lingraphica SGD device effectively and efficiently for work, social interactions, and to improve the quality of his life. The following goals and objectives were outlined for RL:

1. Formulating two- and three-word sentences and short phrases with 80% accuracy on his SGD.
   Outcome: During a treatment session, he was able to use the SGD to answer simple questions during a role-modeling activity. The SLP modeled a client and/or colleague seeking his services as an attorney. On a social level, he successfully communicated with his wife, communicated with a communication partner at the stroke support group, and ordered food at a restaurant.

2. Programming a new page on the SGD with 15 messages independently and syncing the page to the keyboard page.
   Outcome: RL successfully accomplished this goal after 1 week of treatment. He was able to create, store, and retrieve messages pertaining to a number of topics using both pictures and text. He was able to locate pre-stored messages and generate new messages using the keyboard and word-prediction array with both text and symbols.

3. Accessing and using prestored messages he created on specific work-related and social topics appropriately 90% of the time. Outcome: RL successfully completed six interactions and transactions with the SLP present as he ordered take-out food at his favorite fast food restaurant, called a staff member at work, communicated with his children and wife, and ordered a book by telephone at the local Barnes & Noble bookstore.

References

Basilakos, A., Rorden, C., Bonilha, L., Moser, D., & Fridriksson, J. (2015). Patterns of poststroke brain damage that predict speech production errors in apraxia of speech and aphasia dissociate. *Stroke, 46*(6), 1561–1566.

Darley, F. L., Aronson, A. E., & Brown, J. R. (1975). *Motor speech disorders*. Elsevier.

Duffy, J. (2013). *Motor speech disorders, substrates, differential diagnosis, and management*. Elsevier.

Goodglass, H., Kaplan, E., & Barresi, B. (2001). *Boston Diagnostic Aphasia Examination* (BDAE, 3rd ed.). Pro-Ed.

Haley, K. L., Jacks, A., de Riesthal, M., Abou-Khalil, R., & Roth, H. L. (2012). Toward a quantitative basis for assessment and diagnosis of apraxia of speech. *Journal of Speech, Language, and Hearing Research, 55*(5), S1502–S1517.

Kaplan, E., Goodglass, H., & Weintraub, S. (2001). *Boston Naming Test* (BNT, 2nd ed.). Pro-Ed.

Kempster, G. B., Gerratt, B. R., Verdolini Abbott, K., Barkmeier-Kramer, J., & Hillman, R. E. (2009). Consensus Auditory–Perceptual Evaluation of Voice: Development of a standardized clinical protocol. *American Journal of Speech-Language Pathology, 18*, 124–132.

Millar, D., Light, J., & Schlosser, R. (2006). The impact of augmentative and alternative communication intervention on the speech production of individuals with developmental disabilities: A research review. *Journal of Speech, Language, and Hearing Research, 49*, 248–264.

Schlosser, R., & Wendt, O. (2008). Effects of augmentative and alternative communication intervention on speech production in children with autism: A systematic review. *American Journal of Speech-Language Pathology, 17*, 212–230.

Strand, E. A., Duffy, J. R., Clark, H. M., & Josephs, K. (2014). The apraxia of speech rating scale: A tool for diagnosis and description of apraxia of speech. *Journal of Communication Disorders, 51*, 43–50.

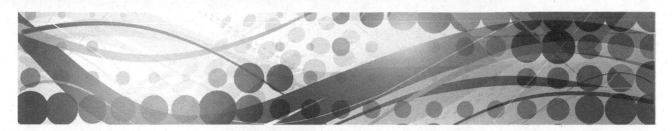

Chapter 27
AAC FOR PERSONS WITH AMYOTROPHIC LATERAL SCLEROSIS

Telina Caudill

Fundamentals

Adults who acquire neurological diseases likely will experience symptoms that will interfere with the individual's motor speech, language, and/or cognitive function. This chapter summarizes intervention approaches to implement with persons with amyotrophic lateral sclerosis (pALS). Although the content is specific to pALS, the treatment methods could be applied to adults with complex communication needs associated with another neurological disease. ALS is a degenerative neurological disorder that leads to profound physical disabilities including weakness, fatigue, and paralysis of the muscles necessary for walking, using our hands, as well as those for respiration, speech, and swallowing (Beukelman et al., 2007). ALS type is diagnosed by site of onset and labeled as bulbar, spinal, or mixed.

Communication impairments common to ALS include dysarthria, anarthria, dysphonia, and aphonia. At some point, pALS will require respiratory support with either noninvasive ventilation or tracheostomy with invasive ventilation. Other sequela of ALS may include cognitive-linguistic impairments associated with frontotemporal dementia. Given the progressive nature of the disease, communication abilities for pALS (persons with ALS) gradually deteriorate, with greater than 75% of pALS unable to use natural speech or writing at some point during the disease progression (Beukelman et al., 2011). As a result, pALS will eventually require and depend on augmentative and alternative communication (AAC) for the basic human need of communication. Beukelman et al. (2011) reported study participants within the Nebraska ALS database benefited from AAC use for up to 31.1 months and until within a few weeks of their deaths. Timing of AAC assessment, acquisition, and intervention, therefore, is vital for this population to ensure a system is in place as their needs change to reduce burden and impact on activities and participation. Frequency of AAC intervention is equally imperative given progressive debility and potential cognitive decline necessitating modified access methods and/or language representations over the course of the disease. This chapter focuses on the role of the speech-language pathologist (SLP) in supporting the complex communicative needs of adults with acquired neurological disease through the implementation of AAC service provision, strategies, and treatment principles.

Communication Symptoms

Planning for scheduled SLP sessions to assess motor, speech, voice, and cognitive functions over time facilitates timely and successful AAC intervention service provision.

Dysarthria

ALS results in mixed flaccid-spastic dysarthria given upper and lower motor neuron involvement. In mild dysarthria, spasticity or flaccidity usually predominates; however, the disease progresses leading to profound impairments and anarthria for most (Beukelman et al., 2011). Bulbar ALS, initially affecting speech and swallowing, is the most aggressive type with rapid progression and commonly associated with pseudobulbar affect (Makkonen et al., 2018). The literature supports that speaking rate, specifically, rate lower than 125 words per minute, is an accurate prediction of eventual intelligibility demise, irrespective of ALS type (Ball et al., 2002).

Voice Disorder

Dysphonia caused by respiratory insufficiency is present in pALS. Poor breath support usually manifests by decreased vocal intensity and short phrasing. Individuals, typically spinal ALS, who require noninvasive ventilation such as bilevel positive airway pressure (BiPAP), often present with relatively intact speech. However, due to the physical barriers associated with the masks that cover the whole face, partial face, or nares, verbal communication becomes laborious, limited, or sometimes impossible. Coordination of speech with the delivery of air through the nose or mouth becomes difficult. Additionally, vocal intensity and resonance are disturbed.

The pALS may be forced to remove the mask to speak, thus becoming rapidly fatigued and short of breath. Moreover, in the presence of upper extremity weakness, they will depend on others to remove the mask for them, in turn, losing the natural spontaneity of communication. As a result, caregivers often take on the role of interpreters and find that they often must stop what they are doing and come into proximity with the pALS for successful communication exchange to occur. Caregivers may assume the responsibility of managing phone calls, household duties, medical care, and supporting social interactions with others. They may become reticent to leave the pALS's side for

fear that they cannot speak for themselves, creating a codependency.

Aphonia is present in pALS following invasive ventilation, either elective or emergent. Invasive ventilation increases the life expectancy of pALS as well as the duration of AAC use (Beukelman et al., 2011). Strategies for the adult with aphonia often include methods such as exaggerated articulation to support lipreading, use of an electrolarynx, or an in-line speaking valve, if indicated.

Cognitive-Communication

Cognitive-linguistic changes do occur in ALS and tend to be more distinct with bulbar involvement, 10% exhibiting frontotemporal dementia (FTD) symptoms and up to 50% demonstrating more global cognitive decline on neuropsychological testing, as reported by Yunusova et al. (2016). There are four variants of FTD, one of which is primarily behavioral deviation with the remaining variants of primary progressive aphasia (PPA) mainly characterized by language impairment.

Dysphagia

Sialorrhea or excessive drooling may result in social isolation and avoidance of communicative interactions. It may interfere with the flow of verbal speech as the pALS will need to swallow more often, frequently wipe their mouths, or even maintain gauze or towels intra-orally to minimize secretion overflow.

Communication Needs

AAC interventions, both high-tech and low-tech, should focus on personally relevant messages within the four purposes of communicative interaction that include expression of needs and wants, information transfer, social closeness, and social etiquette (Light & McNaughton, 2015). Additionally, communicative environments, settings, and partners such as home versus work or school, individual versus groups, in-person versus telephone or computer should be identified by the SLP and incorporated into the AAC treatment plan to maximize carryover.

Intervention Phases

Beukelman, Garrett, and Yorkston (2007) list three general phases of AAC service provision for pALS, as shown in Table 27–1. We delve into each phase

as it relates to the five ALS intervention stages proposed by DeRuyter and colleagues (2004) adapted from the Revised Amyotrophic Lateral Sclerosis Functional Rating Scale (ALSFRS-R) (Cedarbaum et al., 1999). Intervention at each stage may occur via inpatient, outpatient, home-health and/or tele-AAC depending on the needs and abilities of the client. The SLP should involve the caregiver(s) and/or significant other within treatment to support generalization of learned skills within the natural environment(s).

Table 27–1. Intervention Phases by Amyotrophic Lateral Sclerosis (ALS) Stages

Intervention Phase 1			
Staging	**Monitor**	**Prepare**	**Support**
Stage 1: Normal speech processes Stage 2: Detectable speech disturbance	Evaluate speaking rate and intelligibility	• Education on the course of the disease and what to expect • Train compensatory speech strategies • Train caregiver(s) on communication partner tips • Begin voice banking • Begin message banking	Provide access to printed, digital, online, and community resources
Intervention Phase 2			
Staging	**Assess**	**Recommend**	**Implement**
Stage 3: Reduction in speech intelligibility Stage 4: Use of AAC	• Introduce no-tech and low-tech aids • Initiate high-tech evaluation	Develop plan of care with treatment frequency of three times per week for 12 weeks *Inpatient and telehealth allow for increased frequency vs outpatient	• Provide training resources in multiple formats • Caregiver and staff involvement
Intervention Phase 3			
Staging	**Adapt**	**Accommodate**	
Stage 5: No functional speech	• Modify communication system and access modalities to meet changing needs • Adjust treatment frequency as indicated	• Maintain high-tech system with software updates and upgrades as indicated • Maintain low-tech communication system as backup method	

Note. See *Augmentative Communication Strategies for Adults With Acute or Chronic Medical Conditions*, by D. R. Beukelman, K. L. Garrett, and K. M. Yorkston (Eds.), 2007. Copyright Paul H. Brookes. "Speech Pathologist's Clinical Pathway for Communication Changes With ALS," by F. DeRuyter, *ALS Clinical Pathways*, 2004 (http://aac-rerc.psu.edu/index.php/files/list/type/1).

Phase 1: Monitor, Prepare, and Support

At this point in the disease, the speech of the pALS is either intact or functional with perceived changes (Stages 1: Normal Speech Processes and Stage 2: Detectable Speech Disturbances).

Monitor

First, the SLP should routinely evaluate speaking rate and intelligibility during 15-min ALS multidisciplinary clinic visits once every 3 to 4 months.

Prepare

Second, education is key to preparation. Systematic, consistent, individualized, and timely discussion of the known course of the disease, AAC supports available (no-tech to high-tech), and adjustments to new communication norms for PWUAAC are necessary. The SLP should prepare caregivers by discussing role changes (from supporters to translators) and pragmatic changes resulting from energy conservation methods (telegraphic speech) which may appear blunt or rude (Judge et al., 2018). It is paramount to empower the patient and caregiver to recognize changes in speech function to be informed and self-advocate.

Compensatory Speech Strategies and Communication Partner Tips. Although clients with functional speech and their communication partners may deny the need for speech strategy training, SLP counseling and education should emphasize that anticipation of the onset of communication impairment is difficult, thus knowledge is powerful in overcoming the challenges. Strategy training for the client may include the following:

- slow down speaking rate
- exaggerate articulation
- pause between words
- use alphabet supplementation, gestures, writing or communication boards
- avoid talking on residual air
- practice energy conservation such as strategically engaging in anticipated conversations during times when speech tends to be strongest and clearest, speak succinctly, use a voice amplifier, and take breaks
- discourage oral motor exercises and articulation drills that hasten fatigue and worsen dysarthria
- instead educate that normal speaking is enough exercise

Strategy training for the caregiver and/or significant other may include the following:

- optimizing speaking environments by reducing or eliminating background noise
- minimizing distance between communication partners
- speaking face to face, maintaining eye contact, and trying to give your full attention

Voice Banking. Voice banking is the creation of a personalized synthetic voice, modeled after the client's natural speech patterns, which can then be programmed as the default voice on a speech-generating device (SGD), thereby preserving a piece of their identity. Voice banking should be discussed when speech is intact. The pALS may decline given the seemingly nonurgent need due to lack of dysarthria. Others may find it emotionally difficult to hear their premorbid voice, which may contribute to apparent disinterest as found by Judge et al. (2018). It is the responsibility of the SLP to review disease progression and optimal recording situations prior to onset of dysarthria, respiratory impairment, or poor endurance. Should the client communicate interest in voice banking, the SLP should provide education on the following:

- identifying voice banking software options and equipment requirements
- troubleshooting support available through the various companies
- completing the software registration process
- setting up the equipment
- recording processes specific to the selected software company

Although participation in voice banking is optimal when the client's speech is intact, the client may participate when experiencing early onset of speech changes. The SLP should explore various software options that meet the client's needs to ensure voice banking participation and completion. Some software options require as few as only 50 phrase recordings to create a personalized synthetic voice.

Message Banking. Message banking is the term used for creating digitized recordings of vocal utterances of the individual's choosing, sometimes referred to as legacy messages. They are recordings of the person's natural voice that can be stored electronically until an SGD is required and then transferred and programmed within the software at that time. pALS can also message bank directly into an SGD should they already have one. Message banking can also be completed on a handheld voice recorder, a voice recording app, native sound recorders on computers, teddy bears, and children's recordable storybooks. Hurtig and Downey (2009) underscore the value of the personalized voice for both acceptance and use of the AAC device with the pALS and their loved ones. Notably, Oosthuizen and colleagues (2018) found in their study that pALS who chose to message bank, ranked messages related to social closeness as most important to them. Inclusion of idiosyncratic comments, curse words, expressions of anger and sarcasm, pet commands, and absolutely anything personally relevant to the pALS is highly recommended. Typically, the role of the SLP in message banking is to provide the client and significant other/caregiver with education on the following:

- differences between message banking and voice banking
- equipment that could be used to participate in message banking
- resources to secure access to equipment for message banking
- custom sound, vocalization, and phrase identification

Support

Support their learning by providing access to community resources, reputable online content, individualized handouts, and materials that they can explore both with you and on their own, self-paced, when they have reached acceptance. Consider educational materials that meet accessibility standards for those with disabilities.

Phase 2: Assess, Recommend, and Implement

At this stage, the pALS's speech intelligibility is reduced requiring repetition and/or use of AAC (Stages 3: Reduction in Speech Intelligibility and Stage 4: Use of AAC). Functionally, the pALS is now likely compensating by texting or writing instead of calling or speaking. No-tech to low-tech systems such as gestural communication, alphabet and topic supplementation, written aids, communication boards, voice amplifiers, and palatal lifts should be considered while procurement of a high-tech AAC system, for those indicated, is initiated.

Assess

The SLP should provide or assist with the coordination of a comprehensive AAC evaluation with device trials to ensure the client has access to an AAC system that meets their communication needs aligned with those identified in feature-matching analysis. The SLP uses information gathered during the comprehensive evaluation to prepare for intervention following procurement. For example, the client and caregiver are assigned the task of listing favorite web pages, preferred browsers, e-mail accounts, and favorite television channels. Additionally, the SLP provides a list of default categories and phrases from within the selected AAC software and guides the client and caregiver in customizing the list in advance. If upper extremity weakness is present, alternative access methods to direct selection such as partner-assisted scanning, eye-tracking, laser-pointing, switch-scanning and optical tracking are indicated.

Recommend

Immediate, consistent, and frequent training for the pALS and the caregiver to maximize learning of high-tech systems while residual speech remains functional is imperative. A suggested schedule of SLP intervention to achieve competency with an AAC system is three times a week for 12 weeks. The SLP should evaluate the client's barriers to access AAC services and assess potential solutions to mitigate them. For example, transportation to an outpatient clinic may be physically challenging for the client. One solution could be to evaluate if the service is available closer to the client's home or if tele-AAC is a viable option for both the client and the therapist. This can occur during inpatient, outpatient, home health, tele-AAC, or a combination of the above service modalities as well as in conjunction with training from the device vendor, and is discussed in Chapters 35 and 36.

Implement

The focus of intervention should be toward obtaining strategic and communicative competency for not only the client but also the caregiver, now the AAC facilitator. Initial training is typically performed by the device representative upon installation in the home. The SLP provides the device representative with individualized client input as stated earlier to maximize efficiency during setup. The SLP supplements vendor training in the appropriate treatment modality providing hands-on training, ongoing programming and customization, role-playing, and modeling. Training resources developed by the SLP such as picture guides, video tutorials, written step-by-step instructions, and links to online learning content are invaluable and empower caregivers and AAC facilitators to maintain their SGD.

The SLP should determine client preference for AAC facilitators and communication partners to "guess" or complete sentences on their behalf, akin to AAC etiquette training (e.g., allow client time to complete an utterance, maintain eye contact with the client vs. reading from the device). Education on the benefits and challenges of communication partners engaging in anticipatory completion of an utterance is warranted with both the client and the client's communication partners. The client should be provided with a script to navigate requests for communication partners to use and/or to termi-

nate use of anticipatory completion of an utterance. Findings from a study by Bloch (2011) reveal both advantages and disadvantages of anticipatory completion of an utterance that may save time and effort if accurately predicted on one hand or, conversely, increase time and effort if inaccurately predicted.

Phase 3: Adapt and Accommodate

Intervention Staging: Stage 5: No Functional Speech. At this stage, the pALS has no functional speech and is completely dependent on the AAC systems in place to engage with others.

Adapt

In this "maintenance" phase of intervention, the SLP monitors and modifies the communication methods and systems to meet the changing needs of the client associated with disease progression. This may include, though is not limited to, access methods, selection settings, language representations, and page layouts. The SLP should transition from weekly sessions to monthly follow-ups. Once the client demonstrates independence and has no ongoing current needs, follow-up service can now be converted to an as-needed basis as indicated by the client. The SLP should ensure that the client has means to independently contact their provider, if necessary.

Accommodate

Maintaining high-tech systems includes software upgrades, troubleshooting, sustaining contact with device representatives, and technical support and ability to connect with remote assistance. In this phase, the pALS must maintain competency with low-tech backup communication methods as technological issues are inevitable. The SLP can support nonverbal means of communication by training others on partner-assisted scanning, developing a reliable nonverbal yes/no response mechanism, creating a gestural legend for unfamiliar partners and developing a list of frequently used messages or topics to minimize demands on the pALS. Early intervention with recurring treatment sessions specific to the client's communication needs may improve participation in personally relevant activities and quality of life and reduce abandonment of AAC among adults with diseases that cause speech, language, and cognitive impairments.

Expert Tips or Practical Advice

- Consider durability and placement of AAC devices as well as potential waterproofing adaptations for pALS presenting with significant sialorrhea (Beukelman et al., 2007).
- Consider educational materials that meet accessibility standards for those with disabilities.
- Create simplified step-by-step instructions with screenshots to post at bedside for staff education.
- Collaborate with device representatives to compile digital resources including software default phrase banks.
- Encourage caregivers to record video of training sessions as permitted for additional resources.

Case Study: RP

Clinical Profile and Communication Needs

The Individual

RP, a 77-year-old married man, was a veteran and retired construction superintendent who was diagnosed with bulbar-onset ALS in April 2012; symptom onset in 2011 involved speech changes and shortness of breath. He was initially referred to the ALS team including speech pathology/assistive technology (AT) in June 2012 exhibiting mild dysarthria. He was previously evaluated by the

pulmonologist given his respiratory dysfunction. A BiPAP and cough assist were prescribed to him to manage the ALS symptoms. By 2013, the disease had rapidly progressed—RP suffered neuromuscular respiratory failure and required intubation and mechanical ventilation. He underwent a tracheostomy due to ventilator dependence. He continued to be followed as an outpatient by the ALS interdisciplinary team before he was admitted to long-term care in 2015. Interdisciplinary services, including AT, resumed for the long-term care resident and continued until his death in 2019.

RP was prescribed single-vision lens glasses and bilateral hearing aids. He rarely used the equipment because he was able to perform functional activities without them. At initial assessment, RP ambulated without an assistive device and was independent for all activities of daily living (ADLs). However, respiratory impairment was a significant barrier for participation in activities, and he was easily fatigued. His speech was mildly dysarthric characterized by impaired articulation, reduced intensity, and slowed rate, though significantly worsened with fatigue. His performance fell within the range of Stage 2, "Detectable Speech Disturbance," on the ALSFRS-R (Cedarbaum et al., 1999) and Group 1 "Adequate Speech & Adequate Hand Function" per the Classification of Functional Capabilities scale (Yorkston et al., 2013). He endorsed substantial decline in speech function over the past 6 months. He identified the ability to maintain in-person communication, long-distance communication, environmental control, and Internet access as top communication goals. Message and voice banking were discussed with RP in the initial evaluation, and he politely declined participation. Compensatory speech strategies were insufficient to consistently meet his communication needs. Hence, an AAC evaluation was warranted to expedite the procurement process. Language and cognition were within normal limits. RP as well as his spouse had good basic technology skills, and RP was highly motivated to learn novel communication software and access methods in advance of actual need. Within 2 years of initial assessment, his physical abilities had deteriorated to the point of total dependence, complete quadriplegia.

Their Communication Partners

RP's primary and secondary circles of communication partners at diagnosis consisted of his spouse and family members including siblings, children, and grandchildren. Paid workers (medical staff) were considered fourth-circle communication partners (Blackstone & Berg, 2003). As the disease progressed and when he required care at the long-term care facility, his most frequent communicative partners shifted to medical and rehabilitation staff. RP maintained regular contact with his spouse and family members for the remainder of his life while a resident in the long-term care facility. The communicative setting in which he typically interacted (e.g., in-person) shifted to distance communication using e-mail and social media.

Their Environment

Initially, AAC intervention was geared toward use in the home environment primarily, with integration within the community including trips to the store, visiting with family, or attending medical appointments. As such, both indoor and outdoor as well as use while traveling in a car were considered. Given declining endurance, ambulation soon proved problematic, and he was fitted for a power wheelchair to maximize safety and activity participation. Once he became a long-term care resident, his natural environment became the medical setting with occasional passes to his home as well as community outings with recreation therapy. In the advanced stage of his disease, he was primarily bed-bound though could tolerate short periods of sitting in his power wheelchair a few times a week.

AAC Considerations

A dedicated SGD, often bulky and heavy, was ruled out during his initial presentation in 2012 as his primary AAC system given unaided mobility, intact upper extremity function, and integration within the community at initial evaluation. He did not require the multiple access methods available on such devices at the time. Moreover, a dedicated system generally takes significantly longer to receive given procurement processes and purchasing approvals related to high-cost medical devices. In consideration of his then current communicative limitations and rapid progression, this potential delay was an additional reason to consider alternatives to provide near immediate support during the interim of awaiting approval of a dedicated system. Android-based tablets were ruled out not only due to his existing familiarity with iOS but also due to reduced availability of speech-generating apps appropriate for this population.

RP was an iPhone user and very familiar with iOS. Use of a familiar system limited the potential of RP experiencing new learning burden or excessive cognitive burden from a novel system. iOS has a multitude of SGD apps appropriate to meet his communicative needs while allowing access to the Internet as he desired and within a lightweight system that would facilitate ease in portability. Procurement could be expedited with low-cost everyday mobile device apps.

AAC System or Service Considerations

Following app and device trials, RP was asked to rate each app for ease of use for various features such as using word prediction, adding new phrases, navigating among features, and correcting typos given a numeric scale (Bardach, 2017). The ratings for each device across features were totaled, and an average percentage was calculated. Other user feedback was subjectively discussed, such as overall satisfaction with the user interface and access to integrated features that he rated important to him (Bardach, 2017). The data indicated an appropriate match with Predictable for iPhone and the Tobii C12. RP utilized his iPhone SGD for 2 years before transitioning to the C12. When he required a power chair for mobility and alternative access to his SGD, mounting solutions and an infrared (IR) phone were integrated into his AAC system.

The Rationale for Clinical Decision-Making

RP's long-term communication system until his death in April 2019 consisted of the high-tech Tobii C12, floor mount, wheelchair mount, and IR phone. The system was identified as an appropriate AT match following the feature-matching process and comprehensive assessment previously discussed. RP primarily utilized his iPhone SGD via direct selection when access was intact. Once the C12 was approved, purchased, and received (3–4 months later), he was able to access the equipment directly and learn Communicator software at his own pace, without significant burden or fatigue. In fact, RP began training on Communicator software using a C12 demo within the clinic while awaiting receipt of his C12.

Next Steps

RP customized his phrase bank by working with the AT team in editing the default phrases and supplementing with his personalized messages. He selected his preferred home page, features to include/discard from the home page, keyboard settings, and addition of contacts. The AT providers saved the settings to RP's individual user profile and transferred this to a USB thumb drive. Once the SGD was delivered, the vendor who performed the installation within his home was able to transfer RP's user profile directly onto the device. Prior programing and customization increased the vendor's productivity and allowed for more time to provide direct client training. Through a combination of vendor in-home visits, AT in-home visits, as well as SLP service provision during brief hospital admissions, RP participated in multiple scheduled follow-up sessions to ensure his operational and strategic competency. After 2 years from his initial visit, direct select access became impractical, and he transitioned to a modified tracker ball mouse and use of the Permobil R-net Bluetooth module from his power wheelchair for joystick control. Eventually, addition of an eye-tracking camera was required and later installed to accommodate the changes in his access needs. It was around this period when RP was admitted to long-term care at the James A. Haley Veteran's Hospital. Given the physical distance that was imposed with his transfer from home to long-term care, he became more reliant on social media, phone calls, and e-mail to maintain social connectedness.

RP experienced improved access to technology support directly and indirectly from the AT providers with his long-term care admission due to the elimination of the travel burden.

SLP intervention shifted from directly to the patient to consultative/training services of the nursing staff. It was imperative that the nursing staff acknowledged the importance of setting up RP's SGD and eye-tracking device everyday just as one would provide daily respiratory and tracheostomy care. Multiple interactive in-services across nursing shifts to target all staff were vital to RP's communication success. The implementation of a hands-on experience that simulated life without use of extremities, natural voice for self-expression, total dependence on AT to interact with the world, as well as reliance on others to position the device was invaluable to carryover training objectives to RP's daily care. The SLP provided necessary instruction to nursing assistants on the process to ensure RP's SGD was connected to facility guest Wi-Fi. The AT team provided ongoing assistance with SGD customization through equipment programming (i.e., easy access to e-mail and social media pages, adding personal contacts). Assisting with integration of environmental controls in the new medical environment to include control of his television and direct link to the nurse call system at bedside was completed. Regular maintenance including software updates for both Communicator and Windows, Wi-Fi connectivity issues, adjustment of dwell settings, and general technology glitches or accidental setting changes (by patient or staff) were regular occurrences. Training of new staff was required intermittently as was refresher training to educate that even small movements (accidental kicks) of the floor mount or changes in head of bed height, and even fluctuations in mattress inflation for pressure relief can have detrimental effects on accuracy for eye-tracking users. Patient education was required to allow for intermittent rest periods, as increased inaccuracies were evident with fatigue. Backup systems are necessary as technology will inevitably fail at times. Thus, RP was proficient in low-tech methods of communication as needed, albeit slower and less independent. These systems include partner-assisted scanning for either spelling or identifying pre-set messages using low-tech communication boards. It also included a low-tech eye-tracking system again offering spelled communication for spontaneous utterances as well as phrases or general topics pre-arranged. Posted signage at bedside alerting staff and visitors of RP's nonverbal yes/no system (e.g., eyebrow raise for yes and squeeze eyes shut tight for no) was crucial as well as regular updating of this signage as physical abilities and response mechanisms changed over time. Adjustment of dwell settings, selection settings, keyboard layout, and general grid display were also required with disease progression to maximize efficiency, reduce effort, and improve accuracy.

Communication with ALS providers such as hospice, palliative care, and psychology would not have been possible without AAC as RP began to discuss end-of-life desires. It was his wish to be removed from the ventilator when communication was no longer feasible for him, when his eye movements deteriorated, and it became labor intensive. He utilized his AAC system to say goodbye to his family surrounding his bed as he died.

Treatment goals upon admission to long-term care included the following at a frequency of three times a week for 12 weeks:

- Use AAC to repair communication breakdowns and to convey more complex communication needs (i.e., greet others, offer information, ask questions, express feelings, and/or make requests) given setup and moderate cues.
- Demonstrate mastery of basic maintenance and operation of SGD (shutdown, restart, volume, speech/voice adjustments, etc.) with 100% accuracy.
- Collaborate with SLP to program his SGD in order to customize the device for his individualized communication needs 100% of the time.
- Use rate enhancement strategies (i.e., word prediction and abbreviation expansion) on SGD to expedite message production when sharing information or asking questions of caregiver and/or medical personnel independently and with 100% accuracy.

- Compose and respond to electronic messages and social media on SGD given minimum assistance within 8 weeks.

SLP service provision slowly decreased and shifted from weekly sessions to a maintenance, or as needed, schedule (e.g., once a month) once RP neared strategic competency, treatment goals had been met, and he indicated no further direct needs. RP would e-mail AT providers or alert nursing staff when assistance was needed, and we would assist accordingly. Additional support for nursing staff was provided in the form of posted signage (e.g., simplified instructions with screenshots), an AAC binder resource with copies of signage and segments from the website's FAQ, lists of necessary passwords and login info, technical support contact information affixed to the back of the device, and access to short 1- to 2-min video clips on a YouTube site for basic troubleshooting needs.

References

Ball, L. J., Beukelman, D. R., & Pattee, G. L. (2002). Timing of speech deterioration in people with amyotrophic lateral sclerosis. *Journal of Medical Speech-Language Pathology, 10*(4), 231–235.

Bardach, L. G. (2017). *CommNeedsQuestionnaire.pdf.* https://cehs.unl.edu/documents/secd/aac/CommNeedsQuestionnaire.pdf

Beukelman, D., Fager, S., & Nordness, A. (2011). Review article: Communication support for people with ALS. *Neurology Research International*, Article 714693. https://doi.org/10.1155/2011/714693

Beukelman, D. R., Garrett, K. L., & Yorkston, K. M. (Eds.). (2007). *Augmentative communication strategies for adults with acute or chronic medical conditions.* Paul H. Brookes.

Blackstone, S., & Hunt Berg, M. (2003). *Social networks: A communication inventory for individuals with severe communication challenges and their communication partners.* Augmentative Communication, Inc.

Bloch, S. (2011). Anticipatory other-completion of augmentative and alternative communication talk: A conversation analysis study. *Disability and Rehabilitation, 33*(3), 261–269. https://doi.org/10.3109/09638288.2010.491574

Cedarbaum, J. M., Stambler, N., Malta, E., Fuller, C., Hilt, D., Thurmond, B., & Nakanishi, A. (1999). The ALSFRS-R: A revised ALS functional rating scale that incorporates assessments of respiratory function. *Journal of the Neurological Sciences, 169,* 13–21.

DeRuyter, F. (2004). Speech pathologist's clinical pathway for communication changes with ALS. *ALS Clinical Pathways.* http://aac-rerc.psu.edu/index.php/files/list/type/1

Hurtig, R. R., & Downey, D. A. (2009). *Augmentative and alternative communication in acute and critical care settings.* Plural Publishing.

Judge, S., Bloch, S., & McDermott, C. J. (2018). Communication change in ALS: Engaging people living with ALS and their partners in future research. *Disability and Rehabilitation: Assistive Technology, 14*(7), 675–681. https://doi.org/10.1080/17483107.2018.1498924

Light, J., & McNaughton, D. (2015). Designing AAC research and intervention to improve outcomes for individuals with complex communication needs. *Augmentative and Alternative Communication, 31*(2), 85–96. https://doi.org/10.3109/07434618.2015.1036458

Makkonen, T., Ruottinen, H., Puhto, R., Helminen, M., & Palmio, J. (2018). Speech deterioration in amyotrophic lateral sclerosis (ALS) after manifestation of bulbar symptoms. *International Journal of Language and Communication Disorders, 53*(2), 385–392. https://doi.org/10.1111/1460-6984.12357

Oosthuizen, I., Dada, S., Bornman, J., & Koul, R. (2018). Message banking: Perceptions of persons with motor neuron disease, significant others and clinicians. *International Journal of Speech-Language Pathology, 20,* 756–765. https://doi.org/10.1080.17549507.2017.1356377

Yorkston, K. M., Miller, R. M., Strand, E. A., & Britton, D. (2013). *Management of speech and swallowing disorders in degenerative diseases* (3rd ed.). Pro-Ed.

Yunusova, Y., Graham, N. L., Shellikeri, S., Phuong, K., Kulkarni, M., Rochon, E., . . .Green, J. R. (2016). Profiling speech and pausing in amyotrophic lateral sclerosis (ALS) and frontotemporal dementia (FTD). *PLoS ONE, 11*(1). https://doi.org/10.1371/journal.pone.0147573

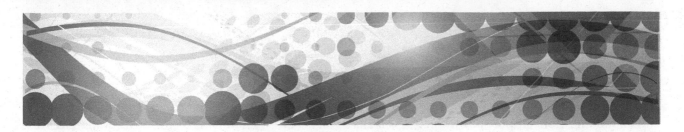

Chapter 28
AAC FOR PERSONS WITH APHASIA

Kimberly A. Eichhorn

Fundamentals

Aphasia can result in impairments across multiple modalities of language including spoken and written expression as well as comprehension of auditory and written information. These impairments can limit independence, social relationships, and employment (Davidson et al., 2008; Graham et al., 2011). High-, low-, or no-technology augmentative and alternative communication (AAC) is one solution that offers innovative methods for supporting communication for a person with aphasia (PWA). The use of AAC can be common practice in building bridges to enhance functional communication, but in the quest to reestablish functional communication for patients following stroke, speech-language pathologists (SLPs) may find themselves rushed to find a solution without the opportunity to fully assess cognitive-communicative functioning. Because the extent of language and cognitive deficits that arise from cerebrovascular accidents (CVAs) can vary widely, a thorough understanding of a PWA's unique needs is paramount in making decisions regarding AAC interventions.

Individualized language assessment is essential in matching a PWA's impaired and preserved linguistic skills to the linguistic demands of an AAC system being considered (Lasker, 2008). Perhaps the most used classification system for aphasia, the Bostonian Classification of Aphasia Types (Murdoch, 1990), is one that clinicians will commonly encounter in both inpatient and outpatient settings. This system is based on landmark work by European anatomists in the late 19th century, Paul Broca and Carl Wernicke. The foundation of this system has roots in the following assumptions: (a) language representations are stored in discrete "centers"; (b) centers are connected to one another by unique and discrete pathways; (c) lesions in specific centers or pathways create specific, differentiable types of aphasia; and (d) the behavioral dimensions of fluency, comprehension, and repetition are unitary, localizable, and bimodally distributed. With advancement in functional magnetic resonance imaging (fMRI), we no longer consider these assumptions as accurate, and classical models of language processing and the assessments associated with these assumptions rarely can provide an understanding of the complex linguistic system of a PWA.

Those who ascribe to a psycholinguistic model of language processing and production assert that communication breakdowns may arise within various interconnected pathways that include visual, phonological, graphemic, and lexical information (Kay et al., 2007). For example, a PWA may recognize an image of a penguin but may be unable to name it to confrontation, write it from seeing the picture, or even be able to choose the picture of the penguin after hearing the name. However, they may be able to match the written word with the picture or even write the initial grapheme "p." Knowledge of the strength or weakness of these pathways along with the strength of input and output buffers (i.e., number of content units) are key considerations in utilizing AAC for rehabilitation and communication support in PWAs. Assessments that consider the notion of interconnected pathways may reveal a relatively preserved modality that can be utilized within an AAC system. Alternatively, the language assessment may identify a significant semantic impairment that limits a PWA's ability to access language across all modalities. The functional impact of this level of impairment directly affects the use of picture supports within a system because recognition of pictures is reliant on the ability to process distinguishing semantic features. With an understanding of **individual** differences in language processing impairments, clinicians can develop treatment plans and AAC systems (no-, low-, or high-tech) to assist in improving linguistic processes and functional communication.

Clinicians and researchers have acknowledged that many PWAs also have deficits in areas of nonverbal cognition including visual working memory, attention, and various executive functions such as cognitive flexibility (Nicholas & Conner, 2017; Purdy & Dietz, 2010). There is a paucity of available literature to definitively outline the effects of attention, memory, and executive functions on a PWA's ability to learn to use AAC devices and strategies effectively (Nicholas & Connor, 2017). Clinicians can address the potential effects by carefully measuring cognitive factors and considering their potential effect on AAC use by using tasks that reduce the linguistic burden of the cognitive task (e.g., abstract design memory tasks) and tasks that closely resemble the functions needed to successfully use AAC devices such as visual-perceptual scanning.

As a clinical picture of a PWA's cognitive language profile emerges, it is the responsibility of the clinician to consider not only personally relevant vocabulary content, but more importantly a structure and organization that the PWA can use successfully. Figure 28–1 provides a review of the traditional frameworks for vocabulary organization in grid-based displays (developed from content from Koul, 2011).

With advances in technology and research that are bringing use of AAC in PWAs to the forefront, system design features are being developed to increase the success with which a PWA can use high-tech AAC (Beukelman et al., 2015; Dietz et al., 2014; Fried-Oken et al., 2012; Wallace & Hux, 2014). For example, when studying the effect of two different layouts on the ability of two PWA to navigate high-tech AAC, Wallace and Hux (2014) demonstrated that participants learned to use both interfaces but that they demonstrated improved efficiency and accuracy of learning when provided with a navigation ring over traditional grid layout.

Clinicians who use AAC regularly in their practice recognize communicator characteristics as an additional key to successful AAC use. These often include age, familiarity with technology, insight, expectations of the technology, and social supports (Taylor et al., 2019). Some PWA may remain dependent on partners for facilitating communication interactions. Table 28–1 outlines key characteristics discussed in the literature of subtypes of communicators within this category (created from content outlined in Koul, 2011).

PWAs who require minimal support for auditory comprehension often are partner-independent users of AAC. Their verbal output deficits secondary to aphasia and/or apraxia require the use of AAC to assist with functional communication. Table 28–2 outlines key characteristics of subtypes of communicators within this category (created from content outlined in Koul, 2011).

Research regarding high-tech AAC as a compensatory tool for PWAs is continuing to emerge with studies documenting positive results (Russo et al., 2017). Additionally, Dietz and colleagues (2018) examined the feasibility of employing an AAC treatment as a dual-purpose tool designed to support language recovery and compensate for aphasia-related deficits in PWAs.

Compared to the usual care group, the AAC intervention group trended toward larger treatment effects. On fMRI, the AAC intervention group showed increased leftward lateralization of language function and increased activation in visual processing regions. This work encourages continued consideration of the role of AAC-based interventions in aphasia recovery.

In summary, the qualitative and quantitative information garnered from an in-depth assessment may assist clinicians in designing AAC language platforms to maximize functional communication,

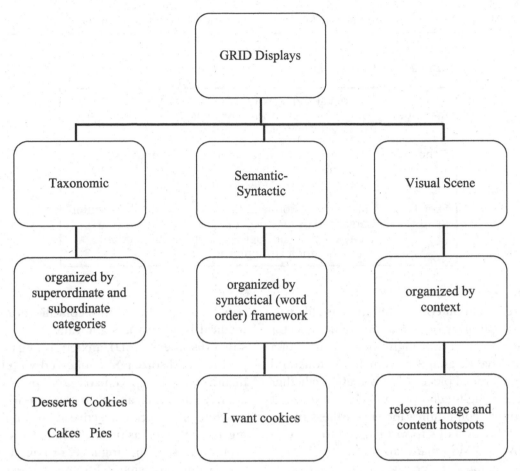

Figure 28–1. Vocabulary organization for grid-based displays. (Content adapted from Koul, 2011.)

Table 28–1. Partner-Dependent Communicators

Subcategory	Communication Characteristics	Partner Involvement	Example Stimuli Ideas
Emerging	Severe deficits across modalities	Systematic instruction to partners to assist with eliciting use of photographs, drawings (as examples) for basic needs	Choice making; reinforce cars/effect of no technology/technology support
Contextual-choice	May not initiate communication, but can identify/point to objects/symbols to identify wants/needs	Train partners in multimodal communication (supported conversation for adults with aphasia—Kagan, 1998, as an example)	Choice making within conversation with options for response; multimodal communication opportunities
Transitional	Use of symbols, words, gestures to augment verbal output—moving toward independence with augmentative and alternative communication (AAC)	Train partner to encourage use of AAC in common and recurring situation	Use of AAC for ordering food, communicating on the phone

Table 28–2. Partner-Independent Communicators

Stored message	Retrieval and use of stored messages in familiar situations—even with dynamic display; limited use in novel situations
Generative	Able to communicate in multiple settings; novel information may be inconsistent and marked by communication breakdowns
Specific need	May or may not need/want AAC but communication breakdowns may occur in specific situations (e.g., may need to consider word/phrase prediction software for a writing need)

enhance treatment outcomes, and increase life participation. Vocabulary organization, communicator characteristics, and a thorough understanding of a PWA's cognitive-language system limitations and strengths are crucial pieces of information whether a no-, low-, or high-tech option is chosen to assist with functional communication. Regardless of the system and the level of support needed to successfully use AAC, a systematic approach to training both the patient and the communication partner is a necessity to ensure positive outcomes.

Case Study: WP

Clinical Profile and Communication Needs

The Individual

In this case, WP is a 33-year-old right-handed female who presented to the emergency department with aphasia and right-sided weakness 10 days after delivering her first baby. Reports of her MRI study stated that there was an infarct in the left middle cerebral artery territory. While in the hospital she underwent thrombectomy for left internal carotid artery terminal occlusion. Her echocardiogram revealed severe cardiomyopathic abnormalities and left ventricular thrombus, the likely cause of her infarct. Due to pneumonia, her course was further complicated by respiratory failure requiring brief intubation, but she was successfully extu-

bated without additional complication. Her past medical history was significant for post-traumatic stress disorder (PTSD), anxiety, and gastroesophageal reflux disorder. She followed with behavioral health services (psychiatry and psychology) for anxiety, insomnia, and PTSD prior to her stroke. At baseline, she wore corrective lenses, but her hearing was reported as normal. There were no known premorbid speech, language, or cognitive deficits.

Initial assessment for this patient was conducted in an in-patient rehabilitation setting and included the following: examination of the strength, symmetry, range, speed, and accuracy/coordination of the movements of cranial nerves V, VII, IX–XII; tasks for assessing nonverbal oral movement control and sequencing (Duffy, 2013); motor speech screening; the Comprehensive Aphasia Test (CAT; Swinburn et al., 2004); subtests from the Psycholinguistic Assessment of Language Processing in Aphasia (PALPA; Kay et al., 2007); Pyramids and Palm Trees (Howard & Patterson, 1992); and surrogate form of the Aphasia Communication Outcome Measure (ACOM, Doyle et al., 2013).

Her oral motor exam showed mild lower central facial weakness noted at rest and with movement. Her tongue deviated mildly to the right upon protrusion with good range and motion and strength bilaterally. Labial strength was intact bilaterally with left greater than right excursion on retraction. She was unable to coordinate movements for the alternation of labial protrusion/retraction, visibly making attempts at movements that were severely reduced for range and delayed in initiation. Inaccurate or off-target attempts were present for all the single-step commands that were presented with a model. She was not able to initiate or sequence two-step commands for oral motor tasks.

Given her paucity of verbal output, motor speech evaluation was limited. She did not initiate any verbal communication without prompting or models. She was unable to complete diadochokinetic tasks (alternating or sequential motion rates). She was unable to repeat any single words, but with a visual model, she was able to repeat the following phonemes: /m/, /ai/, /o/, /i/ (her baseline phonemic inventory). Her phonatory quality in sustained phonation was judged as normal in terms of pitch for her age and gender with steadiness of tone and normal resonance. She did not repeat or complete any automatic/rote speech tasks. No diagnosis of dysarthria was made given the limited sample.

In terms of her cognitive-language function, she was classified as nonfluent with impairments across all modalities: speaking, listening, reading, and writing. She demonstrated strengths in visual and recognition memory. Her input and output span were limited to one content unit, which in addition to limiting her comprehension and expression, would have a significant impact on her ability to retain content and navigate dynamic displays in an AAC system. Repetition of words was poor, but she was able to maintain syllable structure in her attempts at repetition. She was unable to name items to confrontation, but she was able to select correct written word names from a list of semantically unrelated options. Both semantic and phonological error patterns were evident in word retrieval attempts. Comprehension of written material was a strength over auditory comprehension. Length and complexity of written language resulted in breakdown of comprehension. She was able to write her full name and copy letters. However, she was unable to write picture names or write to dictation. All letters were legible, consistent in size, and with no evidence of neglect. Supplemental tests from the PALPA suggested difficulty with phonological segmentation of words and poor ability to recognize graphemes/corresponding phonemes. Finally, given the frequency of her semantically related errors on the CAT, the Pyramids and Palms Test confirmed a significant impairment in retrieval of lexical items that were closely related. On the

ACOM, her husband rated her communication as mostly effective for the following: indicating likes/dislikes in specific contexts, greeting people, indicating a need for help, making her wants/needs known, and understanding a single written word. She was diagnosed with a severe mixed aphasia with concomitant apraxia of speech.

Their Communication Partners

WP's communication partners included her spouse, new baby, mother-in-law, grandmother, multiple medical providers within the facility (doctors, nurses, therapists), psychologist, friends, and work managers/colleagues.

Their Environment

She earned a master's degree in Infectious Disease and was working at a local florist prior to taking time for maternity leave. She was responsible for orders, arranging flowers, and planning weddings; she was to become the manager of the florist on return from leave. She served in the United States Marine Corps for 4 years, and her military occupational specialty was data/communications. She was married and lived with her husband, who worked from home. Her mother-in-law moved into their home to assist with caring for the new baby. Her interests include music, cooking, sports (softball and hockey), and animals.

AAC Considerations

The choice to enhance functional communication with AAC for this nearly nonverbal patient seemed as though it should be the priority in this case. In fact, most providers were pushing for a "communication board." However, her stated goals included a quick return to verbal communication. The complexity of her language deficits coupled with the devasting loss of communication made choosing the correct communication support that could cultivate her recovery imperative. With her semantic and working memory deficits, dynamic, grid-based displays with taxonomic or syntactic-semantic organization were not effective means for communication.

Despite her strength in reading comprehension, her impairments in phoneme-to-grapheme conversion, letter recognition, and spelling rendered a keyboard for text-to-speech output ineffective as well. In addition to her strength in reading comprehension, her visual memory, executive functioning skills, and familiarity with technology were positive prognosticators for designing pagesets with salient vocabulary to increase functional communication and foster recovery. She had normal hearing, and vision was functional with corrective lenses. She was well able to compensate for mild right hemianopsia. She was ambulatory with right ankle foot orthosis and assistive device. Her right upper extremity was spastic and nonfunctional. Taken together, it was clear that one support, a dedicated system or app, would be insufficient to fully meet her needs and that she would benefit from a portable device on which she could use touch access with her nondominant hand.

The AAC System or Service Considerations

Her journey with AAC was designed to be facilitative but also therapeutic. Along with implementation of AAC, she participated in traditional in-person aphasia/apraxia therapy targeting auditory comprehension, lexical retrieval, multimodality sentence generation, and phoneme-level comprehension and production. A commercially available tablet was chosen as the platform for her communication support. After trial and error using no-technology communication boards to manipulate field size and content, an AAC application with flexibility to allow for static grid displays for personally relevant content, such as family names, was chosen (Figure 28–2). This same application was used to create salient visual scenes (photos from her home) with hotspots and to create episodic navigation rings to practice procedures related to infant care (see Figure 28–2).

A flashcard application was used to improve semantic processing and verbal output by (a) encouraging attention to distinguishing semantic features within personally relevant categories and (b) encouraging verbal practice of target words following the model (auditory and video-embedded visual; Figure 28–3). Baseline and treatment probes were collected for vocabulary trained with flashcards. A storytelling application was employed for script training of nursery rhymes and oral reading goals. She used the applications for home practice, and her overall progress for oral reading goals was monitored for independent oral reading (without device support) in sessions. Finally, as her phoneme-to-grapheme correspondence improved through traditional therapy, a keyboard was slowly intro-

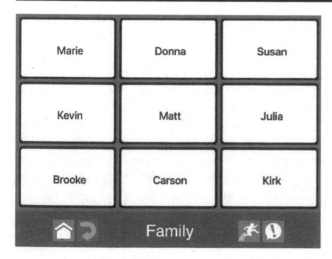
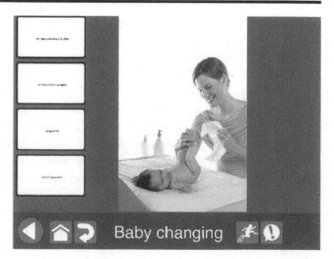

Figure 28–2. GoTalkNow in grid and modified visual scene layouts. Used with permission from Attainment Company, Inc.

Figure 28–3. INKidsLLC Flashcard Application. Used with permission from INKids Education LLC.

duced to assist with first letter self-cueing to prime word retrieval and facilitate verbal responses. Her strengths in visual memory and executive functions resulted in several practice and orientation trials with applications before she achieved independence in navigation of her practice applications. She was hesitant to utilize AAC for functional communication, so portions of therapy sessions were designed to create communication opportunities in which she could practice supplementing communication for relevant topics available on her device. Her husband participated in sessions for training in Supported Conversation for Adults with Aphasia (Kagan, 1998) and AAC applications/implementation, particularly those focused on care needs and home situations.

Next Steps

The flexibility of the communication system chosen has allowed growth and development with the system as the patient has progressed along her recovery. Initially, her communication device primarily served to assist communication partners using Supported Conversation for Adults with Aphasia (Kagan, 1998) in contextual-choice situations to narrow the field of topics or persons about which the patient was attempting to communicate. It continues to serve as a therapeutic tool for her language recovery. Additional functional communication pagesets (designed as episodic navigation rings) with topics of interest were developed. In moving forward, systematic training with the patient and family is planned with the goal for the patient to initiate use as needed in daily conversational exchanges. With the increased complexity and volume of communication support pagesets, the following systematic instruction (Sohlberg & Turkstra, 2011) plan is suggested:

1. Individual therapy sessions with conversational topics paired to communication pagesets to ensure the patient shows clear knowledge of how, when, and why to use AAC to support her message
   a. Minimize errors during drilled practice
   b. Move from massed (one conversation) to distributed practice (multiple/changing topics)

c. Provide sufficient practice

d. Lengthen the distributed practice

e. Correct errors and fade cues, as appropriate

2. Introduce random practice antecedents or triggers for when device use should be initiated

3. Incorporate caregivers and others in naturalistic contexts and situations and ensure opportunities for use

Data collection and treatment outcome measures could include some of the following:

- accuracy and application of using AAC in conversational exchanges with clinician
- effectiveness of overall multimodal message delivery
- accuracy and application of using AAC in conversational exchanges with others
- effectiveness of AAC use in naturalistic, target environments using reports from self and/or significant other

Finally, the clinician could consider repeat and additional self-reported outcome measures for communicative effectiveness (such as the ACOM; Doyle et al., 2013) and satisfaction with the communication device (such as the Psychosocial Impact of Assistive Devices Scale; Jutai & Day, 2002).

Expert Tips or Practical Advice

- Take time to understand a patient's cognitive-language system before choosing an AAC system (no-, low-, or high-tech) for a PWA.
- The device must match the individual patient's needs and goals.
- Incorporate AAC into treatment to enhance outcomes.
- Implement the level of systematic training needed to ensure success with the AAC system.

References

Beukelman, D. R., Hux, K., Dietz, A., McKelvey, M., & Weissling, K. (2015). Using visual scene displays as communication support options for people with chronic, severe aphasia: A summary of AAC research and future research directions. *Augmentative and Alternative Communication, 31*(3), 234–245.

Davidson, B., Worrall, L., & Hickson, L. (2008). Exploring the interactional dimension of social communication: A collective case study of older people with aphasia. *Aphasiology, 22*(3), 235–257.

Dietz, A., Vannest, J., Maloney, T., Altaye, M., Holland, S., & Szaflarski, J. P. (2018). The feasibility of improving discourse in people with aphasia through AAC: Clinical and functional MRI correlates. *Aphasiology, 32*(6), 693–719.

Dietz, A., Weissling, K., Griffith, J., McKelvey, M., & Macke, D. (2014). The impact of interface design during an initial high-technology AAC experience: A collective case study of people with aphasia. *Augmentative and Alternative Communication, 30*(4), 314–328.

Doyle, P. J., Hula, W. D., Hula, S. N. A., Stone, C. A., Wambaugh, J. L., Ross, K. B., & Schumacher, J. G. (2013). Self-and surrogate-reported communication functioning in aphasia. *Quality of Life Research, 22*(5), 957–967.

Duffy, J. R. (2013). *Motor speech disorders: Substrates, differential diagnosis, and management.* Mosby.

Fried-Oken, M., Beukelman, D. R., & Hux, K. (2012). Current and future AAC research considerations for adults with acquired cognitive and communication impairments. *Assistive Technology, 24*(1), 56–66.

Graham, J. R., Pereira, S., & Teasell, R. (2011). Aphasia and return to work in younger stroke survivors. *Aphasiology, 25*(8), 952–960.

Howard, D., & Patterson, K. (1992). *The Pyramids and Palm Trees Test: A test of semantic access from words and pictures.* Thames Valley Test Company.

Jutai, J., & Day, H. (2002). Psychosocial Impact of Assistive Devices Scale (PIADS). *Technology and Disability, 14*(3), 107–111.

Kagan, A. (1998). Supported conversation for adults with aphasia: Methods and resources for training conversation partners. *Aphasiology, 12*(9), 816–830.

Kay, J., Lesser, R., & Coltheart, M. (2007). *Psycholinguistic assessments of language processing in aphasia.* Psychology Press.

Koul, R. (2011). Overview of AAC intervention approaches for persons with aphasia. In R. Koul (Ed.), *Augmentative and alternative communication for adults with aphasia: Science and clinical practice* (pp. 47–63). Brill.

Lasker, J. P. (2008). AAC language assessment: Considerations for adults with aphasia. *Perspectives on Augmentative and Alternative Communication, 17*(3), 105–112.

Murdoch, B. E. (1990). Bostonian and Lurian aphasia syndromes. In B. E. Murdoch (Ed.), *Acquired speech and language disorders* (pp. 60–96). Springer.

Nicholas, M., & Connor, L. T. (2017). People with aphasia using AAC: Are executive functions important? *Aphasiology, 31*(7), 819–836.

Purdy, M., & Dietz, A. (2010). Factors influencing AAC usage by individuals with aphasia. *Perspectives on Augmentative and Alternative Communication, 19*(3), 70–78.

Russo, M. J., Prodan, V., Meda, N. N., Carcavallo, L., Muracioli, A., Sabe, L., & Olmos, L. (2017). High-technology augmentative communication for adults with post-stroke aphasia: A systematic review. *Expert Review of Medical Devices, 14*(5), 355–370.

Sohlberg, M. M., & Turkstra, L. S. (2011). *Optimizing cognitive rehabilitation: Effective instructional methods.* Guilford Press.

Swinburn, K., Porter, G., & Howard, D. (2004). *Comprehensive aphasia test.* Taylor & Francis.

Taylor, S., Wallace, S. J., & Wallace, S. E. (2019). High-technology augmentative and alternative communication in poststroke aphasia: A review of the factors that contribute to successful augmentative and alternative communication use. *Perspectives of the ASHA Special Interest Groups, 4*(3), 464–473.

Wallace, S. E., & Hux, K. (2014). Effect of two layouts on high technology AAC navigation and content location by people with aphasia. *Disability and Rehabilitation: Assistive Technology, 9*(2), 173–182.

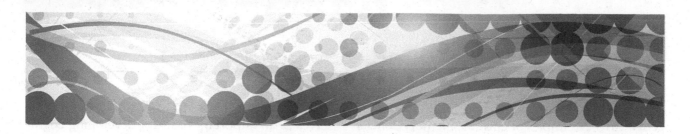

Chapter 29
AAC FOR PERSONS WITH DEMENTIA

Vanessa L. Burshnic-Neal

Fundamentals

Setting the Stage for AAC Use in Dementia

Augmentative and alternative communication (AAC), in the traditional sense, consists of tools and interventions to help people with communication impairments increase communicative participation in preferred activities and social settings. In the context of dementia, however, AAC is not used as a direct intervention for supplementing speech and language. Rather, AAC in this context comprises interventions aimed at strengthening the underlying cognitive systems that support communication (e.g., attention and memory). Interventions often include low-tech written and visual aids, designed to enhance comprehension and stimulate recall. Another way to conceptualize this difference is to expand the definition of AAC in dementia to include not only interventions that enhance communication with others (external communication), but communication with *self* (internal communication) (Beukelman et al., 2007).

Strengths and Deficits in Dementia

Memory

Memory loss is typically the earliest and most defining feature of dementia pathology. The mem-ory system generally consists of three subdivisions, including working (short-term) memory (Baddeley, 1992), declarative (explicit) memory, and nondeclarative (implicit) memory (Squire, 1992). Working memory refers to a function of the brain that provides temporary storage and manipulation of information. Subcomponents of working memory include the central executive (attentional control), phonological loop (storage and processing of auditory information), visuospatial sketch pad (maintenance of visual information), and episodic buffer (integration and interpretation auditory and visual information) (Baddeley, 1992, 2000). Working memory is necessary for complex tasks, such as language comprehension, learning, and reasoning. This memory system is impaired early in dementia, which may lead to rapid forgetting of recent information, difficulty following conversations, and difficulty integrating new with previously learned information (Hickey & Bourgeois, 2018).

Declarative (explicit) memory operates consciously and includes memories for facts and events. It has two subsystems: episodic and semantic memory. Episodic memory is the recall of personal events or experiences. It is distinct from other memory systems in that it relies on a sense of self and subjective position in place and time (Tulving, 2001). Episodic memory works closely with working memory to encode (process), consolidate (store), and later retrieve information from longer-term storage (Harvey, 2019). Episodic memory is impaired early in dementia, largely due to failures at the level of encoding, preventing information from reaching long-term storage (Hickey & Bourgeois, 2018). Examples of episodic memory deficits include being unable to recall the location of a recent vacation or what was eaten for breakfast this morning. Episodic deficits can also occur for spatial information, such as recalling where a car was parked in a parking lot.

Semantic memory refers to a person's acquired knowledge of the world, relationships, facts, and concepts. It also includes memory for words and their meanings. Unlike episodic memories, semantic memories are derived without reference to a specific autobiographical event (Matthews, 2015). Semantic memory is relatively spared in early dementia, as this information is typically overlearned, stored, and repeatedly accessed over time (Bayles & Kim, 2003; Hickey & Bourgeois, 2018). As dementia progresses, access to semantic memory is increasingly compromised, resulting in difficulty retrieving words in conversation or naming common objects (i.e., anomia) (Hickey & Bourgeois, 2018).

Nondeclarative (implicit) memory is defined as the ability to acquire cognitive and behavioral skills, through repetition, that subsequently operate automatically (Matthews, 2015). In contrast to declarative memory, nondeclarative memory does not require active (conscious) recall of concepts or events. Types of nondeclarative memory include procedural memory, priming, habits, and conditioned responses. Procedural memory is memory for motor actions and skills. Examples of procedural memory include knowing how to ride a bicycle or the sequence of buttons to press when turning on the TV. Priming refers to the improved ability to access and retrieve information after previous and repeated exposure to specific or related stimuli, such as retrieving a word after receiving a semantic cue (e.g., "a type of vegetable"). The effect of priming is often measured in units of speed and accuracy (Bayles & Kim, 2003; Hickey & Bourgeois, 2018). The third nondeclarative subtype, habits, includes learned behaviors that become subconscious over time, such as participating in the actions of one's morning routine. Finally, conditioned responses are automatic behaviors that occur in response to a particular stimulus, such as reaching for a phone when it rings. Nondeclar-

ative memory is relatively spared in dementia and serves as an important basis for developing cognitive-communication interventions.

Communication

In early dementia, speech remains relatively intact, and the person is aware of memory and communication breakdowns. Expressive speech is fluent with no articulation or syntactic difficulties. In addition, conversation, oral reading, reading comprehension, and writing remain functional. People with early dementia may struggle to retrieve words used less frequently and have difficulty following complex conversations.

The middle stages of dementia are characterized by increasing anomia, empty speech (e.g., referring to common objects as "things"), auditory comprehension deficits, and pragmatic difficulties (e.g., off-topic or inappropriate comments). As working memory declines, persons in the middle stages of dementia may ask repetitive questions. Strengths at this stage include articulation, grammar, oral reading, reading comprehension for familiar words and phrases, and nondeclarative memory.

The later stages of dementia are characterized by severe impairment of verbal communication (e.g., mutism or unintelligible vocalizations) and auditory comprehension. Alertness and attention may fluctuate, and memory is typically impaired across all domains. Strengths at this stage include appropriate affective responses to sensory stimuli and cooperation with appropriate tactile, visual, and affective cues (Fried-Oken et al., 2015; Hickey & Bourgeois, 2018).

Strengths and Deficits in Dementia: Clinical Implications

As previously described, dementia is characterized by deficits in declarative memory, including the ability to effectively encode, store, and retrieve memories. It was once assumed that people with dementia were unable to learn new information due to these apparent deficits. Research has shown, however, that people with dementia can learn new information when communication partners and clinicians manipulate the conditions at encoding and retrieval. For example, spoken information presented in written and visual (e.g., picture) form reduces demands on working memory, allowing for extended processing time and easier encoding. Other strategies that facilitate encoding include grouping information in themes, pairing information with motor activities, actively involving the person in designing the memory aid, and using tangible and meaningful materials (Bayles & Kim, 2003).

Furthermore, people with dementia have shown better performance on semantic recall tasks (e.g., naming common objects) when primed with information (e.g., semantic or phonemic cues) or when the task relies on recognition (e.g., word-picture matching or multiple choice), versus free recall. Some researchers have theorized that the ability to cue semantic recall (word-finding) suggests that the underlying impairment is not with semantic representations themselves, rather with the ability to *access* these representations from the semantic store (Bayles & Kim, 2003; Nakamura et al., 2000). The effectiveness of cues may differ, however, depending on the type of dementia (e.g., semantic dementia vs. Alzheimer's disease) and word characteristics (e.g., frequency and imageability) (Bonner et al., 2009; Reilly et al., 2011).

Finally, people with dementia can learn information when taught through procedures that capitalize on preserved nondeclarative memory. One such example is spaced retrieval training, which was developed based on principles of priming and classical conditioning. This technique involves asking people with dementia to recall facts and procedures over gradually longer intervals of time to facilitate long-term recall (Brush & Camp, 1999; Hopper et al., 2005).

Guidelines for Developing AAC for People With Dementia

The overarching goals of AAC interventions for people with dementia are to maximize independent functioning to the extent possible and maintain quality of life, using a strengths-based, person-centered approach. Interventions should be designed to reduce demands on impaired memory systems (working and episodic memory) and capitalize on preserved nondeclarative systems (Bayles & Kim, 2003; Hickey & Bourgeois, 2018). The following guidelines provide strategies for accomplishing these goals:

- *Know the person.* Consider the person's level of literacy, cognitive deficits, cognitive strengths, level of awareness of memory deficits, as well as familiarity with and motivation to use compensatory strategies. Also consider the person's ethnic, cultural, linguistic, and educational background. Memory and communication aids must be designed so that they are easy to use and address needs that are important to the person and that person's care partners. Consider how the memory aid fits into the person's daily routine and lifestyle. For example, if the person is mobile, a portable memory aid may be needed, such as a small memory book (i.e., memory wallet) with a lanyard attached to prevent loss (Bourgeois et al., 2001). Finally, consider the extent of training that may be needed to promote use of the memory aid (e.g., cuing from care partners or spaced retrieval training). Presence of the memory aid alone does not guarantee appropriate use (Hickey & Bourgeois, 2018).
- *Support sensory abilities.* Information enters through the sensory systems; therefore, it is vital to optimize vision and hearing abilities to support encoding. Sensory supports may include glasses, magnifying glasses, low-tech assistive listening devices (e.g., pocket talkers), hearing aids, or audio and tactile support for low vision. Clinicians can also support vision by adjusting font sizes, increasing the visual contrast of materials and reducing glare (Brush et al., 2011).
- *Reduce cognitive demands.* The general environment should be relatively free of clutter and unnecessary noise to reduce demands on attention and processing.

Visual and written cues should be in noticeable locations that align with the person's preferred routine. The content of the memory aid should include only the information needed to support comprehension and the desired behavioral response. Semantic and category cues, as well as familiar photographs, reduce the need for effortful (free) recall and support access to semantic storage. Training strategies should include principles of priming and classical conditioning (e.g., spaced retrieval training) to capitalize on strengths in spared nondeclarative memory functions.

■ *Use tangible and meaningful stimuli.* Tangible stimuli, such as objects, realistic dolls, and animals, have been shown to activate recall, increase verbal ability, and maximize alertness during interactions (Bayles & Kim, 2003). When possible, incorporate tangible stimuli in conversations, or increase tangibility by presenting information externally, in the form of printed words and pictures.

■ *Present information in chunks.* Deficits in working and episodic memory impair abilities to meaningfully organize information in the brain, leading to less efficient storage and access of memories. Chunking information within manageable themes or categories helps enhance comprehension and can lead to improved communication interactions. Specific strategies for chunking information might include centering conversation around a printed key word or picture (Beukelman & Mirenda, 2013).

Examples of AAC for People With Dementia

Supported Preference Assessment

Knowing the interests, values, and preferences of individuals with dementia is the cornerstone of person-centered treatment planning. Supported preference assessments were developed to enhance comprehension of preference questions and expression of preference information by persons with dementia. Empirically tested supported preference assessments range in topics from activities and leisure preferences to end-of-life medical decisions. These assessments commonly take the form of labeled picture cards (Figure 29–1) and a sorting mat (Figure 29–2). The person with dementia is asked to place the card in the location on the sorting mat that indicates their preference or feeling (e.g., always, sometimes, never) (Bourgeois et al., 2016). Research shows that supported preference assessments improve comprehension (Burshnic & Bourgeois, 2020), communicative effectiveness (Murphy et al., 2010), and clarity of decision-making (Chang & Bourgeois, 2020) in persons with dementia.

When using supported preference assessments, clinicians must consider the types of questions they will be asking and the level of response the person with dementia is able to give. For persons in earlier stages, clinicians may ask the person to elaborate on the preference rating (e.g., "Why

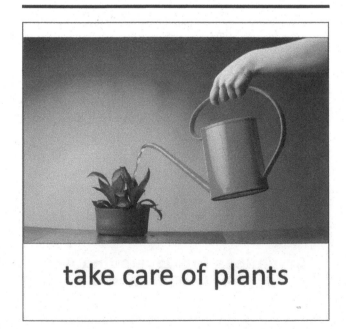

Figure 29–1. Sample preference card.

Important	Somewhat Important	Not Important

Important	Not Important

Always	Sometimes	Never
☺	☺	☹

Happy	Unsure	Unhappy
☺	🧍	☹

Figure 29–2. Example preference sorting mats.

is reading important to you?"). For persons in later stages, response options can be reduced from three to two options (i.e., binary choice) to ease cognitive demands in choice-making. Visual stimuli (cards) should contain clear, high-contrast images with large print, sans serif font (e.g., Arial) (Brush et al., 2015).

Memory Books

Memory books are one of the most researched methods for supporting communication in people with dementia. A memory book is an album consisting of personal photographs with simple declarative sentences (e.g., "I was born on June 1, 1931") on each page. Memory books have been shown to improve comprehension and cooperation in daily care activities (Bourgeois et al., 2002), as well as improve equity in conversations between communication partners and persons with dementia (Bourgeois, 1993; Hoerster et al., 2001). Memory books may take an autobiographical form (life story) or review a singular topic, such as a favorite hobby or vacation. Font size for the memory book can be determined using a brief oral reading screening (e.g., Bourgeois Oral Reading Screening) (Bourgeois, 2014). Photographs with faces should be large and easily visible. Figure 29–3 provides an example of a memory book based around a single topic: personal art.

It is important to consider the communication or cognitive need the memory book will address. For example, persons with dementia who have difficulty recalling the names of grandchildren may benefit from a memory book containing names and photographs. For persons who have strengths in long-term recognition memory, past photos should be placed next to present photos to indicate what the children look like in present time. People with dementia who have difficulty orienting to time and place may benefit from a series of pictures in chronological order, illustrating their early life (e.g., hometown, school, marriage) to where they are today. More specifically, the end of the memory book might say, "I moved to Sunset Senior Living to receive assistance with my care" and other reassuring messages, such as "My family knows I am here and visits me often." Memory books can also serve as a supportive conversation tool, allowing the person to reminisce and share information about their life story without depending on others for facts and information.

As dementia progresses, the memory book can be adapted to support changing cognitive abilities, such as reducing the number of pages in the book and simplifying sentence structure. For persons with severe vision deficits or low literacy levels, talking photo albums may be a helpful alternative to a traditional memory book. Talking photo albums are not recommended for people with functional vision and reading, however, because research has shown that audio messages can be distracting and decrease verbal output in these individuals (Fried-Oken et al., 2009).

J's Book of Memorable Art

About J's Book of Memorable Art

- I have been an artist my whole life.
- I have many family and friends who are also artists.
- This is my book of memorable art.
- I can use this book to share art with others, when I am not in my room.
- I can add to this book whenever I need to.

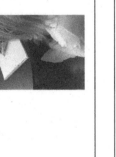

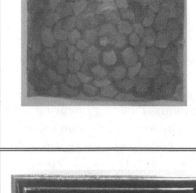

This painting is by my mother, VA.
She painted this after visiting the islands.

This painting is by my daughter, L.

This painting is by my granddaughter, A.
She made this in art school.

This painting is by my brother, B.

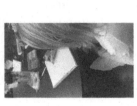

This print is by my friend, HN.

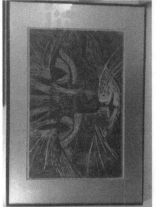

By: JK

This is one of my paintings.

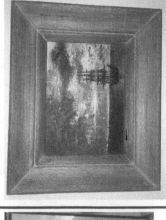

Figure 29–3. Memory book about personal art.

436

Orientation Aids

Orientation aids include clocks, calendars, and wayfinding supports (i.e., directional signage) (Figures 29–4 and 29–5). Like other visual supports, orientation aids should contain large print with high contrast (e.g., white font on a magenta background) and be placed in a noticeable location (Brush et al., 2011). The location of the orientation aid is critically important to its use. For example, a care partner may consider placing the calendar on the refrigerator or next to the coffee machine if the person with dementia is known to visit that location every day. It may also be helpful to create a memory "station" where orientation information is meaningfully organized (i.e., chunking information). The station may include a digital clock, calendar, medication organizer, and "to-do" list. Orientation aids should be reviewed with the person with dementia, to ensure comprehension. And when possible, the person with dementia should have input in designing the attributes of the orientation aid (e.g., color, size, location, wording) to enhance personal relevance.

People who have difficulty remembering to use orientation aids can be trained using spaced retrieval training (SRT). As described previously, SRT is a systematic procedure for helping people with dementia recall information over progressively longer intervals of time. The procedure involves a prompt and conditioned response. For example, in training use of a calendar, the prompt might be, "What do you do when you need to know the schedule today?" and the response would be "I look at my calendar." SRT responses can also be paired with a motor response (e.g., gesturing toward the calendar) to strengthen encoding (Camp, 2006).

Reminder Cards

Reminder cards are used to solve a problem or provide information to a person with dementia. Reminder cards (Figure 29–6) are a particularly effective method for reducing repetitive questions (Bourgeois et al., 1997). When a question

---

Today is:

The weather is:

To Do:

Figure 29–4. Orientation aid.

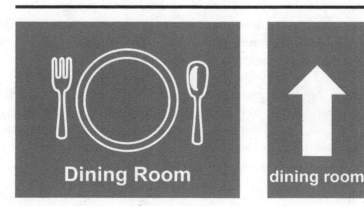

Figure 29–5. Wayfinding signage.

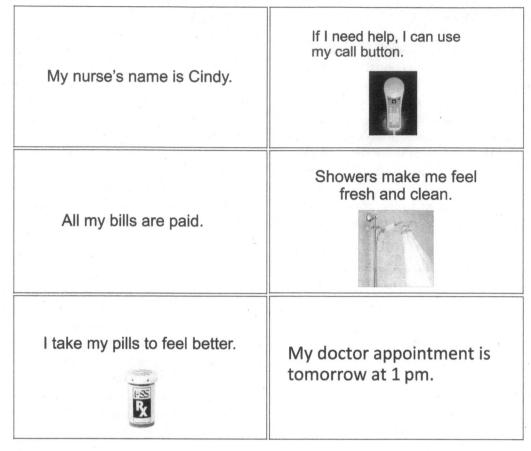

Figure 29–6. Reminder cards./HHA's name included

is repeated (e.g., "When is my doctor appointment?"), the answer to the question (e.g., "My doctor appointment is at 1:00 PM.") is written in large print and normal sentence case on a small piece of paper or note card. Every time the question is repeated, the communication partner points to the card and says, "Read this." Alternatively, the partner might say, "I think the answer to that question is on your card" ("Card" in this context, can also be replaced with another preferred memory aid, such as a whiteboard or memory book). With repetition of this procedure, the person learns to refer to the external cue (e.g., card or whiteboard) for information, rather than depending on the communication partner. Reminder cards may also take the form of invitational signage (Figure 29–7) and can be used to promote independent initiation of meaningful tasks.

Activities of Daily Living Support

Visual and text cues can also be useful for a variety of daily living activities, such as identifying objects and completing multistep tasks. For example, it is common for household items to have small-print labels that may be difficult for the person to read. In addition, bottles may look similar, leading the person to mistake one item for another. Large-print labels on objects, such as liquid soap and lotion, can help the person distinguish these items and use them correctly. Similarly, labels can be affixed on doors, cabinets, and drawers to help persons with dementia efficiently locate items in their environment.

Visual sequencing aids (Figure 29–8) may help increase independence with multistep tasks, such as meal preparation and bathing (Hopper et al.,

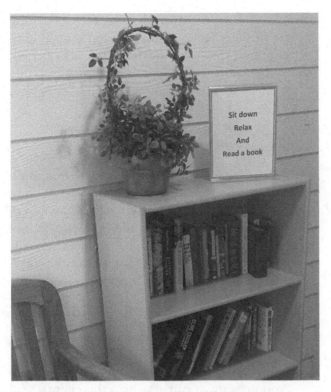 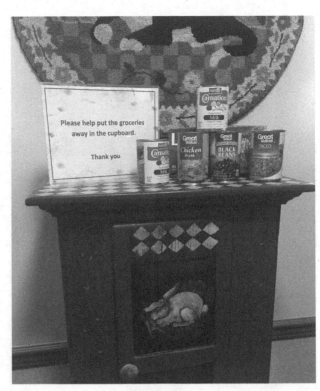

Figure 29–7. Invitational signage examples.

2005). Important considerations for visual sequencing aids include task analysis and the person's ability to follow written commands. The person may require consistent cuing to look at the aid, but this may still enhance the level of independence they would have with verbal cues alone.

Supporting Care Partners

People with dementia will become increasingly dependent on others for care as the disease progresses. Thus, training care partners in effective communication and memory support strategies is vital to helping people with dementia maintain function and quality of life.

Clinicians can train care partners to maximize the person's attention (e.g., speak face-to-face, limit distractions); speak in a tone that is relaxed, calm, and shows interest; provide time for the person to express thoughts; break tasks into small steps; and use short and simple instructions (Hickey &

Bourgeois, 2018; Small & Gutman, 2002; Smith et al., 2011). Clinicians can also provide training on supporting communication with the use of nonverbal and visual aids, such as gestures, modeling, and captioned photographs (Hinshelwood et al., 2016; Smith et al., 2011).

It is common for people with dementia to verbalize information that may be false or inaccurate. Partners should be encouraged not to argue with the person or try to convince them of what is true (Gitlin et al., 2012). Instead, provide validation for feelings, rather than "facts," and, when appropriate, gently redirect the conversation to a more positive topic. For example, if a person with dementia says, "My mother is in the hospital and I'm worried about her," an acceptable response may be "I'm so sorry. It makes sense that you're worried about someone you love." This response validates the person's emotions toward the mother, rather than focusing on the facts (i.e., the mother is deceased). Often false statements or questions are an attempt to communicate needs for connection and meaningful

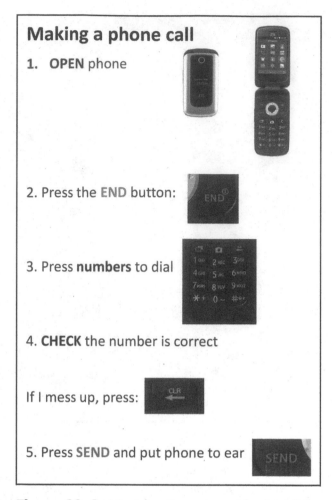

Making a phone call

1. **OPEN** phone

2. Press the **END** button:

3. Press **numbers** to dial

4. **CHECK** the number is correct

If I mess up, press:

5. Press **SEND** and put phone to ear

Figure 29–8. Visual sequencing aid example.

engagement. For example, a person may ask, "when am I going home?" when feeling out of place or bored. In such situations, it is important for care partners to consider the unmet needs of people with dementia and respond accordingly.

Additionally, care partners can learn to adapt memory and communication aids as the disease progresses to support changing abilities. For example, for persons who have difficulty with reading, the text can be replaced with print in a larger font and/or supplemented with pictures. Readability can also be improved with simplified sentence structure and shortened sentence length (Bourgeois, 2014). Finally, it is important to ensure care partners are

providing for their own well-being, such as getting regular health checkups, resting, and engaging in pleasant activities. Care partners may also benefit from connections to local support groups.

Conclusion

AAC for people with dementia is used to strengthen the underlying cognitive systems that support communication. AAC tools must be person centered, address meaningful problems, and capitalize on preserved cognitive-communication abilities. Finally, care partners should be incorporated in the intervention and trained in using supportive strategies.

- Create a binder of example memory aids to show clients and care partners. Examples help to contextualize the suggestions you provide. It can also help the clients know what to expect and can be used as a tool to engage them in a conversation about the design of the memory aid (e.g., appearance, location, etc.).
- Memory books can take a long time to make. Have a Word or PowerPoint template on hand that you can share with care partners, so all they need to do is add pictures and fill in captions. For care partners who do not have access to Word or PowerPoint, the template can be edited in Google Docs.

Case Study: AM[1]

Clinical Profile and Communication Needs

AM is a 90-year-old male who was referred to speech-language pathology by his primary care

---

[1]Names and identifiers have been changed to protect client confidentiality.

doctor due to increasing communication difficulties and resistance during showers. His past medical history is significant for vascular dementia (diagnosed 3 years ago), intracranial hemorrhage (3 years ago), left-side parieto-occipital ischemic stroke (2 years ago), depression, and falls. AM wears glasses and an assistive listening device (ALD) for hearing. A recent cognitive screening indicated AM's level of impairment was "moderate."

AM's wife, JM, reports that AM did not exhibit symptoms of aphasia after his stroke; however, she also states that AM is unable to discuss recent events, and he has difficulty following commands during care routines. Given AM's history of hearing and cognitive impairment, as well as stroke, it is likely his communication challenges are a result of multiple factors.

The Individual

AM has a master's degree in education from a prominent university. He served in the military as a cryptographic officer (no combat) and then held a career teaching math and science. His interests include woodworking, reading, and music.

Their Communication Partners. JM is AM's primary communication partner. He also communicates with his home health aide (HHA), neighbors, and the individuals who lead and attend his day program (see Environment). AM and JM have two adult children who each have families of their own, for a total of five grandchildren. AM likes to chat on the phone weekly with his children. He enjoys engaging playfully with his grandchildren, even though sometimes he forgets their names.

Their Environment

AM lives with his wife, JM, in an independent living retirement community. AM receives care through a visiting HHA for bathing and dressing on weekday mornings. JM helps AM with his care and personal routines at all other times. AM also attends a day program for people with dementia three times per week. AM is largely dependent on his wheelchair for mobility and requires one person to help him transfer.

AAC Considerations

After completing an interview with JM, the speech-language pathologist (SLP) learns that AM often asks questions about autobiographical information, such as "How long have we been married?" and "When are we going home?" (when he is home). JM is younger and functionally more independent; she is very active in her religious community and enjoys social outings with friends. JM states that she wishes she could have "meaningful conversations" with her husband. JM also expresses concern regarding AM's compliance during morning routines. She says he will sometimes nod "yes" in agreement to start the routine, but later shows verbal and physical resistance (e.g., yelling or striking out).

Upon observation of the morning routine, the SLP noticed that AM appeared very anxious when transitioning from bed to the wheelchair as evidenced by increased body tension and trembling. AM's fear causes him to freeze in position during the transfer. The aid and spouse respond with firm commands, asking him to "keep moving" and "sit down" in the wheelchair. These efforts to rush AM's movements appeared to increase his anxiety and agitation, leading him to defend himself with acts of verbal and physical aggression. The SLP also noticed that AM was not wearing his ALD, and there was a TV playing in the background, which may have interfered with his comprehension. During the shower, the aide had to repeat the steps to showering to AM several times, in part due to his hearing impairment (he is unable to wear his ALD in the shower).

The AAC System

Screenings were conducted to further assess AM's deficits and strengths. First, a structured interview was conducted to better understand AM's conversation ability and personal preferences. AM was pleasant and cooperative and maintained good eye contact throughout the interaction. AM verbalized mostly in single words and short sentences. His communication benefited from the communication partner's use of increased response time and supportive cues in the form of text, personal pictures, and tactile stimuli (e.g., holding his woodworking). While looking at pictures of family, AM was able to identify himself, his wife, his brother, and his father correctly, in response to an open-ended prompt ("what can you tell me about this picture?"). He referred to his wife to recall names of his children and grandchildren. AM benefited from binary-choice (e.g., "Do you like A or B?") when answering questions about specific preferences. Next, a reading screening was administered to determine appropriate font size for the communication aids. The screening consisted of five short sentences in 16-pt, 24-pt, 36-pt, 48-pt, and 72-pt font, respectively. AM was able to fluently read all five sentences without signs of vision difficulty (e.g., squinting). Finally, the SLP provided simple written commands to assess AM's reading comprehension. AM was able to follow single-step written commands but was unable to follow those with more complex sentence structure (e.g., "Make a fist, after you point to your left ear").

The Rationale for Clinical Decision-Making

Several AAC systems were recommended based on AM's preferences as well as cognitive-communication abilities identified in the assessment. AM had strengths in oral reading and comprehension for simple written commands. He enjoyed reminiscing about his life history and, although his verbal expression was limited, appeared engaged in conversation and demonstrated appropriate pragmatic behaviors, such as taking turns and topic maintenance. The observation of the care interaction showed a need for educating JM about supporting the communication environment and recognizing possible causes of AM's challenging behaviors (e.g., fear of falling).

Treatment began with care partner training to build a foundation for maintenance. The SLP reviewed the evaluation findings with JM, discussed strategies for supporting communication interactions, and reviewed rationale and use for the AAC systems. Communication strategies included limiting distractions (e.g., turning off the TV), providing one instruction at a time, speaking face-to-face, using an even tone, providing encouragement

and reassurance, and supporting comprehension with written and visual cues. The SLP also praised JM for seeking support from her church community and encouraged her to continue this self-care behavior.

Four AAC systems were used in this intervention including an orientation board, reminder card, visual sequencing aid, and memory book. The orientation board (see Figure 29–4) was used to improve AM's recall of temporal information and prime him for upcoming events (e.g., going to the day program). The orientation board also included the name of his HHA for that day. JM reviewed the board with AM while he was sitting up in bed, then prompted him to read the information out loud. Next, a reminder card (Figure 29–9) was used to prime AM to the activity of showering and ease him into the transition of getting out of bed. JM handed AM the reminder card and said, "Please read this card." After AM read the card, she would ask, "would you like to have a shower now?". After AM agreed, the process of transitioning from bed to shower began. During the shower, a visual sequencing aid (Figure 29–10) was used to improve auditory comprehension and promote task completion. JM or the HHA would point to one step on the list at a time and read the step out loud. If AM was unable to follow instructions with the verbal

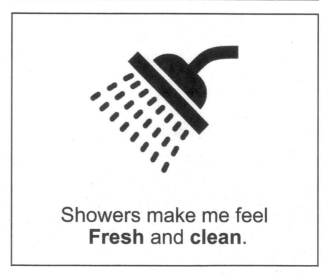

Showers make me feel **Fresh** and **clean**.

Figure 29–9. Reminder card for AM/primer for shower.

My Shower Checklist

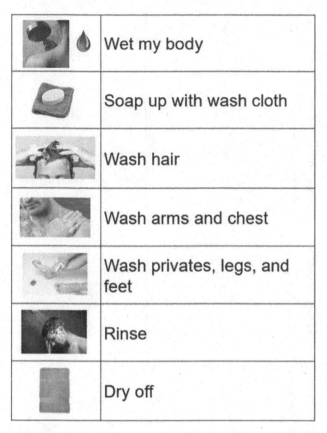

	Wet my body
	Soap up with wash cloth
	Wash hair
	Wash arms and chest
	Wash privates, legs, and feet
	Rinse
	Dry off

Figure 29–10. Visual sequencing shower aid for AM.

and external cue, JM or the HHA would progress to modeling the step using gestures or, if still unsuccessful, providing hand-over-hand guidance (e.g., gently guiding AM's hand to the shampoo bottle). The reason for this hierarchy was to allow AM to complete the activity with the least amount of assistance possible. JM and HHA were also instructed to provide verbal encouragement and reassurance throughout the task to help AM feel capable and successful.

Finally, the SLP worked with the family to create a memory book that would answer AM's repetitive questions regarding marriage and home, and improve the quality of conversations between AM and JM. The pages contained captions with simple sentence structure and 36-pt Arial font Figure 29–11). When AM asked repetitive questions, JM was instructed to say, "I think the answer to that question is in your book", then review the book with AM.

Table 29–1 provides a summary of the intervention components reviewed above, as well as the clinical rationale and implementation strategies.

Next Steps

The AAC tools were reviewed with AM to ensure comprehension. In addition, JM verified the information in the memory book was accurate. After providing training in the use of the AAC tools, the SLP observed care interactions (e.g., waking AM and showering) and provided additional training and feedback as needed. The interventions improved AM's comprehension of the morning routine and increased his compliance with verbal instructions. JM's use of supportive communication strategies was also effective in decreasing AM's agitation and anxiety. Due to frequent HHA turnover, JM had to constantly reeducate new staff on using visual aids, but sometimes forgot or felt she did not have the time. The SLP provided assistance by creating a short instructional video, accompanied by brief instructional handouts, showing how to use the AAC systems with AM. The video was recorded on JM's phone with permission and shown to new HHAs. Finally, the memory book helped decrease repetitive questions about orientation information and became an engaging activity for AM and JM, allowing the couple to reminisce together about happy memories.

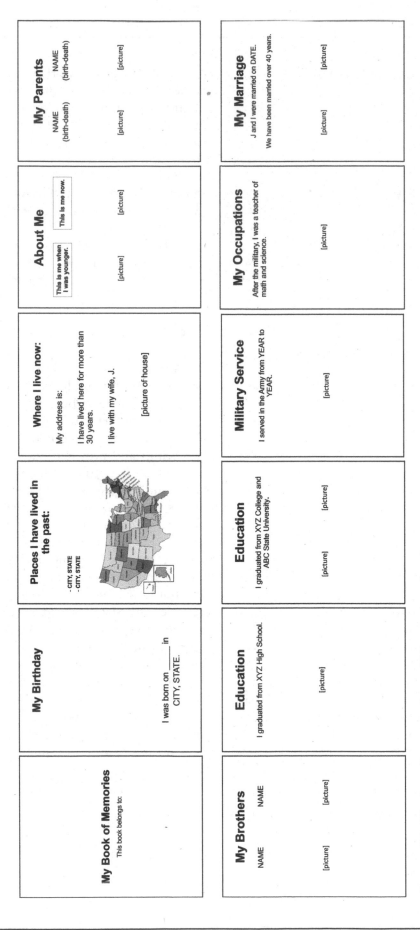

Figure 29–11. Sample pages from AM's memory book.

Table 29–1. AAC System and Service Considerations

Augmentative and Alternative Communication (AAC) System	Rationale	Service Considerations
Orientation board (Figure 29–4)	Improving comprehension of steps in the morning routine and increasing compliance	Board was presented to AM while he was still in bed, along with the prompts, "Let's review the schedule for today. What does this say?"
Reminder card (Figure 29–9)	Orientation to showering activity and support for auditory comprehension	After reviewing the orientation board, JM would hand AM the reminder card and say, "read this." After AM read the card, she would ask, "would you like to have a shower now?"
Memory book (Figure 29–11)	To answer repetitive questions regarding marriage and home; improve meaningful conversations between AM and JM	Font size, sentence structure, content. When AM asked questions about the marriage or home, JM would say "I think the answer to that question is in your book."
Care partner training	Encourage maintenance of communication and memory support strategies; reinforce self-care behaviors	Training consisted of information on supporting sensory abilities (wearing assistive listening device and glasses when possible), reducing background noise, increasing time for response, communicating in an even tone, providing one instruction at a time, providing verbal encouragement, and providing visual and text cues. The speech-language pathologist praised JM for getting support from her church community and friends and encouraged her to continue this self-care behavior.

References

Baddeley, A. (1992). Working memory. *American Association for the Advancement of Science, 255*(5044), 556–561.

Baddeley, A. (2000). The episodic buffer: A new component of working memory? *Trends in Cognitive Sciences, 4*(11), 417–423. https://doi.org/10.1016/S1364-6613(00)01538-2

Bayles, K. A., & Kim, E. S. (2003). Improving the functioning of individuals with Alzheimer's disease: Emergence of behavioral interventions. *Journal of Communication Disorders, 36*(5), 327–343. https://doi.org/10.1016/S0021-9924(03)00047-9

Beukelman, D. R., Fager, S., Ball, L., & Dietz, A. (2007). AAC for adults with acquired neurological conditions: A review. *Augmentative and Alternative Communication, 23*(3), 230–242. https://doi.org/10.1080/07434610701553668

Beukelman, D. R., & Mirenda, P. (2013). *Augmentative & alternative communication: Supporting children and adults with complex communication needs* (4th ed.). Paul H. Brookes.

Bonner, M. F., Vesely, L., Price, C., Anderson, C., Richmond, L., Farag, C., . . . Grossman, M. (2009). Reversal of the concreteness effect in semantic dementia. *Cognitive Neuropsychology, 26*(6), 568–579. https://doi.org/10.1080/02643290903512305

Bourgeois, M. S. (1993). Effects of memory aids on the dyadic conversations of individuals with dementia. *Journal of Applied Behavior Analysis, 26*(1), 77–87. https://doi.org/10.1901/jaba.1993.26-77

Bourgeois, M. S. (2014). *Memory and communication aids for people with dementia.* Health Professions Press.

Bourgeois, M. S., Burgio, L. D., Schulz, R., Beach, S., & Palmer, B. (1997). Modifying repetitive verbalizations of community-dwelling patients with AD. *The Gerontologist, 37*(1), 30–39.

Bourgeois, M. S., Camp, C. J., Antenucci, V., & Fox, K. (2016). Voice my choice: Facilitating understanding of preferences of residents with dementia. *Advances in Aging Research*, *5*(6), 131–141. https://doi.org/10.4236/aar.2016.56013

Bourgeois, M. S., Dijkstra, K., Burgio, L., & Allen-Burge, R. (2001). Memory aids as an augmentative and alternative communication strategy for nursing home residents with dementia. *Augmentative and Alternative Communication*, *17*(3), 196–210. https://doi.org/10.1080/aac.17.3.196.210

Bourgeois, M. S., Schulz, R., Burgio, L. D., & Beach, S. (2002). Skills training for spouses of patients with Alzheimer's disease: Outcomes of an intervention study. *Journal of Clinical Geropsychology*, *8*, 53–73. https://doi.org/10.1023/A:1013098124765

Brush, J. A., & Camp, C. J. (1999). Effective interventions for persons with dementia: Using spaced retrieval and Montessori techniques. *Perspectives on Neurophysiology and Neurogenic Speech and Language Disorders*, *9*(4), 27. https://doi.org/10.1044/nnsld9.4.27

Brush, J. A., Camp, C., Bohach, S., & Gertsberg, N. (2015). Developing signage that supports wayfinding for persons with dementia. *Canadian Nursing Home*, *26*(1). https://brushdevelopment.com/wp-content/uploads/2015/09/CNH_spring_2015.pdf

Brush, J., Sanford, J., Fleder, H., Bruce, C., & Calkins, M. (2011). Evaluating and modifying the communication environment for people with dementia. *Perspectives on Gerontology*, *16*(2), 32. https://doi.org/10.1044/gero16.2.32

Burshnic, V. L., & Bourgeois, M. S. (2020). A seat at the table: Supporting persons with severe dementia in communicating their preferences. *Clinical Gerontologist*. https://doi.org/10.1080/07317115.2020.1764686

Camp, C. J. (2006). Spaced retrieval. In D. K. Attix & K. A. Welsh-Bohmer (Eds.), *Geriatric neuropsychology: Assessment and intervention* (pp. 275–292). Guilford Press.

Chang, W-Z. D., & Bourgeois, M. S. (2020). Effects of visual aids for end-of-life care on decisional capacity of people with dementia. *American Journal of Speech-Language Pathology*, *29*(1), 185–200. https://doi.org/10.1044/2019_AJSLP-19-0028

Fried-Oken, M., Mooney, A., & Peters, B. (2015). Supporting communication for patients with neurodegenerative disease. *NeuroRehabilitation*, *37*(1), 69–87. https://doi.org/10.3233/NRE-151241

Fried-Oken, M., Rowland, C., Baker, G., Dixon, M., Mills, C., Schultz, D., & Oken, B. (2009). The effect of voice output on the AAC-supported conversations of persons with Alzheimer's disease. *ACM Transactions on Accessible Computing*, *1*(3), 15. https://doi.org/10.1145/1497302.1497305

Gitlin, L. N., Kales, H. C., & Lyketsos, C. G. (2012). Non-pharmacologic management of behavioral symptoms in dementia. *JAMA*, *308*(19), 2020–2029. https://doi.org/10.1001/jama.2012.36918

Harvey, P. D. (2019). Domains of cognition and their assessment. *Dialogues in Clinical Neuroscience*, *21*(3), 227–237. https://doi.org/10.31887/DCNS.2019.21.3/pharvey

Hickey, E. M., & Bourgeois, M. S. (2018). *Dementia: Person-centered assessment and intervention* (2nd ed.). Routledge.

Hinshelwood, H., Henry, M., & Fromm, D. (2016). Helping them hold on. *ASHA Leader*, *21*(10). https://doi.org/10.1044/leader.FTR1.21102016.44

Hoerster, L., Hickey, E. M., & Bourgeois, M. S. (2001). Effects of memory aids on conversations between nursing home residents with dementia and nursing assistants. *Neuropsychological Rehabilitation*, *11*(3–4), 399–427. https://doi.org/10.1080/09602010042000051

Hopper, T., Kim, E., Azumo, T., Bayles, K. A., Cleary, S. J., & Tomoeda, C. K. (2005). Evidence-based practice recommendations for working with individuals with dementia: Spaced-retrieval training. *Journal of Medical Speech-Language Pathology*, *13*(4), xxvii–xxxiv.

Matthews, B. R. (2015). Memory dysfunction. *Continuum: Lifelong Learning in Neurology*, *21*(3 Behavioral Neurology and Neuropsychiatry), 613–626. https://doi.org/10.1212/01.CON.0000466656.59413.29

Murphy, J., Gray, C. M., van Achterberg, T., Wyke, S., & Cox, S. (2010). The effectiveness of the Talking Mats framework in helping people with dementia to express their views on well-being. *Dementia*, *9*(4), 454–472. https://doi.org/10.1177/1471301210381776

Nakamura, H., Nakanishi, M., Hamanaka, T., Nakashi, S., & Yoshida, S. (2000). Semantic priming in patients with Alzheimer and semantic dementia. *Cortex*, *36*(2), 151–162. https://doi.org/10.1016/S0010-9452(08)70521-5

Reilly, J., Peelle, J. E., Antonucci, S. M., & Grossman, M. (2011). Anomia as a marker of distinct semantic memory impairments in Alzheimer's disease and semantic dementia. *Neuropsychology*, *25*(4), 413–426. https://doi.org/10.1037/a0022738

Small, J. A., & Gutman, G. (2002). Recommended and reported use of communication strategies in Alzheimer caregiving. *Alzheimer Disease & Associated Disorders*, *16*(4), 270–278. https://doi.org/10.1097/00002093-200210000-00009

Smith, E. R., Broughton, M., Baker, R., Pachana, N. A., Angwin, A. J., Humphreys, M. S., . . . Chenery, H. J. (2011). Memory and communication support in dementia: Research-based strategies for caregivers. *International Psychogeriatrics, 23*(2), 256–263. https://doi.org/10.1017/S1041610210001845

Squire, L. R. (1992). Declarative and nondeclarative memory: Multiple brain systems supporting learning and memory. *Journal of Cognitive Neuroscience, 4*(3), 232–243. https://doi.org/10.1162/jocn.1992.4.3.232

Tulving, E. (2001). Episodic memory and common sense: How far apart? *Philosophical Transactions of the Royal Society of London. Series B: Biological Sciences, 356*(1413), 1505–1515. https://doi.org/10.1098/rstb.2001.0937

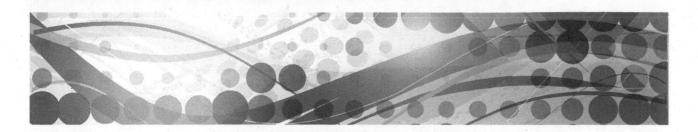

Chapter 30

AAC FOR PERSONS WHO ARE MEDICALLY COMPLEX

Abygail E. Marx and Sarah Marshall

Fundamentals

Introduction

In this chapter, we focus on the factors that contribute to communication success and difficulties for individuals with medically complex diagnoses. We discuss unique barriers and needs created by their medical complexities, as well as augmentative and alternative communication (AAC) considerations and strategies that can help these individuals achieve functional communication throughout their life span. Some of the key diagnoses of individuals who are medically complex are covered in other chapters of this book (e.g., cerebral palsy [CP], traumatic brain injury [TBI], dementia, and degenerative conditions). Additional medically complex diagnoses include genetic syndromes such as Rett and Down syndromes and Trisomy 13 and 18; disorders that impact brain development such as holoprosencephaly, hypoxic ischemic encephalopathy (HIE), congenital cytomegalovirus (CMV) infection, and fetal alcohol effects; and pediatric degenerative conditions, which pose considerations for supporting communication as the child experiences the progression of diagnoses such as Friedreich's ataxia, muscular dystrophy, and Sanfilippo syndrome. Some of these are detailed in Table 30–1.

Within AAC services, it is essential to consider and incorporate expertise from the large interdisciplinary team that inevitably cares for these populations. The team starts with the individual and their family, as their expertise about the person's needs and priorities cannot be overstated. In addition to their primary care team, the person may also work with neurologists, developmental or rehabilitation physicians, geneticists, and health psychologists for management of multiple medical needs. Given complex motor and sensory needs, the therapeutic team may include multiple speech-language pathologists (SLPs), occupational therapists (OTs), physical therapists (PTs), vision specialists, audiologists, and durable medical equipment and assistive technology (AT) professionals. The care team may also include members across the child's natural environments, such as case managers, school teams, and in adulthood, residential and vocational support staff.

Not only is it essential to coordinate with team members to provide exemplary patient- and family-centered care, but their unique expertise provides essential information for decision-making throughout AAC assessment and implementation. When working as part of an extensive team, it is helpful to reference the different roles and responsibilities that each team member plays. In their seminal AAC textbook, Beukelman and Light (2020) reference the different communication partners that an

Table 30–1. Medically Complex Disorders and Relevant Augmentative and Alternative Communication (AAC) Resources

Diagnosis	Considerations	Reference
Spinal muscular atrophy (SMA)	Although children with SMA historically relied heavily on AAC, given significant motor impairment and anarthria, new gene modification and replacement treatments are largely eliminating impacts of SMA.	Ball, L. J., Chavez, S., Perez, G., Bharucha-Goebel, D., Smart, K., Kundrat, K., Carruthers, L., Brady, C., Leach, M., & Evans, S. (2019). Communication skills among children with spinal muscular atrophy type 1: A parent survey. *Assistive Technology*, *33*(1). 38–48. https://doi.org/10.1080/10400435.2019.1586788
Rett syndrome	Individuals with this diagnosis experience severe apraxia, impacting functional hand use. Prior to eye-gaze technologies being widely available, their cognitive skills were estimated to be very low. However, with use of eye gaze for learning and communication, as well as use of alternative testing strategies, individuals have demonstrated they can achieve significantly higher levels of learning and interaction than had been previously estimated. Allowing processing time without continued prompting or questioning supports their ability to demonstrate skills and independence.	Townend, G. S., Marschik, P. B., Smeets, E., Berg, R. V., Berg, M. V., & Curfs, L. M. (2015). Eye gaze technology as a form of augmentative and alternative communication for individuals with Rett syndrome: Experiences of families in the Netherlands. *Journal of Developmental and Physical Disabilities*, *28*(1), 101–112. https://doi.org/10.1007/s10882-015-9455-z Vessoyan, K., Steckle, G., Easton, B., Nichols, M., Siu, V. M., & Mcdougall, J. (2018). Using eye-tracking technology for communication in Rett syndrome: Perceptions of impact. *Augmentative and Alternative Communication*, *34*(3), 230–241. https://doi.org/10.1080/07434618.2018.1462848
Trisomy 18 and 13 syndromes	Children with these syndromes were historically thought to have significant cognitive impairment with limited expectation beyond the 12-month level, but early intervention with AAC and alternative access methods have revealed many more capabilities.	Liang, C. A., Braddock, B. A., Heithaus, J. L., Christensen, K. M., Braddock, S. R., & Carey, J. C. (2013). Reported communication ability of persons with trisomy 18 and trisomy 13. *Developmental Neurorehabilitation*, *18*(5), 322–329. https://doi.org/10.3109/17518423.2013.847980
Cleft and craniofacial anomalies	Children with cleft and craniofacial disorder often do not receive AAC intervention, though they have a wide variety of complex medical diagnoses. This is a population that may be underserved related to AAC and should not be overlooked.	Brown, M. N., Grames, L. M., & Skolnick, G. B. (2021). Augmentative and alternative communication (AAC) use among patients followed by a multidisciplinary cleft and craniofacial team. *Cleft Palate-Craniofacial Journal*, *58*(3), 324–331. https://doi.org/10.1177/1055665620947606
Cornelia de Lange syndrome	Diagnosis has significant impacts on cognitive and motor skills, but speech and language are even more severely impaired than would be expected based on overall development. Early intervention with AAC supports development and reduction of challenging behaviors characteristic of this diagnosis.	Ajmone, P., Rigamonti, C., Dall'Ara, F., Monti, F., Vizziello, P., Milani, D., Cereda, A., Selicorni, A., & Costantino, A. (2014). Communication, cognitive development and behavior in children with Cornelia de Lange syndrome (CdLS): Preliminary results. *American Journal of Medical Genetics, Part B, Neuropsychiatric Genetics*, *165B*(3), 223–229. https://doi.org/10.1002/ajmg.b.32224

individual will interact with, the roles these team members may serve (e.g., as AAC Finders or Daily Facilitators), and the knowledge and skills these partners need to successfully support communication. Use of interprofessional practice guidelines will also help address any differences in opinion about the most essential or "best" approaches for meeting the individual's highly complex and individualized therapeutic and health care needs.

This chapter addresses children who may be facing diagnoses that result in shorter life expectancy, ongoing decline in functioning, recurrent setbacks, or missed opportunities due to sacrifices for medical care. Selecting a tool that will meet an individual's needs after a possible decline in functioning requires open and honest, although difficult, dialogue about expected changes. Knowledge and implementation of appropriate counseling techniques may improve outcomes while maximizing quality of life for individuals and their families (Holland, 2007).

Counseling for this population must abandon the "medical" model, which emphasizes what is wrong with the person. Instead, we must focus on how the unique strengths of the person and their family unit can be mobilized to deal with adversity (Holland, 2007). Finding this balance is truly a dance, as you must not minimize or ignore the overwhelming grief that an individual or their family may be experiencing. Counseling involves an active listening process, in which we aim to help individuals and their families grieve what has been lost, develop coping strategies, increase resilience, make adaptations, capitalize on strengths, and live as fully as possible (Holland, 2007).

Empathy and compassion are achieved when active listening strengthens our relationships with clients. However, we must be mindful of compassionate fatigue and burnout. As AAC providers, we are fortunate that our role focuses on providing positive solutions, while other providers often focus on what has been lost. Knowing that some form of communication remains possible throughout a disease, and that even small changes (e.g., environmental modifications, communication partner training) can enrich lives, may offer hope for clinicians and families alike. When our role of counseling exceeds our own expertise, we must work closely with our colleagues in health psychology for both our clients and ourselves.

Participation Framework

Along with the priorities of strengths-based approaches, interdisciplinary care, counseling, and supporting the individual and their family through their evolving medical and communication needs, our focus as AAC professionals also must emphasize the importance of participation and self-determination to the highest extent possible. The Participation Model is an essential pillar of evidence-based practice in the field of speech-language pathology. In this model, it is recognized that AAC assessment and intervention "are integrally linked, with AAC assessment serving as the information-gathering process required to plan effective AAC intervention" (Beukelman & Light, 2020).

The dynamic nature of moving between assessment and intervention throughout the AAC journey is never more true or essential than for individuals who are medically complex. These individuals experience ongoing changes in their needs related to AAC, whether these changes are connected to illnesses and hospitalization, or a degenerative condition. Given the need to move through the different components of the Participation Model on an ongoing basis, we use this framework to organize the remainder of the content and highlight key considerations and communication approaches for individuals who are medically complex.

Component 1: Assessment of the Individual's Participation Patterns and Communication Needs

The AAC assessment process is highly individualized, and interdisciplinary collaboration is the most effective approach for assessing participation patterns and communication needs. The American Speech-Language-Hearing Association (ASHA) recommends the World Health Organization's (2001) International Classification of Functioning, Disability, and Health (ICF) framework to guide assessment of underlying limitations in body functions and structures, and intervention focused on improving function, activities, and participation in daily life. Similarly, the GENIAL biopsychosocial model is an approach developed in relation to AT needs of individuals with chronic health conditions, that shifts focus away from mitigating impairments, and leverages services that promote overall well-being, success, and health (Figure 30–1). This model is relevant for guiding AAC services given its underlying intent to "facilitate opportunities for positive psychological experiences, positive health behaviors, positive social relationships and community integration," which are all key tenets of successful AAC implementation (Howard et al., 2020). Tools we may use to guide our clinical decision-making include interviews, social networks, communication needs assessments, and participation inventories (Beukelman & Light, 2020).

Evaluating children with complex communication needs also involves dynamic approaches that assess their learning style and environment. Children naturally learn language and world knowledge through exploration, exposure, and interaction within their environment. Medically complex diagnoses are often associated with cognitive, attention, processing, sensory, and/or motor differences. Children with these types of impairments are at an inherent disadvantage for accessing their environment and the experiential learning that is crucial for communication development. Therefore, a key piece of this assessment is identifying meaningful contexts for children with complex communication needs and setting up the environment to support that interaction. As providers, we must be conscientious about how we create learning opportunities, as well as how we coach and support parents to do the same. Educating parents on environmental adaptations and communication partner strategies for interacting with children with complex vision, hearing, motor, and medical needs, can help us further assess participation patterns and communication needs through a "response to intervention" approach that focuses on dynamic assessment principles.

Many interaction strategies come naturally to parents, but there may be response differences from children who are medically complex. For example, some children may not be able to respond in the same ways through vocalizations, facial expression, or eye contact. They may need more time to pro-

cess and respond, or they may experience seizures or alertness differences that render their attention during interactions more intermittent. They may need more repetition to learn before they respond in expected ways. When parents experience limited or unexpected responses from their children, this may diminish their confidence or enthusiasm for providing language input. Encouraging parents to respond to all communication attempts, increase wait time, and provide modeling in repeated and motivating activities and interactions is so important to ensure that participation and communication opportunities are provided consistently for children with complex medical and communication needs.

Component 2: Assessment of Environmental Supports and Opportunity Barriers

Beukelman and Light (2020) list policy, practice, knowledge, skill, and attitude as environmental supports and opportunity barriers to assess during the evaluation process. This aligns closely with societal barriers unique to individuals with chronic conditions discussed by Howard and colleagues (2020). By increasing our awareness of common barriers, AAC providers are better prepared to normalize challenges and equip individuals and their teams with the needed tools and strategies to achieve success

The first theme described by Howard and colleagues (2020) is *design and function* of AT systems. Devices that are reliable, accessible across environments, and customizable are more likely to be consistently implemented. Discussing operational features of devices within the evaluation process is recommended. This ties into the next barrier, *awareness and information* about the AAC system. Providers should prioritize involving the individual and their interdisciplinary team in the setup of the system, provide operational instructions, and encourage relationships with AAC vendors for ongoing support.

Service provision, or timely and local follow-up support after placement of an AAC system, is a priority for successful implementation. The placement of an appropriately matched system is just the beginning of the process. Person-centered,

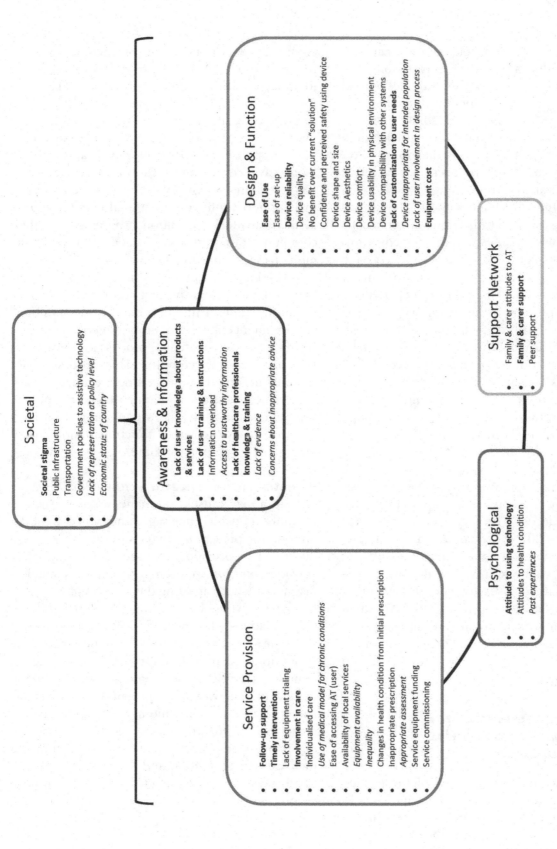

Figure 30–1. From the GENIAL biopsychosocial model for promoting health and well-being of individuals with chronic health conditions, the themes describe common barriers to implementation of assistive technology with this population. (From "Exploring the Barriers to Using Assistive Technology for Individuals With Chronic Conditions: A Meta-Synthesis Review," J. Howard, Z. Fisher, A. H. Kemp, S. Lindsay, L. H. Tasker, and J. J. Tree, 2020, *Disability and Rehabilitation: Assistive Technology.* Used with permission.) These themes align closely with the policy, practice, knowledge, skill, and attitude barriers identified by Beukelman and Light (2020) in the Participation Model. KEY: **Bold themes** were identified 15 times or more. *Italicized themes* were identified fewer than five times.

evidence-based intervention via a service delivery model (e.g., in-person, teletherapy) that best meets the individual's needs is a must for ongoing success. *Psychological barriers*, or attitudes toward using technology, comprise the fourth theme identified by Howard and colleagues (2020). Individuals with chronic conditions must accept their health condition before being open to the use of AAC. A lack of acceptance may be seen in a teenager with Friedreich's ataxia who is not yet ready to augment his dysarthria, or a child with CP who refuses to use her AAC system because none of her friends communicate this way. SLPs are encouraged to provide counseling, seek peer mentors, or encourage individuals to join virtual communities to connect with others with similar diagnoses or experiences.

Equally important is the individual's *support network*, or the attitudes and support of family, friends, and the interdisciplinary team. Like patients who have not yet accepted their condition, family members may also not be ready to consider AAC. For example, a parent of a child with Rett syndrome may refuse trials of eye-gaze technology in the hopes that their daughter could still learn to use her hands, despite stereotypic hand movements being a classic symptom of the disorder. Providing counseling, honoring the grieving process, and highlighting the importance of independence may promote success. The final theme of Howard et al.'s model (2020), *social context*, is the impact of wider environmental context on disability and well-being. For example, many health insurances have exclusionary clauses for speech-generating devices (SGDs), despite approving other AT. Advocacy at the state and national level is within the scope of SLPs, and involving individuals with medical complexity and their families can strengthen advocacy initiatives.

Component 3: Assessment of the Individual's Capabilities and Access Barriers

The goal of the third component of the Participation Model is to capitalize on the individual's current capabilities by matching them to features of AAC systems that leverage those skills and increase opportunity for language growth. This "feature-matching" process for individuals with complex medical needs must include a three-pronged approach that supports decision-making for today, tomorrow, and the future. For today, what AAC solutions are most appropriate and efficient to meet current communication skills and access needs? For tomorrow, how will these AAC solutions support language development and learning more advanced communication skills over time? For the future, which AAC solutions offer features that support continued functional communication as the individual's condition progresses and their communication and access needs change, while minimizing the need for relearning?

Thinking back to the features of AAC systems that were covered in the first section of this book, we now highlight unique changes in conditions that we might expect and important considerations within the feature-matching process for individuals who are medically complex. This process is not typically accomplished in a single evaluation session; rather, it includes ongoing diagnostic therapy throughout the individual's communication journey to support their most functional communication at any given point in time.

Potential Loss of Speech. For individuals whose condition may cause a permanent loss of speech, we must consider message and voice banking options for preserving their natural speech (like discussed in previous chapters). One important consideration for children with complex medical diagnoses is that capturing the recordings for either message or voice banking may be more difficult than for adults who are able to sit and record messages in a structured setting. Families may need to set up a recorder during typical family interactions (e.g., eating dinner, playing a game, talking on the phone with grandparents) to capture as many organic, personal messages as they can. We must also ensure the selected SGD can incorporate banked messages, providing an opportunity to increase personalization and motivation for learning the system before decline occurs, so that messages are ready to use as soon as they are needed.

Sensory or Motor Changes. Many progressive conditions will impact vision, hearing, and/or motor status, so the feature-matching process for these individuals must consider systems that meet their current needs most efficiently but have flexibility to adjust over time. You may initially be selecting a device that the individual points to with their fingers but may later access via eye gaze or auditory scanning, as their motor skills diminish. Similarly, for an individual who may lose vision, the use of visual symbols alone to represent language may be too limiting, so alternatives such as auditory cues, tactile keyguards, or zoom features should be considered. Thinking about potential status changes and incorporating appropriate features from the beginning can help the individual learn and practice the alternative access strategies before they are needed and diminish the need to learn a new system when abilities decline.

Cognitive and Medical Status Changes. Changes in cognitive or processing skills may impact an individual's ability to continue using an AAC system. The more opportunity they have to learn and incorporate AAC prior to these changes, the more likely strategies will become automatic and routine. If we capitalize on learning prior to changes in cognition, attention, and alertness, these skills may be preserved as the individual's condition progresses. Urgent referrals and expedited scheduling of AAC services are essential to take advantage of developmental trajectories before deterioration begins. Communication partner training is likewise essential so that if changes in cognition and medical status impact the individual's ability to independently use their AAC systems over time, these trained partners can scaffold functional communication throughout the life span. For example, transitioning from independent auditory scanning to a partner-assisted scanning strategy can take some of the cognitive burden off the individual.

Mounting/Positioning Considerations. Respiratory conditions may impact an individual's ability to sit upright, requiring mounts to position AAC systems effectively and securely. If an individual must lie flat on their back, we may mount devices directly above their head (if comfortable) or off to a side with their head turned. Individuals with complex medical needs often have an array of necessary equipment, including switches to access communication, to signal for help (e.g., nurse call), or for other environmental controls (e.g., adjusting bed or lights). The feature-matching process involves not only *what* AAC systems the individual will use, but *how* those systems fit into the bigger picture of their AT and medical equipment needs.

Component 4: Planning and Implementation of Intervention With the Individual Who Requires AAC and the Communication Partners

When working with individuals who are medically complex and their families, one intervention consideration is the method and location of service delivery. For in-person services, clinicians must be aware of any emergency protocols (e.g., rescue medication for seizures, suctioning) and who is responsible for executing them. It is essential to advocate that these individuals are present or nearby during treatment sessions. Familiarize yourself with facility emergency procedures and communicate to necessary staff that help may be needed. The use of teletherapy offers an opportunity to continue care when patients are ill, homebound, or staying home to avoid contracting illness. For example, many children with medical complexities will receive virtual schooling and therapies during cold and flu season. The techniques for Tele-AAC assessments, interventions, and consultations in Chapters 35 and 36 of this text are critical for this population.

Another unique intervention consideration for individuals who are medically complex is the need to prepare for planned and emergency hospitalizations. Instruction in health literacy should begin immediately. Ensure that needed vocabulary (e.g., medications, diagnoses, personnel, pain, etc.) is available and that direct instruction in functional use is provided. Create opportunities to role-play and practice this vocabulary in low-stress situations, avoiding the need for all learning to occur when hospitalized. Practice both successful interactions and communication breakdowns, creating opportunities to teach repair and resilience in communication. For routine medical appointments, encourage developmentally appropriate ways to involve individuals (e.g., checking in, identifying pain location or level) and modeling of vocabulary throughout the visit. Self-advocacy, autonomy, and control over medical care should be both taught and respected by involving the individual as much as possible. For example, you might program videos of daily care routines directly within a child's communication device so they can take an active role in training new caregivers.

Blackstone and Pressman (2015) highlight the importance of SLPs providing AAC service in preparing individuals for medical encounters. They suggest developing a "*grab-and-go bag*," or a collection of materials to support communication during hospitalizations, including a description of the individual's communication strategies, health-related communication boards, printed boards from an SGD, and wall signage to highlight essential information (e.g., the person's "yes" signal, how to position the SGD). Outpatient and school SLPs are encouraged to obtain permission to share communication strategies and adaptations with inpatient staff to support successful patient-provider communication and outcomes. Providing information on therapy goals is appropriate for prolonged admissions when inpatient staff may be taking over school instruction to mitigate regression from missed opportunities.

Children who are communicating verbally may also be facing admissions with either a temporary (i.e., endotracheal intubation) or permanent (i.e., tracheostomy placement) loss of speech. The inability to communicate effectively is the leading cause of adverse medical errors and can negatively affect a patient's mood, anxiety, fear, and feelings of connectedness (Santiago et al., 2019). Providing counseling to the child on the temporary or permanent status of this communication change is crucial *prior* to surgery. Proactive AAC consultation and instruction on gaining attention in the room, participating in medical care, and interacting socially can all increase a sense of control and improve outcomes (Santiago et al., 2019). For additional information about supporting communication in the inpatient setting, see the final chapters of this book.

Component 5: Evaluation of the Effectiveness of the Intervention and Follow-Up as Required

The Participation Model emphasizes the importance of ongoing assessment and recognition that "the job is never done." As AAC professionals, we must always be evaluating if our interventions are successful. We must continually question if the person is interacting and participating successfully across all desired partners and environments, meeting their functional communication needs, and achieving goals for learning, participation, and quality of life.

If the answer to these questions is "no," then we must go back through the components of the Participation Model, using the ICF and GENIAL frameworks as applicable, to reevaluate the individual's participation patterns, communication needs, capabilities, and access barriers. Ensure the individual, their family, and the interdisciplinary team are involved in the planning and implementation of AAC interventions to mediate identified barriers and increase success. If the answer is "yes," our work is still not done, as needs may change. The interdisciplinary team serves an essential role in monitoring the effectiveness of AAC systems for meeting long-term needs and making required adjustments through both developmental gains and setbacks.

Thinking back to the roles and responsibilities of the team, our AAC Finders and Daily Facilitators continue to serve an important role, even if specialized care with the AAC expert is on hold for a time. Coaching and counseling about what to look for in terms of changes and progression are essential, not only for appropriate referrals and reevaluation in a timely manner, but also to support the individual and their family through setbacks they may experience with medically complex diagnoses. The relationship between AAC providers, the individual, their family members, and the interdisciplinary team may be difficult and even turbulent at times, but it is rewarding and of paramount importance to building and maintaining the ongoing AAC supports essential for this unique population of individuals.

Case Study: LG

Clinical Profile and Communication Needs

The Individual

LG is a 15-year-old male with Sanfilippo syndrome, subtype A. This is a rare genetic metabolic condition in which the child's body is unable to break down a certain carbohydrate, heparan sulfate. The heparan sulfate accumulates and damages the cells of the central nervous system, leading to progressive loss of cognitive, language, sensory, and motor skills. There are four types of Sanfilippo syndrome (Types A, B, C, and D), with Type A being the most severe. Subtypes vary based on the gene that is mutated, resulting in different rates and severity of progression. In Subtype A, symptoms typically begin between 2 and 6 years of age and include hyperactivity and aggressive behaviors, sleep issues, seizures, vision/hearing impairment, and eventual loss of motor control and speech. Ultimately, the progression leads to premature death at around 20 to 30 years of age (Shapiro et al., 2019). The details of this case study are fictional and represent a compilation of examples commonly experienced by individuals with this diagnosis and their families.

Their Communication Partners

LG's immediate family and care providers include his parents, older sister, and grandparents. He is supported by a large interdisciplinary care team (described later). His individualized education program (IEP) team includes his SLP, OT, PT, special education teacher, and vision specialist.

Their Environments

LG lives with his parents and sister in an adapted home. He attends school in his local district. LG and his family have strong connections with their church and neighborhood. He is also frequently in clinical and hospital settings for therapy and medical care.

AAC System or Service Considerations

LG participated in a dynamic feature-matching process, moving between assessment and intervention throughout his AAC journey. His story began at the age of 2 years after receiving his diagnosis from a geneticist, who referred LG to a complex care program for interdisciplinary medical management, a rehabilitation clinic for interdisciplinary therapeutic management, and our AAC evaluation and treatment center for an urgent assessment given disease progression. LG's mother accepted a visit with both the complex care and rehabilitation clinics but declined to schedule the AAC visit as LG was using some speech to communicate. We quickly contacted the social worker in the rehabilitation clinic and the palliative care nurse practitioner in the complex care clinic to provide information on voice and message banking, the importance of starting early, and available AAC solutions. When social work and palliative care met with LG's family to discuss goals of care and share this information, his family identified goals to maximize quality of life and participation, opening the door for accepting an AAC evaluation.

Coordination of care was established with LG's complex care, rehabilitation, and early intervention (EI) teams to gain a comprehensive picture of his current needs and skills and expected disease progression and timeline. Communication with genetics and palliative care confirmed that the family had been educated in LG's disease, and although still grieving, were ready to engage in needed discussions. LG's initial AAC evaluation was scheduled with the SLP and OT team around his third birthday. Through chart review, parent interview, and interdisciplinary collaboration, a variety of essential SGD language and access features were identified for LG.

To begin, we knew that we needed to start LG with a robust system to prevent the need for relearning skills later. Children with Sanfilippo syndrome have a period of developmental gains prior to regression; thus, we needed to ensure that LG's system would have enough vocabulary to meet his communication needs. The device needed to offer alternative access methods (e.g., use of a keyguard, auditory fishing[1], auditory scanning). Disease progression varies in Sanfilippo, and some children show more decline in vision and hearing than in motor function, while others maintain their sensory status but show decline in motor functioning. LG's family was eager to begin the voice and message banking process, and thus the selected system must also support this feature. We next shifted our focus to LG's unique learning style and communication needs.

Family reported that LG learns best by seeing and doing. Visual supports (e.g., timers, schedules, video models) had already been introduced by his EI team, and the need for a system that integrates these features was prioritized. LG had strengths in social interaction and was motivated by telling jokes, directing play, and quickly sharing his message. Family described LG as a "quick mover" and desired an AAC system that supported access to full-phrase messages organized by topic, as this best aligned with goals for participation and quality of life. Family did not have goals for linguistic development, so although core vocabulary instruction was provided to communicate essential messages related to medical needs (i.e., help, move, up, down), other linguistic features (e.g., grammatical endings, unique syntactic structures) were not prioritized. With fine motor delays and the possibility of further decline, a system with dynamic page branching (e.g., selecting "eat" generates possible food options) or predictive messaging (e.g., selecting "my" generates "turn" or "favorite") might lead to frustration from selection errors resulting in unintended navigation and changing displays. Instead, a consistent and predictable display was selected.

A final consideration was whether off-the-shelf technology (i.e., iPad with speech-generating application) or durable medical equipment (i.e., dedicated SGD) was a better match for LG's needs. Ultimately, family and team agreed that LG would eventually need a dedicated AAC system with ongoing technical support and needed accessories (e.g., keyguard, switches, wheelchair mount). However, insurance funding was not available while

LG was still meeting his functional communication needs and making progress in speech and language development. Therefore, LG's family leveraged state waiver funding to purchase an iPad with a communication application for his immediate use to maximize opportunities for learning the selected system during this period of developmental gains. This application was also available on a dedicated SGD, so his customized pagesets could be transferred later, eliminating the need for relearning.

From 3 to 5 years of age, LG continued to progress in verbal communication and completed voice and message banking. Given his high levels of movement and difficulty participating in structured activities, many of the messages were recorded during natural interactions, with LG's family recording on cell phones and the AAC team later segmenting out specific messages. The family's recordings were imported into sound editing software, and specific words and sentences were saved as separate audio files. His messages were immediately loaded onto his communication device and programmed onto buttons, as LG showed increased engagement when the device was speaking in his own voice. Legacy messages were prioritized, such as LG poking fun at his sister and saying "I love you" to his parents. Intervention focused on communication partner training about the role of aided language stimulation to capitalize on this developmental period. LG showed delays in language comprehension, and use of aided language stimulation and visual supports within his system supported both comprehension and participation in a range of activities (e.g., brushing teeth, getting dressed) with increased independence. Last, health literacy concepts were introduced through the addition of medical vocabulary and targeting body part vocabulary within his favorite activity, Mr. Potato Head!

At age 6 years, LG experienced a plateau and then regression in verbal speech. Simultaneously, and perhaps because of this change, LG began engaging in self-injurious (e.g., head banging) and aggressive behaviors (e.g., hitting, biting). Although LG was previously engaged in using the AAC device, he began to throw or push it away when it was pre-

---

[1]A direct selection method that allows the user to browse through the items on display by touching locations and listening to auditory cues.

sented. We implemented a functional communication training (FCT) approach in which challenging behaviors were replaced with use of AAC. Video modeling, visual schedules, and first/then prompts were prioritized. His most motivating communication partner, his sister, continued to provide aided language stimulation and encouragement to engage with his SGD. Additionally, LG began work with health psychology for developmentally appropriate counseling on the changes he was experiencing with his speech, as this was likely very scary for him. Simultaneously, his parents were meeting with counselors about how best to support LG and their family through this difficult period of progression. With this interdisciplinary approach, LG reengaged with his system and ultimately completed the funding process for a dedicated SGD, as he then met medical necessity standards due to declines in his speech.

LG's physical skills continued to deteriorate. At age 8 years, he was preparing for a 2-week admission for an electroencephalogram (EEG) to monitor for new seizure activity, the placement of a gastrostomy tube (G-Tube), and surgery to repair his scoliosis. Leading up to his admission, we created a hospital-specific topic area on his SGD. Vocabulary was added related to upcoming medical procedures and the new professionals he would be interacting with. Additionally, visual scene displays (VSDs) were introduced as LG's SGD offered both grid-based and VSD communication options. His mom arranged with complex care and the admitting unit to take a picture of LG's room before admission. We worked to create "hot spots" within the room, to help LG both visualize what to expect and provide another means of communication when admitted, for example, touching the picture of the TV in the room to request the TV be turned on. An extra SGD charger, low-tech backups of his hospital topic area, and a variety of visual schedules were prepared for LG's "grab-and-go" bag. LG's school and outpatient SLPs both provided "helpful tips" sheets for the inpatient SLP and other staff to support his communication during his stay.

Between ages 8 and 10 years, LG experienced more motor, visual, and cognitive decline. His fine motor and vision skills no longer supported direct selection with a keyguard, and the concept of two-switch auditory scanning was introduced. With the extent of LG's cognitive decline, learning the scanning process was tiresome and frustrating. Discussion with family revealed that pursuing this access method did not align with their goals of quality of life and participation. We all questioned if introducing the concept of scanning earlier in LG's disease progression would have led to a more positive outcome. Instead of teaching LG two-switch scanning, we instead provided instruction to both LG and his communication partners on partner-assisted auditory scanning (PAAS). LG had already established a "yes, that's my choice" response by clapping and a "no" response by shaking his head. LG's team was instructed to use his current system and present each item on the display sequentially, allowing for his needed 5s processing time, and wait for LG to signal "yes, that's my choice" to communicate his message. Use of PAAS was successful for LG and offered an efficient and less taxing means of accessing his current SGD.

Today, LG is 15 years old, and his sister is still his favorite person. He still laughs at favorite jokes and benefits from his established routines. Unfortunately, LG has experienced continued motor and cognitive decline, along with an increase in seizure activity. As a result, he is more agitated, confused, and distressed throughout his day. Keeping his goals for quality of life and participation in the forefront of all clinical decision-making, intervention shifted exclusively to communication-partner training. Strategies commonly used for individuals with dementia (e.g., giving fewer choices, repeating key information, and environmental modifications) were introduced. We helped LG maintain participation in family activities via additional AT solutions (e.g., telling a joke via a simple voice output device, turning on the lights with an adapted switch). LG's banked messages continue to provide a sense of comfort for his family and garner a positive reaction from LG each time they are played.

Next Steps

As we look toward the future, the focus is on maintaining LG's ability to use functional communication strategies that match his unique language, sensory, and motor needs. As we think about appropriate treatment goals, given the life expectancy for most individuals with Sanfilippo syndrome, we are not looking at expanding grammar or syntax skills, nor are we focusing on communication for the purposes of college or vocational settings. Instead, LG and his family will benefit most from a focus on maintaining social closeness and expressing essential medical and care needs. Providing supports to mitigate the aggressive behaviors and anxiety associated with his diagnosis is essential for safety and quality of life for both LG and his family and team. As his cognitive and motor skills may continue to decline, his AAC systems will be adapted, and further communication partner training and scaffolding will continue to be the focus in order to offer functional means for LG to communicate to the end of his life.

References

Beukelman, D. R., & Light, J. C. (2020). *Augmentative & alternative communication: Supporting children and adults with complex communication needs*. Paul H. Brookes.

Blackstone, S. W., & Pressman, H. (2015). Patient communication in health care settings: New opportunities for augmentative and alternative communication. *Augmentative and Alternative Communication, 32*(1), 69–79. https://doi.org/10.3109/07434618.2015.1125947

Holland, A. L. (2007). *Counseling in communication disorders: A wellness perspective*. Plural Publishing.

Howard, J., Fisher, Z., Kemp, A. H., Lindsay, S., Tasker, L. H., & Tree, J. J. (2020). Exploring the barriers to using assistive technology for individuals with chronic conditions: A meta-synthesis review. *Disability and Rehabilitation: Assistive Technology*, 1–19. https://doi.org/10.1080/17483107.2020.1788181

Santiago, R., Howard, M., Dombrowski, N. D., Watters, K., Volk, M. S., Nuss, R., . . . Rahbar, R. (2019). Preoperative augmentative and alternative communication enhancement in pediatric tracheostomy. *Laryngoscope, 130*(7), 1817–1822. https://doi.org/10.1002/lary.28288

Shapiro, E., Lourenço, C. M., Mungan, N. O., Muschol, N., O'Neill, C., & Vijayaraghavan, S. (2019). Analysis of the caregiver burden associated with Sanfilippo syndrome type B: Panel recommendations based on qualitative and quantitative data. *Orphanet Journal of Rare Diseases, 14*(1). https://doi.org/10.1186/s13023-019-1150-1

World Health Organization. (2001). *International classification of functioning, disability, and health (ICF)*. https://apps.who.int/iris/handle/10665/42407

SECTION VII
AAC Services for Stakeholders

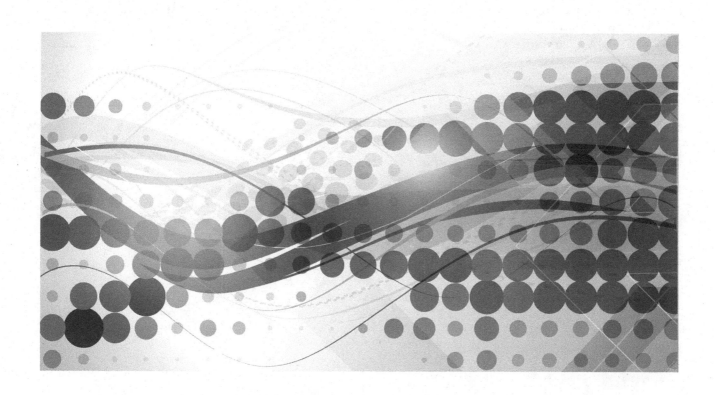

The final section of this text focuses on the communication partners and stakeholders essential to the success of augmentative and alternative communication (AAC). Chapter 31 discusses AAC consultation detailing the process of shared and collaborative decision-making. As Chapter 32 shifts to communication partner training for families, the need for careful family- and person-centered planning is detailed, and ways of supporting authentic communication and connection are offered.

Chapter 33 essentially shifts to training a trainer. The need for clinicians with specific and sufficient knowledge and experience to effectively support persons who use AAC (PWUAAC) and their teams persists, and this chapter reviews how to train clinicians to be able to train others while maintaining their role as a critical communication partner. Chapter 34 also reviews communication partner training but details supporting educational staff with the goal of increasing the partner's use of augmented input (or AAC modeling).

The final two chapters of this text cover the basics of tele-AAC and tele-AAC services, in Chapters 35 and 36. Although effective service delivery methods exist for individuals using AAC, tele-AAC has the unique ability to seamlessly and effectively involve pertinent team members in a range of settings, for a number of purposes.

Key Terms Reviewed in This Section

- AAC consultation
- Active listening
- Asynchronous
- Circles of support
- Coaching model
- Collaboration
- Consultation
- Family centered
- Hybrid
- Informative feedback
- Mind-Brain Education (MBE)
- Opportunity barriers
- Person centered
- Professional development
- School staff instruction
- Self-determination
- Special education
- Synchronous
- Tele-AAC
- Telepractice
- Visual access

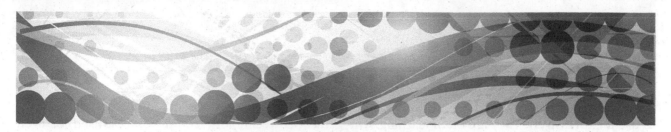

Chapter 31
AAC CONSULTATION

Erin S. Sheldon

Introduction

Augmentative and alternative communication (AAC) consultation has shifted away from an expert-led process, toward greater collaboration with AAC users and their communication partners. This chapter begins by explaining this shift. Next, it explores five aspects of the collaborative consultation process: learning, teaching, building consensus on the problem, shared decision-making, and building capacity for AAC implementation. Each aspect is paired with simple tools and strategies to assist the speech-language pathologist (SLP) at each step. Finally, the chapter concludes with a case study to illustrate the impact of collaborative approaches to consultation.

Terminology

This chapter is intended for anyone working in a role to provide AAC technology to those who need it, including SLPs, AAC consultants, or assistive technology (AT) specialists. For simplicity, in this chapter, anyone in this role will be referred to as the **SLP**. AAC users are very diverse, can be any age, and can have emergent to sophisticated language skills. **AAC learner** will distinguish any user still developing symbolic language skills, such as children. This distinction matters when exploring the role of families in the AAC consulta-

tion process. **Family** will refer broadly to anyone in an AAC user's closest circle of relationships, including caregivers.

The Fundamentals of AAC Consultation

Consultation is the process of gathering stakeholders for the purpose of making a decision. A consultant is a professional tasked with giving expert advice. Historically, the consultation process occurred when the SLP conducted detailed assessments and trials to match the needs of the person who uses AAC (PWUAAC) to the features of available technology. AAC was provided after the SLP determined which technology was the best fit. Once AAC was provided, the therapy team could move to the question of how the technology would be implemented.

Limits of the Traditional AAC Consultation Process

The expert-led process generally worked well to describe a person's access needs for AAC and to match them with an appropriate, accessible technology. But the process could fail AAC learners with early language skills, such as young children or some individuals with multiple disabilities. They need AAC long before they have the competence to use it expressively. They are often learning symbolic language while simultaneously developing joint attention, turn-taking, motor control, sensory regulation, and mobility. It may take them years to develop the language, motor skills, and motor memory to access AAC technology. In the meantime, they need frequent demonstrations of how alternative forms of language (such as graphic symbols or manual signs) are used pragmatically in natural environments. AAC consultation for these populations has to encompass both what the user can communicate independently, and what communication partners can teach and scaffold over time. Old, narrow approaches to feature matching, focused only on the AAC user's current skills and apparent abilities, provided a snapshot of the user's current development. But this snapshot could lead to faulty assumptions about the learner's potential to learn language and overlooked the role of communication partners. As a result, many children and adults with developmental disabilities were provided with inadequate AAC, or no AAC at all. Some received only simple tools to meet a narrow range of communication needs, such as requesting toys or food during specific daily routines. Many of these AAC tools could not support growth in symbolic language or communication functions. As a result, a child's AAC system could change multiple times, resulting in new symbol sets, vocabulary organization, and access patterns with each new AAC consultation. Many of these systems could not support the range of communication needs that occur over the life span. Few supported the development of language with both graphic symbols and the alphabet.

The traditional expert-led model of AAC assessment could also fail PWUAACs with fluent language skills but challenges in comprehension or written expression. Historically, AAC assessments have emphasized synchronous face-to-face interaction. Consultation could overlook an individual's unique patterns of communication with their closest communication partners and across environments. Many did not provide the tools needed to enhance comprehension, communicate asynchronously, or communicate on a range of platforms, such as through text messages, instant messaging,

social media, or videoconferencing. Carefully prescribed technology could be underused, or even abandoned, when it was inconsistent with the user's preferences and unique communication patterns and contexts.

Finally, AAC implementation was often an afterthought. AAC was underutilized without preparing the user's environments and communication partners to facilitate the individual's access to AAC and support successful communication. This preparation could include everything from ensuring AAC was charged and available, to training partners to model use of the device, support the user to focus on a topic and participate in a discussion, respect the user's privacy when maintaining the device, or prompt use of AAC when an individual's speech was unintelligible or when a repair strategy was needed.

Collaborative Consultation

The limits of the expert model have led to the adoption of new approaches to consultation. Planning for AAC has broadened, becoming more inclusive of the user and their communication partners. These new approaches focus on *collaboration* and *reciprocity*.

Reciprocity refers to approaching AAC consultation as a dialogue. The SLP is the expert on the content of AAC information. The SLP contributes their knowledge of language development, communication disorders, ATs, and implementation strategies. The SLP teaches the AAC user and their partners to consciously plan for the different functions and modes of communication, as well as the various skills and competencies needed to meet all of a person's communication needs. In contrast, the AAC user and their partners are the experts on the context of how communication actually occurs for this individual. The context of communication includes who they communicate with, how they communicate, for which communication functions, and how they participate in activities. It includes how well they are understood and where breakdowns in communication occur. But it also includes the individuality of the user, including personal identity, interests, preferences, culture, and background.

SLPs collaborate with PWUAACs and their communication partners to elicit this contextual information. Reciprocity allows the SLP's content knowledge to inform the context knowledge of the AAC user and their partners to select the best-fit AAC supports. Dunst and colleagues (2007) describe these as relational practices necessary for reciprocity between SLPs and families. These practices include beliefs that value the knowledge of users and families, and clinical skills that foster sharing, such as active listening, trustworthiness, and empathy.

Collaboration recognizes that communication is highly contextual and deeply personal. SLPs partner with users and their social network to understand how communication is currently happening, then involve them in all aspects of AAC decision-making. Collaboration builds on reciprocal dialogue to identify and prioritize the user's unmet communication needs, select AAC, and commit to an implementation plan. It recognizes that communication is only as good as the countless interactions between a PWUAAC and their regular partners. Collaboration helps ensure that the selected technology builds the capacity of the PWUAAC and their partners to be better understood, and to better understand the other. Dunst and colleagues (2007) describe these as participatory practices, including SLP responsiveness to family priorities and needs, and active involvement of users and families in AAC decision-making.

Collaborative consultation is even more important when the AAC learner has emerging language skills. Families and caregivers are the most important influence in early language development. Every daily interaction is an opportunity for the AAC learner and their family to attend closely to what the other is expressing, and to respond with sensitivity and encouragement. The messages exchanged in each routine, activity, or unexpected event are how children learn to share ideas and information, ask questions, protest, make requests, and begin to comment and develop narrative skills. Families know how their learner participates in ordinary activities, and where this participation is least successful. They must be enlisted to help map symbolic language to the communication demands of daily life. The best AAC technology is only as good

as its implementation by caring adults in the learner's life. Collaborative consultation recognizes that families are the most important actors to develop a learner's language and communication skills. Collaborative consultation is a commitment to build the capacity of the entire family by providing sufficient support, information, skill development, and technology.

The collaborative approach is widely recognized for improving AAC outcomes. It is consistent with the values and beliefs of most SLPs (Mandak & Light, 2018) and is enshrined in professional practice guidance (e.g., American Speech-Language-Hearing Association [ASHA], n.d.) and legislation (e.g., Individuals with Disabilities Education Improvement Act [IDEA], 2004). IDEA requires the provision of services in natural environments rather than clinical settings. This allows PWUAACs and their families to learn and practice skills in the same setting where those skills will be used and generalized to new contexts. Intervention processes have shifted from the clinician providing direct therapy to the child, to the clinician supporting the child's communication partners to embed intervention in ordinary daily routines and activities. This intensifies the effect of AAC intervention, by distributing opportunities for learning across an entire day with multiple partners, rather than assuming all AAC learning can occur primarily in clinical settings. It also builds the capacity and efficacy of families, educators, and communication partners as well as the PWUAAC. Table 31–1 compares and contrasts expert-led versus collaborative consultation practices.

The challenge of collaboration, however, is in its application (Mandak & Light, 2018). The remainder of this chapter focuses on the professional practices that foster authentic collaborative consultation.

The Collaborative Consultation Process

There are five essential tasks for the SLP in the collaborative consultation process: (a) learn from the PWUAAC and their partners, (b) teach the PWUAAC and their partners, (c) develop consensus

Table 31–1. Observable Signs of Expert-Led Versus Collaborative Consultation

Expert-Led Approach	Collaborative Approach
Clinic or therapy room setting	In family home or classroom, preschool, or community
Special one-off activity	Regular daily routines and activities
Special materials (e.g., symbol board for a single book or activity)	Incorporate materials that are already in place, such as the books already in the house
Speech-language pathologist (SLP) working 1:1 with student; parent or educator passively observing or not present	SLP observes and supports from the sidelines, stepping in to support parent or partner
SLP problem-solves and enacts strategies without explanation	SLP uses "I wonder" statements and questions like "what do you think would happen if . . ." to teach problem-solving
The form of AAC use is more important than function	Function of communication more important than the form: Was it understood? Could anyone understand it?
"Homework" activities make caregivers a proxy for SLP	"Homework" activities are to practice different routines for feedback and self-reflection
SLP describes new strategies without demonstration or feedback	SLP demonstrates new strategies or technologies, explains the purpose, and invites the partner to give it a try on their own and brainstorm when/if it might be helpful; SLP provides additional demonstrations as needed

on the problem(s) we are trying to solve with AAC, (d) share the decision-making in selecting AAC solutions and strategies, and (e) build capacity for AAC implementation. These five tasks are drawn from the literature addressing family-centered services and intervention (e.g., Mandak & Light, 2018; Starble et al., 2005) and collaborative consultation (e.g., Woods et al., 2011). Each role demands more of the SLP than the traditional consultation approach because of the need for these reciprocal collaborative practices. Before, an SLP might conduct evaluations without needing to explain what they were assessing or what criteria they used to select a technology. Assessment results were often shared as data points, rather than as insights into what is working or not working in the user's communicative interactions. Now, SLPs need to share what they are considering and why it matters. They involve PWUAACs and their partners in evaluating different options so they can make informed judgements on what works or does not work in their particular context. This means that SLPs must move beyond the role of experts to become learners, teachers, coaches, and facilitators.

Speech-Language Pathologists as Learners

SLPs must start the AAC consultation process from a place of discovery and curiosity about the values and priorities of the user and their partners. These may differ from those of the SLP, and the SLP should be prepared to suspend their personal assumptions about what priorities should guide AAC implementation. Learning from users and their partners often starts with gathering background information and interviewing stakeholders. Then it goes further, by investing time to observe the user during their communicative interactions to notice patterns of participation, observe current problem-solving strategies, and identify where breakdowns are occurring.

SLPs learn from the PWUAAC and their partners in part to gauge each stakeholder's background knowledge and familiarity with AAC technology and implementation strategies. Many families need time to process new information and wrap their heads around the need for AAC intervention. The SLP learns what methods and formats the user and their partners prefer to receive new information. These formats include hands-on observation of in-person demonstrations or role-plays, viewing recorded video demonstrations or presentations, reading print articles or websites, or participating in social media groups or following influencers. This information helps the SLP consider issues like format and text readability when deciding what information to share at any given time.

SLPs should also invite the PWUAAC and their family members to share the resources they have already discovered on their own. Many have researched AAC extensively before the AAC evaluation has even started. They may be well-informed on emerging technologies or evidence-based strategies within a particular population. Knowledge sharing must be reciprocal and part of a dialogue, so that SLPs are eliciting and learning as much from PWUAACs and their families as they are teaching in return.

Speech-Language Pathologists as Teachers

SLPs empower PWUAACs and their families to collaborate when they level the information playing field so that all parties can contribute. Collaborative AAC consultation respects users, families, and communication partners wherever they may be in this process. For SLPs, this means thinking more like an educator than a clinician, considering how to prepare users and their families to become informed members of a collaborative team. Families who try to learn AAC implementation on their own are often bombarded with competing information on different devices and strategies. SLPs can curate this information to prevent being overwhelmed.

They can individualize information for families and provide it in preferred formats and in manageable doses. This involves sharing expert knowledge and expertise in plain language that feels accessible to PWUAAC, families, and educators. It means expecting that users and families can learn the terminology, technologies, strategies, and communication partner skills necessary for effective AAC use, but they need to learn it over time and at their own pace.

Many families approach AAC as though they are just starting to work on communication with their nonspeaking child; they may not realize how much communication is already happening. SLPs as educators teach families how much communication is already taking place. Whenever possible, maximize and build on what is already familiar and natural. This may mean introducing a single new technology or strategy into only the most familiar contexts, such as natural environments with familiar partners during ordinary daily routines. If a family member is already responsive and attentive to their child, then SLPs should name this responsivity and explain its importance to the child's language development. If a caregiver is actively problem-solving the function behind a child's gestures or behavior, then SLPs can celebrate their initiative while expanding the strategies or tools the caregiver uses to respond. This builds confidence and self-efficacy by helping families realize how much they already know. If communication partners are not yet responsive to the AAC learner, then the SLP might first teach responsive skills before adding on new technology. In these cases, consider working with the family to develop a gesture inventory and dictionary to help the partners correctly interpret and respond to all current communication attempts.

Teaching PWUAACs and their communication partners includes scaffolding their experiences with new technologies in ways that build confidence and efficacy. SLPs can predict that AAC technologies (e.g., speech-generating devices [SGDs] and symbol displays), and intervention strategies (e.g., aided language stimulation), may be unfamiliar and intimidating to new users and their partners. SLPs can ease this discomfort by using the plainest language to describe and demonstrate them. SLPs should define new terminology and explain new strategies each time they use them, knowing that most users and their families will need to hear new terms many times before their meaning becomes familiar.

SLPs are expert problem-solvers in the area of communication breakdowns. SLPs need to model and teach these problem-solving strategies to PWUAACs and their partners. Use teaching strategies such as think-alouds to make the SLP's internal problem-solving process more transparent to families. This can include reflecting aloud on what worked or did not work, asking questions, and using "I wonder" statements to provoke users and their communication partners to notice patterns, visualize how a learner might respond to a strategy, or imagine how a technology could fit into an activity. This supports families to become stronger problem-solvers themselves.

Developing Consensus on the Problem

PWUAACs and their partners may disagree with the SLP (and each other) about which technology or strategy is the most appropriate. Disagreement can result from a lack of consensus about the problem we are trying to solve with AAC. Do we agree about which communication needs are currently met, and which needs are unmet? Do we agree on the highest priorities for intervention? Have we considered all the different contexts where communication occurs before setting priorities? Do we agree that partners also need to learn new strategies, or does the family expect that only the AAC learner needs to be taught new skills? Disagreement is common when there is a mismatch between expectations and understanding about the nature of the problem.

SLPs can support consensus by encouraging the user and their partners to thoughtfully set priorities. What does the user most want to change in their communication outcomes, as evidenced in everything from their formal communication to their behaviors and mood or affect? What do partners know is important for the user, in how they participate and interact with others over a day or week? What is most important right now? What is important in the future, as the learner grows and

requires more independence with more communication partners? Is there any conflict between different stakeholder perspectives?

Families and partners may need explicit support to separate their priorities from those of their AAC learner. For example, the AAC learner may have early language skills but demonstrate through their behavior that participating in peer social interactions is important to them. The AAC learner may feel that an AAC device is cumbersome and interferes with those peer interactions. The whole team will need to consider how to respect and balance this concern with the need to foster AAC adoption.

It is essential to collect the AAC user's perspective on what is working and not working in their communication, in which contexts, and with which partners. Many PWUAACs may participate more effectively in this process using a Talking Mats approach. Talking Mats is a structured conversation designed to elicit the AAC user's perspective. The interviewer asks open-ended questions about a specific target topic, using visual supports and a simple rating scale to help the PWUAAC express their views (Cameron & Matthews, 2017). The process of Talking Mats is designed to level the communication playing field by situating the PWUAAC at the center of their own planning. PWUAACs with a range of underlying communication disorders may find it easier to organize their thoughts, participate in discussion, express critical opinions, and evaluate the quality of their existing supports during a Talking Mats interview. See the case study and Figure 31–1 for an example of the visual supports provided by Talking Mats.

Shared Decision-Making

AAC consultation is most effective when it brings users and their families into the decision-making process of selecting and implementing the best-fit AAC technology. Clinical practice guidelines encourage SLPs to involve users and their families in this decision-making to the greatest extent possible (ASHA, n.d.). Shared decision-making requires strong consensus on the problem, as well as a shared knowledge base about the technologies and strategies that might be selected to solve

Top Scale

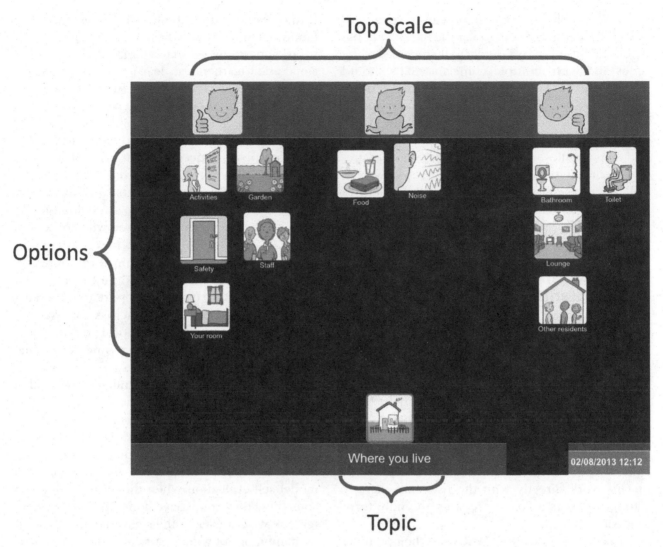

Options

Topic

Figure 31–1. An example of a Talking Mat visual support. © Talking Mats LTD

it. Shared decision-making fosters self-determination and self-advocacy by creating new space for the PWUAAC or learner to participate in decisions about their own AT and accommodations.

Stakeholders may disagree about the best-fit AAC for an individual user. SLPs can foster effective shared decision-making by helping the team develop the criteria by which they will judge success before a final decision is made. For example, if one stakeholder had a strong preference for a particular solution, the team might agree to trial that option for a set period of time, then evaluate its success based on criteria the team developed ahead

of that trial. Criteria can include data such as the rate of initiation and use of the AAC device by the user, patterns of use with new and existing communication partners or for different communication functions, or PWUAACs and partner satisfaction with the features of the technology. Establishing the criteria for success before the trial builds commitment regarding what data need to be collected and builds understanding for how that data will be used in decision-making. This approach encourages PWUAACs and their partners to take ownership of AAC implementation by respecting their preferences in device and strategy trials.

AAC consultation often appears to end with device selection. However, over the life span of the AAC user, this process is likely to be repeated many times and with multiple clinicians. SLPs should understand AAC selection as an iterative process that will evolve along with the AAC user, and in sync with changes in technology and the user's environments. For better or for worse, PWUAACs and their families will bring the experiences of previous consultations with them to each new one. Collaborative consultation prepares them both to implement AAC decisions, and to participate more effectively and openly in future consultations.

Building Capacity for AAC Implementation

The final goal of AAC consultation is not simply to provide AAC technology to those who need it. Rather, it is to see that technology is effectively implemented to expand the AAC user's participation in all aspects of life. Consultation must build the capacity of PWUAACs and their partners to implement new technology and strategies in ordinary daily life. This collaboration requires SLPs to shift from the role of clinicians to coaches. Clinicians work directly with the user in a therapy setting, whereas a coach prepares an entire team as a cohesive unit.

Coaches support PWUAACs and their partners as active learners. SLPs demonstrate new strategies and tools, then encourage users and their partners to observe, explore, and practice. Coaches provide informative feedback, support problem-solving, and help users and their families reflect on what worked. Some families may appear to be passive observers. SLPs can explicitly tell them what to look for and why it matters. Give specific instructions, such as "watch me highlight symbols on this display while I talk, so you can try it yourself next." Some families are more engaged when the SLP helps them draft a short checklist of practices to look for as they observe the SLP. Family members can notice how many times the SLP used an expectant pause or count how many seconds the SLP allowed that pause to last. They can observe in order to give examples of how the SLP followed the learner's

lead or expanded on the learner's message. If the family member is still hesitant, encourage them to ask questions or share their concerns. While some adult learners can learn just from watching or reading, most adult learners need to see multiple demonstrations, then receive support while they practice. Avoid leaving family members with homework to practice a skill independently if they have not first practiced with a coach. If only one communication partner is actively engaged, consider inviting additional partners to observe them and provide feedback, using the same "look-for" or "look-at" that the first partner used when observing the SLP. After demonstrating a new strategy, ask users and their partners to brainstorm more routines or activities when it could be helpful. Some families need this explicit support to generalize how a strategy could be used across contexts.

Self-evaluation is also a critical step in coaching and active learning. PWUAACs need to reflect on their own communication successes and failures to learn effective repair strategies when they are misunderstood. Families and partners need to engage in self-evaluation to become more responsive supporters of the PWUAAC. Coaches create a safe space for self-reflection when they encourage feedback on their own practice and teaching. SLPs model self-evaluation when they reflect aloud on something they could have done differently or better. Ask what a user or their partners thinks could be helpful or not with a particular strategy or tool. If a family expresses doubt about its value, treat this information as a form of assessment data. Consider shifting the focus to a skill the family feels confident using, then revisit the new strategy at a later date. Some families may simply need more time to process the new information. They may benefit from materials they can study on their own, such as videos or articles, then discuss again at the next session. Other families may find that new strategies make them question if they have been doing everything wrong up until this point. Help families celebrate all their communication success to date. SLPs can share stories of how their own practice has changed as they have learned new information. At the end of a meeting, ask users and their partners to reflect on what was most helpful. Use this feedback to inform how you approach the next session.

Coaches help users and their partners set realistic time frames within which to see growth. Many families wish for a quick fix with AAC technology. Reciprocity and collaboration include helping families understand that communication skills develop over a lifetime. If a learner is making slow progress, encourage partners to focus on their own growth and success as they develop new skills. Effective AAC implementation is often as much about improving communication partner skills as it is about the user adopting new technologies. Help partners measure success by how often they fostered authentic choice-making, demonstrated the use of a device, ensured the SGD was charged and available, or waited patiently for the user to express an idea. When communication partners seem unmotivated or intimidated, consider ways to help them identify the barriers they are facing so they can start addressing them. For example, some SLPs assign homework-style tasks for families to do between therapy visits. These kinds of tasks can be motivating when the family is successful but can have the opposite effect when the task reinforces the family's feeling of failure. Instead, ask families to notice what got in their way. For example, what interfered with having AAC available during mealtimes this week? The list may be long, but unpacking these barriers can become the focus of collaborative problem-solving as the SLP and family slowly work through them. Maybe the family will decide that bath time is a better routine to practice new skills with AAC than dinner. Maybe they will notice that while the caregivers are busy at mealtime, a sibling is available to take on the role of making AAC available. Each problem that made success difficult can lead to an insight that teaches problem-solving and fosters later success.

Collaborative consultation might appear cumbersome and time-consuming. It often is, but the alternative to collaboration is worse. SLPs have prescribed too many devices that were abandoned, while families and users have tried to go it alone selecting iOS apps with no clinical guidance or support. Many support teams invest countless hours troubleshooting challenging behaviors without establishing an effective communication system or consistently responsive communication partners. The final task of collaboration is often advocacy to

ensure that SLPs have the time and resources they need to do AAC consultation correctly. As a field, SLPs need to push back against AAC evaluation processes that leave users and their families out of key decisions. Expert-led consultations cut corners in important areas where stakeholder investment is crucial to long-term success. The following case study illustrates how investing in the practices of collaborative consultation builds a cohesive team.

Case Study: JE

Clinical Profile and Communication Needs

JE is a 14-year-old female with multiple disabilities who was diagnosed with a neurogenetic disorder, Angelman syndrome, at age 2 years. Her epilepsy was controlled with medication throughout most of childhood, but absence seizures returned at puberty. She experiences migraines, a sleep disorder, and gastroesophageal reflux. Her family carefully observes JE for signs of pain or seizures, such as rising agitation, holding her head, and rapid eye blinking.

JE produces some consonant sounds but no recognizable words. She regularly uses a handful of idiosyncratic manual signs to refer to favorite people or items. JE has been monitored by speech-language pathology since age 2 years. She had limited success with the Picture Exchange Communication System (PECS) at age 4 years. At age 7 years, JE was prescribed an iPad with the app GoTalk NOW. Her mother has been the primary person responsible for adding words to the app and feels the system is currently working because JE direct selects to navigate between sections. She was referred for AAC evaluation by her special educator out of concern that JE had outgrown the AAC system she has used for 7 years. JE's special educator describes her current AAC vocabulary as a large, unwieldy hodgepodge of over 80 unrelated activity-based pages. Each page includes a few relevant core words combined with photographs of nouns. For example, the word "eat" appears on the food page along with photos of JE's regular meal and snack options. JE has old pages that date back to her old Scouting days, with prerecorded messages for everything from the Brownie promise to complete camp songs.

In preparation for transition planning, the school psychologist recently completed the *Supports Intensity Scale* (SIS) (Shogren et al., 2017). Overall, the SIS indicates that JE's support needs have stayed consistent since the time she first moved to the school system from early intervention. At age 3 years, JE's scores on the *Bayley Scales of Infant Development, Third Edition* (Weiss et al., 2010) assigned her an age equivalency of 10 months for cognition, 11 months for receptive and expressive communication, 8 months for fine motor skills, and 18 months for gross motor skills. Now, at age 14 years, JE's overall *Support Needs Index* score on the SIS was 123. This indicates a Support Needs Index Percentile Rank of 90. This means that JE has more intense support needs than 90% of the standardized sample of individuals with developmental disability. Across all areas of daily living, the SIS indicates that JE requires full or partial physical assistance on a frequent basis for much of the day. JE requires the most support in the domains of home living (e.g., personal care, eating and preparing food) and lifelong learning (e.g., problem-solving, self-determination, functional academics). She has relative strengths in the areas of community living (e.g., participating in preferred community activities, visiting friends and family) and social activities (e.g., making and keeping friends, participating in leisure activities, socializing within the household). JE's pattern of support needs indicates that there are significant concerns regarding her safety due to medical issues, including extensive support to stimulate swallowing and prevent choking, and to monitor and treat her epilepsy. JE has extensive support needs to prevent a range of behaviors, including emotional outbursts, injuries to others, damage to property, wandering, and pica.

The Individual

JE is a sociable teenager. During observation of a typical afternoon routine at home, the SLP noticed JE use a variety of activity-specific pages to request preferred items for a snack and to mention spe-

cific people at school. JE's family expanded on her messages verbally by repeating her utterance and commenting. JE often responded with vigorous head nods but did not always respond. JE spontaneously used social pagesets recorded by her sisters to engage the SLP in joke telling. She did not, however, have the vocabulary necessary to help her respond to the SLP's jokes. JE successfully used photographs and activity pages to set the topic of conversation with family. Specifically, JE used a scene display from a visit to an amusement park and combined it with an adapted sign (lifting her flat hand in a rising gesture) to set the topic of roller coasters. JE's love of roller coasters is legendary in her family. JE's family members were very responsive and correctly interpreted this as a cue to talk about an amusement park trip. JE became frustrated, however, when her stepfather apparently told the wrong story associated with that park. JE shook her head vigorously, vocalized, and beat on her head with her palm. Her mother used the prompt "show me," and JE scrolled through her iPad photo app to find a photograph of the specific event she was recalling. This repair strategy was successful, and JE's stepfather told a different story about a roller-coaster misadventure. JE clapped her hands and jumped in pleasure as the story was shared. While the desired story was eventually shared, the SLP noticed that the entire family experienced stress managing JE's participation in the story. She waited for a relaxed opportunity to discuss this stress with JE's mother and stepfather. She praised them for their problem-solving and responsiveness before encouraging them to imagine what it could look like for JE to share more of her own stories herself.

Their Communication Partners

JE lives with her family, including her mother, stepfather, and an older brother. Two stepsisters are attending college and come home periodically. JE is close to her sisters, and they FaceTime daily. These calls are a highlight of JE's day, but her participation is limited to vocalizations, gestures, facial expressions, and idiosyncratic signs. JE's father lives 2 hours away and visits infrequently. JE's mother reports that her ex-husband does not feel comfortable visiting JE without a support worker. She would like to support JE to be closer to her father.

Their Environment

JE has attended school with the same cohort of students since preschool. She is in ninth grade and receives special education support in both regular and special contexts. In childhood, she attended summer camp and Scouts and frequently had friends over for playdates. JE's sisters helped facilitate these friendships. Her family, however, has been at a loss to support JE to maintain these friendships in adolescence, especially once her sisters left home. Her mother reports JE's old friends message her rather than JE. She is exploring options for JE to engage with same-age peers in a local youth activity.

AAC Considerations

JE's family and school team have started transition planning. She was referred for AAC evaluation by her special education teacher. The special educator has tried to introduce JE to both Proloquo2Go® and Language Acquisition through Motor Planning (LAMP) (systems she currently uses with other students) but finds JE will not even look at the displays. She has also noticed that JE is drawn to another student's high-contrast Picture Communication Symbols (PCS). The special educator would like to evaluate the symbol set and teach JE to generate novel sentences with a core word vocabulary.

The SLP interviewed the family (mother, stepfather, brother) and the special education teacher to complete the *Pragmatics Profile for People who use AAC* (Martin et al., 2017). She selected this free structured interview in order to elicit as much information as possible about the range of nonlinguistic methods JE uses to meet a variety of communication needs. She felt the Pragmatics Profile would prepare the team (especially JE's mother) for conversations about JE's unmet communication needs. The *Pragmatics Profile* asks a series of strengths-based open-ended questions, such as, "If JE doesn't want something to happen, something

that she doesn't have an option about, how does she tell you?" The SLP then charted the responses in summary tables so the team could discuss JE's overall communication methods and identify unmet communication needs. See Figure 31–2 for a sample page of a summary chart.

The chart showed that JE's most common communication methods are eye pointing or eye contact, and body movements and gestures. Her AAC device is used when gaining or drawing attention, naming, and requesting. While her gestures and use of eye gaze are easily interpreted by all communication partners, only her most familiar partners can interpret her vocalizations and signs. JE has few methods of sharing information, commenting, or asking questions. She has many ways to reject, but these are only understood by familiar partners and can be perceived as challenging behaviors.

The special educator had reported that JE was drawn to the high-contrast PCS symbols used by another student. The SLP requested information on JE's functional vision. JE's mother says JE was prescribed prescription lenses in the past but refused to wear them. JE's visual acuity indicated significant astigmatism and near-sightedness. JE had not been screened for cortical visual impairment (CVI). The SLP observed JE's special education classroom and noticed that she was drawn to bold visuals on a backlit screen and to visuals that moved (such as videos or animations) but avoided engaging with a range of other visuals. The SLP requested a screening for CVI from the teacher for the visually impaired, who conducted an assessment and found JE to have mild CVI. JE has largely integrated her vision with movement and demonstrates visual curiosity, along with regard for most high-contrast colors. She has difficulty with visual complexity and isolating novel items from a busy array. She warms up quickly to novel materials presented in isolation against a black background.

The SLP set up multiple, short opportunities to interview JE directly using a Talking Mats format. She used Talking Mats as a form of dynamic assessment, to determine how well JE could engage with graphic symbols and participate in multiple turns in a structured conversation on a high-interest topic. The SLP was particularly interested in how

Appendix 1: Methods of communication chart

*FO = Understood by familiar only
ALL = Understood by all

		Uses AAC resource: single words	Uses AAC resource: sentence or phrase	Eye pointing, eye contact		Body movement		Vocalisation, sound, word or word approximation		Sign		Gesture		Facial expression		Other
				FO*	ALL	FO	ALL	FO	ALL	FO	ALL	FO	ALL	FO	ALL	
1	**Context and motivation**															
1.1	Shows likes	☒	☐	☐	☒	☐	☒	☒	☐	☐	☐	☐	☒	☐	☒	☐
1.2	Shows dislikes	☒	☐	☐	☒	☐	☒	☒	☐	☐	☐	☐	☒	☒	☒	☐
2	**Gaining attention**															
2.1	Interest in interaction	☐	☐	☐	☐	☐	☒	☒	☐	☐	☐	☐	☒	☐	☒	☐
2.4	Gaining attention to prepare for an interaction	☒	☐	☐	☐	☐	☒	☒	☐	☐	☐	☐	☒	☐	☒	☐
3	**Drawing attention**															
3.1	... to self	☒	☐	☐	☒	☐	☒	☐	☒	☐	☐	☐	☒	☐	☒	☐
3.2	... to an event or action	☒	☐	☐	☒	☐	☒	☐	☒	☐	☒	☐	☒	☐	☐	☐
3.3	... to an object	☒	☐	☐	☒	☐	☒	☐	☒	☐	☐	☐	☐	☐	☐	☐
3.4	... to other people	☒	☐	☐	☒	☐	☒	☐	☐	☒	☐	☐	☐	☐	☐	☐
4	**Requesting**															
4.1	... a person	☒	☐	☐	☐	☐	☐	☒	☐	☒	☐	☒	☐	☐	☐	☐
4.2	... recurrence	☐	☐	☐	☐	☐	☐	☒	☐	☐	☐	☐	☐	☐	☐	☐
4.3	... cessation	☐	☐	☐	☐	☐	☐	☒	☐	☐	☒	☐	☒	☐	☐	☐
4.4	... assistance	☒	☐	☐	☐	☐	☐	☒	☒	☐	☐	☐	☐	☐	☐	☐
4.5	... an object	☒	☐	☐	☒	☐	☐	☒	☒	☐	☐	☐	☐	☐	☐	☐
4.6	Responding to direct request for action	☐	☐	☐	☐	☐	☐	☐	☐	☐	☐	☐	☐	☐	☐	☐
4.7	... an event or action	☒	☐	☐	☒	☐	☐	☒	☒	☐	☐	☐	☐	☐	☐	☐
4.8	... information	☒	☐	☐	☐	☐	☐	☒	☐	☐	☐	☐	☐	☐	☒	☐
4.9	Responding to a request for information	☐	☐	☐	☐	☐	☐	☐	☐	☐	☐	☐	☐	☐	☐	☐
4.10	... confirmation of information	☐	☐	☐	☐	☐	☐	☐	☐	☐	☐	☐	☐	☐	☐	☐
5	**Rejecting**															
5.1	... a person	☐	☐	☐	☒	☐	☐	☒	☐	☒	☐	☐	☒	☐	☒	☐

Figure 31–2. Sample page of a Summary Chart, included in the Pragmatics Profile for People who use AAC (Martin et al., 2017). © Ace Centre

JE might demonstrate her comprehension of the topics of conversation. She scheduled these interviews as short interactions distributed over several weeks in order to see if JE built skills used in Talking Mats across sessions. The SLP also viewed these interviews as training opportunities for JE's partners. She scheduled them at times when both JE's mother and special educator could observe.

The SLP prepared for the Talking Mats interviews by first identifying topics where JE has well-established preferences such as food, animals, and amusement park rides. The SLP printed a selection of high-contrast symbols of animals, along with the symbols for LIKE, DON'T LIKE, and ANIMALS. She displayed LIKE and DON'T LIKE in each corner of a large black slanting felt board. She put the symbol for ANIMALS at the bottom. She reserved a stack of symbols for various common animals. JE was immediately curious about the symbols. She moved her face close to the symbols and listened intently as the symbols were named. The SLP explained that they were going to talk about animals. Different people like different animals, and she wanted to know what animals JE liked. The SLP demonstrated the use of the symbols by saying, "We will talk about one animal at a time. This picture is for dogs. I'll ask you how you feel about dogs. If you LIKE dogs (as she moved the symbol to the LIKE button) or if you do NOT LIKE dogs (as she moved the symbol to the NOT LIKE side)." JE observed closely while her mother and special educator used the symbols to demonstrate their own preferences. They compared how their opinions about animals were the same or different, to reinforce the idea that there were no right answers in this exercise. When it was her turn, JE pointed to the symbols for dog and cat but did not try to move them to the LIKE or NOT LIKE columns, then quit the activity. One week later, the same set of symbols was used a second time. After observing several models by the adults, JE moved the symbols to indicate her preferences with respect to both foods and animals.

The AAC System. With the information about CVI, the SLP knew that JE was engaged by large, high-contrast symbols. She did not attend to a variety of symbol displays, including those with over 20 symbols on one array, or to displays with symbols that were highly detailed or difficult to distinguish. Given JE's resistance to corrective lenses, the SLP determined that a visually simple AAC display using an array of 20 or less high-contrast symbols was appropriate.

JE's mother felt that the activity-based system in the GoTalk NOW app helped her daughter be successful. She preferred to keep the same app but add additional words. JE's special educator agreed that there was a role for some activity-specific pages but felt the current system was not tenable. She gave examples of how JE has to jump between different pages to combine ordinary high-frequency core words. JE's special educator already models large displays of the Proloquo2Go app and LAMP in her classroom. She had hoped that one of those could be used with JE but now realized they were not visually accessible. JE's mother and special educator agreed that they could use a well-organized system with a combination of core vocabulary and some activity-specific pages to scaffold participation in ordinary routines.

The SLP shared examples of early Pragmatic Organization Dynamic Display (PODD) books to demonstrate how core vocabulary, categories, and activity-themed pages could be organized into one system. The family had heard about PODD from within their online parent community. JE's mother was reassured to know other families who felt it was successful. The SLP felt that a 12-per-page one-page opening PODD with high-contrast PCS symbols would provide manageable visual complexity. She felt it would be relatively simple to move JE to a 20-per-page book once she understood the navigation and was initiating use of PODD for multiple purposes. JE's mother wondered if they could program PODD into the current app. They explored this idea but decided it was too onerous and prone to problems. They agreed to compare commercial options for the PODD vocabulary.

JE's special educator wanted to shift her to using more symbols rather than photographs. But JE's mother was concerned that photographs are a key support to JE's communication. The SLP suggested that memory books or social media could help JE better use visuals to share experiences and explore narratives. JE's mother and sisters were active on Instagram and Facebook, so they began to plan how to support JE to share on those platforms. JE's mother was reassured that changing AAC systems would not mean taking away JE's rich library of photos and videos.

The SLP agreed with the special educator that JE's current and future communication needs cannot be met using her existing AAC. JE requires AAC that can express a range of communication functions, novel utterances, and repair strategies. The team decided to do the following:

1. Continue using and teaching the Talking Mats process to involve JE in her transition planning. The special educator was enthusiastic about the Talking Mats framework. Photos of completed mats and written captions could also be the basis of conversation starters with JE's friends and family. Every time JE participated in a mat, her school team or family would help her draft a summary statement to caption it, such as "I like dogs, cats, and chickens. I do not like insects, lizards, and spiders." Talking Mats was also an opportunity for direct instruction on the meaning of the new high-contrast PCS symbols.
2. Introduce a 12-per-page PODD light-tech pageset with high-contrast PCS arrayed on a black background. The team felt this was the best fit for JE's need for bold visuals, reduced visual complexity, and supportive communication partners. JE's mother, sisters, and special educator would attend a PODD training. The SLP and special educator would train JE's school staff.
3. Within the year, introduce PODD on an SGD through the Grid iOS app. The team felt this was the best fit for JE to explore independently and continue her experience with speech output. The new app would be offered on a loaner iPad, alongside JE's current GoTalk NOW app, as she transitioned to the larger vocabulary.
4. Continue to explore social media. JE's mother and sister would set up a cloud-based shared photo album to support distance sharing of photos. JE's sisters would set up social media accounts for JE and support her to invite friends and share content.

The Rationale for the Clinical Decision-Making

Careful attention to JE's strengths, unmet communication needs, and visual considerations yielded a plan and a workable and growable AAC system. Importantly, the SLP listened to all stakeholders and elicited the most important information from JE using Talking Mats to facilitate conversations and with careful observations of JE in her common environments. Owing to JE's diagnosis of CVI, use of LAMP and the Proloquo2Go app was ruled out due to the visual complexity of the displays and JE's need for large symbols.

The agreed-upon system provided avenues for growth while capitalizing on JE's strengths and interests, and involved the entire team in the process of assessment and decision-making.

Next Steps

JE's special educator extended the Talking Mats framework of a rating scale and open-ended questions to a range of instruction for all her students. JE's long-term transition goals reflected the Talking Mats process, with goals to use increasingly sophisticated rating scales to participate in her own decision-making and evaluate critical areas of her life.

The family and school team prioritized modeling the pathways in PODD to ask questions, comment, and give information. JE's first expressive use was to indicate 'Something's Wrong' to express discomfort from headache, and to ask when her sisters were next coming home.

Over summer break, JE's sisters helped her set up social media accounts and a shared iCloud photo library. The sisters modeled possible comments and helped her post photos on her social media. JE enjoyed deciding which family or friends to tag in each photo. The sisters made a habit of tagging JE's father so that he had more to talk with her about when he visited.

Collaborative AAC consultation starts with listening and learning, to build agreement about the nature of the problem. Invest the time to bring the whole team on board to identify unmet communication needs.

Level the playing field so that everyone on the team has the same information.

Do not be afraid to not have the answer. Model how to find out more information and experiment with different options.

Be willing to trial AAC systems or strategies that would not be the SLP's first choice. Help the team set objective, measurable criteria for how they will measure success.

Dynamic assessment can achieve dual purposes, such as learning from the AAC user while simultaneously teaching partners new skills.

The best AAC system is the one that is used most often with the most people to improve how the AAC user participates in ordinary life.

References

American Speech-Language-Hearing Association (ASHA). (n.d.). *Augmentative and alternative communication* [Practice portal]. https://www.asha.org/Practice-Portal/Professional-Issues/Augmentative-and-Alternative-Communication/

Cameron, L., & Matthews, R. (2017). More than pictures: Developing an accessible resource. *Tizard Learning Disability Review, 22*(2), 57–65. https://doi.org/10.1108/TLDR-10-2016-0028

Dunst, C., Trivette, C., & Hamby, D. (2007). Meta-analysis of family-centered help-giving practices research. *Mental Retardation and Developmental Disabilities Research Reviews, 13,* 370–378. https://doi.org/10.1002/mrdd.20176

Individuals with Disabilities Education Improvement Act of 2004, Pub. L. No. 108-446 § 118 Stat. 2647 (2004).

Mandak, K., & Light, J. (2018). Family-centered services for children with complex communication needs: The practices and beliefs of school-based speech-language pathologists. *Augmentative and Alternative Communication, 34*(2), 130–142. https://doi.org/10.1080/07434618.2018.1438513

Martin, S., Small, K., & Stevens, R. (2017). *The Pragmatics Profile for People who use AAC.* https://acecentre.org.uk/resources/pragmatics-profile-people-use-aac/

Shogren, K., Wehmeyer, M., Seo, H., Thompson, J., Schalock, R., Hughes, C., . . . Palmer, S. (2017). Examining the reliability and validity of the Supports Intensity Scale–Children's Version in children with autism and intellectual disability. *Focus on Autism and Other Developmental Disabilities, 32*(4), 293–304. https://doi.org/10.1177/1088357615625060

Starble, A., Hutchins, T., Favro, M., Prelock, P., & Bitner, B. (2005). Family-centered intervention and satisfaction with AAC device training. *Communication Disorders Quarterly, 25*(47), 47–54. https://doi.org/10.1177/15257401050270010501

Weiss, L., Oakland, T., & Aylward, G. (2010). *Bayley-III clinical use and interpretation.* Academic.

Woods, J., Wilcox, M., Friedman, M., & Murch, T. (2011). Collaborative consultation in natural environments: Strategies to enhance family-centered supports and services. *Language, Speech, and Hearing Services in Schools, 42,* 379–392. https://doi.org/10.1044/0161-1461(2011/10-0016)

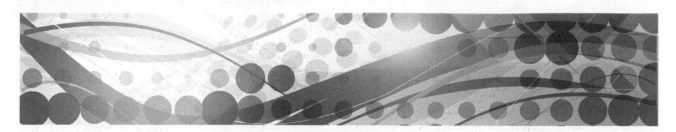

Chapter 32

COMMUNICATION PARTNER TRAINING FOR FAMILIES

Tabitha Jones-Wohleber

Fundamentals

Communication partners are a substantial and essential part of the communication equation for individuals learning to use augmentative and alternative communication (AAC). Transactional by nature, the intrinsically motivated dynamic of authentic communication begs us to enrich our discourse around supporting communication partners to engage in the emotional work of understanding the essence of communication as part of the human experience. Yet this work must also be manageable and empowering, so that families and practitioners can embrace it. Influenced by a myriad of factors, including time, resources, personnel, knowledge, skills, understanding of roles and expectations of team members, reimbursement and other policy factors, as well as perceptions and biases, effective implementation of AAC can be challenging. Well-defined and often executed elements of the implementation process may include procuring an AAC tool and training on the tool. Key ideas for teaching AAC such as using core words and aided language input may also be reviewed. But learning AAC is a journey, not a moment in time. When examining the needs of communication partners learning to use and teach AAC, it is worth reflecting on, and noting the parallels of, the needs of the persons who use AAC (PWUAAC): instruction, time, repetition, relevant (motivating) topics to interact

about, meaningful connection, acknowledgment of effort, a supportive community, and the freedom to make mistakes and receive informative feedback. These considerations (and perhaps others) highlight the need for implementation planning that moves beyond introductory training sessions and addresses the need for ongoing discourse to develop knowledge and skills, problem-solve, and build community around the PWUAAC and their family and, perhaps most important of all, the need to empower communication partners to understand their role as an imperative part of the transaction that is authentic and meaningful communication. This chapter explores considerations and practices for supporting family members and caregivers of individuals learning AAC, with a goal of equipping the reader with the tools to consider the characteristics and components of a thoughtful and responsive implementation process respectfully and creatively.

Person-centered planning constructs can orient and anchor us to our purpose when developing the practices for supporting communication partners. A look at the *Circles of Support* (Snow, 1998), one element of person-centered planning, places communication partners that surround an individual in context. The first and closest circle is the *Circle of Intimacy*. It includes close family members, such as those with whom the individual lives. It may also include grandparents, cousins, or other valued familial relationships, close peers, or family friends. While this chapter specifically discusses implementation support for parents or immediate caregivers, including others from the child's circle of intimacy is a worthwhile endeavor. Collectively, the efforts exerted, and connections, challenges, and joys experienced within the *circle of intimacy* will become an integral part of the journey of the PWUAAC and their family.

The second circle is the *Circle of Friendship* and may include friends and family members with whom an individual enjoys spending time, but they are not as close as those in the circle of intimacy. The *Circle of Participation* is third and includes club memberships, school and workplace connections, sports groups, faith communities, and other such groups. The outermost circle, the *Circle of Exchange*, encompasses those individuals who are paid to be part of an individual's life, such as teachers, doctors, therapists, hairdressers, and so forth. Supporting speech-language pathologists (SLPs) and other professionals as communication partners, who are included in the *Circle of Exchange*, is discussed in Chapters 33 and 34 of this book. It is worth noting that fluidity exists between circles; as relationships develop and roles shift, those in outer circles may move to inner circles. Additionally, the number of individuals in the circle of exchange for individuals with disabilities may be far greater than those in the circles of friendship or participation when compared to nondisabled peers. Limited mobility and communication skills, and the resulting isolation that many people experience can impact opportunities for participation and development of friendships. However, when those in the *circle of intimacy*, and the *circle of exchange*, come together to consider the whole individual, a network of support for AAC implementation that fosters increased participation and opportunities to develop connections with others across circles can emerge. Connection is the essence of communication.

Family Characteristics

Supporting families with AAC implementation is a humbling journey. Guiding families through explo-

ration of options, decision-making, learning, asking, questioning, shifting gears, defining priorities, and discovering their skills and needs in support of being the most effective communication partner they can become, is, for many, a lifelong endeavor. Forging trust is an important first step. However, facilitating a spirit of collaboration is equally imperative. Practitioners must understand that their role in the life of an individual and their family is short-term, even when supporting a family over many years. Expertise is an important resource to families but, ultimately, we are tasked with empowering families to take ownership of their AAC journey and develop *their* expertise such that lifelong advocacy for the communicative rights and opportunities of their loved one is part and parcel to development of the individual's communication skills.

As families are as varied as snowflakes, family dynamics, prerogatives, resources, and needs of individual members inform the AAC implementation process. Considerations may be shaped by cultural influences, socioeconomic factors, geography, family history with disability, and other influences, which may include the following:

- Perceptions (of): AAC, disability, inclusion
- Resources: time, financial, educational, technology
- Support systems: emotional support network, help from family/friends, agency support
- Individual characteristics of caregivers: level of confidence, background knowledge and experiences, capacity for new information and experiences
- Family dynamics and parenting style
- Family priorities and expectations for the individual's participation and development of communication skills
- Characteristics of the individual who uses AAC: verbal and nonverbal communication skills, motor skills, sensory skills and needs, social interaction styles influenced by affect and attention, language and learning skills, medical factors

Often, this information is dynamic and gleaned as relationships with families are developed, anecdotal stories of celebration and challenge are shared, skills are discussed and discovered, and frustrations and concerns are expressed. While "getting started" may be somewhat formulaic, and include an overview of the AAC tool and an introduction to using AAC, *active listening* is a key element that enlightens the subsequent components of AAC implementation; it ensures ongoing support and strategies are responsive and relevant to the family's characteristics and needs, which contributes to family satisfaction with AAC supports and services (Starble et al., 2005). It also fosters pacing of collaboration and resource sharing that is conducive to the family's capacity to utilize information and develop skills over time to support their loved one.

In addition to being responsive to a family's immediate and evolving concerns, the implementation process can also serve the purpose of providing families with valuable resources to shift and shape their understanding of the potential and possibilities for achievement and opportunity for their PWUAAC. Discourse that highlights the characteristics of authentic communication and autonomy, as well as blogs, videos, and social media posts of individuals who use AAC and are thriving with disability, invites families to envision a path toward self-determination and informed advocacy. Such a perspective can inspire deliberate and creative decision-making that puts quality of life at the center of their purpose throughout their journey.

AAC in Everyday Life

Coaching, a service delivery model widely used in Early Intervention, is also useful for supporting families with loved ones of all ages who are learning to use AAC. It is a process by which families are valued as the expert of their child. Practitioners then facilitate a multipart process of inquiry in which caregivers are supported to gain knowledge and nurture skills and habits to facilitate skill development in their child. The combination of strategies utilized includes joint planning, observation, practice, reflection, and feedback (Rush & Shelden, 2020). The relationship with the family

is at the center of this process. Jim Knight (2016) specifies in great detail beliefs and behaviors that foster connection with others through dialogue. Among these, *listening with empathy*, *being non-judgmental with open questions*, and *facilitating back-and-forth conversations that are life-giving* seem especially useful in forging equitable learning relationships between practitioners and families.

Another notable component of the coaching model when supporting families is an emphasis that skills and strategies such as teaching AAC be embedded in the child's and family's natural environment. Natural contexts may include *activities* such as daily routines, self-care routines, and leisure activities; *familiar places* such as home, the grocery store, library, playground, or grandma's house; and *interactions with familiar people* such as mom, brother, peers, bus driver, or teammates. Providing "right-size" strategies that reflect a family's immediate needs and priorities, such as those described in the following sections, can be integrated into everyday life to build confidence with AAC implementation.

All-the-Time Access

Helping families articulate and problem-solve logistical limitations of AAC use can foster awareness of those limitations and investment in ensuring ample communication opportunities. Aided language tools are an added physical item in the environment. Use of a strap, harness, handle, or mount may be needed for portability and positioning. At home, a device may not move from room to room with a child all day long. Having paper-based AAC on the fridge, on the coffee table, or next to the bathtub (laminated of course) creates easy access and reduces the logistical burden of aided language. It may also be useful for communication partners to wear AAC lanyards providing easy access across environments. Keeping paper-based copies of AAC layouts in the family vehicle ensures AAC is available with little planning when on the go. Paper-based tools may be a copy of the core page of an individual's technology-based system, targeted vocabulary for a location or activity, or a combination.

Leverage Requesting

Choice-making and requesting is the communicative function for which many families readily provide opportunities. Building on what they are already doing, requesting can be leveraged to include comments and descriptive language, as well as help families understand the importance of refusal. A strict focus on repeated requests can limit turns, compromise engagement, and minimize the range of communicative functions used. Following up a request with a comment such as *"that is a good choice," "you really like that,"* or *"I'm surprised you chose that"* extends opportunities to model AAC and adds interest to the interaction. Similarly, using AAC to model descriptive language can add richness to the exchange. For instance, when selecting music, it may be described as loud, fast, crazy, or beautiful. Refusal may be an under-recognized component of choice-making. Whether conscious or unconscious, not choosing or refusing the choices presented may be perceived as lack of ability, lack of cooperation, or noncompliance. Reframing disinterest and refusal as the individual's way of communicating "that is not what I want" can create a powerful shift toward a more productive and respectful dynamic.

"Something Different"— All-the-Time Choice

"Something different" can be incorporated as an all-the-time choice (Erin Sheldon, personal communication, February 2019). Adding "something different" to an array of choices provides the PWUAAC the opportunity to express that they want something different than the options presented. For instance, if *apple, crackers, yogurt,* and *something different* are presented, and the individual selects *something different,* additional choices can be offered. Of course, communication partners will likely need to teach *something different.* Following the child's lead, when no choice is made, frustration is expressed, or the PWUAAC is expressing a request but not related to the choices presented, the communication partner points to *something different,* and says "maybe you want something different," and proceeds to offer other choices. In addition to offering more choices, selecting *something different* may invite the communication partner to offer *no thanks* as an alternative choice. Ensuring that individuals who use AAC can assert their preferences, absent an expectation of compliance, is an important form of advocacy to ensure their unique voice is heard and valued.

Referencing

Verbal referencing is a form of think-aloud where caregivers observe their child, describe nonverbal language, and label what it means. For instance, while watching a show, mom may say, "I see you smiling, I think you find that funny," while demonstrating "it funny" with AAC. Seeing a child go to the door and get upset that it will not open, dad could say, "You look frustrated. I think you want to go out. Let me help you." This strategy helps families recognize and begin to add language to the multimodal communication strategies their loved one uses, and provides embedded opportunities to use AAC in everyday interactions. Verbal referencing may need to be practiced without AAC before adding AAC to the equation.

Before, During, and After

Some activities do not lend themselves to ample opportunities to use AAC, such as playing on the playground or at the water park, sledding, going for a hayride, or other such activities. However, these experiences may be among the most meaningful and motivating to talk about. Discussing the role of AAC before, during, and after the activity is of great utility in empowering families to enjoy and embrace the moment, yet still provide meaningful opportunities to use AAC to talk about the experience. Before the activity, use AAC to talk about where, who, and what. Encourage families to ensure some form of AAC is available, technology or paper-based, during the activity, if possible. But if demonstrating AAC is too cumbersome, suggest they take a few photos and just have fun. Afterward, review the photos and use AAC to talk about it. To extend this natural and motivated interaction, share the photos with others, and continue to use AAC to talk about the experience, providing repeated practice and opportunities for connection.

Addressing current concerns and discussing communication strategies in everyday activities makes use of AAC immediately tangible. Clinicians who model skills and interaction personally or through video examples show "what it looks like." As families begin to make AAC a part of their daily practice, the need for additional information, often shaped by new questions, may arise to continue to move their AAC adventure forward. Connecting with or learning about the experiences of other families who use AAC may also be beneficial. Ongoing discourse brings awareness to what is needed to support families to actualize the communicative potential of their loved one who uses AAC.

Spiraling Learning Experiences for AAC Communication Partners: Four Key Elements

In addition to right-size strategies, a big picture perspective is also needed to effectively support families. Revisiting topics repeatedly in different contexts over time, also known as spiraling, is useful for addressing four key elements of AAC implementation: Information, Technology/Tools, Skills, and Habits (Erin Sheldon, personal conversation, May 2020). Some caregivers seek out information and put themselves to the task of becoming an expert before taking action to apply the information. Others are eager for hands-on practice. Still others are focused on the technology or tool—how it works and how to manage or customize it. Regardless of the focal point of initial energies, integrating all four elements equips families with a well-rounded toolbox for engaging with and advocating for the communicative needs of their loved one. The four elements are outlined next.

Information

Exploring an array of topics can serve as a springboard for informing and inspiring families as they get started and move forward on their AAC journey. While key points such as the role of core vocabulary and the importance of aided language input are prioritized, discussions about language development and AAC, honoring multimodal communication, and the necessity of motivation to foster authentic interactions, among others, are also imperative to establish a robust foundation for implementing AAC. Timely and relevant information to provide answers to questions, or to specifically address a family's frustrations is also needed. For instance, myths about the hierarchical nature of symbol representation abound; explaining the limitations of photos may be necessary to facilitate an openness to using a symbol set that will allow an AAC system to grow with a child.

Where to start and how to continue should align with a family's needs. As first steps with AAC can feel overwhelming, distilling new and often complex information into manageable chunks is vital to invite families into the full power of their role as communication partners and advocates, as well as to lay the foundation for future learning. It is also notable that the more accessible the information, the more shareable it becomes. When a mom of a PWUAAC articulates her evolving understandings about AAC to her brother, friend, and child's teacher, she expands the circle around her child and gains ownership of what she has learned. Though much information is readily available online with a few keystrokes, engaging families in discourse enhances understanding and makes it relatable to their child. Additionally, sharing information iteratively, over time and in different contexts, enhances proficiency with that knowledge, and empowers caregivers to be full partners at the table where decisions for their child are made.

Tools/Technology

The relevance of information about AAC implementation principles is increasingly applicable when

AAC tools are "in-hand." These may include paper-based communication boards or books, communication apps on mobile devices, or high-tech AAC devices. In addition to learning about the organization and navigation of the tool, customization and use of supportive strategies such as masking may also be investigated. When embarking on their AAC journey, families benefit from seeing how tools will fit into their daily activities, allow their loved one to engage about topics or with individuals who are important to the family, and help the family navigate everyday interactions related to caring for and interacting with one another. Similarly, when the individual who uses AAC presents with vision or motor impairment, exploring and troubleshooting alternative access modalities such as scanning, eye gaze, or head-pointing influences the tool selected, or how it is used.

Due to the often lengthy and involved process of procuring high-tech AAC tools, it is worth noting that more accessible tools such as paper-based communication displays, perhaps paired with simple voice output devices, are useful for getting families started with AAC, as well as for making evident the multifaceted nature of an AAC system; it is not just an app or device, but a compilation of tools and strategies that allow an individual to communicate for a variety of purposes and across environments. Additionally, these tools may enable practitioners to guide families who are resistant to AAC; when perceived as less intrusive, easier, or even temporary, AAC exploration can shift from overwhelming to manageable, and worth a try. Targeting specific needs of the family can also foster an openness to trying AAC. For instance, families often identify mealtime as an activity in which they would like to support their loved one's communication skills. Because the family has identified the need, buy-in exists. The practitioner can then provide a communication display that reflects key features of AAC tools such as use of core words, as well as fringe words specific to the family and activity; and words that allow communication for a variety of purposes such as requesting, commenting, and social words. Such tools overtly demonstrate the need for more than just labels, and provide tangible insight into using AAC to engage in naturalistic interactions. Over time, the limitations also become evident and,

when an inquiry-based coaching model is applied, open the door to conversations about expanding the individual's AAC system.

Skills

Developing communication partner skills persistently evolves as new knowledge is gained, proficiency with technology increases, interactions become learning experiences, and communication partners engage in community with one another. A skilled communication partner is one whose interaction style encourages naturalistic, motivating, and authentic interaction. Often their behaviors and responses are subtle or nuanced and seem to manifest a mindset of presumed potential of the individual who uses AAC. Such skills may include the following (among others):

- uses AAC to express a variety of communicative functions (requesting, refusing, commenting, social closeness, sharing information, and asking questions)
- uses think-alouds with AAC to comment, describe, and problem-solve
- facilitates intrinsically motivated communication opportunities
- notices and responds to multiple modalities, including nonverbal communication
- respects and accepts "no" and "no response" (avoids power struggles, and keeps the conversation going)
- provides appropriate wait or pause time
- co-constructs messages for efficiency or clarity, in a manner acceptable to the PWUAAC
- uses AAC even when it is not perfect, and is ok with making mistakes

The gradual and evolving nature of skill development highlights the need to acquire (and revisit) information over time to make it one's own. Communication partner skills can be shaped by feedback, as well as by seeing examples of others engaging with AAC. Feedback may manifest as a reaction from the PWUAAC, come about as part of the coaching process, or arise from the communication partner's own reflection or emotional experience of using AAC. Social media and video sharing platforms connect families and professionals across geography, who may or may not be known to one another, and can be incredibly useful for providing examples of what it looks like to speak AAC.

Developing communication partner skills also encompasses accounting for the individual's long-term needs and taking action to support the range of communicative competencies, which include linguistic, social, operational, and strategic competence and also consider factors related to psychosocial factors as outlined by Light and McNaughton (2014). Linguistic competencies are often the primary target of AAC implementation and focus on using words, expanding vocabulary, and developing language skills. Operational competency speaks to managing AAC tools. This may include navigating tabs or buttons, managing the message by clearing the message window, and controlling the volume of messages. It may also include noticing and alerting another when their AAC system needs to be charged, or learning to charge it themselves. Independence with device programming is also an important operational skill for many PWUAACs. Using AAC to develop and sustain relationships falls in the domain of social competency. As mentioned earlier in this chapter, those in the circle of intimacy and the circle of exchange often have ample opportunities to use AAC to build memories and rapport. However, cultivating circles of friendship and circles of participation around individuals with disabilities, including those who use AAC, may be limited when compared to same-age peers. As such, teams may consider planning and advocating to identify opportunities for the PWUAAC to engage with peers and members of the community as valued partners. Strategic competency is problem-solving in action. It may include attention-getting strategies or messages, repairing communication breakdowns, or using synonyms or linguistically similar words available in their AAC system to convey messages that are not available. For instance, a PWUAAC I once knew requested marshmallows by combining *March + yellow*. Psychosocial factors that may also impact communicative competencies include motivation, attitude, confidence, and resilience.

Habits

Establishing habits of AAC use conveys that communication is a priority and facilitates ease of use. Habits and routines cultivate patterns of behavior that decrease the cognitive load of planning for and executing that behavior. Engaging families to identify their goals related to creating an AAC habit invites them to take stock of where they are on their journey and identify a next step. Habit-creating goals such as *making sure AAC is always available* provides the specific opportunity for caregivers to become aware of the barriers that may be impeding that habit. For instance, a strap, stand, or more durable case may be needed. Identifying and addressing barriers sets communication partners up for success by bringing focus to a component of the AAC implementation process that is meaningful to them, and supports them to trouble-shoot and prepare. Other examples of habit-forming goals may include the following:

- use AAC during five activities each day
- use comments each time when watching TV
- post paper-based core boards in each room of the house
- use AAC to tell where we are going, what we will do, and who we will see before going out
- facilitate AAC use with other family members (pass it around the dinner table)
- pause and make time for AAC when reading books each night

As goals are established, it is appropriate to discuss the barriers that may interfere with success, and determine how to address them. Barriers may be related to the communication partner, the environment, or others in the environment, and may include factors related to mindset, knowledge, skill, logistics, time, durability, and opportunity.

Responsive implementation support weaves these components together to create the unique fabric of each family's experience of learning and connecting with AAC. Knowledge provides context for tools/technology features and informs skill development; tools/technology provide a platform to bring skills to life; the process of acquiring skills evokes a need for more knowledge and provides insights for more effective use of technology; establishing habits of AAC use gives families a focal point to practice and refine how speaking AAC looks and feels in the context of their family dynamic.

Case Study: PH

Clinical Profile and Communication Needs

The Individual

PH is a 10-year-old girl with cerebral palsy who loves animals and dance music. She uses a manual wheelchair, though powered mobility is currently being explored. Upon obtaining her first technology-based AAC device, her mom, dad, and 12-year-old brother were excited for her to finally be able to say more than "yeah" and "nah." Her body language and facial expression were quite expressive, and they always felt she had much to say.

Their Communication Partners

As a fourth grader at her neighborhood school, PH was a social student. She was included with her peers, supported by a paraprofessional, much of the day. She worked with the special education teacher in a small group for reading and math each morning and afternoon. Music was her favorite class. School staff appreciated her sense of humor; her peers were patient and kind though she had not yet forged close friendships with many classmates. She joined playdates with her brother and his friends, and with neighborhood kids of family friends who had known her since preschool. Her grandmother visited weekly, and often took her to the park, movies, or other such fun outings.

PH's school team was instrumental in recognizing her need for AAC and helping the family navigate the process of procuring a device through their health insurance. Admittedly, the family was overwhelmed by the device. Though she also received speech therapy at school, when the device arrived, they sought additional support through private speech therapy with a speech-language pathologist (SLP).

Their Environment

PH and her family live in a small neighborhood in a rural-suburban community that is part of a largely suburban school district. Their one-level accessible rancher accommodates her wheelchair and newly mounted AAC device, though the recent addition of an accessible bathroom in her bedroom has been an improvement. Their home has a large yard and is situated on a street with two other families with similarly aged children. A personal assistant gets PH off the bus and helps her with her homework and personal care needs for a few hours after school 2 days per week while mom and dad are at work. She also participates in therapeutic horseback riding each week.

AAC Service Considerations

At their intake session, it was evident to SLP1 that the family was eager to help PH reach her potential but were intimidated by the AAC technology. They were able to anticipate her needs, and as a family had a positive social dynamic. They also recognized she had more to say than body language and photos on the fridge would allow her to express. Getting started felt daunting, and SLP1 quickly recognized that she needed to work with PH's mother to increase her understanding of AAC and help her feel successful supporting her daughter. Together, SLP1 and PH's mother drafted a plan for how they could work together to build PH's communication skills, cognizant of the need to facilitate familiarity with the device, develop foundational knowledge about AAC, cultivate PH's mother's skills as a communication partner, and help her establish habits around using AAC in everyday interactions. Finding ways to engage PH's dad, brother, and grandmother were also considered.

The Rationale for Clinical Decision-Making

To empower the family to take ownership of the device and the resources available to them as a device owner, SLP1 put them in contact with their vendor representative to arrange training on the device. To prepare for the training by the vendor,

SLP1 reviewed terminology with PH's mother and helped her generate a list of questions for the training. Links to the vendor's website and YouTube channel were provided as well.

SLP1 also reviewed a set of one-page handouts with PH's mother on key AAC implementation topics such as communicative functions, aided language input, and core vocabulary. Mindful of the cognitive load of so much new information, she also provided a list of recorded webinars and encouraged PH's mother to view a few over the next several weeks to learn more about these topics at her own pace. She suggested that the handouts could be used as a guideline to share what she was learning with PH's dad, brother, and grandmother. When SLP1 offered to continue providing resources, PH's mother requested she do so only once a month, as she juggled the demands of work and family that would give her a clear idea of what to explore over the course of the month, and allow her to approach the information in a more organized fashion than if resources came to her at random intervals. Monthly resource lists included links to a combination of informational handouts and websites, explainer videos, videos of individuals using AAC, and stories from PWUAACs. The family was encouraged to share the latter with PH. With PH's mother's approval, these resources were shared with PH's school team who were also invited to contribute to the monthly resource document for the family.

SLP1 emphasized the importance of communication partners across environments engaging with PH to teach her to use her AAC; it was determined that PH's mother would take part in therapy sessions, for at least part of the time, so she could see her daughter's AAC in action, and they could learn together. In addition to practicing AAC with motivating activities during each session, a weekly follow-up task was set collaboratively based on the family's priorities or activities for that week. Over time, tasks included a range of practice opportunities from using five targeted words in four different activities each day, to following up requests and choice-making with a comment, to enlisting her brother and cousins to generate a list of jokes to add to her device to prepare for joke week at school. Weekly tasks were also shared with PH's

school team. Though these did not always align with individualized education program (IEP) goals, it created open dialogue about PH's AAC journey.

Each session began with SLP1 using AAC to greet PH, telling her something about her week or sharing a bit of animal trivia, and inviting PH and her mom to also share. This routine provided authentic opportunities to use greetings and establish rapport. It also motivated PH and her mom to pre-think about something to share, creating a routine for practicing novel messages with AAC. They then discussed the previous week's task. SLP1 used guided questions and reflection to bring specificity to the discourse, celebrating successes and addressing challenges and barriers. The following week's task was then decided upon. PH was then given the choice of having her mom stay as she and SLP1 played games, read books, and went on virtual field trips with AAC, or having mom join for the last 10 min when PH would "tell all about it." Both were encouraged, as they provided different opportunities for PH's mother to learn how to support her daughter. By joining in these activities, PH's mother observed aided language input in action, often in the context of activities they also did at home. Getting a summary of the activities showed her how to follow her daughter's lead to co-construct messages, which she could then use to support PH to tell her dad and brother about activities and events of her day.

PH's mother was also encouraged to periodically take videos of herself and her family using AAC, for two purposes. First, documenting their AAC journey would allow them to see success over time, even when progress seemed slow. Second, videos would allow them to review what AAC actually looks like, share examples of using AAC with others, and make them aware of pitfalls in their interactions.

Due to scheduling conflicts, PH's dad was rarely available to participate in sessions, though her brother and grandmother did attend periodically. However, her dad appreciated SLP1's informative feedback when PH's mother shared videos of him using AAC with PH. As those closest to PH increased their competence as communication partners, they were motivated to create opportunities for PH to expand her circle and participate in activities such as nature club and dance classes.

Next Steps

This purposeful and responsive approach was instrumental in shaping PH's mother's understanding of communication and AAC, as well as her skills as a communication partner. She was better able to articulate her goals for her daughter at IEP team meetings, and engage as an informed participant in discussions about PH's potential as a learner and communicator. She was also increasingly confident when advocating and planning for PH to participate in community activities.

Initially, PH's family thought a device would be a bit like magic in helping PH be a better communicator. They quickly learned that learning AAC would be a journey for all of them, not just PH. Through "right-size" information and engagement in targeted practice opportunities with feedback, PH's family embraced their roles as communication partners.

References

Knight, J. (2016). *Better conversations: Coaching ourselves and each other to be more credible, caring and connected.* Corwin.

Light, J., & McNaughton, D. (2014). Communicative competence for individuals who require augmentative and alternative communication: A new definition for a new era of communication? *Augmentative and Alternative Communication, 30*(1), 1–18. https://doi.org/10.3109/07434618.2014.885080

Rush, D. D., & Shelden, M. L. (2020). *The early childhood coaching handbook* (2nd ed.). Brookes Publishing.

Snow, J. A. (1998). *What's really worth doing and how to do it—A book for people who love someone labeled disabled (possibly yourself).* Inclusion Press.

Starble, A., Hutchins, T., Favro, M. A., Prelock, P., & Bitner, B. (2005). Family-centered intervention and satisfaction with AAC device training. *Communication Disorders Quarterly, 7,* 47–54. https://doi.org/10.1177/15257401050270010501

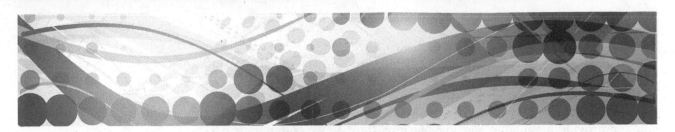

Chapter 33

COMMUNICATION PARTNER TRAINING FOR CLINICIANS

Tabitha Jones-Wohleber

Fundamentals

Communication partner training is as important to augmentative and alternative communication (AAC) implementation as the tools and technology, likely more so. AAC implementation is a responsive and dynamic process shaped by the priorities, skills, and needs of persons who use AAC (PWUAAC), as well as the contributions, skills, and needs of their interdisciplinary teams, composed of professionals and caregivers. A speech-language pathologist (SLP) is a key team member guiding decision-making, providing information, coordinating tools and strategies, and often fostering collaboration among team members. In the field of speech-language pathology, a need for clinicians with specific and sufficient knowledge and experience to effectively support PWUAACs and their teams persists. SLPs may be positioned to take on instrumental roles such as supporting team members in planning for AAC implementation; training caregivers and other professionals on AAC-related topics; and, of course, being a communication partner with individuals who use AAC. This chapter weaves together information and considerations relevant to each of these roles.

Communication-Partner Training

In a meta-analysis of the literature, Kent-Walsh, Murza, Malani, and Binger (2015) underscore the importance of including communication-partner training in AAC implementation planning. They specifically note positive outcomes from strategy and skill-based instructional approaches. In their review, frequently targeted strategies included aided language input, expectant delay, and use of open-ended questions. The need for communication-partner training is evident when considering typical characteristics of exchanges between PWUAACs and their communication partners. Interactions tend to be dominated by the communication partner in terms of initiations, turns, and topic setting. Kent-Walsh et al. (2015) note that these well-documented patterns of interactions also contribute to device abandonment. They poignantly suggest that "provision of instruction should be routinely provided unless there is clear evidence that typical partners in a full range of environments are regularly demonstrating the skills needed for a successful interaction" (p. 280).

Communication-partner training can take many forms and may be based on a predetermined sequence or evolve entirely in response to the needs of individual teams. The resources outlined in this chapter provide a valuable starting place as they specifically address communication-partner training.

Kent-Walsh and McNaughton (2005) outline a multistep process in which communication partners learn target skills through instruction, verbal rehearsal, role-play, and feedback. Focusing specifically on the verbal rehearsal step of the process, Senner and Baud (2017) specified the ingredients to successful partner-augmented input with the acronym SMoRRES: slow rate, model, respect and reflect, repeat, expand, and stop to provide an expectant pause. Implemented across home and community settings, they note this efficient strategy supports generalization of effective communication partner skills (Senner & Baud, 2018).

Model as a MASTER PAL is another acronym and training series that outlines communication-partner strategies, with a focus on behaviors and belief systems that foster meaningful interactions. The modules included in this series are Model, Motivate, Accept Multiple Modalities, Statements more than Questions, Time (wait time and time for language development), Engage Naturally, Response not Required, Presume Potential, Appropriate Prompting, and Let the Child Lead. Components of Model as a MASTER PAL are explored in the following section to heighten the clinician's understanding of its constituent parts and how they facilitate responsive and engaging interactions.

These models for communication-partner training highlight the necessity of providing partners with similar support to that which is required by PWUAACs learning to communicate with their tools: explicit and specific instruction, paired with opportunities to practice and receive informative feedback, in the context of high-value interactions. Building community across stakeholders, inclusive of professionals, caregivers, and peers, can be a key factor in establishing and sustaining knowledge, skills, and habits across communication partners.

Responsive and Engaging Communication Partners

Communication modalities may be symbolic or nonsymbolic, aided or unaided, but by its very nature, communication is intrinsically motivated. We communicate to

- advocate for our wants and needs, including refusal
- connect with and build relationships with others
- express what we are thinking and learning, and how we perceive our world.

Responsive and engaged communication partners embrace the transactional nature of communication and facilitate authentic interactions prioritizing a person-centered rather than task-oriented focus. Often nuanced or barely perceived behaviors or strategies, some of which are described next, contribute to the naturalistic style of skilled communication partners.

Speak AAC

Aided language input is one of many terms applied to the well-documented practice of using AAC to teach AAC, in which communication partners touch symbols *to compose their side of the conversation.* Though simple in definition, using aided language input readily draws out the complexity of language, communication, and interaction. The automaticity of spoken language does not intuitively translate to aided language tools. Communicating with symbols requires familiarity with the symbols that are available, knowledge of the organization of those symbols, as well as ability to use symbols flexibly. For instance, adjusting the complexity of the aided language message to reflect the language skills of the AAC user (use AAC to say "go out," while verbalizing "we are going out") or selecting synonyms for unavailable words adds to the cognitive load of using AAC for communication partners. Practice or preplanning can be useful. A helpful technique to build comfort and familiarity using AAC for families and clinicians is a *language walk-through* in which two or more team members brainstorm words and phrases that can be used to participate in a selected activity, exploring to locate symbols as they are discussed. Speaking AAC is rarely intuitive at the start, but with modeling and practice it can become second nature.

Accept Multiple Modalities and Attribute Meaning to Communicative Attempts

Communication partners are tasked with being responsive to all communicative intents in their endeavor to teach language through AAC. This is not a burden, it is an invitation; capitalizing on the individual's intrinsic motivation to communicate provides frequent, embedded, and naturalistic opportunities to use AAC to teach language, no planning required. However, communication partners often need to be taught to recognize communication opportunities. When a toddler smiles as a favorite toy spins, using AAC to say "like," "it turns," or some variation allows the child to experience those words authentically. A child verbalizes "water" while reaching for a water bottle. On her AAC system, a communication partner models "you want drink" or "need water" while passing her the water bottle, seizing the opportunity to expand her utterance using her AAC. A teen moving toward peers playing a game expresses a desire to join. A peer modeling "want to play?" with AAC, to invite him to join, shows him how he may initiate in the future. It is not necessary for the AAC user to then use AAC to express the message, again. The cumulative experiences of AAC demonstrated are part of the process of learning AAC. A turn may be offered, but the utility of accepting multiple modalities is that it (a) shows the individual that they are a communicator, (b) validates verbal speech (many PWUAACs also have some verbal skills), and (c) shows them how to use their AAC to convey messages expressed through other means, the latter mapping nonsymbolic communication to symbolic modalities.

Wait Time

Extended wait or pause time is beneficial to many PWUAACs, though the amount of wait time needed is unique to each individual. Fractions of a second elapse between many exchanges, such that a mere 5 s may feel excessive. However, for individuals who require wait time or "think time" to support cognitive, visual, or motor processing skills, or perhaps a combination of these, it is an imperative strategy in shaping their communication opportunities. Insufficient wait time can generate misperceptions about what an individual understands and is able to communicate. Video is a useful tool for determining how much wait time an individual may need. Reference the video progress bar and average wait time across several communicative exchanges to better understand the needs of individual PWUAACs.

Model AAC Without Expectation of a Response

Think-aloud is an anytime strategy in which a communication partner provides language input in the context of everyday interactions. It may include describing what one is thinking, feeling, or doing; commenting; or problem-solving aloud. Descriptive language is the practice of using familiar and accessible words (core words) to describe concepts that may not be available in an AAC system. Descriptive language facilitates concept development and demonstrates flexible use of AAC. In learning environments, use of descriptive language shifts discourse from recall of potentially obscure vocabulary words to focusing on meaning. For instance, *photosynthesis* may be described using core vocabulary as *"green color uses sun/light to make food."* Developing habits of thinking aloud with AAC and using descriptive language provides PWUAACs valuable language input that is not reliant on their initiation or response. Inviting a turn may take the form of an expectant pause, an expectant look, or posing a question. However, the AAC user may not respond. The communication partner can continue thinking aloud to provide language input. Integrating these elements creates a responsive low-demand interaction that supports both receptive and expressive language.

Ask Open-Ended Questions

Open-ended questions foster balanced exchanges by not limiting the AAC user to a specific or contrived response. Open-ended questions may be general or may ask the individual to relate to a topic. Examples of open-ended questions may include the following: *what do you think about that, what does it make you think of, what is your idea, tell* *me about __, tell me something that happened,* or *what part did you find interesting?* The power of open-ended questions is that they invite reciprocity and value the authentic communicative attempts of the AAC user. Any response, or even no response, in turn, invites the communication partner to continue providing language input by also weighing in on the question. In this way, interactions are sustained and serve the purpose of fostering connection, maintaining a respectful tone, placing low demands on the AAC user, and continuing to support receptive and expressive language skills by modeling AAC.

Presume Potential

A belief system that assumes all individuals will continue to learn, expand their communication and literacy skills, and contribute to the communities in which they exist manifests in words, actions, and the tone of interactions. Opportunities for inclusive experiences with peers, use of age-respectful learning materials, and engagement in interesting topics convey presumed potential. Ability-positive language describes an individual's skills without judgement. For example, whereas a presumptive tone may say "he is not a reader," ability-positive language says "he enjoys exploring books, and is learning to hold the book right side up while turning the pages." The former dismisses the potential of gaining literacy skills, while the latter describes where the child is on his literacy journey. Communication partners who presume potential recognize that learning is a lifelong endeavor for themselves and the individuals whom they support. They engage respectfully and take responsibility for providing opportunities for the individual to continue developing skills, however incremental, in pursuit of realizing their unique potential.

Supporting Adult Learners to Teach AAC

The charge of supporting adult learners as communication partners, inevitable to many SLPs working with those who use AAC, is worthy of discussion.

Understanding models of support as well as elements of design that maximize learning informs the process.

Models of Support

Differentiating consultation, coaching, and collaboration brings focus to roles and outcomes of each. Reed and Bowser (2012) contrast these approaches by outlining the assumptions brought to each process including perceived relationship, goals, and locus of accountability.

Consultation

Focused on specific procedures, behavior, or strategies, a consultative model calls on a specialist to provide information and recommendations, and to demonstrate processes and strategies. Viewed as an expert, the consultant carries influence but does not have the power to change programming.

Collaboration

Working toward a common goal, collaborators (which may include a specialist) engage in voluntary shared decision-making. Through discourse that includes brainstorming, questioning, clarifying, and action planning, collaboration is characterized by shared contribution and responsibility for outcomes.

Coaching

Coaching processes value the skills and contributions of the adult learner and engage the learner to refine their skills through questioning, observation, goal-setting, and self-reflection. A coach guides meta-cognitive awareness to empower the learner to take ownership of their ability to improve their practice.

While a consultative approach may serve the purpose of addressing foundational needs, collaborative relationships and coaching create the necessary opportunities for communication partners to engage with and practice skills to achieve enduring proficiency. By valuing the contributions of all parties, collaboration fosters consensus in action planning. Coaching extends the learning of individuals by providing the tools and structure for communication partners to be the agent of their own growth and learning.

Designing Effective Learning Opportunities for Communication Partners

In addition to approach, design is another consideration. Mind-Brain Education (MBE) is an emerging field of study that seeks to understand how we best learn, and integrates the sciences of pedagogy, neuroscience, and psychology. MBE practices are relevant to learners of all ages, and familiarity with these strategies is useful when designing a broad range of opportunities to teach others to teach AAC.

Whitman and Kelleher (2016) emphasize that relationship building is a pedagogical strategy; emotional connection is the junction where learning happens. Building on that sense of relevance, MBE strategies create *desirable difficulties* in the learning process to ensure sufficient cognitive engagement and to foster durable learning. For instance, *retrieval practice* is recall of information that after some time has lapsed, and forgetting has occurred. By engaging the brain to re-remember, the durability of that learning is strengthened. Content that is represented through *dual coding* also strengthens learning. Dual coding is a multimodal representation of information and may include a combination of text, graphics, tables, video, or other means. *Spaced practice* occurs when information is shared in bite-size chunks and is progressively reviewed or practiced over time rather than all at once. *Interleaving* is the process of integrating previously introduced topics in new contexts, repeatedly and over time. This allows learners to both relearn information and extend their understanding to include new knowledge. *Managing cognitive load* and *building metacognition* also contribute to a learner's ability to gain insights and integrate what they have learned. While only a few are described here, the many strategies that comprise MBE informed practices may seem familiar, or even obvious. But purposefully and thoughtfully integrating them can enrich engagement in communication-partner training and positively impact its effectiveness.

The "event-like" nature of many AAC trainings limits opportunities for collaboration and coaching as well as application of MBE strategies to enable communication partners to sustain and deepen their understanding. This is an invitation to creatively consider a variety of models for training, supporting, and engaging communication partners.

Barriers to AAC Implementation

Fraught with misperceptions that provision of an AAC tool makes one an AAC user, or that an AAC user will learn to use their tool by being told which messages to touch, or by simply imitating others, AAC implementation practices too often fall short. These misperceptions may be held by service providers who do not yet understand the need to teach AAC outside of speech sessions; by families who are able to anticipate the needs of their loved one and therefore do not fully understand the power of AAC in improving quality of life; or by administrators who have the power to allocate time and personnel resources to meet the needs of individuals with complex communication needs, though they do not adequately understand that need. Beukelman and Mirenda (1998) proposed a framework, the Participation Model for AAC, that identifies opportunity barriers as well as access barriers that interfere with teaching and learning AAC. Access barriers are factors related to the AAC user and the nature of their disability, such as motor skills, sensory needs, or environmental access. Of particular relevance to supporting communication partners, reflecting on opportunity barriers provides valuable insight to inform and guide the AAC implementation process.

Opportunity Barriers Include Attitude, Knowledge, Skill, Practice, and Policy Barriers

Limiting perceptions of disability or AAC and the potential of individuals who use AAC manifests as attitude barriers and may be overt or subtle, conscious or unconscious. Knowledge barriers exist when teams have insufficient understanding of AAC and the myriad factors that contribute to effective implementation. But knowledge alone does not make communication partners effective. Implementing AAC requires practice, feedback, and continued acquisition of knowledge. Skill barriers exist when teams have an understanding of *what* they need to do to implement AAC, but do not yet understand *how* to do it. Practice and policy barriers may present as unspoken rules of practice, whether official or unofficial. For instance, providing speech services in a separate therapy room rather than in the classroom in collaboration with a teacher, because that is how it has always been, may be a practice barrier. It can be changed, though there may be some resistance to that change. Policy barriers, by contrast, can only be changed by policy makers. Lack of infrastructure to facilitate and fund communication-partner training in schools, programs, and from insurance companies is a substantive policy barrier.

Taking inventory of stakeholders, resources (both tangible and intangible), and the infrastructure within a setting is needed to thoughtfully identify, target, and ultimately dismantle these barriers. It is worth noting that they do not occur in a vacuum, and each opportunity barrier inevitably impacts additional opportunity barriers. Sheldon, Cummings, Langley, and Jones-Wohleber (2020) emphasize the pervasive influence of attitude barriers, whether positive or negative, on a team's effectiveness. Notably, attitude barriers cannot be mandated, and information alone does little to shift a mindset. Personal experiences, meaningful accounts from others (videos are a great tool), and moments of success are needed to impact attitudinal barriers. Often a necessary first step, collating and sharing resources and opportunities to cultivate positive attitudes and experiences should also be an *ongoing* component of supporting communication partners within teams and institutions.

As teams begin to define and sharpen their focus on the barriers that impact the AAC journeys of those whom they support, accounting for human nature is necessary. Self-determination theory, a motivational theory, as defined by Ryan and Deci (2000), outlines three needs of individuals:

- competence: a sense of gaining proficiency or accomplishment
- relatedness: being part of a group, community, or experience
- autonomy: freedom to make decisions, choose a course of action, or have control over one's resources.

Transparent discussion about these needs is beneficial as they are relevant when supporting both communication partners and PWUAACs. Actualizing positive attitudes, expanding knowledge, growing skills, and developing habits of practice that yield positive outcomes for AAC learners rely on varied, perpetual, and meaningful opportunities to cultivate communication partners who connect and engage competently with PWUAACs.

Case Study: JT

Clinical Profile and Communication Needs

The Individual

JT is an SLP at the local elementary school, a rural-suburban school in a mid-sized district. Her caseload consists of students with a range of speech-language disorders, and includes seven students who use AAC, out of 12 total students, across two self-contained special education classrooms, each with a teacher and three paraprofessionals.

The Communication Partners and Their Environment

Over the last several years, JT has seen an increase in the number of students on her caseload who use AAC. AAC tools are being procured by families through private means, and *assistive technology consideration* through the individualized education program (IEP) process is identifying an increasing number of students who benefit from AAC. JT loved her AAC class in graduate school, but that was quite a few years ago. After spending the first semester of the school year working with the special education teachers to learn the tools and seeking out resources to incorporate AAC throughout the day, she was frustrated. Knowledge about and perceived value of AAC across families and other staff members was highly variable. While some families ensured devices arrived at school charged and ready to go, several arrived with little or no charge, or were inconsistently sent to school. Two paraprofessionals stood out as having exceptional rapport with students and engaged with them respectfully and with a sense of humor, though they rarely used AAC tools in their interactions. However, several staff members used a condescending tone when talking to students with disabilities. Students who use AAC were especially vulnerable to being talked about in their presence without including them in the conversation. Throughout the school day, AAC tools were often reserved for choice-making. When staff did use AAC to provide language input, it was often to tell a student what to do. During instruction, individualized AAC tools were usually put aside and replaced with a choice board of vocabulary items related to the content topic. Each week, JT taught a lesson in each of the self-contained classrooms and provided services to a few students during teacher-taught lessons, in part to model use of AAC to classroom staff. However, with another adult in the room, classroom staff often became passive or used that time to go to the workroom to prepare the next day's lesson materials. Furthermore, school duty schedules (lunch, dismissal, etc.) made it impossible for the teachers, SLP, and paraprofessionals to come together for training and to collaborate around AAC implementation.

AAC Considerations for Training

JT partnered with one of the special education teachers who shared her frustrations to brainstorm how to begin to address these issues. They recognized they would need the support of their principal to shift expectations as well as address logistical barriers of staff time. After discussing their concerns with their principal, it was agreed that their efforts should focus on building an infrastructure around AAC implementation that would be sustainable through staff turnover and student attrition. Collectively, they set the following targets focused on communication-partner training.

Ensure All Stakeholders Are Familiar With the Organization, Navigation, and Customization of AAC Tools, and That Students Have Consistent Access to Their Tools

Across PWUAACs, three different communication systems were used. To build capacity around the tools, paraprofessionals were paired up to become "trainers" on one of the systems. JT provided the paraprofessionals with links to video tutorials, quick guides, as well as checklists of features to explore and customizations to make. They were then tasked with partnering up with JT to teach staff and families to use the AAC tool. Equipping each classroom with someone knowledgeable about and comfortable with each tool provided answers to "in the moment" questions, offered quick troubleshooting support, and facilitated ownership of the AAC systems used by their students. Additionally, an awareness arose for the need to (a) establish a routine for ensuring devices were charged and backed up, (b) create paper-based backup systems for each student, and (c) provide staff with low-tech AAC that reflected student devices. Explicit communication with families around charging devices yielded clear expectations about the need for a student's AAC tools to be ready for the school day and established when and by whom the device would be charged. A digital folder was created for each student, and on the first Monday of each month, paraprofessionals backed up each student's AAC to their folder. In turn, JT sleuthed out or created printable backup systems for each student, which the paraprofessionals had backed up to each student's folder. Screenshots of the home page and chat pages of each AAC system were printed front and back and put on lanyards that were provided to each staff member.

At the start of each quarter, technology support needs were reviewed with a focus on the following:

- Families and staff were invited to request support with AAC tools, if needed.
- New paraprofessionals were given the opportunity to become device trainers.
- Well-used paper-based tools were replaced.

Provide Ongoing Opportunities for Staff and Families to Learn About AAC

Foundational information about communication and AAC was necessary to build a shared knowledge base. Monthly training sessions were facilitated by the SLP in partnership with the special education teachers who alternated months. The principal committed to attend the sessions, even if only for part of the time, both to learn and to show support for the value of AAC implementation. Each month, a 60-min session was held twice, first thing in the morning or immediately after school, on designated days. Families were invited to join these sessions, and the content portion of each session was recorded for those unable to attend. The principal ensured school duty and student supervision coverage for staff members who chose to attend the morning session and allocated funds to pay staff who chose to attend the after-school session. Alternatively, staff could opt to receive microcredentials that could be applied to certifications that allowed them to advance on the salary scale, in lieu of pay. Participation was required for special education staff supporting students who use AAC, and encouraged for all school staff.

Each session began with 5 to 10 min of sharing student success stories from the past month and/or reviewing a video or article of an AAC user's perspective or experience. This was followed by a brief review of previous content through retrieval practice. AAC topics such as core vocabulary, communicative function, multimodal communication, wait time, and appropriate prompting, among others, were covered with direct, specific information, and easy to understand examples. Through these conversations, interleaving was achieved by interweaving concepts such as the importance of intrinsic motivation, attributing meaning, and cre-

ating connection through naturalistic interactions. Role-play or interactive practice opportunities with paper-based AAC were provided, and each session concluded with participants drafting a brief but specific goal to bring focus to their AAC implementation practices over the next month. Within a week after each session, a follow-up e-mail was sent to all participants capturing key ideas and discussion points, and included a related resource such as a handout, website, or video link.

Maintain Focus on Improving AAC Implementation Practices by Embedding Goal Setting in Teaming and Job-Embedded Learning Opportunities

Collaboration through monthly co-planning and weekly co-teaching between JT and the special education teachers was employed to develop intentional habits of AAC implementation. It included brainstorming communication opportunities for each student and outlining language targets for content-based lessons with a focus on integrating student AAC systems rather than just using vocabulary-focused choice boards. Goals set by classroom staff during monthly trainings were reviewed by the SLP (JT) to ensure opportunities to work toward those goals. To build on this collaboration, coaching was introduced after several months based on two different but specific needs. First, it was quickly evident that one staff member, Ms. X, was not influenced by incidental modeling to shift her behaviors as a communication partner. Second, a few staff members, passionate about expanding and refining their skills, were eager to engage in richer conversations about AAC implementation. Coaching was offered to all staff members on a voluntary basis, though Ms. X was specifically encouraged to participate by the principal. Coaching opportunities were initially facilitated by the SLP (JT), though in time peer coaching also occurred. Coaching practices included goal-setting, observing, practicing, reflecting, and responding to feedback. Those being coached were videotaped at multiple intervals to facilitate this process. Videos of exemplar practices were compiled for others to view and learn from.

Build Community Around Using AAC Throughout the School

The human need for connection underlies the imperative of building community around use of AAC and normalizing AAC across environments. The team at the local elementary school addressed this need in multiple ways. First, language boards were posted in various environments throughout the school, including in the lobby and front office, in the cultural arts classrooms (gym, music, art) and media center, and in the cafeteria. Second, peers in classrooms where students who used AAC were included at various times throughout the day were engaged to learn about their communication devices and were provided with opportunities to use communication boards during fun activities. Peers were encouraged to use the paper-based communication boards at any time to interact with students who use AAC, and each other. Last, an AAC social was held for staff in the teacher's lounge during the half hour before students arrived on the last Friday of each month. Paper-based communication boards were picked up at the door and used for the duration. Staff used their AAC to engage with one another in general and related to the specific topic or task for that social. Donuts were provided, and each participant's name was entered into a drawing for a coffee gift card. This motivated staff to experience AAC authentically for themselves and thereby inform and improve their interactions with students.

Next Steps

Though it took 2 years for JT and her team to identify, organize, and implement these practices, they were ultimately successful at shifting the school culture to support students who used AAC by prioritizing (a) all the time access to AAC, (b) the role of communication partners in teaching AAC, and (c) connection through community. Factors that contributed to the sustainability of supporting staff and peers to become skilled communication partners of students who use AAC included staff and leadership changes and engagement in scheduled revisiting, revision, and refocusing on the goals initially set forth by the team.

References

Beukelman, D. R., & Mirenda, P. (1998). *Augmentative and alternative communication: Management of severe communication disorders in children and adults* (2nd ed.). Paul H. Brookes.

Jones-Wohleber, T. (2018). *Model as a MASTER PAL.* https://bit.ly/ModelasaMASTERPALtrainingmodule

Kent-Walsh, J., & McNaughton, D. (2005). Communication partner instruction in AAC: Present practices and future directions. *Augmentative and Alternative Communication, 21*(3), 195–204. https://doi.org/10.1080/07434610400006646

Kent-Walsh, J., Murza, K. A., Malani, M. D., & Binger, C. (2015). Effects of communication partner instruction on the communication of individuals using AAC: A meta-analysis. *Augmentative and Alternative Communication, 31*(4), 271–284. https://doi.org/10.3109/07434618.2015.1052153

Reed, P., & Bowser, G. (2012). Consultation, collaboration, and coaching: Essential techniques for integrating assistive technology use in schools and early intervention programs. *Journal of Occupational Therapy, Schools, & Early Intervention, 5*(1), 15–30. https://doi.org/10.1080/19411243.2012.675757

Ryan, R., & Deci, E. (2000). Self-determination theory and the facilitation of intrinsic motivation, social development, and well-being. *American Psychologist, 55*(1), 68–78.

Senner, J., & Baud, M. (2017). The use of an eight-step instructional model to train school staff in partner-augmented input. *Communication Disorders Quarterly, 38*, 89–95.

Senner, J. E., & Baud, M. R. (2018). *Ingredients to successful modeling: SMoRRES and partner-augmented input* [Webinar]. International Society for Augmentative and Alternative Communication. https://youtu.be/3RtWBvTWEXU

Sheldon, E., Cummings, M., Langley, R., & Jones-Wohleber, T. (2020). *Re-frame it to change it: Reframing barriers to AAC implementation* [Pre-conference session]. Closing the Gap Virtual Conference.

Whitman, G., & Kelleher, I. (2016). *NeuroTeach: Brain science and the future of education.* Rowman & Littlefield.

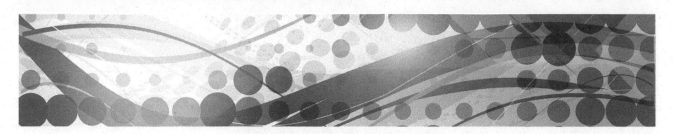

Chapter 34

COMMUNICATION PARTNER TRAINING FOR STAFF

Jill E. Senner and Matthew R. Baud

Fundamentals

Communication involves two or more individuals, and both an individual using augmentative and alternative communication (AAC) and their communication partner need to adjust to each other's skills and needs for a conversation to be successful. In fact, the success of communication between a child using AAC and a communication partner will depend heavily on the skills of the communication partner (Kent-Walsh & McNaughton, 2005). School-aged children spend roughly 30 hours a week attending classes, making school staff members (e.g., therapists, teachers, paraprofessionals) key communication partners in the academic environment (Senner & Baud, 2017). Partner-dominated interactions are often seen at schools with untrained staff, with children using AAC serving as respondents in as high as 91% of communicative opportunities. Furthermore, during naturally occurring events at school, students tend to interact primarily with adults rather than peers. Even in inclusive classrooms where peers are in frequent proximity, students using AAC interact primarily with an assigned staff member, most frequently instructional assistants or special educators (Andzik et al., 2016; Chung et al., 2012).

Many speech-language pathologists (SLPs) and special education teachers "may graduate from preservice training with minimal or no exposure to AAC" (Costigan & Light, 2010, p. 202). Therefore, classroom staff are likely to require professional development (PD) opportunities to further knowledge and skills in AAC (Senner & Baud, 2017). Analyses of communication-partner training programs suggest that there is consistent evidence that communication-partner instruction not only improves the skills of communication partners but also has a positive impact on the communication of people who use AAC (Kent-Walsh et al., 2015; Shire & Jones, 2015). Communication-partner education can be used effectively as an intervention strategy for individuals using AAC. Furthermore, communication-partner training is an essential part of AAC evaluation and implementation and should routinely be delivered when a child receives a speech-generating device (SGD; Kent-Walsh et al., 2015; Senner & Baud, 2016, 2017; Senner et al., 2019). Unfortunately, traditional training approaches such as lectures are frequently insufficient in enabling school staff to change their behavior in the classroom.

The use of a combination of training elements is correlated with maximal positive results. In 2015, Carl Dunst identified key features of PD associated with positive student and staff outcomes, including the following: (a) explicit explanation and illustration of the specific content knowledge and practice to be learned; (b) active and job-embedded practitioner opportunities to learn to use a practice and engage in evaluation of their experiences; (c) reflection (i.e., helping staff think about their own performance); (d) coaching, mentoring, or performance feedback by a PD specialist; (e) follow-up supports by PD specialists; and (f) sufficient duration and intensity (i.e., learning opportunities distributed over time).

Coaching is collaborative and requires live observation and feedback in the natural environment (e.g., the classroom). Many skills needed by educators can be introduced in training but must really be learned on the job with the help of a coach. Kent-Walsh and McNaughton (2005) proposed an eight-step instruction model for communication partners of persons who use AAC (PWUAACs). Their model includes all of the key features of successful PD as follows:

- Pre-test and Commitment to Instructional Program
- Strategy Description
- Strategy Demonstration
- Verbal Practice of Strategy Steps
- Controlled Practice and Feedback
- Advanced Practice and Feedback
- Post-test and Commitment of Long-Term Strategy Use
- Generalization of Targeted Strategy Use

The Kent-Walsh and McNaughton (2005) model has been used successfully to train instructional assistants in school environments. Increases in child AAC use following partner training were reported. However, this model has primarily (a) focused on a single activity, storybook reading, an activity that may not occur frequently in all classrooms; and (b) incorporated activity-based communication displays (ABCDs) created specifically for the reading activities rather than the child's existing SGD, thus limiting the likelihood of generalization (Binger et al., 2010; Sennott & Mason, 2016). The SMoRRES training program is based on the aforementioned eight-step instructional model; however, it was specifically designed to be used within naturally occurring activities in the classroom and to promote use of partner-augmented input (PAI) on a child's current SGD.

PAI, also referred to as natural aided language, aided language modeling, or aided language stimulation, is a modeling strategy in which one or more key words from a staff member's utterance are activated on a child's SGD immediately before, during, or after a spoken message. "Augmented input can be broadly defined as an umbrella term for systematic modeling input from two or more modalities, one of which must include the learner's AAC system" (Allen et al., 2017, p.157). Overall, PAI is an evidence-based strategy associated with gains in pragmatics, semantics, syntax, and morphology, and is effective in individuals of varying ages, disabilities, and language skills (Sennott et al., 2016).

Although pointing to pictures while talking may be a familiar idea for some, having awareness about a strategy alone does not typically result in being able to implement it in the classroom. Joyce and Showers (1980) differentiated between levels of impact of training including (a) awareness, (b) concepts and organized knowledge, (c) principles and skills, and (d) application and problem-solving. Only when school staff reach the application and problem-solving level can they transfer modeling skills to the natural environment and use them along with other strategies in their repertoires.

The SMoRRES training program was created to help communication partners reach the application and problem-solving level with PAI. In 2017, Senner and Baud used this model to teach instructional assistants, a teacher, and an SLP to provide PAI in a self-contained classroom throughout the school day. All staff increased the percentage of utterances modeled following staff participation in this training program. "Outcomes of this study extend the research by training school personnel and applying the strategy across activities within a natural classroom environment with minimal disruption to the daily routines of the staff involved. This study strengthens and extends the literature by demonstrating that using participants from the same context (e.g., self-contained classroom) regardless of their backgrounds and experiences can be beneficial in increasing augmented input of partners across activities." (Alant et al., 2017, p. 12)

The following case study illustrates the implementation of the SMoRRES communication partner training program within an educational setting.

Case Study: BT

Clinical Profile and Communication Needs

The Individual

BT was a 9-year, 10-month-old male with autism who had used a NovaChat 8[1] SGD with WordPower[2] 60 for approximately 2 years via direct selection (i.e., pointing with an index finger). He was referred by the District Special Education Program Supervisor for an AAC consultation to improve his ability to communicate in the classroom. He had been receiving 90 min of speech and language services per week, but his expressive communication remained limited to two sign approximations (e.g., help, more), vocally imitating a variety of one-syllable words (e.g., "pop," "too," "toy," "boy"), and limited use of his NovaChat 8™.

On a recent Receptive One-Word Picture Vocabulary Test, Fourth Edition (ROWPVT-4), he had a standard score below 55, which put him below the first percentile for his age. His language age equivalent on this test was 2 years, 8 months. During testing, BT accurately pointed to a variety of familiar nouns, verbs, and adjectives (e.g., hand, shoe, hat, cookie, open, jump, happy) on the test plates.

The district assistive technology (AT) coordinator implemented the SMoRRES training program to teach staff to better incorporate device modeling into the existing classroom schedule (Kent-Walsh & McNaughton, 2005; Senner & Baud, 2016, 2017). As part of Step 1, Pre-test and Commitment to Instructional Program, staff were videotaped using the device with the student in the classroom during three regularly occurring, 30-min class periods: (a) speech therapy, (b) snack, and (c) reading. Language samples were transcribed from the pretest videotapes. Analysis revealed that 80% of his SGD selections were prompted verbally (i.e., an adult telling BT to say a word), gesturally (i.e., an adult pointing to icon and telling BT to touch it), or

physically (i.e., hand-over-hand assistance) across classes. Only about 20% of his utterances were produced independently. He produced fewer than two messages per minute across activities. There was little lexical variety in his samples, with the primary communicative function being requesting objects (e.g., puzzle, iPad) and actions (e.g., squeeze). He demonstrated decreased joint attention to educational materials and his device, in other words, poor focus on the same thing as each staff member (i.e., looking up at the ceiling during the lesson instead of his device or book) and reduced mutual engagement during activities. In addition, he was noted to elope (i.e., leave the work area without permission) an average of four times per activity.

The Communication Partners and Their Environment

Three paraprofessionals, a teacher, and an SLP were regularly in BT's self-contained classroom in a public, community-based elementary school. There were a total of six students with developmental disabilities in the class, two of whom used SGDs. School staff had a minimum of a bachelor's degree, and two staff members had obtained master's degrees in their fields. Three of the four staff members held sate teaching certificates. Length of work experience ranged from 4 months to 15 years.

AAC Considerations

The AAC System or Service

The week following pretest videotaping, communication partner training began with staff participating in a 3-hour group instruction session. This was the only step of the training that required staff time outside of the classroom. During this in-service, staff completed Step 1. Each of the staff members was asked to individually watch a pretest videotape of her interaction with the student and to reflect on her own use of the student's SGD. Staff discussed their strengths and weaknesses in providing PAI on

---

[1]NOVA Chat is a product of Saltillo Corporation of Millersburg, Ohio.
[2]WordPower is a product of Inman Innovations of Baltimore, Maryland.

the device with the AT coordinator. Staff also signed a written statement acknowledging that they were committed to the entire training process. On the written commitment form, they also set personal goals (e.g., "Give more/longer pauses as opposed to prompting"). Step 2, Strategy Description, was also conducted during the group training session via a PowerPoint presentation that outlined what PAI is, why it can be useful, and the SMoRRES ingredients to modeling language on SGDs. Step 3, Strategy Demonstration, was conducted via presentation of videotaped samples of PAI being used in classrooms.

During the in-service, Step 4, Verbal Practice of the Strategy Steps, was completed using the SMoRRES (slow rate, model, respect and reflect, repeat, expand, stop) mnemonic (Senner et al., 2019), as shown in Table 34–1.

The staff labeled and described each step aloud during the training with guidance from the instructors to confirm that they understood the strategies. The AT coordinator also led staff through rehearsal (i.e., vocal repetition of the strategy steps) to aid in memorizing steps involved. Each staff member had

a communication device or app with the student's pageset to participate in Controlled Practice and Feedback (Step 5). During controlled practice, staff were asked to generate a variety of practice phrases on the devices as well as to generate phrases to model based on scenarios presented. The scenarios related to activities at school and required staff to think about what types of models they might provide in the situations described (e.g., "The student pushes away an activity you are doing. What could you respect and reflect on your student's device to convey his or her intent?")

Following the group training session, staff participated in eight, once-weekly, 30-min coaching sessions in the classroom. During these sessions, the AT coordinator modeled SMoRRES ingredients during each of the three classes (Step 4). For example, when the student was in snack, parallel talk was demonstrated by modeling things like "eat more crackers" and "I like it." In addition, staff had an opportunity to participate in Controlled Practice (Step 5) and Advanced Practice (Step 6) with the AT coordinator providing coaching. During coaching, the SMoRRES Observation Tool, a checklist with

Table 34–1. SMoRRES Mnemonic

Letter(s)	Meaning	Definition
S	Slow rate	Speak in a slow, clearly articulated manner.
Mo	Model	Point to the symbol on the child's device while simultaneously providing parallel-talk or self-talk.
R	Respect and reflect	When the child communicates something through another modality (e.g., gesture, word approximation, sign), *respect*, honor the communication, and *reflect,* model a word or phrase to communicate the same thought or feeling *without making the child repeat himself.*
R	Repeat	Provide multiple models of targeted words in a variety of contexts.
E	Expand	Build on the child's communication, adding one to two words and fixing any errors.
S	Stop	Stop—Provide an *expectant pause* before, during, or after your model to provide the child an opportunity to communicate.

each of the mnemonic letters listed, was used to tally the number of times staff used each behavior. For example, if a child said "bubble," and the staff member modeled, "a big bubble," then the coach made a tally mark under E for expand. If the child signed "more," and the staff member honored the request while modeling "more" on the SGD, the tally mark was placed under the first R for Respect and Reflect. Coaching was gradually faded between Controlled and Advanced Practice. Figure 34–1 shows an AT coordinator demonstrating a strategy in the classroom environment.

School staff received access to one of their post-test videos to watch on their own, and they discussed their PAI use with the AT coordinator (Step 7). During the last two coaching sessions, the AT coordinator pushed into a fourth classroom activity which had not previously been practiced during coaching sessions (Step 8). The generalization activity was social skills group. The staff also discussed strategies for long-term PAI use in the classroom with the AT coordinator during their final coaching session.

Language sampling and analysis of post-test videos revealed that all staff significantly increased frequency of modeling. All staff reported increased familiarity with BT's device. Positive changes were also seen in BT. At post-test, greater than half of his utterances were produced spontaneously and independently, possibly due to increased communication opportunities created by staff incorporating regular expectant pauses. In addition, his frequency of communication increased to greater than three utterances per minute. Furthermore, his lexical variety (i.e., number of unique words used) increased by 150%. While he may have learned new vocabulary words, it is also possible that the increased modeling allowed him to better locate words that he already knew on his SGD. Finally, staff reported an increase in BT's joint attention and a decrease in eloping following training.

Next Steps

The AT coordinator scheduled a follow-up visit with the team 8 weeks later to monitor staff maintenance of PAI. Typically, staff use of SMoRRES will be maintained or slightly increase over time; however, some staff may demonstrate decreases over time (Senner & Baud, 2017). BT's parents were invited to a parent academy, an evening group parent training series at the school, where a similar eight-step instructional model for parents was being implemented (Senner et al., 2019).

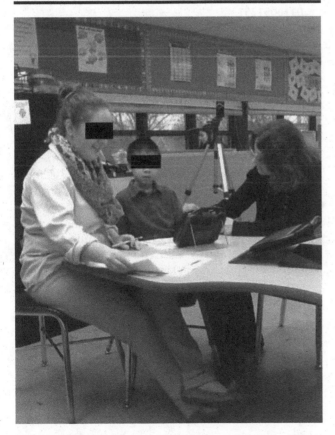

Figure 34–1. AT Coordinator providing strategy demonstration in the classroom. Technology & Language Center, Inc. © 2013–2021.

> SLPs must align what they *know* (i.e., theory and science) with what they *do* (i.e., policy and practice). One must use *both* effective training elements (i.e., implementation features) and effective methodologies (i.e., intervention features) to establish evidence-based practices (EBPs). In other words, *how* one teaches is as important as *what* one teaches for EBP.

References

Alant, E., Alshubrumi, A., & Sun, L. (2017). Use of an eight-step instructional model to train school staff in partner-augmented input shows potential. *Evidence-Based Communication Assessment and Intervention, 11*(1–2), 9–13. https://doi.org/10.1080/17489539.2017.1317100

Allen, A. A., Schlosser, R. W., Brock, K. L., & Shane, H. C. (2017). The effectiveness of aided augmented input techniques for persons with developmental disabilities: A systematic review. *Augmentative and Alternative Communication, 33*(3), 149–159. https://doi.org/10.1080/07434618.2017.1338752

Andzik, N. R., Chung, Y., & Kranak, M. P. (2016). Communication opportunities for elementary students who use augmentative and alternative communication. *Augmentative and Alternative Communication, 32*(4), 272–281.

Binger, C., Kent-Walsh, J., Ewing, C., & Taylor, S. (2010). Teaching educational assistants to facilitate the multi symbol message productions of young students who require augmentative and alternative communication. *American Journal of Speech-Language Pathology, 19*(2), 108–120. https://doi.org/10.1044/1058-0360(2009/09-001e5)

Chung, Y., Carter, E. W., & Sisco, L. G. (2012). Social interactions of students with disabilities who use augmentative and alternative communication in inclusive classrooms. *American Journal on Intellectual and Developmental Disabilities, 117*(5), 349–367.

Costigan, F. A., & Light, J. (2010). A review of preservice training in augmentative and alternative communication for speech-language pathologists, special education teachers, and occupational therapists. *Assistive Technology, 22*, 200–212.

Dunst, C. J. (2015). Improving the design and implementation of in-service professional development in early childhood intervention. *Infants & Young Children, 28*, 210–219. https://doi.org/10.1097/IYC.0000000000000042

Joyce, B. R., & Showers, B. (1980). Improving inservice training: The message of research. *Educational Leadership, 37*, 379–385.

Kent-Walsh, J., & McNaughton, D. (2005). Communication partner instruction in AAC: Present practices and future directions. *Augmentative and Alternative Communication, 21*, 195–204.

Kent-Walsh, J., Murza, K. A., Malani, M. D., & Binger, C. (2015). Effects of communication partner instruction on the communication of individuals using AAC: A meta-analysis. *Augmentative and Alternative Communication, 31*, 271–284.

Senner, J. E., & Baud, M. R. (2016). Pre-service training in AAC: Lessons from school staff instruction. *Perspectives of the ASHA Special Interest Groups, 1*(SIG 12), 24–31. https://doi.org/10.1044/persp1.SIG12.24

Senner, J. E., & Baud, M. R. (2017). The use of an 8-step instructional model to train school staff in partner-augmented input. *Communication Disorders Quarterly, 38*(2), 89–95. https://doi.org/10.1177/1525740116651251

Senner, J. E., Post, K. A., Baud, M. R., Patterson, B., Bolin, B., Lopez, J,. & Williams, E. (2019). Effects of parent instruction in partner-augmented input on parent and child speech generating device use. *Technology and Disability, 31*, 27–38. https://doi.org/10.3233/TAD-190228

Sennott, S. C., Light, J. C., & McNaughton, D. (2016). AAC modeling intervention research review. *Research and Practice for Persons with Severe Disabilities, 41*, 101–115. https://doi.org/10.1177/1540796916638822

Sennott, S. C., & Mason, L. H. (2016). AAC modeling with the iPad during storybook reading pilot study. *Communication Disorders Quarterly, 37*, 242–254.

Shire, S. Y., & Jones, N. (2015). Communication partners supporting children with complex communication needs who use AAC: A systematic review. *Communication Disorders Quarterly, 37*, 3–15.

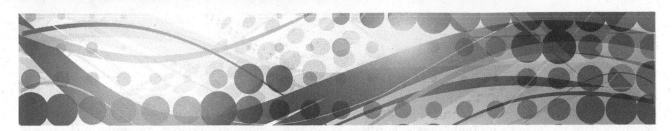

Chapter 35
TELE-AAC: THE BASICS

Michelle Boisvert

Fundamentals

Tele-AAC is the strategic combination of video-conferencing technology and augmentative and alternative communication (AAC) tools to deliver direct and indirect AAC services to clients with complex communication needs (CCNs) regardless of geographical location. In general, the term "telepractice" refers to the use of technology to enable specialists to provide clinical services over a geographical distance (Dudding & Justice, 2004), and it is an appropriate model of service delivery by speech-language pathologists (SLPs; Brown, 2011). This method of service delivery can be used for direct and indirect AAC services. This application of telepractice is called "tele-AAC." There are many reasons why clinicians and clients might seek out tele-AAC services. For example, some clients with CCNs have limited access to providers willing to travel long distances, lack transportation to the specialist's location, or reside in areas where highly specialized clinical services are difficult to obtain (Burke et al., 2008; Demiris et al., 2005). Inconsistent services also occur in cases where the client is homebound due to immobility, and in-person therapy may induce increased anxiety (Harwood et al., 2011). Furthermore, some clients require significant monitoring (Harwood et al., 2011) or their caregivers need frequent professional assistance (Kolb, 2009). Finally, some clinical plans stipulate consultative and collaborative services with providers in several different locations, making it challenging for specialists to coordinate frequent in-person meetings. Given the critical need to accommodate and provide clinical services, clinicians can use tele-AAC as a viable option to deliver services.

By its very nature, telepractice reduces geographical barriers and extends clinical expertise on an ongoing or acute consultation basis, and this holds true for tele-AAC as well. When sensibly implemented, a tele-AAC service delivery model creates additional or more consistent direct and indirect service opportunities, enables real-time collaboration with team members, and complements traditional, on-site service delivery models (Juenger, 2009). Tele-AAC empowers teams to be creative with technology and includes the client's communication partners in authentic activities and functional daily living tasks. The ability to use mobile technology provides many opportunities to support the communication using AAC across the client's day in varying activities and with different communication partners. As communication partners gain more exposure to clinical strategies, they may feel more confident to model the use of AAC, provide scaffolds, and help the client transfer the skills and use AAC to communicate with others.

While the benefits of tele-AAC are clear, teams must also be aware of the considerations that must be addressed prior to implementing a tele-AAC program. The barriers that are typically encountered include access to high-speed Internet, appropriate space, infrastructure, and on-site support. Additional technology is required for tele-AAC, and as such, a workspace must accommodate extra computers, laptops, and webcams as well as provide space to accommodate the client's mobility needs. Furthermore, specific equipment or technology is required for tele-AAC. While most technology is readily available (i.e., laptops, smartphones, etc.), the client and their communication partners must be aware of the specific types of hardware and software that are best suited for this service. The communication partner must also be available during the times of direct, synchronous services to support the client and address any technical issues that arise.

Methods of Tele-AAC Service Delivery

There are various methods of tele-AAC that can be implemented to provide high-quality services. Typically, service delivery in telepractice falls under two broad headings: synchronous (in real time) and asynchronous (offline or store-and-forward). Synchronous services are conducted with an interactive audio and video connection in real time to create an in-person experience, like more traditional on-site services. A live, interactive videoconference session is one in which the specialist and the client are present at the same time, but not in the same location. The specialist is often located either in their office, home, or facility, and the client is in a different location, such as a clinic, school, nursing home, or hospital. The client's caregiver is generally present with the client and supports the services from a technical standpoint and is the client's primary communication partner. Synchronous tele-AAC services are used to provide real-time assessments, interventions, and team consultations and collaborations. It is important to note that even if synchronous telepractice cannot occur due to barriers such as lack of high-speed Internet, available infrastructure, on-site support personnel, or technical knowledge, asynchronous telepractice and store-and-forward methods (i.e., audio or video recordings) can still take place.

Asynchronous services are used when images or data are captured via video, audio recordings, pictures, or data and transmitted (i.e., stored and forwarded) for viewing or interpretation by a professional. This method of telepractice allows the AAC specialist to accurately monitor the client and provide strategies and recommendations outside of a direct intervention session. Store-and-forward methods are particularly useful to enhance a communication partner's ability to utilize AAC tools, model language, and engage with a client when live and in-the-moment tele-AAC services cannot occur.

The combination of the two approaches can be applied in tele-AAC to provide hybrid sessions. Hybrid sessions use components of live, interactive, and store-and-forward methods to best support clients with CCNs. A hybrid tele-AAC model has the advantage of making use of all technologies that are available to diagnose, treat, and consult the client and their team and is not limited to a single communications approach. Examples of hybrid approaches include remote monitoring, distance supervision, and active consultation.

Prior to the initiation of any direct or indirect services, it is essential that teams have access to hardware and software that support tele-AAC, and that the infrastructure is configured in a way that supports robust services. Given a location that has access to stable high-speed Internet and commonly used hardware and software, there are no inherent limits as to where telepractice can be implemented, if the services comply with national, state, institutional, and professional regulations and policies (Cason & Cohn, 2014). Planning and testing out the systems not only ensures that clinicians are more confident in the use of technology to deliver tele-AAC services but also enhances clinical flexibility so that the sessions are focused on reliable clinician exchanges, targeted goals and objectives, and transfer of skills, rather than on technical glitches, issues, or troubleshooting.

The type of preparation that is typically used for on-site services should be consistent with tele-AAC services. This includes determining the most appropriate tools and placement to ensure client privacy, comfort, and utility along with material presentation using evidence-based AAC intervention methods. In addition, there are several elements that exist that are unique to tele-AAC. For live, interactive services, the environment needs to be designed to enhance the quality of the video and audio interactions and support the context of communication, accommodate the AAC tools and activities, as well as account for the client's physical and sensory needs as shown in Figure 35–1. Additionally, the client and clinician often need to have access to two video inputs, either through the videoconferencing system or through an additional computer, to maintain visual and auditory communication with each other while at the same time using a secondary webcam or document camera to share physical items (i.e., a speech-generating device [SGD], low-tech [paper-based] communication boards, visuals, etc.).

Hardware and Software Considerations

The hardware and software recommended at each site to deliver and receive tele-AAC include a computer or laptop, videoconferencing software, webcams (internal and supplemental cameras that are positioned above a SGD or material), SGD simulation software or similar procedures for SGD screen sharing (i.e., Screen Mirroring App), and a secondary mode of communication (i.e., cell phone). The visual infrastructure of the equipment must support the clinician's ability to provide visual cues and models as well as use of nonverbal body language (i.e., gestures and facial expressions) via videoconferencing. External webcams (versus a built-in webcam) often provide a wider visual field of the remote environment and provide freedom of movement as the camera can be repositioned in any direction. While not mandatory, it is recommended that the computer or laptop used can support the use of two webcams (i.e., one integrated and the other external) or that the clinician use two separate computers—one to maintain a consistent audio and video connection and the other to share content. The use of two webcams offers the clinician the ability to simultaneously view the client and use a document camera to display a device, low-tech communication boards, or any other tangible items. This allows the clinician to provide and share tangible content without the need to create a digital format of the material or simulation of the device.

> ### Expert Tip: Two Computers to Deliver Tele-AAC Services
>
> The use of two computers supports the clinician-client exchanges and allows for more options related to sharing online and tangible assessments and material, in-the-moment modeling, and training. In addition, dedicating one device for content sharing helps organize shared content when screen sharing. The second webcam can be utilized to share SGDs, paper-based material, visuals, and cue cards, while the other computer provides a consistent visual/audio connection. In addition, the use of two computers enables the clinician to monitor the client view and make any changes to the presentation of material as needed. It also serves as a backup computer if technical issues arise.

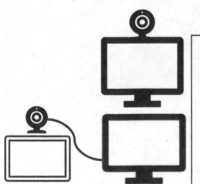

1 – Computer for audio and video

2 – Computer to share content through screen share or external device.

Figure 35–1. The tele-AAC configuration of technology. Symbols used with permission from n2y.com.

Videoconferencing software is needed to deliver synchronous tele-AAC services. There are several options available that clinicians can use for telepractice that range from free web conferencing systems to far more expensive options. However, it is essential that the videoconference system being used has the needed Health Insurance Portability and Accountability Act (HIPAA, 1996), Family Educational Rights and Privacy Act (FERPA, 1974), and security protocols in place to protect client confidentiality and records. Moreover, there are specific features that a videoconferencing system must have to best support tele-AAC. These include the ability to screenshare, share keyboard and mouse controls, take back control as needed, minimize the self-view of the video screen, change position of the video screen on the computer, use accessibility features (i.e., enlarged font size in chat), use closed captioning, and use scheduling capabilities as shown in Figure 35–2. It is also helpful if the video software allows the clinician to use two webcam inputs at the same time. As previously mentioned,

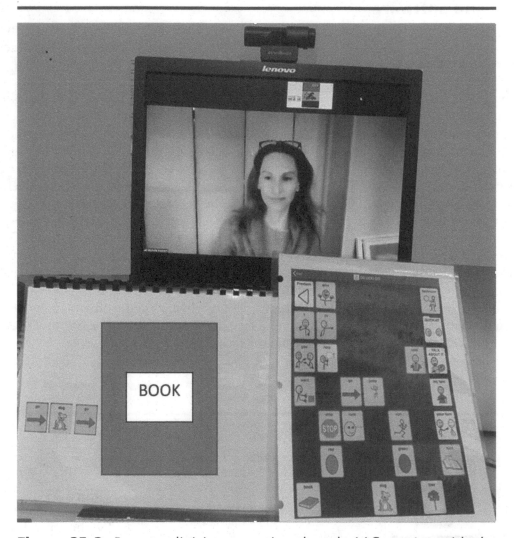

Figure 35–2. Remote clinician preparing the tele-AAC session with the on-site team utilizing videoconferencing and online material along with tangible material. Symbols used with permission from n2y.com. Copyright © 2021 SymbolStix, LLC. All rights reserved. Screenshots of Proloquo2Go pages customized for this project. Images used with permission.

this feature allows the clinician to share content while, at the same time, maintaining visual and verbal and nonverbal communication. Depending on the material that is being presented, some videoconferencing systems also have a "green screen" option. There are many different activities and materials that use green screens that offer exciting and engaging games for some clients.

The best approach for a successful tele-AAC program is to ensure that both the client and the clinician have access to the needed infrastructure, technology, on-site support, and training. With the foundation in place and strategies to support communication between on- and offsite personnel, tele-AAC is a viable method for delivery of clinical services to clients who have complex communication needs.

Case Study: JS

Clinical Profile and Communication Needs

The Individual

JS is a 9-year-old female student in the third grade who participates in an intensive program embedded into the public-school setting. She has an individualized education plan (IEP) due to Multiple Disabilities including Intellectual Impairment, Autism, and Health (Down Syndrome). Her medical history is significant for celiac disease, congenital heart disease, epilepsy, and visual and auditory impairments. Her communication is characterized by sign language, vocalic vocalizations, gestures, and behaviors to direct her communication partners. She is socially motivated and seeks out interactions with peers and adults. Her communication intent is a relative strength but is severely limited by her ability to produce sounds and overall receptive and expressive language abilities, which results in frequent communication breakdowns. JS has a 1:1 aide who is with her throughout the day and supports her behaviors, routine-based communication (i.e., greetings) through gestures (i.e., waving, pointing), vocalizations (i.e., "mmm," "ba-ba"),

language through lite-tech tools (i.e., paper-based communication overlays, visual choice icons), social interactions, and functional daily living skills. She receives discrete trial instruction, and her program includes safety directions, receptive and expressive identification, manding, two-step gross motor imitation with verbal prompts, responding to her name, and following directions.

Their Communication Partners

JS's primary communication partners are her family members (mom, dad, and older sister), 1:1, service providers at home and school, and some peers.

Their Environment

JS participates in class-based activities such as art, music, gym, and lunch. When engaging in those settings, the amount of communication she exhibits with peers is limited.

The AAC Service Considerations

JS attends school in a district where an SLP trained in AAC is not employed; therefore, the district contracted a specialist who was geographically located 50 miles away from the physical school building. The school-based team was interested in using telepractice to access services, increase the frequency and consistency of services, as well as provide team consultation. An AAC evaluation was conducted through a hybrid of on-site and asynchronous methods. Based on the outcomes from the assessment, a high-tech AAC device was recommended. An iPad with Proloquo2Go® was identified as the most appropriate high-tech tool as it provides a wide range of customizable vocabulary using a folder-based system, and JS was already familiar with the use of an iPad. JS's main page included core words in consistent locations, and activity-specific vocabulary words were put into separate folders (i.e., vocabulary for preferred books and music activities), as shown in Figure 35–3. While this tool was recommended for JS, her school-based team and family were unfamiliar with the device and requested significant training on the use and application of the device to support JS's

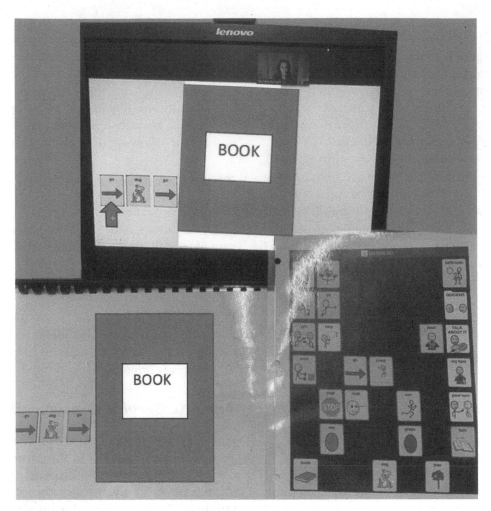

Figure 35–3. On-site view of tele-AAC session using screen sharing, annotation tools, and tangible material. Symbols used with permission from n2y.com. Copyright © 2021 SymbolStix, LLC. All rights reserved. Screenshots of Proloquo2Go pages customized for this project. Images used with permission.

communication throughout her school day. Moreover, the school-based team and family did not have experience with online services and required basic training on the technology and methods to access the clinician as well.

Tele-AAC Setup for Optimal Visual Access

Prior to the start of tele-AAC services, the school-based team required training on the setup of the

telepractice technology and how to best position the computers for optimal visual access of the AAC device. On-site, JS and her communication partner used one laptop computer and had the device with them for each session. The clinician recommended that they use an external webcam rather than the internal one built into the laptop as external webcams provided a wider visual field of the remote environment along with extra freedom of movement as the camera can be repositioned in any direction (i.e., directly pointing at the device). They had access to the videoconferencing site (i.e.,

Zoom) and practiced logging in and changing the features to best support tele-AAC: hiding nonvideo participants, enabling the gallery view, displaying screen-share in a side-by-side mode, and increasing the size of the text in the chat by 200%.

The clinician used two laptops during the training to deliver the services. Both computers were logged into the same videoconferencing meeting at the same time (one as the host and the other as a participant). The clinician's first laptop was used to sustain all communication using an internal webcam, microphone, and headset. The computer was elevated somewhat so that the webcam was in line with the clinician's head placement. This created a more natural head and body position and supported expected nonverbal interpersonal behaviors. It also provided a slightly wider view so the clinician could use more nonverbal language, sign language, and gestures during the session. When interacting with JS and her communication partner during the training, the clinician looked at the internal webcam as much as possible, as this established approximate and more appropriate eye gaze. The second computer, or content computer, was used to screen-share all material and was in an easily accessed and utilized workspace right below the first computer. The document camera was attached to the second computer so that the clinician could easily share, or model a SGD, applications, tangible objects, or material (i.e., low-tech communication boards).

The on-site team practiced connecting to the online meeting several times and confirmed that they could see and hear the clinician along with the presented material both through screen-share and the document camera.

Next Steps

Once the on-site team was comfortable connecting with the clinician in an online format, times were scheduled for team consultation as well as intervention sessions. The sessions were scheduled using Google calendar, and a notification reminder was set up for the team. The notification was sent 30 min prior to the session each day using the automatic notification feature built into Google calen-

dar. The e-mail included confirmation information such as the date and time of the session, the meeting link, and the clinician's contact information.

The team determined the initial target vocabulary based on JS's preferred interests. The vocabulary for each activity was located on one page, and the school-based team and family practiced accessing the vocabulary prior to the first intervention session. In addition to activity-specific vocabulary, interpersonal and familiar action symbols and core words (i.e., more, all done, turn page) were also visible on the screen. As the AAC device was being introduced to JS, the AAC specialist asked that her communication partners model the language on the device rather than require her to activate the icons. The goal was to increase JS's exposure to the language system and gradually aid her language during the activities. The AAC specialist met with the family once a week to review the same procedures that the school-based team was using to promote carryover in the home setting. While the device was with JS throughout her day, initially it was used during content-specific activities at school and at home. The procedures and strategies used for tele-AAC intervention and consultation are described in Chapter 36.

References

Brown, J. (2011). ASHA and the evolution of telepractice. *Perspectives on Telepractice, 1*(1), 4–9.

Burke, B. Jr., Bynum, A., Hall-Barrow, J., Ott, R., & Albright, M. (2008). Rural school-based telehealth: How to make it happen. *Clinical Pediatrics, 47*(9), 926–929.

Cason, J., & Cohn, E. R. (2014). Telepractice: An overview and best practices. *Perspectives on Augmentative and Alternative Communication, 23*(1), 4–17.

Demiris, G., Shigaki, C. L., & Schopp, L. H. (2005). An evaluation framework for a rural home-based tele-rehabilitation network. *Journal of Medical Systems, 29*(6), 595–603.

Dudding, C. C., & Justice, L. M. (2004). An e-supervision model: Videoconferencing as a clinical training tool. *Communication Disorders Quarterly, 25*(3), 145–151.

Family Educational Rights and Privacy Act of 1974, 20 U.S.C. § 1232g. (1974).

Harwood, M. T., Pratt, D., Beutler, L. E., Bongar, B. M., Lenore, S., & Forrester, B. T. (2011). Technology, telehealth, treatment enhancement, and selection. *Professional Psychology: Research and Practice, 42*(6), 448–454.

Health Insurance Portability and Accountability Act of 1996 (HIPAA; Pub. L. 104–191, 110 Stat.

Juenger, J. M. (2009). Telepractice in the schools. *ASHA Leader, 14*(12), 20–21.

Kolb, M. J. (2009). An online training program for parents of children with autism. Dissertation Abstracts International (PsychINFO, UMI No. 3316404).

Zoom. (n.d.). https://zoom.us

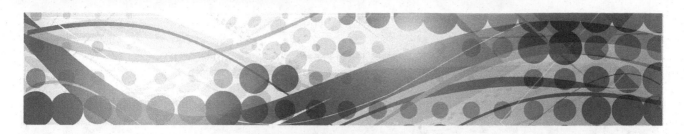

Chapter 36
TELE-AAC FOR SERVICE DELIVERY

Michelle Boisvert

Fundamentals

Tele-AAC is an exciting method that can be used to deliver both synchronous and asynchronous services. As described in the previous chapter, tele-AAC is an application of telepractice that uses technology to deliver evidence-based clinical services regardless of the client's and clinicians' geographical location. It is a growing method of service delivery and can be used for assessments, direct and indirect services for clients with complex communication needs (CCNs), as well as team consultation and collaboration. Without a doubt, the integration of telepractice into an augmentative and alternative communication (AAC) implementation plan adds extra organizational, technical, and training components for the entire team but is feasible, especially given the critical need for this service. Online assessment, intervention, and consultation are becoming more prevalent and widely accepted, and this is arguably necessary during nationwide or statewide travel restrictions, in cases whereby the access to highly qualified professionals is hard to attain, to compliment in-person services, or as a method to support high workload demands that services providers are often faced with.

In most cases, there will be a need for on-site support to facilitate tele-AAC services. The on-site support personnel are typically the primary communication partner for the client in that environment. The communication partner works closely with the clinician during the clinical sessions while interacting with client and embeds the learned strategies, modeling, and cues into the session and, ideally, throughout the client's day. The role of the communication partner can be filled by one or several trained individuals, paraprofessionals, or caregivers as shown in Figure 36–1. They are directly involved in the session; therefore, frequent communication with the clinician is essential to promote effective use of the technology required for telepractice, effective communication using AAC, and to facilitate the AAC tools, materials, and strategies during an assessment, intervention session, or consultation. Often, direct training in the implementation of telepractice methods and ongoing AAC guidance are necessary as the needs of the client and goals of the AAC tools may fluctuate.

To provide optimal support for a tele-AAC session, the training for the communication partner should be twofold. First, they must be able to set up the basic technology required for tele-AAC (i.e., hardware and software), and second, they must understand the target objectives or goals for the session related to the AAC tool. They should also have access to all materials that will be utilized during the session, and the clinician should guide specific action steps needed for the materials (i.e., print out material, send links, give access to files, etc.), as demonstrated in Figure 36–2. In most cases, the communication partner is responsible for scheduling, preparing, and bringing the client to and from services. While they are not responsible for primarily directing any part of the clinical services, they are asked to model language, support

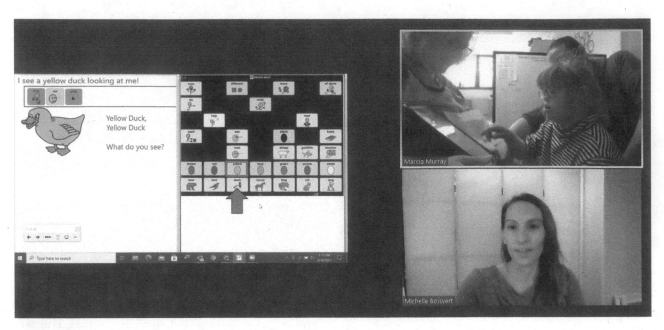

Figure 36–1. On-site communication partner during tele-AAC session. Symbols used with permission from n2y.com. Copyright © 2021 SymbolStix, LLC. All rights reserved.

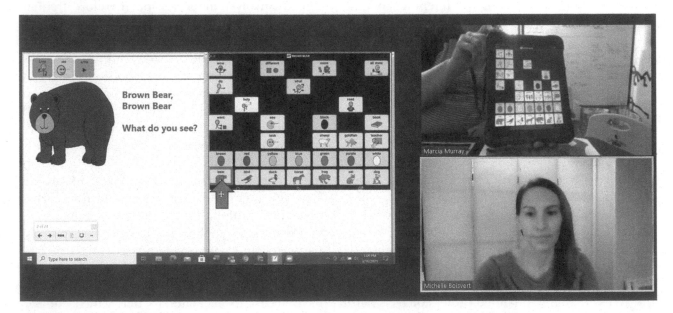

Figure 36–2. On-site communication partner preparing material for the session. Symbols used with permission from n2y.com. Copyright © 2021 SymbolStix, LLC. All rights reserved. Screenshots of Proloquo2Go pages customized for this project. Images used with permission.

communication opportunities, and generalize certain skills that have been reviewed by the clinician. This person facilitates communication between the remote clinician and other members of the client's team such as educators, support staff, family members, or caregivers. At times, the communication partner provides support for behavior modification as needed and should be able to handle basic troubleshooting of the technology and equipment used during the sessions.

One of the major hurdles associated with tele-AAC assessment and service delivery is the added variable of needing to view and access the output of the speech-generating device (SGD). While advancements in technology have made the digitized voice output of SGDs easier to understand, the ability to view a client's device and overlay in an interactive and virtual clinical setting requires careful configuration and use of technology (Hall & Boisvert, 2014). Regardless of the method used for AAC intervention (i.e., on-site or online), the clinician's ability to observe the client's communication method, irrespective if it is high-, mid-, or low-tech, as well as the message that is generated from the tool, is highly beneficial (Boisvert & Hall, 2018). There are some specific strategies that can be implemented to share SGD's, mid- or low-tech communication boards, or any other tangible materials used to enhance or model communication in real-time synchronous sessions. These approaches are described later in this chapter.

Both synchronous and asynchronous tele-AAC methods can be implemented when conducting assessments. As discussed in prior chapters, an AAC assessment is a comprehensive review of the client's current method of communication and provides appropriate strategies and recommendations for enhancing their future communication and linguistic growth. Information that drives the outcome of the AAC assessment is typically obtained in a variety of methods, including observations, interviews, feature matching, formal and informal testing, and device trials. Depending on the nature and severity of a client's profile, an AAC evaluation may examine the form and structure of a client's speech and language as well as the use of language in a variety of functional and social settings, and across different communication partners. A comprehensive assessment requires the clinician to be current on the expanding technical advancements that support augmentative communication (Dietz et al., 2012), evidence-based evaluation approaches, and the identification of the appropriate AAC system that best meets the client's needs.

Conducting an AAC assessment through telepractice adds another layer of technical knowledge on the part of the clinician and their ability to train or guide the communication partner (i.e., family member, caregiver, paraprofessional) through the process. Without a doubt, the clinician must be knowledgeable of the online platforms that are used to conduct a tele-AAC evaluation and be able to troubleshoot minor technical issues as they occur. The added component of telepractice typically requires additional training for the individual with CCNs and their communication partner to prepare for the evaluation. This type of training and preparation should be considered when factoring in the amount of time needed to conduct the assessment. To that end, the use of online methods may also open different scheduling times and enable the clinician to view and observe the client more frequently or in several settings. While many aspects that comprise a tele-AAC assessment can be completed using asynchronous methods or through access to prior information, recorded observations, language analysis, or samples, some portions may also enable the clinician to utilize synchronous telepractice approaches to obtain additional assessment and observational data.

Synchronous assessment sessions give opportunities for the clinician to provide AAC instruction, ask the communication partner to carry out certain strategies to identify a client's ability to access AAC devices throughout the day or when presented with cognitive demanding tasks, probe multimodal approaches during highly motivating, preferred, or functional activities, or determine necessary positional modifications based on the environmental setting. Synchronous assessments may also provide increased opportunities to view functional tasks along with the varying expectations of the client engaged in the tasks. This helps the clinician determine barriers associated with more complex access needs and how these needs may change based on the expectations. For example, some clients with significant motor challenges will benefit from an eye-gaze input method to access to their SGD. This can be trialed in a tele-AAC synchronous method by using a secondary computer and external webcam that is logged into the videoconference meeting, so that it provides a "birds-eye view" of the client as they interact with the device. The remote clinician must work closely and guide the communication partner(s) to ensure consistent placement of the device, perhaps through a mounting system, as well as the various seating, standing, or lying positions that are best for the client. Providing this support through synchronous tele-AAC methods gives the clinician more in-the-moment opportunities to see and modify the environment (i.e., lighting), symbol target size, and device positioning or placement based on the client's motor control, visual acuity, visual processing skills, as well as the available mounting equipment. In some cases, this may be challenging and might be more easily conducted in an in-person/on-site setting.

Expert Tip: Use a Checklist for Evaluation Information Gathering

A tele-AAC evaluation plan or checklist helps the clinician organize and obtain necessary information, identify specific action steps, schedule assessment sessions, collect language analysis data, and provide follow-up AAC instructions. Many established AAC checklists or evaluation plans can be used and modified to include the added telepractice elements. When conducting a tele-AAC evaluation, additional factors include communication partner training on how to log in and set up the technology required for telepractice (i.e., computer, webcam placement, etc.); how the AAC tools will be sent to the client, what tools will be sent, and when; methods to obtain trial device data logs; and follow-up AAC instruction.

Methods of data collection, language activity monitoring, or language analysis can be collected and obtained through asynchronous methods. As the clinician cannot be physically with the client, caregivers or communication partners may need training on how to activate automatic data log features in an AAC system and then send the logfiles through e-mail, upload them to a shared folder, or send them to the clinician using another format. If language data are collected over a period of time, the clinician may ask the primary communication partner to upload the logfiles on a weekly basis, after an assessment session, or following a series of daily activities as the information will help guide future recommendations and other potential device trials. During a tele-AAC evaluation session, the clinician may also objectively collect data on client access to the AAC tool, visual and physical access, attention, motor planning skills, and navigation abilities through either asynchronous or synchronous telepractice methods.

When providing direct intervention, the goal of any tele-AAC service is to optimize the client-clinician interaction, target specific skills, and provide reliable and effective services that directly benefit the client. Establishing a systematic routine that the client and the on-site communication partner follow each time they join the tele-AAC session is helpful to reduce any additional stress or technical issues that may come up. It is also recommended that these steps are reviewed and practiced prior to the first tele-AAC clinical session. Providing clear and consistent supports, along with concrete strategies and examples of the procedures used to successfully implement tele-AAC will maintain the client's and caregivers' confidence and assurance that tele-AAC is comparable to on-site services.

Evidenced-based AAC interventions, as outlined in other chapters of this book, can be provided in an online setting using a strategic setup of hardware and use of videoconferencing software. Tele-AAC services are provided using built-in features supported by the videoconferencing software, specifically screen sharing and shared mouse, and keyboard control. The delivery of activity-based material can be screen shared, and both the client and/or communication partner and clinician can interact with the material through joint mouse and keyboard control. The shared screen can also display simulated SGDs, overlays, or other tools needed to model the use of the AAC tool. Communication is facilitated through the videoconferencing features, audio output of the SGD, text or chat messaging, or other modes (i.e., gestures, sign language, visual icons). If the clinician uses the screen sharing for activity-based material and verbally cues the communication partner to model or aid language on the device, the communication partner must be familiar and comfortable with navigation and use of the AAC tools.

Specific strategies can be used to view the client's AAC device and provide direct modeling in a tele-AAC environment. These approaches can be implemented to share SGDs, mid- or low-tech communication boards, or any other tangible materials used to enhance or model communication in real-time synchronous sessions. They include text-based tele-AAC and tele-AAC with shared SGDs using an external webcam or mirroring software. These approaches are described in more detail in the book *Tele-AAC: Augmentative and Alternative Communication through Telepractice* (Hall et al., 2019). There are benefits and limitations to each tele-AAC method, and these need to be carefully considered prior to the start of services.

Implementing direct text-based tele-AAC refers to the ability to engage in services using text-based screen sharing. To achieve this, the client needs to have an SGD with an output feature that will send data from the SGD to a computer, serving as an external keyboard for a computer (Hall & Boisvert, 2014). With the device connected to the client's computer, anything input into the device will present as text in a word-processing program, shared document, chat, or text box on the client's computer. Using the screen-sharing feature in the videoconferencing software, the client and the clinician can simultaneously interact with the same activity and engage in reciprocal exchanges (Boisvert & Hall, 2018; Hall & Boisvert, 2014; Hall et al., 2019). This method of synchronous tele-AAC requires that shared activities be formatted for text input (i.e., text box, shared word-processing document, chat feature, etc.). This approach restricts client candidacy to individuals who are literate, and relatively proficient AAC users. Additionally, this form of tele-AAC does not easily allow the clinician to offer direct AAC modeling or icon selection, or engage in augmented input without a similar device at their personal workstation along with the use of a secondary webcam to broadcast their use of the device through the videoconferencing software (Hall & Boisvert, 2014).

For most individuals using AAC, the ability for the clinician to directly model augmented input is an essential feature and supports evidence-based intervention, such as aided language stimulation. Furthermore, the clinician's ability to "see" how the client is navigating their device, overlay, or communication board is of paramount importance when teaching the client and their communication partner or caregiver how to best use the AAC system (Hall & Boisvert, 2014; Hall et al., 2019). One approach to provide in-the-moment modeling and demonstrate regular use of a system in a telepractice environment is with a secondary computer with an external webcam pointed at the communication tool (like shown in Figure 36–3). This method enables streaming video of the device as it is being used. The use of an external webcam pointed at the client and clinician's device provides a view of the AAC tool as well as how they are navigating it. To use this method, the client and clinician must use two computers that are logged into the same online meeting room or utilize a videoconferencing tool that allows for the concurrent display of two webcam views. This configuration and use of technology allow the clinician to model specific targets on their SGD at the same time as viewing the client navigation of their SGD and therefore provides AAC modeling and augmented input. While this setup enables both the client and clinician to see each other's devices, it does require the clinician to have a device that is comparable to that of the client. Other options to share SGDs include screen mirroring or simulation programs that are then shared via the screen-sharing feature. However, this eliminates the ability to use the screen-sharing feature for materials. In this case, the client, their communication partner, and the clinician may need to utilize resources that allow for joint access, such as cloud-based programs, like Google Docs.

Activity-based materials can be consistent with the types of materials that would be used for on-site intervention sessions. These include websites, books, interactive materials, online games, photos, or any item(s) that are of interest to the client and that will be a motivator to assess their skill set, competency, and use of the selected AAC tools (i.e., using text, selecting one or two icons, sequencing icons, navigating pages, etc.). Clinicians must carefully consider the material used for

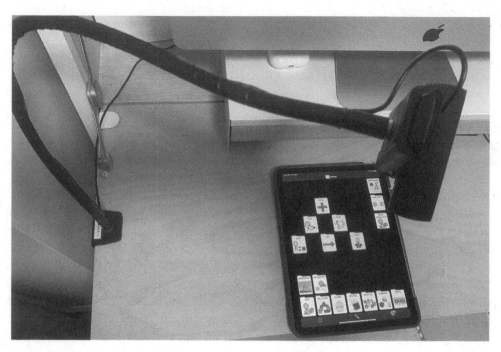

Figure 36–3. Configuration for synchronous tele-AAC with external webcam. Symbols used with permission from n2y.com. Copyright © 2021 SymbolStix, LLC. All rights reserved. Screenshots of Proloquo2Go pages customized for this project. Images used with permission.

tele-AAC with respect to the usability and content. The focus of any telepractice session should continue the clinical relationship and have a usable, goal-oriented purpose rather than the presentation of complicated and/or flashy activities.

A successful tele-AAC program will involve the client's communication partners from the beginning to help support all services. As a team, the methods and strategies that will provide the most effective services for the client with a complex communication profile are identified, implemented, and modified as the client's needs change. In addition, clear communication should occur around the quality of the telepractice services. This includes the audio and video connection, strategies to address technical issues, access to the technology, and ability to model and share AAC tools. Frequent and ongoing training or consultation with the communication partner and caregiver enables the team to take a proactive approach to any barriers, increase awareness of upcoming functional activities that can be pre-taught, continue to grow intervention

approaches, and discuss skill transfer and curriculum-related modifications. Strong communication between the treating clinician and the on-site team enables transfer of approaches that have been successful within an on-site setting to be carried over into the tele-AAC sessions. Additionally, communication partners who accompany the client can provide consistent modeling, redirections, and prompting within a tele-AAC session as required.

The American Speech-Language-Hearing Association requires that therapy provided through telepractice should be evaluated for quality assurance, clinical effectiveness, and client, caregiver, and provider satisfaction regardless of the equipment, tools, or services that are utilized (Theodoros, 2011). Therefore, the treating clinician must ensure that they uphold this standard, monitor client access and progress, and recognize when additional support is needed or situations that may not be appropriate for tele-AAC. To support quality services that are comparable to on-site services, the clinician and the client's team should incorporate quality monitoring techniques that will provide information regarding the various procedural, structural, and instructional components that are needed for tele-AAC.

Approaches to monitor quality control, document clinical outcomes, facilitate on-site and remote team collaboration, incorporate clinical flexibility, and use evidence-based intervention approaches must be systematically assessed on an ongoing basis. Tele-AAC readiness refers to the specific infrastructure, environmental setting, and support personnel available to support tele-AAC services. The tele-AAC team should determine if the necessary hardware and software are available and set up, if training has been provided, and that the communication partner has access to the AAC tools and is aware of the benefits and limitations associated with tele-AAC.

Data collection and documentation are crucial components of any clinical service. Due to the need to accurately validate and report client services, share client information with team members, and use information to guide recommendations, both qualitative and quantitative data are typically collected. In addition to the type of data collection that is consistent with on-site services, the clinician should continue to identify the most appropriate methods and activity-based materials that target goals and objectives, and the responsiveness of the client during the session (including external behavior, distractions, and AAC access). Documenting the amount and type of support that the communication is providing and the team's overall satisfaction with tele-AAC services is important as well. With respect to the additional layer of technology required for tele-AAC services, clinicians should monitor the type of technical difficulties that are being experienced and provide procedures to login and troubleshoot to the communication partners.

Evaluating the tele-AAC sessions helps teams determine if the client is demonstrating adequate progress and if they are responding to tele-AAC in a way that is expected. Bringing this information to team consultations supports the overall collaboration process as team members can assess the success of the tele-AAC program and make appropriate adjustments, modifications, or shifts in the tele-AAC approach to better benefit the client. The

increased engagement of communication partners increases the opportunities for language to be embedded into the client's life in many ways. Teams that frequently meet to collaborate, discuss success, brainstorm barriers, share material, and provide direction for future intervention sessions impact the quality of services and provide a robust communication environment for the client.

Case Study: JS

Clinical Profile and Communication Needs

As first described in the previous chapter, JS is a 9-year-old female student who primarily communicates through sign language, gestures, behaviors, and limited vocalizations. She enjoys dancing, playing with toys, reading books, and listening to music, and has high social interest. JS is motivated by her peers and will often learn certain motor skills more quickly when observing peers rather than in an individual setting. JS qualified for services with a diagnosis of Intellectual Impairment, Autism, and Health. She has Down syndrome and a history of celiac disease, congenital heart disease, epilepsy, as well as visual and auditory impairments.

While primarily in an intensive program, she spends time with her class during music, gym, and art, and has lunch each day with one peer and with adult support. Her primary mode of communication is through approximated sign language, and with adult support she can communicate basic greetings, as well as her wants and needs (i.e., "my turn," "more," "all done," "music," "go," and "water"). She has also been provided with communication boards and visual choice icons to help her identify functional items, social interactions, and choices within activities and music. She receives discrete trial instruction under the supervision of a board-certified behavior analyst (BCBA), and her current discrete trial programs include safety directions, receptive and expressive tacting, manding, motor imitations, and attention to task. Following an evaluation, she was prescribed a high-tech AAC device, specifically an iPad with Proloquo2Go®.

This device was recommended, as Proloquo2Go provides a folder-based vocabulary system and JS was familiar with an iPad for other uses (i.e., listening to music). Specific pages were developed within the app with target vocabulary based on her preferred interests and motivators. As the device was being introduced, her communication partners were encouraged to model language during activity-specific times both at school and at home. Over several months, JS was shown her AAC device as an adult communication partner modeled using the device to request to watch, listen to music, turn the page [of a book], and read. Gradually, JS was prompted to select the vocabulary symbols through tactile and visual cues and demonstrated an increased accuracy of target button selection. Direct services and modeling were provided through a tele-AAC synchronous method that utilized two computers and a screen capture of JS's SGD page. The specific activity was presented on half of the screen, and the SGD capture was presented on the other half. Annotation tools were used to provide modeling for the correct button selection for JS's communication partners, as seen in Figure 36–4.

Their Communication Partners

JS's communication partners include her family members (i.e., parents and older sister), along with her 1:1 paraprofessional, service providers, and peers at school.

Their Environment

JS communicates within her home and school-based environment. Her social interactions are primarily supported by an adult during school-based activities such as art, music, gym, and lunch.

AAC System or Service Considerations

Recently, JS received a tri-annual evaluation by an SLP who specializes in AAC. Following an on-site assessment and observation, in conjunction with asynchronous assessment procedures, an iPad with Proloquo2Go was identified as the most appropriate high-tech tool for her at this time. Proloquo2Go was recommended as it is easily customizable, supports beginning communicators, and has the capacity to grow with her as her language acquisition

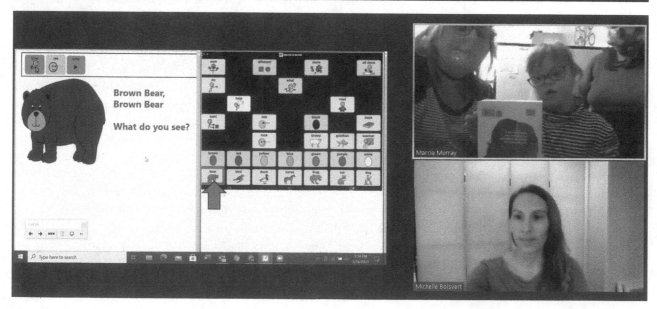

Figure 36–4. Presentation of activity and speech-generating device through tele-AAC. Symbols used with permission from n2y.com. Copyright © 2021 SymbolStix, LLC. All rights reserved. Screenshots of Proloquo2Go pages customized for this project. Images used with permission.

evolves over the years. While this AAC tool was identified as being most appropriate for JS's communication profile and there was high motivation to use the tool from both her family and school-based team, her primary communication partners and school-based team did not have experience using Proloquo2Go; therefore, training, consultation, and direct intervention with JS and her communication partners were provided.

Initial training on Proloquo2Go was provided by an SLP who specialized in AAC to JS's school-based team, specifically her 1:1 paraprofessional and service providers (SLP, occupational therapist, physical therapist, vision specialist) through tele-AAC. First, the AAC specialist ensured that the school-based team was ready for tele-AAC and could access the technology needed for telepractice and provided an initial tutorial. Following the tele-AAC readiness check and during the first AAC device training session, the specialist used two computers that were logged into the same videoconferencing meeting. The first computer was used to establish audio and video communication with the team, and the second, equipped with an external webcam that was directed at the AAC tool, was used to model use of the device. The on-site team had a replica of JS's iPad system with them and practiced the steps that were presented to them to increase familiarity and comfort with the device. With guidance from the AAC specialist, the team determined the initial core vocabulary that would be modeled and presented to JS.

The AAC System or Service

At first, the team identified specific activities that would be presented to JS during certain times of the day and incorporated the use of the device during those times. Throughout the rest of the day, the device was present, and slowly JS's 1:1 started using the device in more natural settings to model vocabulary targets throughout the day. As JS's primary school-based communication partner became more comfortable with the device, it was used more and therefore provided an increase of access and use for JS. The team continued to meet for a weekly check-in with the AAC specialist to discuss challenges as well as brainstorm additional

opportunities for AAC use. New vocabulary was frequently added, and the team's procedure for exposure, modeling, and prompting was repeated. The consistent team collaborations fostered trust and willingness to troubleshoot when technical glitches occurred. Teamwork was essential, especially when the tele-AAC program was initiated given the many layers of technology, training, and modifications that are embedded in intervention sessions, and ultimately generalization of usage of the system.

The AAC specialist also provided weekly consultation with the family to support the use of the AAC device at home. Again, the specialist used two computers with one webcam used to sustain video and audio communication between the client and the family members, and the other with a webcam directed to her own device to provide modeling as needed, especially when new vocabulary targets were introduced. This empowered the family to receive in-the-moment training and enhanced JS's opportunities for communication during fun and relaxing activities (such as watching movies, reading books, and dancing to music). The skill level of the family to navigate the device drastically increased, and JS's accuracy with button use and her overall communication grew in ways that were exciting for the family.

The AAC specialist provided weekly direct intervention tele-AAC sessions at school with JS and her communication partner, who was her 1:1 paraprofessional. The AAC specialist had a similar device for direct modeling. For the first several months, the specialist used two computers: one to present activity-based material while at the same time using the second computer to also share the device via an external webcam (or share a simulation of the SGD so that annotation tools could be used to provide more direct visual modeling with arrows and highlighted shapes). JS and the paraprofessional used one computer with an external webcam to view the clinician and the shared material and positioned themselves so that the clinician could see the navigation and use of the device.

Activities consisting of books with repetitive phrases (i.e., Brown Bear, Hungry Caterpillar), music and preferred activities, and modeling of core words such as "read," "more," "go," "no," and "yes" were practiced with high repetition. Once JS's communication partner became familiar and comfortable navigating the device, the AAC specialist used one computer to present the activities and then brought up specific overlays to help the communication partner sequence or navigate to new words or concepts as needed. The AAC specialist would provide verbal cues (i.e., "Look," "Touch _____."), and JS's communication partner would immediately provide the verbal prompt to JS and pair the prompt with a gestural cue as needed. This fading of direct language modeling to verbal cuing from the AAC specialist empowered JS's communication partner and helped her take on an active role in the session, as well as increase the amount of language exchanges in the sessions. The same approach was used for home-based intervention, and the family experienced an even quicker feeling of comfort and usability with the device. The increased level of communication opportunities transferred into JS's school and home life as her communication partners realized the benefit and power that the AAC device gave to JS to help her communicate and engage in various functional and social experiences.

Next Steps

The team continues to meet on a weekly basis to identify updated vocabulary targets, concepts, and social uses for the device. The overarching goal continues to support JS's interaction with her communication partners using the AAC device to support her language for increasing purposes throughout the day.

References

Boisvert, M. K., & Hall, N. (2018). *School-based telepractice services who are AAC users: Lessons learned*. American Speech-Language-Hearing Association, Boston, MA.

Dietz, A., Quach, W., Lund, S. K., & McKelvey, M. (2012). AAC assessment and clinical-decision making: The impact of experience. *Augmentative and Alternative Communication, 28*(3), 148–159.

Hall, N., & Boisvert, M. (2014). Clinical aspects related to tele-AAC: A technical report. *Perspectives on Augmentative and Alternative Communication, 23*(1), 18–33.

Hall, N., Juengling-Sudkamp, J., Gutmann, M. L., & Cohn, E. R. (Eds.). (2019). *Tele-AAC: Augmentative and alternative communication through telepractice*. Plural Publishing.

SMART Notebook. (2021). https://support.smarttech.com/en/downloads/notebook

Theodoros, D. (2011). Telepractice in speech-language pathology: The evidence, the challenges, and the future. *Perspectives on Telepractice, 1*(1), 10–21.

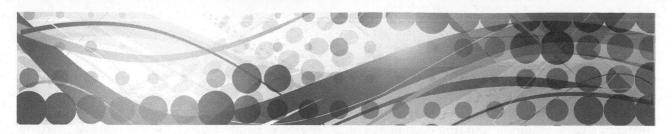

Essay 20

CLINICAL CONSIDERATIONS AND AAC: BUILDING MY AAC VILLAGE

Tannalynn Neufeld

When it comes to preservice augmentative and alternative communication (AAC) education, I got the golden ticket of sorts. My university not only offered a four-credit course entirely devoted to AAC principles but also had a faculty of leading professionals in the field, and some incredible clinical learning opportunities. I was more equipped (and interested, for that matter) than most of the professionals in my cohort, but it still took me years to really have a solid framework to approach complex cases, and in many ways, I am still learning every day. Our scope as speech-language pathologists (SLPs) is unimaginably broad, and it truly is impossible to leave your graduate program knowing all you need to know to do the work being asked of you. So, what do you do when that complex case strolls into your therapy room? I decided to build my AAC village and continue to lean on them daily for support, knowledge, and growth as an AAC professional who will never know everything to help every communicator, all of the time.

I left my graduate program with a treasure trove of resources. Although none of them could walk me from start to finish through what only clinical experience would offer, at least I had a starting point to approach assessment and intervention. I keep my AAC textbooks handy and borrow or purchase books that add practical application to my theoretical foundations. I look for manuals that help me develop activities with my AAC users, and with each text, I learn something new that makes

my practice a bit easier and a lot more effective. It is an exciting time to be an AAC professional. With new and more engaging texts coming out regularly on AAC and related topics, and technology to make reading easier on-the-go, I continue to seek new information and perspectives to add to my toolbox through books.

Discussion and practice are such an important part of learning. I actively reach out to connect and stay connected to professionals who are seasoned in the field of AAC, in my local community and abroad. I keep in touch with my mentors from graduate school, asking questions as they come up, and seek new mentorship connections through my workplace, workshops, conferences, and membership in professional organizations. As social media has entered the professional networking and learning atmosphere, it has been wonderful to connect with even more mentors from around the globe, offering diverse perspectives and backgrounds. Mentoring really is the most effective tool in easing my nerves and building my skills and confidence, and I continue to lean on my mentors for new challenges that arise regularly in my professional life. I also pay it forward, by offering mentorship to professionals in a different season of practice. I find that I learn just as much as I share with each mentoring relationship.

For a more interactive and immersive learning experience, I seek out continuing education in topics related to AAC at local and national conferences,

523

and online. At these events, I can take a deeper dive into a particular topic and find even more colleagues to connect to my village. With the incredible growth in courses through online platforms and social media, it has never been easier to gain continuing education in AAC, at a time and on a budget that works for a busy SLP. When looking for quality professional development, I read the learning objectives and the testimonials from other students and think about how each lines up with my learning needs and what I know of best practice in the field.

We all know how important evidence-based practice is, and we get a bit of this guidance from mentoring and engaging with the resources mentioned earlier. However, I find that the best way for me to stay engaged with evidence is to make time to connect with the evidence directly. I find ways to engage with readable research that helps me get the gist and leads me to other avenues of learning that are more my flavor. When looking for articles to review, I start with the bibliographies of the texts I have read and the references provided by speakers at the workshops I have attended to find topics I want to know more about. Although accessing published articles is not always as easy as reading a blog post, the current tech era makes it easier than ever before to get our hands on this valuable knowledge. Having at least a basic understanding of the research principles behind AAC practice not only helps me help my students and clients, but also helps me discuss my approach to care with families.

Sometimes you just want a highly readable, visually supported avenue to gain some practical information and strategies. I found a few credible blogs and websites and started building a book-marks folder on my web browser to keep these resources handy. I subscribe to those that have subscription options and love the efficiency of new research and clinical information coming straight to my inbox. I ask questions in the comments when they come up, and if a blogger or author presents a topic I am particularly interested in (or feel pretty confused by), I seek out other resources produced by that expert to continue my learning.

We are all lifetime learners and with that, understand the value of asking questions when we do not get something or feel overwhelmed. Initially in my practice, I found it easy to identify the questions I had, but a bit more work to find someone to ask. This is where making those mentoring connections is important. For me, I benefit most from asking questions about my cases to those personal mentors I have a relationship with, whether it be during a staff meeting, a Friday night happy hour, or a quick phone call during my commute. I have encountered others who appreciate connecting with online groups and forums to dialogue about tough cases and points of confusion in the field. I learn volumes from the responses of my colleagues; sometimes it is purely validation that I am on the right track, other times it is guidance to get me onto a different track. I encourage you to find a village you trust and respect, and that trusts and respects you, and ask about the things that are gnawing at you each day. In a service as important as the one we provide, everyone benefits when we ask questions of ourselves and others. I am patient with myself and my colleagues, extending grace and assuming best intentions, understanding that we cannot all know everything, about everything, all of the time. You *can* do AAC, with your village by your side.

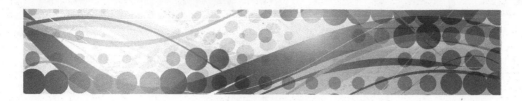

INDEX

Note: Page numbers in **bold** reference non-text material.